SPECIAL FEATURES

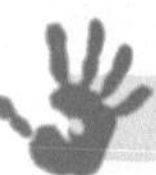

Considerations for Children

Chapter 6 Iron, 44
Chapter 7 Unnecessary Antibiotics, 49
Chapter 7 Antibiotics and Ototoxicity (Auditory Damage), 55
Chapter 9 Hexachlorophene, 72
Chapter 12 Methylphenidate (Ritalin), 106
Chapter 15 Aspirin, 141
Chapter 20 Immunizations, 188

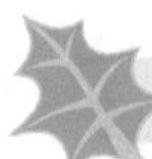

Considerations for Older Adults

Chapter 6 Calcium, 45
Chapter 8 Antihistamines, 67
Chapter 10 Epinephrine, 84
Chapter 11 Digitalis Preparations, 90
Chapter 11 Antiplatelet Agents and Proton Pump Inhibitors, 100
Chapter 12 Hypnotics and Sedatives, 108
Chapter 14 Paroxetine (Paxil), 134
Chapter 14 Buspirone, 136
Chapter 17 Cimetidine (Tagamet), 155

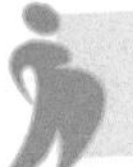

Considerations for Pregnant and Nursing Women

Chapter 6 Folic Acid, 43
Chapter 11 Antilipidemic Drugs, 101
Chapter 14 Lithium, 132
Chapter 17 Orlistat (Xenical), 158
Chapter 18 Thyroid Agents, 166
Chapter 18 Antithyroid Agents, 166
Chapter 19 Thiazide Diuretics, 182

Herb Alert

Chapter 7 Goldenseal, 62
Chapter 9 Aloe, 75
Chapter 10 Red Clover, 82
Chapter 10 Ephedra (Ma Huang), 83
Chapter 11 Horse Chestnut, 93
Chapter 11 Garlic, 95
Chapter 11 *Ginkgo biloba,* 99
Chapter 12 Ginseng, 105
Chapter 12 Valerian, 108
Chapter 12 Feverfew, 112
Chapter 12 Kava Kava, 116
Chapter 14 St. John's Wort, 133
Chapter 15 White Willow, 141
Chapter 17 Comfrey, 154
Chapter 17 Ginger, 156
Chapter 17 Cayenne (Capsicum), 157
Chapter 17 Chamomile, 158
Chapter 18 Black Cohosh, 174
Chapter 19 Juniper, 183
Chapter 19 Saw Palmetto, 185
Chapter 20 Echinacea, 192

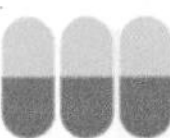

Special Considerations

Chapter 11 Calcium Channel Blockers, 96
Chapter 14 Benzodiazepines, 130
Chapter 15 NSAIDs, 142
Chapter 17 Antisecretory Agents, 156
Chapter 20 Immunizations, 189
Chapter 21 Immunity, 198

Twelfth Edition

Introduction to Pharmacology

Mary Kaye Asperheim, BS, MS, MD
Staff Physician
Little River Medical Center
Myrtle Beach, South Carolina;
Formerly, Instructor of Pharmacology
St. Louis University School of Nursing and Health Services
St. Louis, Missouri

Justin P. Favaro, BS, MD, PhD
Hematologist/Oncologist
Oncology Specialists of Charlotte
Charlotte, North Carolina

ELSEVIER

ELSEVIER
SAUNDERS

3251 Riverport Lane
St. Louis, Missouri 63043

INTRODUCTION TO PHARMACOLOGY, 12TH EDITION ISBN: 978-1-4377-1706-8

Notice

Knowledge and best practice in this field are constantly changing. As new research and experience broaden our understanding, changes in research methods, professional practices, or medical treatment may become necessary. Practitioners and researchers must always rely on their own experience and knowledge in evaluating and using any information, methods, compounds, or experiments described herein. In using such information or methods they should be mindful of their own safety and the safety of others, including parties for whom they have a professional responsibility.

With respect to any drug or pharmaceutical products identified, readers are advised to check the most current information provided (i) on procedures featured or (ii) by the manufacturer of each product to be administered, to verify the recommended dose or formula, the method and duration of administration, and contraindications. It is the responsibility of practitioners, relying on their own experience and knowledge of their patients, to make diagnoses, to determine dosages and the best treatment for each individual patient, and to take all appropriate safety precautions.

To the fullest extent of the law, neither the Publisher nor the authors, contributors, or editors, assume any liability for any injury and/or damage to persons or property as a matter of products liability, negligence or otherwise, or from any use or operation of any methods, products, instructions, or ideas contained in the material herein.

The Publisher

Library of Congress Cataloging-in-Publication Data

Asperheim, Mary Kaye.
Introduction to pharmacology/Mary Kaye Asperheim, Justin Favaro. –12th ed.
p. ; cm.
Includes bibliographical references and indexes.
ISBN 978-1-4377-1706-8 (pbk. : alk. paper)
1. Pharmacology. 2. Pharmaceutical arithmetic. 3. Nursing. I. Favaro, Justin. II. Title.
[DNLM: 1. Pharmacological Phenomena–Nurses' Instruction. 2. Pharmaceutical Preparations–Nurses' Instruction. QV 4]
RM300.A8 2012
615'.1–dc23

2011017156

Acquisitions Editor: Teri Hines Burnham
Senior Developmental Editor: Laura M. Selkirk
Publishing Services Manager: Jeff Patterson/Pallamparthy Radhika
Project Manager: Tracey Schriefer/Vijay Antony Raj Vincent
Designer: Karen Pauls

Printed in the United States of America

Last digit is the print number: 10 9 8 7 6

Reviewers

Maryanne Barra, DNP, FNP-C
Faculty, School of Nursing
Union County College
Plainfield, New Jersey

Michael Dorich, CST, CAHI, DBS
Program Director, Surgical Technology
Pittsburgh Technical Institute
Oakdale, Pennsylvania

Tim Dunn, BS, MA
Mathematics Teacher
St. Louis Public School District
St. Louis, Missouri

Cheri Goretti, MA, MT (ASCP), CMA (AAMA)
Professor and Coordinator, Medical Assisting and Allied Health Programs
Quinebaug Valley Community College
Danielson, Connecticut

Carol Healey, DNP, APN, C
Associate Professor of Nursing
Union County College
Plainfield, New Jersey

Beth Outland Jones, PharmD
Clinical Pharmacist
Missouri Baptist Medical Center
St. Louis, Missouri

Cathy Sermon Maddry, RN, MSN
Health Occupations Department Head
Northwest Louisiana Technical College
Minden, Louisiana

Carolyn McCormick, RN, BSN
Practical Nursing Program Coordinator
Cape Fear Community College
Wilmington, North Carolina

Helena J. Moissant, RN, MSN, PHN
Instructor of Pharmacology
American College of Nursing
Concord, California

Philip Penrod, BS, AA
Program Director, Pharmacy Technicians & MIBC
Everest University
Tampa, Florida

Sandra Reider, RN, BA, BSN, MSN
Associate Professor Emerita
Reading Area Community College
Reading, Pennsylvania

Karen Snipe, CphT, Med
Department Head, Program Coordinator
Trident Technical College
Charleston, South Carolina

Travis E. Sonnett, PharmD
Clinical Assistant Professor
Washington State University
Pullman, Washington

Mary Stassi, RN, C
Health Occupations Coordinator
St. Charles Community College
Cottleville, Missouri

Patricia W. Thompson, RN, BA
Program Director, Practical Nursing
West Georgia Technical College
Waco, Georgia

Brenda Tilton, RN, MSN, FNP-BC
Assistant Professor of Nursing
Southern State Community College
Hillsboro, Ohio

To the Instructor

Introduction to Pharmacology, 12th edition, is a concise, easy-to-understand pharmacology book written to appeal to a wide variety of health profession programs. After providing students with a thorough review of mathematics and dosage calculation, *Introduction to Pharmacology* presents basic pharmacology principles and monographs of the most widely used drugs in a clear, easy-to-read format. The many features included in this textbook make it both an excellent learning tool and a practical reference as students make the transition into clinical practice.

Changes to this edition feature the consolidation of the math chapters into Chapter 1; expanded content on women in Chapter 23; a new chapter on Drug Therapy in Children (Chapter 25), which integrates information on drug dosage for children; and a new chapter on Interactions (Chapter 29), which discusses drug toxicity and drug-drug, drug-herb, drug-food, and drug-consideration interactions. Additionally, all chapters have been thoroughly revised and updated to reflect current U.S. Food and Drug Administration (FDA) labeling and drug withdrawals.

ORGANIZATION OF THE TEXT

As in previous editions, the text is divided into four units: Mathematics of Drug Dosage, Principles of Pharmacology, Drug Classifications, and Special Situations in Pharmacology. Unit One introduces students to the basic mathematical symbols and calculations they will need to administer medications safely. Unit Two provides a background in drug legislation and drug terminology. Unit Three provides need-to-know drug content, organized by drug class or body system. Finally, Unit Four presents students with knowledge of special situations that they are likely to encounter in clinical practice.

FEATURES OF THE TWELFTH EDITION

- **Full-color design** and **illustrations** are useful and visually appealing.
- **Key Terms with phonetic pronunciations and text page references** help improve and supplement terminology and language skills of all students, including English-as-a-Second-Language (ESL) students and students with limited proficiency in English, before they enter clinical practice. Key Terms are in color at first mention in the text and can also be found in the Glossary.
- **Objectives** at the beginning of each chapter guide student learning and assist faculty in knowing what students should gain from the content.
- **Drug Monographs** throughout the text feature generic and trade names, essential information about how the drug works and how it is used, and typical drug dosages.
- **Critical Thinking Questions** and **Review Questions** at the end of the chapters provide opportunities for students to hone their critical thinking skills and test their knowledge of the information presented in the chapter. Answers can be found on the Evolve Resources with TEACH Instructor Resource or in the back of the book.

SPECIAL FEATURES

- **Clinical Implications** at the end of each chapter provide guidance and advice related to safe and effective drug administration and patient teaching for each drug category.
- **Considerations for Children, Considerations for Pregnant and Nursing Women,** and **Considerations for Older Adults** boxes throughout the text address the unique pharmacologic issues for each of these critical stages.
- **Special Considerations** boxes provide students with important information to keep in mind when considering specific drug classes.
- **Herb Alert** boxes highlight herb-drug interactions and contraindications, which is important information for a population that uses complementary and alternative therapies at an ever-increasing rate.
- **Disorders Index and Therapeutic Index** (separate from the General Index) refers the reader to information about medications used for specific disorders and prescribing categories.

TEACHING AND LEARNING PACKAGE

The following supplemental resources for both instructors and students can be found at http://evolve.elsevier.com/asperheim/pharmacology.

FOR THE INSTRUCTOR

- **Test Bank** features more than 400 multiple-choice questions and alternate-format questions so that you can create customized examinations.
- **TEACH Lesson Plans and Lecture Outlines** provide ready-to-use lesson plans based on the textbook learning objectives that tie together all of the text and ancillary components for *Introduction to Pharmacology*.
- **PowerPoint Lecture Slides** feature more than 900 slides that are specific to the text.
- **Image Collection** contains every illustration from the text. Images are suitable for incorporation into classroom lectures, PowerPoint presentations, or distance-learning applications.

FOR THE STUDENT

- **Interactive Bonus Questions** contain more than 250 additional questions that provide immediate feedback.
- **Open-Book Quizzes** feature more than 400 multiple-choice questions, short-answer questions, and math problems to test your knowledge of the content.
- **Animations** depict how drugs and diseases work through the body.
- **Audio Glossary** pronounces terms in English.
- **Answers to Critical Thinking Questions** provide answers to questions found in the textbook.

ACKNOWLEDGMENTS

We would also like to thank the people at Elsevier: Teri Hines Burnham, Executive Editor; Laura Selkirk, Senior Developmental Editor; and Tracey Schriefer, Project Manager.

We are confident that this new edition will be a useful resource in understanding the basics of pharmacology.

Mary Kaye Asperheim Favaro, MD
Justin P. Favaro, BS, MD, PhD

Contents

Unit One MATHEMATICS OF DRUG DOSAGE

1 Basic Math Review, 1
Roman Numerals, 1
Fractions, 2
Decimals, 7
Percentage, 10
Proportion, 12
Fahrenheit and Celsius, 12
Systems of Measurement, 13

Unit Two PRINCIPLES OF PHARMACOLOGY

2 Introduction to Pharmacology, 16
Definitions, 17

3 Drug Legislation and Drug Standards, 20
American Drug Legislation, 20
Drug Standards, 21
Canadian Drug Legislation, 22
Proprietary (Trade) Names, 22

4 Introduction to Drug Dosage, 24
Drug Dosage in Standardized Units, 25
The Prescription, 26

5 Administration of Medications, 29
Guidelines for Safety in Drug Administration, 29
Methods of Drug Administration, 29
Proper Disposal of Unwanted Medicine, 37

6 Vitamins, Minerals, and General Nutrition, 39
Nomenclature of Vitamins, 40
Characteristics of Vitamins, 41
Fat-Soluble Vitamins, 41
Water-Soluble Vitamins, 42
Minerals, 43
Changes in Nutritional Information, 46

Unit Three DRUG CLASSIFICATIONS

7 Antibiotics and Antifungal, Antiviral, and Antiparasitic Agents, 49
Antibiotics, 49
Sulfonamide Drugs, 55
Antifungal Agents, 57
Antiviral Agents, 58
Antiparasitic Agents, 62

8 Antihistamines, 65
Allergic Reactions, 65
Determining the Cause of Allergies, 66
Adverse Drug Reactions and Drug Allergies, 66
Treatment of Allergies, 67
Role of Immunotherapy, 69

9 Drugs That Affect the Skin and Mucous Membranes, 71
Soothing Substances, 71
Astringents, 72
Irritants, 72
Keratolytics, 72
Local Anesthetics, 72
Antifungal Agents, 72
Antimonilial Preparations, 73
General Anti-Infective Agents, 74
Wound Care Products, 75
Sun Damage to Skin, 75
Acne Preparations, 76
Agents Used in the Treatment of Atopic Dermatitis (Eczema), 77
Agents Used in the Treatment of Warts, 77
Topical Corticosteroids, 78

10 Drugs That Affect the Respiratory System, 81
Drugs That Act on the Respiratory Center in the Brain, 82
Drugs That Affect the Mucous Membrane Lining of the Respiratory Tract, 82
Asthma and Allergic Disorders, 83
Drugs That Affect the Size of the Bronchioles, 83
Administration of Drugs by Inhalation, 84
Other Agents Used in the Treatment of Asthma, 85
Other Agents That Act on the Respiratory Tract, 86

11 Drugs That Affect the Circulatory System, 88
Drugs That Affect the Heart, 89
Drugs That Affect the Blood Vessels, 93
Drugs That Affect the Blood, 97

12 Drugs That Affect the Central Nervous System, 104
Central Nervous System Stimulants, 105
Central Nervous System Depressants, 106
Epilepsy, 113
Anticonvulsants and Other Drugs Used to Treat Epilepsy, 113
Antiparkinsonian Agents, 115
Agents Used to Treat Fibromyalgia, 116

13 Pain Medications, 119
Etiology of Pain, 120
Investigation of Causes of Pain, 120
Assessment of Pain, 120
Progressive Levels of Pain Relief, 121
Opiates and Opioids, 123
Neuropathic Pain, 124
Depression and Pain, 124
Coanalgesics, 124
Patient Medication Use Agreement, 125

14 Tranquilizers and Antidepressants, 129
Tranquilizers, 130
Antidepressants, 133
Anxiolytic Agents, 136
Use of Anticonvulsants in Anxiety Disorders, 136

15 Prostaglandins and Prostaglandin Inhibitors, 139
Actions of the Prostaglandins, 139
Prostaglandin Inhibitors, 140

16 Drugs That Affect the Autonomic Nervous System, 145
Sympathetic and Parasympathetic Systems, 145
Sympathomimetic (Adrenergic) Agents, 146
Sympatholytic (Adrenergic Blocking) Agents, 147
Parasympathomimetic (Cholinergic) Agents, 149
Parasympatholytic (Cholinergic Blocking) Agents, 150
Neuromuscular Blocking Agents, 150

17 Drugs That Affect the Digestive System, 153
Helicobacter pylori and Peptic Ulcer Disease, 154
Antisecretory Agents, 155
Antacids, 156
Digestants, 157
Appetite Stimulant, 157
Absorption Inhibitor, 157
Emetics, 158
Antiemetics, 158
Cathartics, 159
Antidiarrheals, 161

18 The Endocrine Glands and Hormones, 164
Pituitary Gland, 164
Thyroid Gland, 164
Parathyroid Glands, 166
Adrenal Glands, 167
Pancreas, 168
Gonads, 172

19 Diuretics and Other Drugs That Affect the Urinary System, 180
Diuretics, 181
Urinary Antiseptics, 183
Drugs Used to Treat Enuresis, 184
Drugs Used to Treat Incontinence, 185
Drugs Used to Treat Benign Prostatic Hypertrophy, 185
Drugs Used to Treat Erectile Dysfunction, 186

20 Immunizing Agents and Immunosuppressives, 188
Immunizing Agents, 188
Immunosuppressive Agents, 192
Immunomodulating Agents in the Treatment of Multiple Sclerosis, 193

21 Antineoplastic Drugs, 198
Alkylating Agents, 199
Antimetabolites, 200
Hormones, 202
Antitumor Antibiotics, 204
Enzyme Inhibitors, 205
Immunomodulating Agents in Cancer, 205
Molecular and Targeted Therapies, 206
Platinum-Containing Agents, 206
Vaccines Used in the Treatment or Prevention of Cancer, 206
Miscellaneous Cancer Treatment Agents, 207
Supportive Agents, 208

22 Molecular and Targeted Therapies, 211
Genetic Basis of Disease, 211
Gene Therapy, 212
Stem Cells, 212

Targeted Therapy, 212
Monoclonal Antibodies, 212
Agents Used to Suppress the Immune System, 213
Agents Used to Treat Rheumatoid Arthritis and Crohn's Disease, 214
Agents Used to Treat Cancer, 214
Miscellaneous Agents, 215

Unit Four SPECIAL SITUATIONS IN PHARMACOLOGY

23 Drug Therapy in Women, 218
Cardiovascular Disease in Women, 218
Osteoarthritis, 219
Osteoporosis, 220
Fibromyalgia Syndrome, 220
Chronic Fatigue Syndrome, 221
Insomnia, 221
Depression, 222
Menstrual and Perimenopausal Migraines, 223
Menstrual Abnormalities, 224
Menopause, 224

24 Drug Therapy in Older Adults, 227
Drug Therapy in Older Adults, 228
Nutrition in Older Adults, 229
Arthritis in Older Adults, 231
Osteoporosis in Older Adults, 231
Pain and Aging, 232
The Aging Thyroid and How It Affects Older Adults, 232
Hypertension in Older Adults, 233
Anti-Infective Therapy in Older Adults, 233
Anxiety in Older Adults, 234
Drugs Used to Treat Alzheimer's Disease, 234
Family Care of Older Adults and Caregiver Stress, 234

25 Drug Therapy in Children, 237
Medications and Fetal Development, 237
Medications Used to Treat Children, 238
Calculating Children's Doses, 238
Body Surface Area Nomogram, 240

26 Home Health and End-of-Life Care, 242
Home Infusion Therapy, 242
Home Therapy for Bone Marrow Transplant Patients, 243
Home Care for Diabetic Patients, 243
Psychiatric Home Care, 244
End-of-Life Care, 244

27 Substance Abuse, 251
Seven Signs of Possible Drug Involvement, 252
Dependence on Narcotics, 252
Sedative-Hypnotic Abuse, 252
Marijuana Abuse, 252
Cocaine Abuse, 253
Alcohol Abuse, 254
Nicotine Abuse, 254
Symptoms of Drug Abuse, 255

28 Herbal Therapies and Drug-Herb Interactions, 257
Herbal Therapies, 258
Drug-Herb Interactions, 263

29 Interactions, 266
Three Broad Classes of Interactions, 266
Drugs with the Highest Potential for Harm, 267
How to Avoid Drug Toxicity Reactions, 267

Glossary, 270
Answers to Exercises and Review Questions, 279
Therapeutic Index, 282
General Index, 283
Disorders Index, Inside Back Cover

Basic Math Review

CHAPTER 1

Objectives

After completing this chapter, you should be able to do the following:

1. Read and write the basic Roman numerals for their Arabic equivalents and vice versa.
2. Explain the meaning of a fraction, give an example of each type of fraction, and convert between improper fractions and whole or mixed numbers.
3. Give the fundamental principles used in computing with fractions and demonstrate accurately the addition, subtraction, multiplication, and division of fractions and mixed numbers.
4. Read, write, add, subtract, multiply, and divide decimals.
5. Convert decimals to fractions and vice versa, percents to decimals and vice versa, and fractions to percents and vice versa.
6. Solve for an unknown term in a proportion.
7. Convert temperature from the Fahrenheit scale to the Celsius scale and vice versa.
8. Convert units of measure within the metric system and from the Avoirdupois system to the metric system.

Key Terms

Arabic (ĂR-é-bîk) **numeral system,** p. 1
Avoirdupois (Ăv-ĕr-dĕ-POIZ) **system,** p. 14
Celsius (SĔL-sē-ĕs) **scale,** p. 12
Complex fraction, p. 3
Decimal, p. 7
Equivalent (ĭ-kwĬV-ĕ-lĕnt) **fraction,** p. 4
Extremes, p. 12
Fahrenheit (FĂR-ĕn-HĪT) **scale,** p. 12
Fraction, p. 2
Gram, p. 13
Improper fraction, p. 2
Liter, p. 13
Lowest common denominator, p. 4
Means, p. 12
Meter, p. 13
Metric system, p. 13
Mixed number, p. 2
Percent, p. 10
Place value, p. 7
Proper fraction, p. 2
Proportion, p. 12
Reduced fraction, p. 3
Roman numeral system, p. 1

In contrast to the **Arabic numeral system,** which uses symbols and decimal places to express numbers, the **Roman numeral system** uses letters to designate numbers. Their use is obviously restricted because mathematical procedures would become extremely complicated if the attempt was made to use these numerals in calculations. Lowercase Roman numerals are occasionally used in prescriptions (see Chapter 4).

Basic Roman numerals are expressed as follows:

Roman Numeral	Arabic Number
I	1
V	5
X	10
L	50
C	100
D	500
M	1000

PROCEDURE FOR READING AND WRITING ROMAN NUMERALS

1. When a Roman numeral precedes one of larger value, its value is subtracted from the larger. When a numeral follows one of larger value, its value is added to the larger.

EXAMPLES

a. IV = (5 − 1) = 4
b. XI = (10 + 1) = 11
c. LXI = (50 + 10 + 1) = 61

2. When two numerals of identical value are reported in sequence, their values are added. (Numerals may never be repeated more than three times in sequence.)

EXAMPLES

a. XXX = 30
b. MMXXVIII = 2028

3. When a numeral is placed between two numerals of greater value, the lesser is subtracted from the numeral following it.

EXAMPLES

a. XIV = (10 + 5 − 1) = 14
b. XIX = (10 + 10 − 1) = 19
c. CXLIX = (100 + 50 −10 + 10 −1) = 149

EXERCISES

A. Express the following in Roman numerals:

1. 35 ______
2. 89 ______
3. 72 ______
4. 55 ______
5. 101 ______
6. 92 ______
7. 135 ______
8. 1580 ______
9. 341 ______
10. 729 ______

B. Express the following in Arabic numbers:

1. MCCXI ______
2. DCCXX ______
3. CLXVI ______
4. DXXIX ______
5. MMMVI ______
6. DCCC ______
7. LVI ______
8. LXXV ______
9. MMDCLXXIII ______
10. LXI ______

A **fraction** indicates division and expresses the number of equal parts into which a whole is divided. If a whole is divided into equal parts, then one or more of this number of equal parts is called a fraction.

EXAMPLE

The fraction ⅜ means 3 of 8 equal parts (Fig. 1-1). This could also be written 3 ÷ 8 because it indicates division into 8 equal parts.

In the above example, the numbers 3 and 8 are called the "terms of the fraction." The lower number of a fraction is called the *denominator*, or the divisor, and tells into how many parts the unit is divided. The upper number of the fraction is called the *numerator*, or the dividend, and tells how many parts of the unit are taken.

KINDS OF FRACTIONS

Proper fraction. Sometimes called a common fraction, or just "fraction," a **proper fraction** has a numerator that is smaller than the denominator and designates less than one whole unit.

EXAMPLES

$$\frac{1}{3}, \frac{2}{5}, \frac{3}{17}$$

Improper fraction. An **improper fraction** is one in which the numerator is larger than the denominator and designates more than one unit (Fig. 1-2).

EXAMPLES

$$\frac{5}{4}, \frac{13}{8}$$

Mixed number. A **mixed number** consists of a whole number and a fraction. A mixed number can also be written as an improper fraction.

EXAMPLES

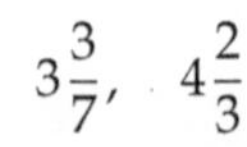

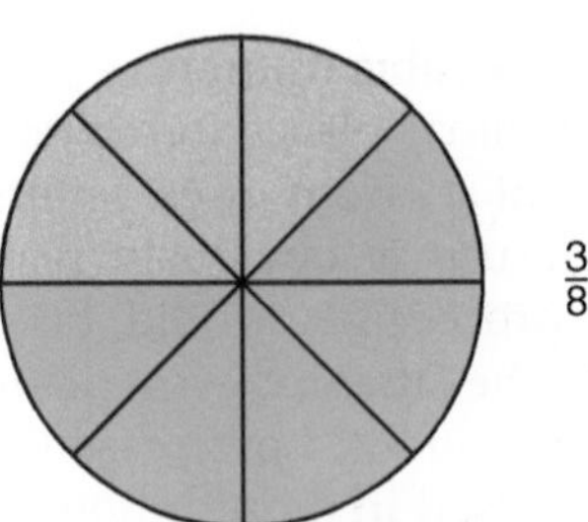

FIGURE 1-1 The fraction $\frac{3}{8}$ means 3 of 8 equal parts.

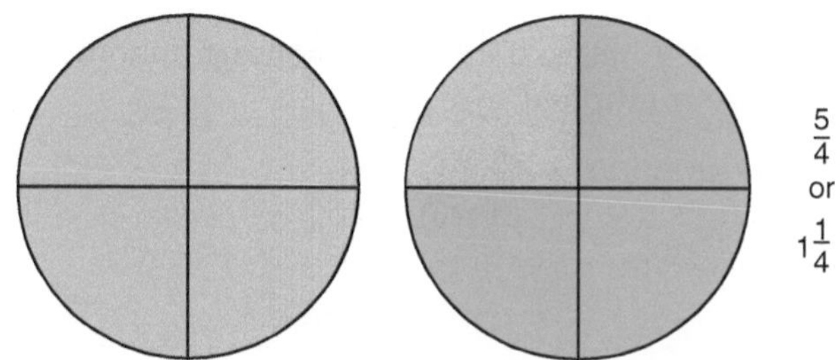

FIGURE 1-2 Example of an improper fraction or a mixed number.

Complex fraction. When both the numerator and the denominator (or just one of these) are in fraction form, we refer to the term as a **complex fraction** (Fig. 1-3).

EXAMPLES

$$\frac{\frac{2}{3}}{\frac{3}{8}}, \quad \frac{\frac{4}{3}}{7}$$

Reduced fraction. A fraction is said to be reduced to its lowest terms when the numerator and denominator cannot be divided exactly by the same number (except 1).

EXAMPLE

$\frac{6}{8}$ This fraction is not reduced because both numerator and denominator can be divided by 2.

$\frac{6(\div 2)}{8(\div 2)} = \frac{3}{4}$ This is the **reduced fraction.**

PROCEDURE FOR CONVERTING BETWEEN IMPROPER FRACTIONS AND WHOLE OR MIXED NUMBERS

CHANGING AN IMPROPER FRACTION INTO A WHOLE OR MIXED NUMBER

1. Divide the numerator by the denominator.
2. Write the remainder, if any, as a fraction reduced to the lowest terms.

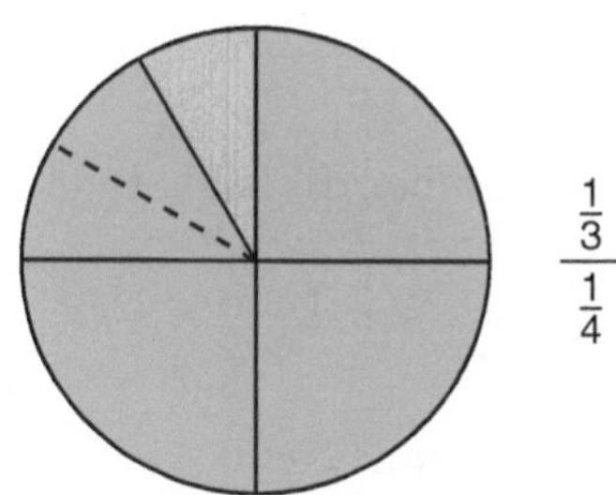

FIGURE 1-3 Example of a complex fraction.

EXAMPLES

a. Change $\frac{8}{4}$ to a whole number.

$8 \div 4 = 2$

b. Change $\frac{16}{6}$ to a mixed number.

$16 \div 6 = 2\frac{4}{6}$, or reduced $= 2\frac{2}{3}$

CHANGING MIXED NUMBERS INTO IMPROPER FRACTIONS

1. Multiply the whole number by the denominator of the fraction.
2. Add this product to the numerator of the fraction.
3. Write the sum as the numerator of the improper fraction; the denominator remains the same.

EXAMPLES

a. Change $2\frac{3}{8}$ to an improper fraction.

$2 \times 8 = 16,\ 16 + 3 = 19 \therefore \frac{19}{8}$

b. Change $4\frac{2}{5}$ to an improper fraction.

$4 \times 5 = 20,\ 20 + 2 = 22 \therefore \frac{22}{5}$

c. Change $9\frac{1}{6}$ to an improper fraction.

$9 \times 6 = 54,\ 54 + 1 = 55 \therefore \frac{55}{6}$

EXERCISES

A. Change the following to whole or mixed numbers:

1. $\frac{12}{8}$ ______
2. $\frac{7}{5}$ ______
3. $\frac{20}{10}$ ______
4. $\frac{12}{4}$ ______
5. $\frac{17}{9}$ ______
6. $\frac{25}{8}$ ______
7. $\frac{79}{5}$ ______
8. $\frac{64}{9}$ ______
9. $\frac{26}{3}$ ______
10. $\frac{410}{100}$ ______

B. Change the following to whole or mixed numbers:

1. $1\frac{1}{3}$ ______
2. $4\frac{1}{2}$ ______
3. $100\frac{3}{7}$ ______
4. $9\frac{1}{8}$ ______
5. $10\frac{4}{5}$ ______
6. $6\frac{4}{5}$ ______
7. $2\frac{1}{8}$ ______
8. $17\frac{1}{4}$ ______
9. $80\frac{5}{12}$ ______
10. $110\frac{1}{4}$ ______

EQUIVALENT FRACTIONS

Equivalent fractions are fractions whose terms are different but that may be reduced to the same fraction. Equivalent fractions may be made by multiplying or dividing both terms of a fraction by the same number. Any number may be used, as long as the numerator and denominator are treated in the same way.

EXAMPLES

a. $\frac{1(\times 2)}{8(\times 2)} = \frac{2}{16}$

b. $\frac{2(\times 32)}{3(\times 32)} = \frac{64}{96}$

c. $\frac{4(\div 2)}{6(\div 2)} = \frac{2}{3}$

Fractions may be changed to obtain a new fraction of any desired denominator by determining what number the present denominator must be multiplied by to give the desired denominator. Both numerator and denominator are then multiplied by this number.

EXAMPLES

a. $\frac{1}{2} = \frac{?}{8}$

$8 \div 2 = 4$, so both numerator and denominator are multiplied by 4.

$\frac{1(\times 4)}{2(\times 4)} = \frac{4}{8}$

b. $\frac{5}{9} = \frac{?}{72}$

$72 \div 9 = 8$, so both numerator and denominator are multiplied by 8.

$\frac{5(\times 8)}{9(\times 8)} = \frac{40}{72}$

EXERCISES

Change the following fractions to equivalent fractions having the specified denominator:

1. $\frac{1}{4} = \frac{?}{20}$ ______
2. $\frac{6}{13} = \frac{?}{39}$ ______
3. $\frac{6}{15} = \frac{?}{60}$ ______
4. $\frac{7}{18} = \frac{?}{36}$ ______
5. $\frac{5}{4} = \frac{?}{32}$ ______
6. $\frac{8}{17} = \frac{?}{51}$ ______
7. $\frac{7}{9} = \frac{?}{63}$ ______
8. $\frac{9}{8} = \frac{?}{16}$ ______
9. $\frac{6}{7} = \frac{?}{21}$ ______
10. $\frac{63}{30} = \frac{?}{10}$ ______

PROCEDURE FOR FINDING THE LOWEST COMMON DENOMINATOR

1. Find the lowest possible number that is divisible by all the denominators, that is, the **lowest common denominator.**
2. Change the fractions to equivalent fractions using this denominator.

EXAMPLES

Find the lowest common denominator for the following:

a. $\frac{1}{3}$ and $\frac{2}{5}$

The lowest number divisible by 3 and 5 is 15, so this will be the new denominator.

$\frac{1}{3} = \frac{?}{15} = \frac{5}{15}$

$\frac{2}{5} = \frac{?}{15} = \frac{6}{15}$

b. $\frac{2}{3}, \frac{7}{8},$ and $\frac{1}{6}$

The lowest number divisible by 3, 8, and 6 is 24.

$\frac{2}{3} = \frac{?}{24} = \frac{16}{24}$

$\frac{7}{8}=\frac{?}{24}=\frac{21}{24}$

$\frac{1}{6}=\frac{?}{24}=\frac{4}{24}$

c. $\frac{2}{4}$ and $\frac{6}{8}$

The lowest common denominator is 8, so only the $\frac{2}{4}$ must be changed.

$\frac{2}{4}=\frac{4}{8}$

$\frac{6}{8}=\frac{6}{8}$

EXERCISES

Change the following to fractions having the lowest common denominator:

1. $\frac{7}{12}$ and $\frac{3}{6}$ ______
2. $\frac{6}{7}$ and $\frac{2}{3}$ ______
3. $\frac{1}{3}$ and $\frac{2}{9}$ ______
4. $\frac{2}{5}$ and $\frac{8}{20}$ ______
5. $\frac{1}{8}$ and $\frac{8}{24}$ ______
6. $\frac{1}{4}, \frac{1}{5},$ and $\frac{1}{6}$ ______
7. $\frac{2}{3}, \frac{1}{2},$ and $\frac{3}{4}$ ______
8. $\frac{3}{4}, \frac{5}{6},$ and $\frac{7}{8}$ ______
9. $\frac{8}{9}, \frac{9}{10},$ and $\frac{1}{3}$ ______
10. $\frac{4}{15}, \frac{3}{5},$ and $\frac{4}{25}$ ______
11. $1\frac{1}{3}, \frac{3}{6},$ and $\frac{1}{4}$ ______
12. $\frac{3}{5}, \frac{4}{6}$ and $\frac{4}{10}$ ______

PROCEDURE FOR ADDITION OF FRACTIONS AND MIXED NUMBERS

1. If the fractions have the same denominator, add the numerators, write the sum over the common denominator, and reduce to the lowest terms.
2. If the fractions have unlike denominators, first find their lowest common denominator, then add the numerators as in step 1.
3. To add mixed numbers, first add the fractions as just described, then add this result to the sum of the whole numbers.

EXAMPLES

a.
$$\begin{array}{r} \frac{1}{5} \\ +\frac{2}{5} \\ \hline \frac{3}{5} \end{array}$$

b.
$$\begin{array}{rl} \frac{3}{5} = & \frac{9}{15} \\ +\frac{2}{3} = & +\frac{10}{15} \\ \hline & \frac{19}{15}=1\frac{4}{15} \end{array}$$

c.
$$\begin{array}{rl} 6\frac{1}{6} = & 6\frac{8}{48} \\ +9\frac{5}{8} = & +9\frac{30}{48} \\ \hline & 15\frac{38}{48}=15\frac{19}{24} \end{array}$$

d.
$$\begin{array}{rl} 1\frac{3}{8} = & 1\frac{15}{40} \\ +9\frac{9}{10} = & +9\frac{36}{40} \\ \hline & 10\frac{51}{40}\left(\frac{51}{40}=1\frac{11}{40}\right)=11\frac{11}{40} \end{array}$$

EXERCISES

Add the following numbers:

1. $\frac{1}{12}+\frac{2}{3}+\frac{4}{9}$ ______
2. $\frac{3}{5}+\frac{2}{3}+\frac{4}{10}$ ______
3. $2\frac{1}{3}+4\frac{1}{8}$ ______
4. $7\frac{1}{4}+6\frac{2}{8}+4\frac{5}{6}$ ______
5. $\frac{2}{3}+\frac{1}{2}+\frac{1}{4}$ ______
6. $3\frac{1}{2}+2\frac{3}{10}+5\frac{2}{5}$ ______
7. $5+\frac{7}{12}$ ______
8. $2+1\frac{4}{4}+2\frac{5}{6}$ ______
9. $24\frac{3}{8}+12\frac{6}{7}+\frac{5}{14}$ ______
10. $4\frac{1}{2}+2\frac{3}{8}+3\frac{1}{4}$ ______

PROCEDURE FOR SUBTRACTION OF FRACTIONS AND MIXED NUMBERS

1. If the fractions have the same denominator, find the difference between the numerators and write it over the common denominator. Reduce to the lowest terms.
2. If the fractions have unlike denominators, first find the lowest common denominator, then proceed as in step 1.
3. To subtract mixed numbers, first subtract the fractions as just described, and then find the difference between the whole numbers. If the fraction in the subtrahend (bottom number) is larger than the fraction in the minuend (top number), it is necessary to borrow from the whole number before subtracting the fractions.

EXAMPLES

a. $\frac{4}{5} = \frac{8}{10}$

$-\frac{1}{2} = -\frac{5}{10}$

$= \frac{3}{10}$

b. $7\frac{16}{24} = 7\frac{16}{24}$

$-3\frac{1}{8} = -3\frac{3}{24}$

$= 4\frac{13}{24}$

c. $21\frac{7}{16} = 20\frac{16}{16} + \frac{7}{16} = 20\frac{23}{16}$

$-7\frac{12}{16}$ $\quad -7\frac{12}{16}$

$= 13\frac{11}{16}$

EXERCISES

Subtract the following:

1. $\frac{8}{18} - \frac{3}{18}$ ________
2. $\frac{5}{7} - \frac{2}{3}$ ________
3. $\frac{7}{8} - \frac{1}{4}$ ________
4. $2\frac{4}{7} - 1\frac{1}{7}$ ________
5. $4\frac{2}{8} - 2\frac{7}{8}$ ________
6. $3\frac{10}{15} - \frac{7}{15}$ ________
7. $6 - 2\frac{2}{3}$ ________
8. $25\frac{4}{5} - 11$ ________
9. $20 - 16\frac{11}{12}$ ________
10. $4\frac{2}{3} - 1\frac{1}{2}$ ________

PROCEDURE FOR MULTIPLICATION OF FRACTIONS AND MIXED NUMBERS

1. Change mixed numbers to improper fractions.
2. Reduce, if possible, by dividing any numerator and denominator by the largest number contained in each.
3. Multiply remaining numerators to find numerator of answer.
4. Multiply remaining denominators to find denominator of answer.

EXAMPLES

a. $\frac{4}{5} \times \frac{15}{16} = \frac{\overset{1}{\cancel{4}}}{\underset{1}{\cancel{5}}} \times \frac{\overset{3}{\cancel{15}}}{\underset{4}{\cancel{16}}} = \frac{3}{4}$

b. $6 \times \frac{3}{8} = \frac{\overset{3}{\cancel{6}}}{1} \times \frac{3}{\underset{4}{\cancel{8}}} = \frac{9}{4} = 2\frac{1}{4}$

EXERCISES

Multiply the following:

1. $\frac{1}{3} \times \frac{1}{4}$ ________
2. $\frac{7}{8} \times \frac{5}{9}$ ________
3. $3\frac{1}{3} \times 1\frac{1}{5}$ ________
4. $\frac{4}{5} \times 1\frac{8}{15}$ ________
5. $1\frac{1}{2} \times 2\frac{5}{6} \times 3\frac{1}{3}$ ________
6. $12 \times 2\frac{3}{4}$ ________
7. $\frac{2}{3} \times 6$ ________
8. $\frac{4}{200} \times 1000$ ________
9. $\frac{1}{3} \times \frac{4}{12} \times \frac{4}{6}$ ________
10. $\frac{3}{4} \times \frac{2}{5} \times \frac{2}{15}$ ________

PROCEDURE FOR DIVISION OF FRACTIONS AND MIXED NUMBERS

1. Change mixed numbers to improper fractions.
2. Invert the divisor (the number after the division sign).
3. Follow the steps for multiplication of fractions.

EXAMPLES

a. $\frac{2}{5} \div \frac{5}{8} = \frac{2}{5} \times \frac{8}{5} = \frac{16}{25}$ b. $8\frac{3}{4} \div 15 = \frac{\overset{7}{\cancel{35}}}{4} \times \frac{1}{\underset{3}{\cancel{15}}} = \frac{7}{12}$

EXERCISES

Divide the following:

1. $\frac{3}{5} \div \frac{7}{8}$ __________
2. $\frac{1}{12} \div \frac{1}{3}$ __________
3. $\frac{4}{5} \div \frac{6}{7}$ __________
4. $\frac{2}{3} \div 4$ __________
5. $3 \div \frac{1}{2}$ __________
6. $\frac{3}{4} \div \frac{4}{6}$ __________
7. $3\frac{1}{2} \div 1\frac{3}{4}$ __________
8. $1\frac{3}{4} \div 2$ __________
9. $1\frac{1}{2} \div 1\frac{1}{4}$ __________
10. $20\frac{1}{2} \div 50$ __________

RATIO

A ratio indicates the relationship of one quantity to another. It indicates division and may be expressed in fraction form.

EXAMPLES

a. $\frac{3}{9}$ may be expressed as a ratio: 3: 9

b. 1:1000 may be expressed as a fraction: $\frac{1}{1000}$

EXERCISES

Express the following ratios as fractions reduced to lowest terms:

1. 1 : 3 __________
2. 5 : 7 __________
3. 2 : 1000 __________
4. 7 : 63 __________
5. 42 : 83 __________
6. 2 : 17 __________
7. 7 : 56 __________
8. 1 : 11 __________
9. 2 : 150 __________
10. 4 : 9 __________

A **decimal** is a fraction whose denominator is 10 or any multiple of 10, such as 100, 1000, and 10,000. However, it differs from a common fraction in that the denominator is not written but instead is expressed by the proper placement of the decimal point. Usually decimal fractions and mixed decimals are just called "decimals."

PROCEDURE FOR READING AND WRITING DECIMALS

1. Observe the scale of place values (Fig. 1-4). The **place value** of a digit is its value based on its position relative to the decimal point. All whole numbers are to the left of the decimal point; all fractions are to the right.
2. In reading a decimal fraction, read the number to the right of the decimal point and use the name that applies to the place value of the last figure.

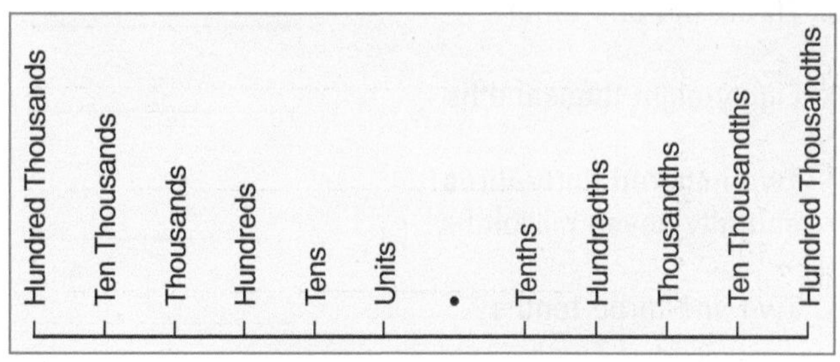

FIGURE 1-4 Place value scale.

EXAMPLE

0.257 = two hundred fifty-seven thousandths

3. In reading a mixed decimal, first read the whole number, then the decimal fraction. The word "and" shows the place of the decimal point.

EXAMPLE

327.006 = three hundred twenty-seven and six thousandths

EXERCISES

A. Write the following:

1. 0.03 ____________
2. 0.089 ____________
3. 23.5 ____________
4. 5.21 ____________
5. 0.0029 ____________
6. 200.09 ____________
7. 37.282 ____________
8. 4256.353 ____________
9. 256.01 ____________
10. 0.0008 ____________

B. Express the following as decimal fractions:

1. Four thousandths ____________
2. Twenty-six hundredths ____________
3. Five and three millionths ____________
4. Seven hundredths ____________
5. Three and one tenth ____________
6. Eighty-eight thousandths ____________
7. Two hundred thirty-three and fifty-seven millionths ____________
8. Two and three tenths ____________
9. Eight and four hundredths ____________
10. Twenty-five and three thousandths ____________

PROCEDURE FOR ADDITION OF DECIMALS

1. Write the decimals in a column, placing the decimal points directly under each other.
2. Add as in the addition of whole numbers. (Zeros may be added after the decimal point as place holders to prevent errors in addition; this does not change the value of the decimal.)
3. Place the decimal point in the sum directly under the decimal points in the addends (the numbers that are being added).

EXAMPLES

a. 0.8 + 0.5 =

$$\begin{array}{r} 0.8 \\ +0.5 \\ \hline 1.3 \end{array}$$

b. 3.27 + 0.06 + 2 =

$$\begin{array}{r} 3.27 \\ +0.06 \\ +2.00 \\ \hline 5.33 \end{array}$$

EXERCISES

Add the following:

1. 7.01 + 3.888 ____________
2. 26.78 + 6.28 + 16.53 ____________
3. 7.52 + 4.9 ____________
4. 0.72 + 0.81 + 5 ____________
5. 0.76 + 2 + 300 ____________
6. 0.81 + 0.973 ____________
7. 6 + 0.09 ____________
8. 0.8 + 6 + 0.245 ____________
9. 77.1 + 0.27 + 0.31 ____________
10. 0.3 + 0.37 + 1.8 ____________

PROCEDURE FOR SUBTRACTION OF DECIMALS

1. Write the decimals in columns, keeping the decimal points under each other.
2. Subtract as with whole numbers. (Zeros may be added after the decimal point as place holders to prevent errors in subtraction; this does not change the value of the decimal.)
3. Place the decimal point in the remainder directly under the decimal point in the subtrahend (bottom number) and minuend (top number).

EXAMPLE

$$0.6 - 0.524 = \begin{array}{r} 0.600 \\ -0.524 \\ \hline 0.076 \end{array}$$

EXERCISES

Subtract the following:

1. 1.65 − 1.004 __________
2. 0.21 − 0.17 __________
3. 64.28 − 23 __________
4. 756.824 − 28.127 __________
5. 0.07 − 0.052 __________
6. 10 − 6.78 __________
7. 5 − 0.3 __________
8. 36 − 1.5 __________
9. 3 − 0.163 __________
10. 109 − 3.29 __________

PROCEDURE FOR MULTIPLICATION OF DECIMALS

1. Multiply as in the multiplication of whole numbers.
2. Find the total number of decimal places in the *multiplier* (bottom number) and *multiplicand* (top number).
3. Starting from the right and moving left, count off in the product this total number of decimal places. Put the decimal point at the left of the last of these.
4. If the product contains fewer figures than the required decimal places, add as many zeros as necessary to the left of the product.

EXAMPLE

$$2.6 \times 0.0002 = \begin{array}{r} 2.6 \\ \times 0.0002 \\ \hline 0.00052 \end{array}$$

EXERCISES

Multiply the following:

1. 4 × 0.8 __________
2. 0.005 × 2.2 __________
3. 3.15 × 0.03 __________
4. 200 × 0.7 __________
5. 59.38 × 0.015 __________
6. 400 × 0.6 __________
7. 0.003 × 0.03 __________
8. 26.17 × 3.8 __________
9. 100 × 1.2 __________
10. 7.302 × 1.54 __________

PROCEDURE FOR DIVISION OF DECIMALS

1. If the divisor is a whole number, divide as in the division of whole numbers and place the decimal point in the quotient directly above the decimal point in the dividend.
2. If the divisor is a decimal, make it a whole number by moving the decimal point to the right of the last number. Move the decimal point in the dividend the same number of places; proceed in division as in Step 1. (If the dividend contains fewer places than required, zeros may be added.)

EXAMPLE

$$15 \div 0.625 = 625\overline{)15.000.}$$

$$\begin{array}{r} 24 \\ 12\,50 \\ \hline 2\,500 \\ 2\,500 \\ \hline 0 \end{array}$$

EXERCISES

Divide the following and carry to the third decimal place. Round to the nearest thousandth when necessary:

1. 300 ÷ 5 __________
2. 14.03 ÷ 6 __________
3. 69.4 ÷ 0.52 __________
4. 24.78 ÷ 4 __________
5. 48 ÷ 2.4 __________

6. 0.2482 ÷ 0.068 ______
7. 84 ÷ 4.2 ______
8. 270.6 ÷ 32 ______
9. 96.2 ÷ 28 ______
10. 0.06128 ÷ 0.72 ______

PROCEDURE FOR CHANGING DECIMALS TO FRACTIONS

1. Express the decimal as it is written in fraction form.
2. Reduce to lowest terms.

EXAMPLES

a. $0.375 = \frac{375}{1000} = \frac{3}{8}$

b. $0.40 = \frac{40}{100} = \frac{2}{5}$

c. $0.8 = \frac{8}{10} = \frac{4}{5}$

PROCEDURE FOR CHANGING COMMON FRACTIONS TO DECIMALS

1. Divide the numerator by the denominator.
2. Place decimal point in proper position.

EXAMPLES

a. $\frac{2}{5} = 5\overline{)2.00}$ (quotient 0.4) $= 0.4$

b. $\frac{19}{100} = 100\overline{)19.00}$ (quotient 0.19) $= 0.19$

c. $\frac{9}{7} = 7\overline{)9.000}$ (quotient 1.285) $= 1.285$

EXERCISES

A. Change the following to decimals. Round to the nearest thousandth when necessary:

1. $\frac{8}{10}$ ______
2. $\frac{1}{6}$ ______
3. $\frac{22}{100}$ ______
4. $\frac{13}{15}$ ______
5. $4\frac{2}{5}$ ______
6. $7\frac{1}{8}$ ______
7. $\frac{38}{54}$ ______
8. $\frac{6754}{10,000}$ ______
9. $4\frac{23}{32}$ ______
10. $\frac{94}{36}$ ______

B. Change the following to fractions or mixed numbers:

1. 0.28 ______
2. 5.07 ______
3. 0.0022 ______
4. 1.28 ______
5. 3.04 ______
6. 0.575 ______
7. 0.76 ______
8. 0.15325 ______
9. 6.09 ______
10. 0.01 ______

The term **percent** and its symbol % mean hundredths. A percent number is a fraction whose numerator is expressed and whose denominator is understood to be 100. It can be changed to a decimal by moving the decimal point two places to the left to signify hundredths or to a fraction by expressing the denominator as 100.

EXAMPLES

a. 5% means $\frac{5}{100}$ or 0.05

b. $\frac{1}{2}$% means $\frac{\frac{1}{2}}{100}$ or 0.005

EXERCISES

Complete the following:

	Fraction	Decimal	Percent
1.	$\frac{1}{4}$	______	______
2.	______	1.25	______
3.	______	______	0.5%
4.	$\frac{1}{8}$	______	______
5.	______	0.56	______
6.	$\frac{6}{1000}$	______	______
7.	______	______	6%
8.	______	0.75	______
9.	______	______	20%
10.	______	______	12%
11.	______	0.05	______
12.	______	______	72%

PROCEDURE FOR FINDING PERCENT OF A NUMBER

1. Change the percent to a decimal or common fraction.
2. Multiply the number by this decimal.

EXAMPLES

a. 23% of 64 = ?
   $0.23 \times 64 = 14.72$

b. 114% of 240 = ?
   $1.14 \times 240 = 273.6$

EXERCISES

Find the following percents. Round to the nearest thousandth when necessary.

1. 6% of 300 ______
2. $\frac{1}{2}$% of 840 ______
3. 5% of 15 ______
4. 8% of 2700 ______
5. 200% of 6.7 ______
6. 0.2% of 10 ______
7. 50% of 75 ______
8. 3% of 200 ______
9. $\frac{1}{3}$% of 360 ______
10. 15.6% of 324 ______
11. $5\frac{1}{2}$% of 2500 ______
12. 35% of 9.25 ______

PROCEDURE FOR FINDING WHAT PERCENT ONE NUMBER IS OF ANOTHER

1. Make a fraction of the two numbers using the number after the word "of" as the denominator.
2. Reduce the fraction to lowest terms.
3. Change the reduced fraction to a percent.

EXAMPLES

a. 27 is what percent of 36?
   $\frac{27}{36} = \frac{3}{4} = 75\%$

b. 9 is what percent of 20?
   $\frac{9}{20} = 0.45 = 45\%$

EXERCISES

Find the following percents. Round to the nearest tenth of a percent.

1. 2 is ? % of 20? ______
2. 10 is ? % of 25? ______
3. 15 is ? % of 85? ______
4. $2\frac{1}{2}$ is ? % of 8? ______
5. What % of 25 is 15? ______
6. 45 is ? % of 80? ______
7. $1\frac{1}{2}$ is ? % of $8\frac{1}{2}$? ______
8. What % of 25 is 50? ______
9. 60 is ? % of 15? ______
10. 3 is ? % of 15? ______
11. 240 is ? % of 1200? ______
12. What % of 15 is 30? ______

A **proportion** shows the relationship between two equal ratios. A proportion may be expressed as:

$$8:16 :: 1:2$$

or

$$8:16 = 1:2$$

The first and fourth terms of a proportion are called the **extremes,** and the second and third terms are the **means.** In a proportion, the product of the means equals the product of the extremes.

It can be seen from the above sample proportion that the product of the extremes $(8 \times 2) = 16$; the product of the means $(16 \times 1) = 16$.

When one term of the proportion is unknown, it can easily be found.

PROCEDURE TO SOLVE FOR AN UNKNOWN TERM IN A PROPORTION

1. Multiply the means and the extremes, letting x signify the unknown term.
2. Divide the known product by the coefficient of x to solve for the unknown term.

EXAMPLES

a. $3:5 = x:10$

$$5x = 30$$

$$x = \frac{30}{5} = 6$$

b. $\frac{1}{2} : x :: 1:8$

$$1x = \frac{1}{2} \times 8$$

$$x = 4$$

EXERCISES

Solve the following proportions for x:

1. 2 : *x* :: 10 : 20 __________
2. 20 : *x* :: 30 : 600 __________
3. 10 : 15 :: *x* : 30 __________
4. *x* : 300 :: 2 : 60 __________
5. 6 : 3000 :: 10 : *x* __________
6. 8 : 24 :: 16 : *x* __________
7. 2.5 : *x* :: 50 : 60 __________
8. 3.4 : *x* :: 17 : 25 __________
9. 4 : 8 :: *x* : 72 __________
10. 3 : 28 :: 6 : *x* __________
11. 4 : 18 :: 20 : *x* __________
12. 7 : 30 :: *x* : 60 __________
13. 4 : 7 :: *x* : 49 __________
14. *x* : 5.2 :: 1.6 : 8 __________
15. 20 : 100 :: 5 : *x* __________

Two scales are commonly used to measure temperature: the **Fahrenheit scale** and the **Celsius,** or centigrade, **scale.** The inner tube of a thermometer contains mercury, which expands and rises in the tube as heat increases, showing the temperatures on the scale (Fig. 1-5).

The Fahrenheit (F) scale is used on most clinical thermometers in the United States, but because the

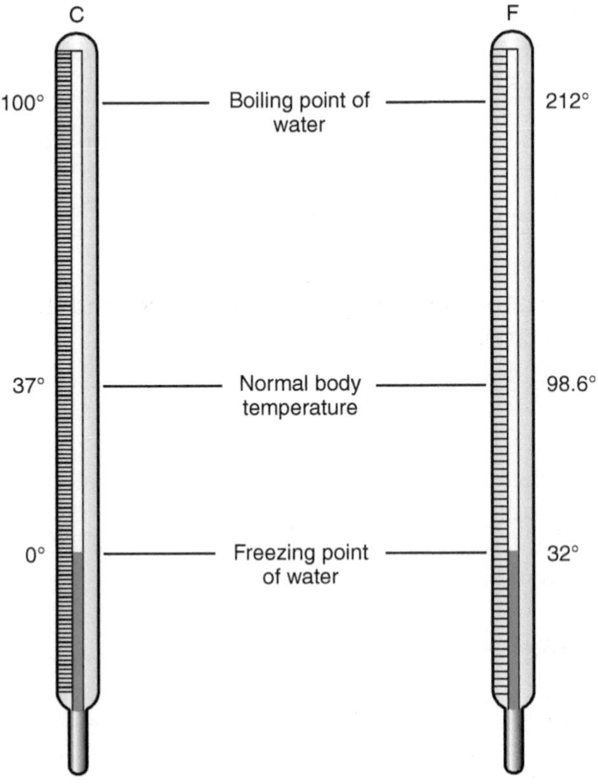

FIGURE 1-5 Celsius *(left)* and Fahrenheit *(right)* scales used to measure temperature.

Celsius (C) scale is also in common use in medical practice, a health care professional should be able to convert from one scale to the other.

Five degrees on the Celsius scale correspond to nine degrees on the Fahrenheit scale, so the ratio is 5 : 9. Also, 0° C corresponds to 32° F, so 32° must be subtracted from the Fahrenheit temperature in addition to considering the simple ratio.

PROCEDURE FOR CONVERTING BETWEEN FAHRENHEIT AND CELSIUS

1. Use the proportion formula C : F–32 :: 5 : 9.
2. Substitute the known temperature in its proper place in the formula.
3. Solve for the unknown temperature as for the fourth term of a proportion.

EXAMPLES

a. Change 50° F to C

$$C : F - 32 :: 5 : 9$$
$$C : 50 - 32 :: 5 : 9$$
$$C : 18 :: 5 : 9$$
$$9C = 18 \times 5$$
$$C = \frac{90}{9} = 10° \text{ on the Celsius scale}$$

b. Change 75° C to F

$$C : F - 32 :: 5 : 9$$
$$75 : F - 32 :: 5 : 9$$
$$5(F - 32) = 675$$
$$5F - 160 = 675$$
$$5F = 835$$
$$F = 167° \text{ on the Fahrenheit scale}$$

EXERCISES

Convert the following temperatures. Round to the nearest tenth.

1. 20° C = ________° F
2. 60° C = ________° F
3. 102° C = ________° F
4. 35° C = ________° F
5. 40° C = ________° F
6. 101° F = ________° C
7. 70° F = ________° C
8. 120° F = ________° C
9. 104° F = ________° C
10. 96.8° F = ________° C

The system of weights and measures used in medicine is the **metric system**. It is essential that the healthcare professional become familiar with this system and be able to use it accurately.

METRIC SYSTEM

The metric system is now used exclusively in the *United States Pharmacopeia-National Formulary* (USP-NF). Arabic numbers and decimals are used with this system.

The units used in the metric system are:

liter for volume (fluids)

gram for weight (solids)

meter for measure (length)

These basic units are multiplied and divided by 10 or a multiple of 10 to form the entire system. There are only a few equivalents that are used in medicine, however. These are:

Volume	Weight
1000 mL = 1 liter (L)	1000 mg = 1 gram (gm)
	1000 gm = 1 kilogram (kg)

Milliliter (mL) is the correct unit for liquid measurements. Common usage, however, interchanges milliliter with cubic centimeter (cc) in a 1:1 ratio, with 1000 cc = 1000 mL = 1 L. Centimeter is actually a linear measurement, and cubic centimeter is a measure of area. Milliliter and cubic centimeter should not be used interchangeably. Instead, cubic centimeters should be converted to milliliters or liters.

PROCEDURE FOR CONVERSION AMONG METRIC UNITS

1. To change milligrams to grams, to change milliliters to liters, or to change grams to kilograms, divide by 1000.
2. To change liters to milliliters, grams to milligrams, or kilograms to grams, multiply by 1000.

EXAMPLES

a. 64 mg = ? gm

$$1000 \text{ mg} : 1 \text{ gm} = 64 \text{ mg} : x \text{ gm}$$
$$1000\,x = 64$$
$$x = \frac{64}{1000} = 0.064 \text{ gm}$$

b. 325 mL = ? L

$$1000 \text{ mL} : 1 \text{ L} = 325 \text{ mL} : x \text{ L}$$
$$1000\,x = 325$$
$$x = \frac{325}{1000} = 0.325 \text{ L}$$

c. 3.5 L = ? mL

$$1000 \text{ mL} : 1 \text{ L} = x \text{ mL} : 3.5 \text{ L}$$
$$1\,x = 3500$$
$$x = 3500 \text{ mL}$$

Note: These rules may be used without use of the ratio and proportion method. The use of the proportion serves to clarify the reasoning behind multiplying or dividing.

EXERCISES

Change to equivalents within the metric system:

1. 1000 mg = ______ gm
2. 500 mg = ______ gm
3. 2000 mL = ______ L
4. 1500 mg = ______ gm
5. 0.1L = ______ mL
6. 750 mg = ______ gm
7. 1 kg = ______ gm
8. 5 L = ______ mL
9. 4 mg = ______ gm
10. 100 gm = ______ kg
11. 0.25 L = ______ mL
12. 0.006 gm = ______ mg
13. 250 mg = ______ gm
14. 2.5 L = ______ mL
15. 0.05 gm = ______ mg

SYSTEM OF HOUSEHOLD MEASUREMENTS

The **Avoirdupois system** of common household measurements, a more familiar system in the United States, may be compared with the metric system. Household measurements include teaspoons, tablespoons, cups, pints, and quarts. These measurements, although more familiar, are not as accurate and should be avoided in the administration of medication.

The American standard teaspoon has been established by the American Standards Association as containing approximately 5 mL, and this measurement is accepted in the USP-NF.

Drugs dispensed by the teaspoonful (i.e., cough syrups, antihistamines, liquid vitamins) generally do not require exactly precise measurements. The household teaspoon may vary considerably in its milliliter equivalent, in some cases ranging from 3.5 to 5 mL. Exact doses for drugs such as digoxin or doses for very young children should be measured using an oral syringe, a calibrated dropper, or a pediatric dosing spoon available from pharmacies. Antibiotic suspensions may generally be administered using the teaspoon.

Some approximate equivalents to household measurements are as follows:

1 teaspoon	$= \frac{1}{6}$ fluid ounce = 5 mL
1 tablespoon	$= \frac{1}{2}$ fluid ounce = 15 mL
2 tablespoons	= 1 fluid ounce = 30 mL
1 cup	= 8 ounces = 240 mL
1 pint	= 500 mL
1 quart	= 1000 mL = 1 L
1 ounce	= 30 gm
2.2 pounds (lb)	= 1 kg

EXAMPLES

a. 45 gm = ? oz

$$30 \text{ gm} : 1 \text{ oz} = 45 \text{ gm} : x \text{ oz}$$
$$30\,x = 45 \times 1$$
$$x = \frac{45}{30} = 1\frac{1}{2} \text{ oz}$$

b. 150 lb = ? kg

$$2.2 \text{ lb} : 1 \text{ kg} = 150 \text{ lb} : x \text{ kg}$$
$$2.2\,x = 150 \times 1$$
$$x = \frac{50}{2.2} = 68.2 \text{ kg}$$

EXERCISES

A. Change to approximate equivalents in household measurements. Round to the nearest tenth

1. 10 mL = ______ teaspoons
2. 2 cups = ______ ounces
3. 10 lb = ______ kg
4. 60 mL = ______ ounces
5. 22 pounds = ______ kg
6. 3 ounces = ______ gm
7. 60 mL = ______ teaspoons
8. 6 teaspoons = ______ fluid ounces
9. 3 fluid ounces = ______ teaspoons
10. 70 kg = ______ lb

B. Convert the following:

1. 0.5 L = _______ mL
2. 4 mL = _______ cc
3. $\frac{1}{2}$ ounce = _______ gm
4. 0.1 gm = _______ mg
5. 500 mL = _______ pint
6. $\frac{1}{2}$ ounce = _______ mL
7. 30 lb = _______ kg
8. 30 mL = _______ teaspoons
9. 1500 mg = _______ gm
10. 2 ounces = _______ gm
11. 5 tablespoons = _______ mL
12. 5 tablespoons = _______ ounces
13. 1 gram = _______ mg
14. 10 mL = _______ teaspoons
15. 15 mL = _______ ounce
16. $2\frac{1}{2}$ quarts = _______ mL
17. 30 gm = _______ ounce
18. 3 kg = _______ lb
19. 165 lb = _______ kg
20. 3 pints = _______ quart

Answers to the Exercises can be found at the back of the book.

evolve Additional math problems and activities can be found at *http://evolve.elsevier.com/asperheim/pharmacology.*

CHAPTER 2 Introduction to Pharmacology

Objectives

After completing this chapter, you should be able to do the following:

1. Name four sources of drugs, and give an example of each.
2. List the responsibilities of the health care provider for drug administration.
3. Name all of the various pharmaceutical preparations.
4. Distinguish between an elixir and a tincture, and give an example of each.
5. Discuss the advantage of administering a capsule instead of a tablet.
6. Distinguish between a lotion and a liniment, and give an example of each.

The administration of medications is one of the most important responsibilities of a health care professional. It is most important that the health care professional apply himself or herself diligently in acquiring all possible knowledge of medicines, their use or abuse, correct dosage, methods of administration (Fig. 2-1), symptoms of overdosage, and abnormal reactions that may arise in the treatment of various conditions. Because of the various properties of the different drugs and their many uses, it is also necessary to know the different ways of preparing them for patient use. This knowledge is an indispensable aid in giving the best possible patient care.

The attitude of a health care professional toward drug administration is important to the effectiveness of the drug. Ideally, the body functions best when given adequate food, rest, relaxation, and freedom from undue emotional stress. However, because of physical or mental abnormalities, it is necessary sometimes to resort to drugs to produce a near-normal state of body function. At best, drugs are crutches, and undue dependence on them can be very dangerous. Used intelligently, drugs are a lifesaving boon; used unwisely, they can produce irreparable harm. A health care professional who combines diligent and intelligent observation with moral integrity and plain common sense in administering drugs can make many lasting contributions to the profession and to the patients in his or her care.

Pharmacology has undergone tremendous changes during the past few decades. Many new agents on the market today were totally unknown a generation ago, and scarcely a day goes by that literature is not received on new agents or medicines and new techniques and theories of drug administration. The

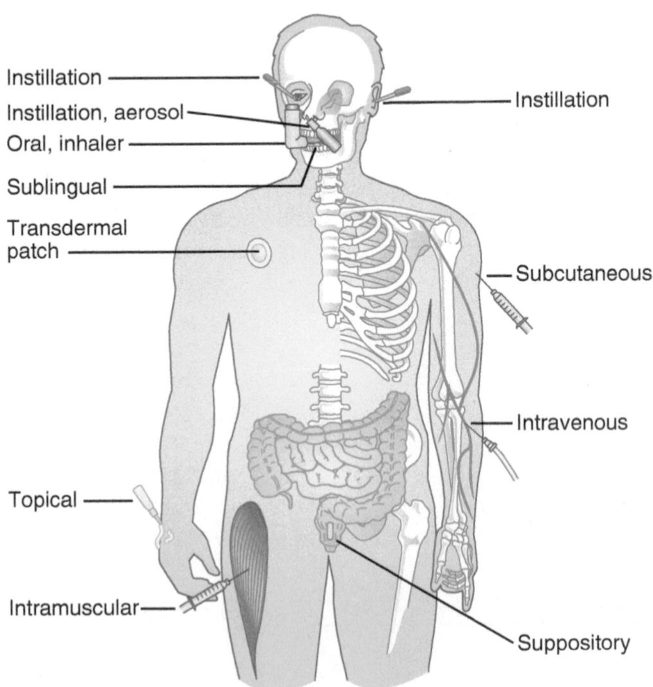

FIGURE 2-1 Some routes for medication administration. (From Kee JL, et al: *Pharmacology: a nursing process approach*, ed 6, St. Louis, 2009, Saunders.)

newest advances are always a source of interest and intrigue to beginning students, but students first need to obtain a well-rounded background in drug therapy before they can begin to appreciate these new "miracles of the modern age."

The information presented in this text lays the foundation for this well-rounded background, but as in all other areas of health care, the responsibility for making this knowledge one's own rests with the students themselves. A true dedication to the profession places the student in the starting position of a lifelong pursuit—a pursuit that, although admittedly arduous, promises the unfailing reward of continuous new horizons.

DEFINITIONS

GENERAL TERMINOLOGY

Animal products: Primarily glandular products that are currently obtained from animal sources (e.g., thyroid hormone, insulin).

Biotechnology: Field of pharmacology that involves using living cells, usually altered cultures of *Escherichia coli,* to manufacture drugs.

Certain food substances: Substances that under some conditions serve both as foods and as medicinal substances (i.e., vitamins and minerals in various foods).

Chemical substances: Agents that may be made synthetically (e.g., sulfonamides, aspirin, sodium bicarbonate).

Drug: Any substance used as medicine (e.g., used to diagnose, cure, mitigate, treat, or prevent disease). Drugs include chemical substances, plant parts or products, animal products, and certain food substances.

Pharmacology: Broad term that includes the study of drugs and their actions in the body.

Pharmacy: Art of preparing, compounding, and dispensing drugs for medicinal use.

Plant parts or products: Crude drugs that may be obtained from any part of various plants and used medicinally; leaves, bark, fruit, roots, rhizomes, resin, and other parts may be used (e.g., ergot, digitalis, opium).

Toxicology: Science that deals with poisons—their detection and the symptoms, diagnosis, and treatment of conditions caused by them.

SPECIFIC PHARMACOLOGY TERMS

Additive effect: Combined effect of two drugs that is equal to the sum of the effects of each drug taken alone.

Adverse or untoward effect: Action, usually negative, that is different from the planned effect.

Allergic reaction: Untoward reaction that develops after an individual has taken a drug.

Analog: Chemical compound that resembles another in structure but has different effects.

Antagonism: Combined effect of two drugs that is less than the effect of either drug taken alone.

Biosynthesis: Formation of a chemical compound by enzymes, either within an organism (in vivo) or in vitro by fragments of cells.

Depression: Decrease in activity of cells caused by the action of a drug.

Diagnostic: Pertaining to the art or act of determining the nature of a patient's disease.

Idiosyncrasy (ID-e-o-SIN-kre-se): Abnormal sensitivity to a drug or a reaction not intended.

Palliative: Agent or measure that relieves symptoms.

Potentiation: Effect that occurs when a drug increases or prolongs the action of another drug, the total effect being greater than the sum of the effects of each used alone.

Prophylactic (PRO-fi-LAK-tik): Agent or measure used to prevent disease.

Side effect: Unpredictable effect that is not related to the main action of a drug.

Stimulation: Increase in the activity of cells produced by drugs.

Synergism: Joint action of agents in which their combined effect is more intense or longer in duration than the sum of their individual effects.

Therapeutic: Pertaining to treatment of disease.

Tolerance: Increasing resistance to the usual effects of an established dosage of a drug as a result of continued use.

PHARMACEUTICAL PREPARATIONS

Aerosols: Active pharmaceutical agents in a pressurized container.

Capsules: Powdered drugs within a gelatin container. Liquids may be placed in soft gelatin capsules (e.g., cod liver oil capsules, diphenhydramine hydrochloride [Benadryl] capsules).

Elixirs: Solutions containing alcohol, sugar, and water. Elixirs may or may not be aromatic and may or may not have active medicinals. Most frequently, they are used as flavoring agents or solvents (e.g., terpin hydrate elixir, phenobarbital elixir).

Emulsions: Suspensions of fat globules in water (or water globules in fat) with an emulsifying agent (e.g., Haley's M-O, Petrogalar). (Homogenized milk is also an emulsion.)

Fluid extracts: Alcoholic liquid extracts of a drug made by percolation so that 1 mL of the fluid extract contains 1 gm of the drug. Only vegetable-based drugs are used (e.g., glycyrrhiza fluid extract).

Gels: Aqueous suspensions of insoluble drugs in hydrated form. Aluminum hydroxide gel, USP-NF, is an example.

Liniments: Mixtures of drugs with oil, soap, water, or alcohol, intended for external application with rubbing (e.g., camphor liniment, chloroform liniment).

Long-acting or sustained-release dosage forms: Active pharmaceutical agents that are either layered in tablet form for release over several hours or placed in pellets within a capsule. The pellets are of varying size and disintegrate over 8 to 24 hours. Sustained-release dosage forms must not be broken or crushed because their efficacy depends on the release of the various layers over time.

Lotions: Aqueous preparations containing suspended materials intended for soothing, using local application. Most are patted on rather than rubbed (e.g., calamine [Caladryl] lotion).

Ointments: Mixtures of drugs with a fatty base for external application, usually by rubbing (e.g., zinc oxide ointment, Ben-Gay ointment).

Pills: Single-dose units made by mixing a powdered drug with a liquid such as syrup and rolling it into a round or oval shape. Pills are largely replaced by other dosage forms today.

Powders: Single-dose quantities of a drug or mixture of drugs in powdered form wrapped separately in powder papers (e.g., Seidlitz powder).

Solutions: Aqueous liquid preparations containing one or more substances completely dissolved. Every solution has two parts: the solute (the dissolved substance) and the solvent (the substance, usually a liquid, in which the solute is dissolved).

Spirits: Alcoholic solutions of volatile substances. These are also known as essences (e.g., essence of peppermint, camphor spirit).

Suppositories: Mixtures of drugs with some firm base such as cocoa butter, which can be molded into shape for insertion into a body orifice. Rectal, vaginal, and urethral suppositories are the most common types (e.g., nitrofurazone [Furacin] vaginal suppositories, magnesium hydroxide [Dulcolax] suppositories), but nasal or ear (otic) suppositories may be made.

Syrups: Aqueous solutions of a sugar. These may or may not have medicinal substances added (e.g., simple syrup, ipecac syrup).

Tablets: Single-dose units made by compressing powdered drugs in a suitable mold (e.g., aspirin tablets). Special forms of tablets include sublingual tablets (to be held under the tongue until dissolved) and enteric-coated tablets (with a coating that prevents their absorption until they reach the intestinal tract). 20-30 min breakdown

Tinctures: Alcoholic or hydroalcoholic solutions prepared from drugs (e.g., iodine tincture, digitalis tincture).

Troches (TRO-kes) **or lozenges**: Flat, round, or rectangular preparations that are held in the mouth until dissolved.

Waters: Saturated solutions of volatile oils (e.g., peppermint water, camphor water).

REVIEW QUESTIONS

1. The study of the effects of a poisonous substance is called:
   a. pharmacology.
   b. pharmacy.
   c. toxicology.
   d. biotechnology.

2. The study of how drugs work in the body is called:
   a. pharmacology.
   b. pharmacy.
   c. toxicology.
   d. biotechnology.

3. A drug is something that is:
   a. made from an animal source.
   b. made synthetically.
   c. made from a plant.
   d. all of the above.

4. An antibiotic can be prescribed as ____ therapy to prevent an infection.
   a. prophylactic
   b. diagnostic
   c. palliative
   d. idiosyncratic

5. Increasing the dose of a drug may be necessary because of:
   a. patient tolerance.
   b. an adverse effect.
   c. a side effect.
   d. an allergic reaction.

6. A suspension of fat globules in an aqueous preparation is called a(n):
   a. elixir.
   b. emulsion.
   c. syrup.
   d. spirit.

7. A solution containing alcohol is called a(n):
   a. syrup.
   b. solution.
   c. elixir.
   d. liniment.

8. A preparation that can be used rectally is called a(n):
   a. gel.
   b. aerosol.
   c. suppository.
   d. powder.

9. Sustained-release capsules may release the drug over:
   a. 30 to 60 minutes.
   b. 1 to 4 hours.
   c. 6 to 10 hours.
   d. 8 to 24 hours.

10. Which dosage form is intended to be given orally?
    a. Gel
    b. Suppository
    c. Aerosol
    d. Elixir

Answers to the review questions can be found at the back of the book.

evolve Additional questions and activities can be found at *http://evolve.elsevier.com/asperheim/pharmacology.*

CHAPTER 3

Drug Legislation and Drug Standards

Objectives

After completing this chapter, you should be able to do the following:

1. Identify drugs according to the current schedule of the Controlled Substances Act.
2. List official drug standards.
3. Use the *Physicians' Desk Reference* to identify a selected list of drugs according to generic and proprietary names.

Key Terms

Controlled Substances Act, p. 20
Drug standards, p. 21
Schedules of controlled substances, p. 20

AMERICAN DRUG LEGISLATION

Drug legislation in the United States underwent major revisions as of May 1, 1971, when the **Controlled Substances Act** became effective. This law requires that every person who manufactures, dispenses, prescribes, or administers any controlled substance be registered annually with the Attorney General; this registration function is the responsibility of the Drug Enforcement Administration (DEA).

Legislation and controls were revised to establish a classification system that categorizes drugs by the potential for abuse, which resulted in five **schedules of controlled substances.** Drugs in the original schedules are subject to revision on an annual basis on notification by the DEA, and many changes have been made within the schedules since the legislation first went into effect.

To get the complete and current schedule of controlled substances, go to the DEA website at http://www.justice.gov/dea/pubs/scheduling.html. Only a few examples of the more well-known drugs in each schedule are included here.

SCHEDULE I

1. The drug or other substance has a high potential for abuse.
2. The drug or other substance has no currently accepted medical use in treatment in the United States.
3. Accepted safety for use of the drug or other substance under medical supervision is lacking.

EXAMPLES OF DRUGS INCLUDED

- Opioids: ketobemidone, allylprodine
- Certain opium derivatives: heroin
- Hallucinogens: lysergic acid diethylamide (LSD), marijuana, mescaline, peyote

SCHEDULE II

1. The drug or other substance has a high potential for abuse.
2. The drug or other substance has a currently accepted medical use in treatment in the United States or a currently accepted medical use with severe restrictions.
3. Abuse of the drug or other substance may lead to severe psychological or physical dependence.

EXAMPLES OF DRUGS INCLUDED

- Many derivatives of opium (e.g., raw opium, morphine, codeine, ethylmorphine, hydrocodone, metopon, thebaine)

- Coca leaves and derivatives (e.g., cocaine)
- Opioids: anileridine, dihydrocodeine, diphenoxylate, levomethorphan, methadone, meperidine, oxycodone
- Stimulants: methamphetamine, amphetamine, phenmetrazine, methylphenidate
- Depressants: amobarbital, secobarbital, pentobarbital

SCHEDULE III

1. The drug or other substance has a potential for abuse less than drugs in Schedules I or II.
2. The drug or other substance has a currently accepted medical use in treatment in the United States.
3. Abuse of the drug or other substance may lead to moderate or low physical dependence or high psychological dependence.

EXAMPLES OF DRUGS INCLUDED

- Phendimetrazine, methyprylon, nalorphine
- Combinations of amobarbital, secobarbital, or pentobarbital with other active ingredients
- Compounds containing limited concentrations of codeine, hydrocodone, ethylmorphine, opium, or morphine with one or more active nonnarcotic ingredients in recognized therapeutic amounts

SCHEDULE IV

1. The drug or other substance has a low potential for abuse relative to the drugs or other substances in Schedule III.
2. The drug or other substance has a currently accepted medical use in treatment in the United States.
3. Abuse of the drug or other substance may lead to limited physical or psychological dependence relative to the drugs in Schedule III.

EXAMPLES OF DRUGS INCLUDED

- Chloral hydrate, chloral betaine, ethchlorvynol, meprobamate, paraldehyde, phenobarbital, chlordiazepoxide, diazepam, flurazepam, chlorazepate, pemoline, pentazocine, oxazepam

SCHEDULE V

1. The drug or other substance has a low potential for abuse relative to the drugs in Schedule IV.
2. The drug or other substance has a currently accepted medical use in treatment in the United States.
3. Abuse of the drug or other substance may lead to limited physical or psychological dependence relative to the drugs in Schedule IV.

EXAMPLES OF DRUGS INCLUDED

- Compounds containing limited amounts of codeine, dihydrocodeine, ethylmorphine, opium, or diphenoxylate in combination with other nonnarcotic active ingredients. (In all cases, the allowable concentration of these agents is lower than the compounds included in Schedule III.)
- Diphenoxylate and atropine preparations (e.g., Lomotil).

DRUG STANDARDS

Several organizations worldwide publish reference texts describing **drug standards** (lists of the known value, strength, quality, and ingredients of various drugs) for quality and strength. Before official standards were published, drugs, particularly those from plant sources, could vary in strength from being ineffective to providing almost a fatal dose, depending on the quality of the plant, the soil, and the growing conditions. The most prominent drug standard texts are listed next.

AMERICAN DRUG STANDARDS

United States Pharmacopeia–National Formulary (USP-NF)

Formerly two standards, the *United States Pharmacopeia* and the *National Formulary* have been combined into one official volume, *United States Pharmacopeia–National Formulary* (USP-NF). The USP-NF includes a list of approved drugs and defines them with respect to source, chemistry, physical properties, tests for identity, method of assay, storage, and dosage. It also provides directions for compounding and general use. The USP-NF is revised periodically by an appointed committee to include new drugs and exclude drugs no longer in general use.

ADDITIONAL SOURCES OF DRUG INFORMATION

Physicians' Desk Reference (PDR)

Revised annually and readily supplied to all hospitals and physicians, the *Physicians' Desk Reference* (PDR) is a widely used reference source. The PDR is not intended as an official standard. Each manufacturer supplies information for inclusion, usually by trade name, and gives the accepted uses, side effects, and doses for commercially available pharmaceutical agents.

Facts and Comparisons

Facts and Comparisons is continuously updated and is available by subscription. The website is www.factsandcomparisons.com and may be accessed by individuals with a subscription to the text.

Epocrates

Drug information is available by subscription through Epocrates.com. This drug information may be downloaded onto personal data assistant devices such as a Blackberry or iPod. It is updated wirelessly.

American Hospital Formulary Service (AHFS) Drug Information

The American Hospital Formulary Service (AHFS) Drug Information is an annual publication by the American Society of Health System Pharmacists that contains useful and current information on drugs. Individual copies may be ordered from the American Society of Health System Pharmacists.

INTERNATIONAL DRUG STANDARDS

International Pharmacopeia

The World Health Organization was originally responsible for the publication of the *International Pharmacopeia* to standardize drugs for many European nations. The names of drugs are in Latin; all doses are in the metric system.

BRITISH DRUG STANDARDS

British Pharmacopeia

Similar in content to the USP-NF, the *British Pharmacopeia* sets the standards for drugs that are official in the United Kingdom and its dominions and colonies. It is published by the British Pharmacopeia Commission under the direction of the General Medical Council.

Pharmaceutical Codex

The *Pharmaceutical Codex* is a text similar to the *British Pharmacopeia* published by the Pharmaceutical Society of Great Britain that gives drug information and standards.

CANADIAN DRUG LEGISLATION

CANADIAN FOOD AND DRUGS ACT

The Food and Drugs Act, passed in 1941, empowers the Governor-in-Council to prescribe drug standards and limit variation in any food or drug. It contains the following schedules:

Schedule A: This schedule contains a list of diseases or disorders for which a cure may not be advertised. It includes diseases such as gangrene, influenza, and appendicitis.

Schedule B: This schedule contains lists of official drug standard texts, such as the USP-NF and the *British Pharmacopeia*.

Schedule C: This schedule contains a list of drugs derived from animal tissues, such as liver extract and insulin, for which special standards of quality and purity apply.

Schedule D: This schedule contains a list of drugs obtained from microorganisms, such as antibiotics, and their requirements for manufacture.

Schedule E: This schedule does not currently contain any drugs.

Schedule F: This schedule lists all prescription drugs not included in the Controlled Drugs and Substances Act.

CANADIAN CONTROLLED DRUGS AND SUBSTANCES ACT

The Controlled Drugs and Substances Act, passed in 1996, repealed the Narcotic Control Act and Parts III and IV of the Food and Drugs Act. This act regulates the possession, production, distribution, and sale of controlled drugs, including narcotics. With this legislation, controlled substances are assigned to eight schedules. For more information, see the Appendix: Canadian Drug Information.

PROPRIETARY (TRADE) NAMES

Most pharmaceutical houses market their drugs primarily under trade names, although some drugs are available under their generic names. A single drug may be sold under numerous trade names. The practice of using these trade names is often confusing to nurses and physicians, to say nothing of the inconvenience to the pharmacist, who must stock four or five different brands of the same drug.

There is a trend to return to the use of official or generic names on prescriptions. In many cases, this is a significant cost issue, with the price of a name-brand drug being much higher compared with the generic form of the drug. Some insurance companies pay only for the generic form of a drug if that is available, or they pay for the brand-name drug only if the patient is responsible for a significantly higher copayment for the prescription. Many hospital pharmacies provide nursing divisions with a formulary that lists the official or generic names for the commercial products stocked in the pharmacy.

REVIEW QUESTIONS

1. Under the Controlled Substances Act, individuals who manufacture, dispense, prescribe, or administer controlled substances are required to register annually with what agency?
   - **a.** FBI
   - **b.** USP-NF
   - **c.** CIA
   - **d.** DEA

2. A complete up-to-date list of controlled substances can be found in or requested from:
   - **a.** *Merck Manual.*
   - **b.** District DEA office.
   - **c.** USP-NF.
   - **d.** *International Pharmacopeia.*

3. An example of a Schedule I medication is:
   - **a.** methadone.
   - **b.** heroin.
   - **c.** cocaine.
   - **d.** methylphenidate.

4. An example of a Schedule II medication is:
   - **a.** heroin.
   - **b.** nalorphine.
   - **c.** diazepam.
   - **d.** codeine.

5. Pemoline is an example of what schedule of medication?
   - **a.** Schedule I
   - **b.** Schedule II
   - **c.** Schedule III
   - **d.** Schedule IV

6. The drug standard text originally compiled by the World Health Organization is:
   - **a.** *International Pharmacopeia.*
   - **b.** *British Pharmacopeia.*
   - **c.** *Pharmaceutical Codex.*
   - **d.** *Canadian Pharmacopeia.*

7. A drug in which schedule would have the highest potential for abuse?
   - **a.** Schedule I
   - **b.** Schedule II
   - **c.** Schedule III
   - **d.** Schedule IV

8. An example of a drug in Schedule III is:
   - **a.** nalorphine.
   - **b.** morphine.
   - **c.** heroin.
   - **d.** opium.

9. The main American drug standard text is the:
   - **a.** PDR.
   - **b.** *British Pharmacopeia.*
   - **c.** *Merck Manual.*
   - **d.** USP-NF.

10. Compounds with limited amounts of codeine in a cough preparation would be in:
    - **a.** Schedule II.
    - **b.** Schedule III.
    - **c.** Schedule IV.
    - **d.** Schedule V.

Answers to the review questions can be found at the back of the book.

evolve Additional questions and activities can be found at *http://evolve.elsevier.com/asperheim/pharmacology.*

Introduction to Drug Dosage

CHAPTER

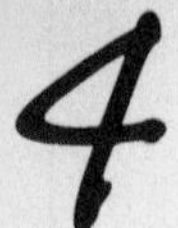

Objectives

After completing this chapter, you should be able to do the following:

1 List the factors influencing dosage.
2 Understand the concept of units per milliliter.
3 Accurately measure the contents of insulin and tuberculin syringes.
4 Convert insulin dosage to milliliters for injection by tuberculin syringe.
5 Calculate the desired concentration of antibiotic.
6 Interpret a medication order and prescription.
7 Use accepted abbreviations.

Key Terms

Automatic stop policy, p. 27
Dosage, p. 24
Dose, p. 24
Drug order, p. 27
Inscription, p. 26
Insulin syringe, p. 25
Prescription, p. 26
Signatura (Sig), p. 26
Subscription, p. 26
Superscription, p. 26
Tuberculin (tū-BŭR-kyĕ-lĭn) **syringe,** p. 25
Units per milliliter, p. 25

Dosage is the proper amount of a medicine or agent prescribed for a given patient or condition. **Dose** is the quantity of medicine to be taken at one time or in divided amounts within a given period of time. The following factors influence dosage:

Age: The age of a patient affects his or her response to drugs. Children and the elderly may require less than the usual adult dose.

Sex: The sex of a patient sometimes affects the response to drugs. Women are more susceptible to the action of certain drugs and are usually given smaller doses. The administration of medication to women in the early weeks of pregnancy may cause damage to the fetus. During the third trimester, premature labor may be caused by drugs that may stimulate muscular contractions.

Condition of the patient: Smaller doses are indicated when resistance in the patient is lowered. Impaired kidney and liver function may cause drugs to accumulate to toxic levels.

Psychological factors: An individual's personality often plays an important part in his or her response to certain drugs.

Environmental factors: The setting in which drugs are given and the attitude of the health care professional who administers the medication may influence the effects of drugs.

Temperature: Heat and cold affect the response to drugs. It may be necessary to decrease the dosage of certain drugs during hot weather.

Method of administration: Generally, larger doses are ordered when a medication is given orally or rectally, and smaller doses are ordered when the parenteral route is used.

Genetic factors: A drug idiosyncrasy is an abnormal or unusual reaction to a drug. It is thought to be due to genetic factors.

Body weight: Because a drug is generally distributed in all body tissues after absorption, the weight of the individual is very important in calculating the proper dose. Many drugs are dosed as milligrams per kilogram of body weight or dosed by the square meters of body surface area.

DRUG DOSAGE IN STANDARDIZED UNITS

INSULIN DOSAGE

Insulin and many other drugs that are obtained from animal sources are standardized in units based on their strengths rather than on weight measures such as milligrams and grams. The reason for this is that the strength of these animal drugs varies greatly, depending on the sources, conditions, and manner in which they are obtained. Many of the hormones (e.g., insulin) are too complex to be completely purified to obtain an exact weight of the drug per unit volume.

Insulin is supplied in 10-mL vials labeled in the number of **units per milliliter**—100-unit insulin means there are 100 units per milliliter. In the past, insulin was administered in 40-unit and 80-unit dosage forms. However, the 100-unit form has almost totally replaced the weaker strengths. The smaller volume required per dose decreases local reactions at the injection site, and mathematical calculations when a fraction of a milliliter is required are simplified.

The simplest and most accurate way to measure insulin is within an **insulin syringe**. The syringe is calibrated in units, and the desired dose may be read directly on the syringe. In Figure 4-1, 35 units are shown drawn up in a 100-unit syringe. If an insulin syringe is unavailable, a **tuberculin syringe** may be used; the unit dosage is converted to the equivalent number of milliliters, using the proportion method.

EXAMPLE

Give 60 units of insulin, using 100-unit insulin and a tuberculin syringe.

$$\frac{60}{100} \times 1 \text{ mL} = 0.6 \text{ mL}$$

Figure 4-2 shows a tuberculin syringe with 0.6 mL drawn up.

HEPARIN DOSAGE

Similar to insulin, heparin is derived from animal sources and is standardized for its activity as an anticoagulant. Heparin is supplied in unit-dose or multiple-dose vials and in strengths ranging from 1000 to 20,000 units per milliliter. There is often no set dose for the use of heparin; the individual's requirements are obtained from blood clotting studies done initially every 4 hours and less frequently as the dosage is stabilized. Blood clotting time is generally maintained at about twice the normal clotting rate to provide a safe yet effective way to decrease the formation of blood clots in the body. Heparin is often given intravenously at first to produce a rapid effect and then later by deep subcutaneous injection in larger and less frequent doses.

ANTIBIOTIC DOSAGE

Many antibiotics are still standardized in units. These may be prepared for injection in the form of a liquid containing a specified number of units per cubic centimeter. The entire amount in the vial may be ordered, but sometimes only part of the contents is used. It is important always to read the label carefully. Antibiotics are also available in the form of a dry powder in a vial that first must be diluted with water or another diluent. The powder should be diluted so that the desired dose is in 1 or 2 mL if the dose is to be given

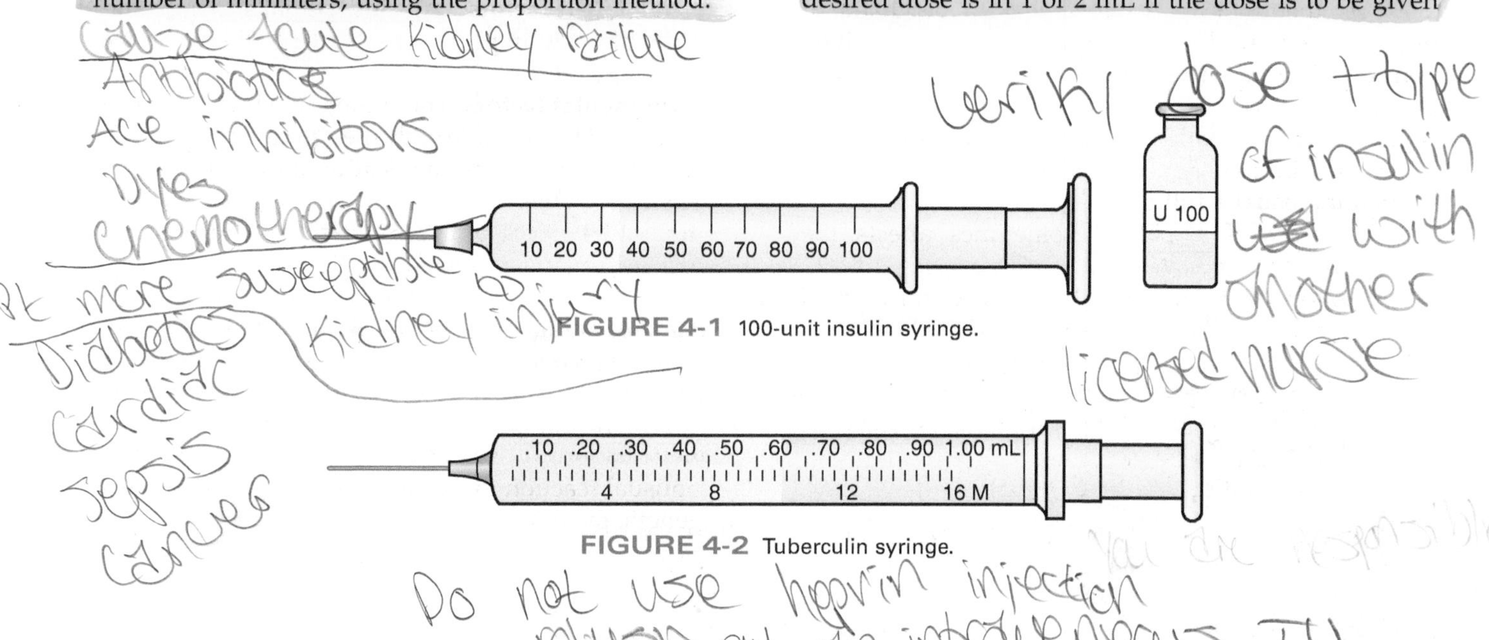

FIGURE 4-1 100-unit insulin syringe.

FIGURE 4-2 Tuberculin syringe.

intramuscularly. If it is to be given intravenously, a larger amount of diluent may be used.

PROCEDURE FOR OBTAINING THE DESIRED CONCENTRATION OF ANTIBIOTIC

1. Using the proportion method, state the desired concentration as the first two terms of the proportion.
2. The total number of units in the vial is the third term; the unknown volume of diluent is the fourth term.

EXAMPLES

a. You have a vial of powdered penicillin G containing 1,000,000 units. How much diluent should be added to obtain a solution containing 100,000 units/mL?

$$100,000: 1 \text{ mL} = 1,000,000: x \text{ mL}$$
$$100,000x = 1,000,000 \times 1$$
$$x = \frac{1,000,000}{100,000}$$
$$x = 10 \text{ mL}$$

b. If a 5,000,000-unit vial of penicillin powder is reconstituted with 10 mL of diluent, how many units will it contain per milliliter?

$$x : 1 \text{ mL} = 5,000,000 : 10 \text{ mL}$$
$$10x = 5,000,000 \times 1$$
$$x = \frac{5,000,000}{10}$$
$$x = 500,000 \text{ units/mL}$$

THE PRESCRIPTION

The prescription is probably as old as the written history of humankind. The first real literature dealing with pharmacy was a scroll called the Ebers Papyrus, which included methods of conjuring away diseases and lists of medicinal agents and methods of compounding.

A **prescription** is an order written by a practitioner, to be filled by a pharmacist, indicating the medication needed by the patient and containing all the necessary directions for the pharmacist and the patient (Fig. 4-3). The prescription consists of several parts, as follows:

1. The **superscription**, which states the date and the name and address of the patient
2. The **inscription**, which states the name and quantities of ingredients
3. The **subscription**, which gives directions to the pharmacist
4. The **signatura (Sig)**, which gives directions to the patient
5. The signature, address, and registry number of the physician
6. If a controlled substance, the physician DEA number

PARTS OF AN ORDER

A physician, dentist, or other qualified practitioner writes orders for the administration of drugs. A health care professional who administers drugs must be familiar with the laws of the state in which he or she is licensed to practice and with the policies of the

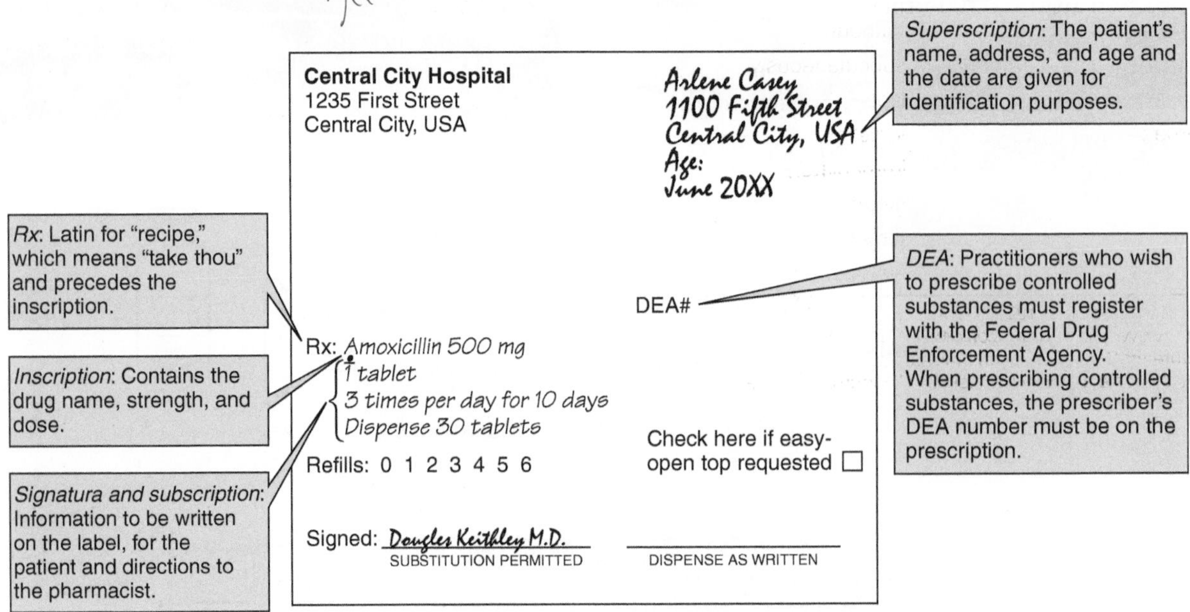

Central City Hospital
1235 First Street
Central City, USA
Arlene Casey
1100 Fifth Street
Central City, USA
Age:
June 20XX
Superscription: The patient's name, address, and age and the date are given for identification purposes.
Rx: Latin for "recipe," which means "take thou" and precedes the inscription.
DEA#
DEA: Practitioners who wish to prescribe controlled substances must register with the Federal Drug Enforcement Agency. When prescribing controlled substances, the prescriber's DEA number must be on the prescription.
Rx: Amoxicillin 500 mg
1 tablet
3 times per day for 10 days
Dispense 30 tablets
Inscription: Contains the drug name, strength, and dose.
Refills: 0 1 2 3 4 5 6
Check here if easy-open top requested
Signatura and subscription: Information to be written on the label, for the patient and directions to the pharmacist.
Signed: Douglas Keithley M.D.
SUBSTITUTION PERMITTED
DISPENSE AS WRITTEN

FIGURE 4-3 Example of a medication prescription. (From Potter PA, et al: *Basic nursing*, ed 7, St. Louis, 2011, Mosby.)

Table 4-1 Common Prescription Abbreviations

Abbreviation	Meaning
aa	of each
ac	before meals
ad lib	as much as desired
bid	twice a day
c̄	with
caps	a capsule
elix	elixir
et	and
fldxt	fluid extract
gm	gram
gr	grain
gt	a drop
hr	hour(s)
HT	hypodermic tablet
IM	intramuscularly
IV	intravenously
L	liter
mcg	microgram
mg	milligram
mL	milliliter
pc	after meals
PO	by mouth
prn	as needed
q	at or every
q2h	every 2 hours
q3h	every 3 hours
qid	4 times a day
qs	quantity sufficient
Rx	take
s̄	without
subcut	subcutaneously
Sig	label
sp frumenti	whiskey
stat	immediately
syr	syrup
tab	tablet
tid	3 times a day

The Joint Commission's (TJC) "Do Not Use" list of abbreviations is available at www.jointcommission.org/Do_Not_Use_List_of_Abbreviations. The Institute for Safe Medication Practices (ISMP) list of error-prone abbreviations is available at www.ismp.org/Tools/errorproneabbreviations.pdf.

employing agency. A typical **drug order** consists of the following: patient name, hospital number, and birth date; date and time of the order; name of the drug; the dosage, how it is to be given, and how many times it is to be given; and the signature of the physician who wrote the order.

Antibiotics and narcotics are examples of drugs that have an **automatic stop policy**. A new order is required for the drug to be continued after a specified time that has been established by the institution.

PRESCRIPTION ABBREVIATIONS

To administer medications safely, it is necessary to become thoroughly familiar with medically accepted or "approved" prescription abbreviations. The amount of a drug to be given is generally written in the metric system. In the metric system, the quantity of the drug is written in Arabic numbers, using decimals, before the abbreviation for the metric unit of measure. Some examples are 100 mg, 2500 mL, 0.5 gm, and 2 L.

The list of abbreviations in Table 4-1 includes those most often found in prescriptions and physicians' orders.

REVIEW QUESTIONS

1. Which of the following would *not* affect the dose of a drug given to an individual?
   - **a.** Age
   - **b.** Weight
   - **c.** Impaired kidney function
   - **d.** Time of day the medicine is administered

2. Unit-100 insulin contains 100 units of insulin in each 1 mL of solution. A 10-mL vial of unit-100 insulin contains how many units of insulin?
   - **a.** 10 units
   - **b.** 100 units
   - **c.** 1000 units
   - **d.** 10,000 units

3. A patient needs 30 units of unit-100 insulin. Considering that there are 100 units of insulin in each 1 mL of unit-100 insulin, how many milliliters would the patient need to inject?
   - **a.** 0.03 mL
   - **b.** 0.3 mL
   - **c.** 3 mL
   - **d.** 30 mL

4. For injection, 20,000,000 units of penicillin G is mixed in 200 mL of solution. How many units of penicillin are in each 1 mL of solution?
   - **a.** 1000 units
   - **b.** 10,000 units
   - **c.** 100,000 units
   - **d.** 1,000,000 units

5. Which part of the prescription indicates the directions to the patient?
   - **a.** The body of the prescription
   - **b.** The dosage form
   - **c.** The signatura (sig)
   - **d.** The subscription

6. The measured portion of medicine to be given to the patient is called the:
   - **a.** mode of administration.
   - **b.** dosage form.
   - **c.** dose.
   - **d.** toxic level.

7. When an individual reacts unusually to a drug, it is termed a(n):
   - **a.** drug overdose.
   - **b.** allergic reaction.
   - **c.** environmental factor.
   - **d.** idiosyncrasy.

8. The abbreviation for "by mouth" is:
   - **a.** ou.
   - **b.** od.
   - **c.** os.
   - **d.** PO.

9. The abbreviation "bid" stands for:
   - **a.** twice daily.
   - **b.** one every other day.
   - **c.** twice weekly.
   - **d.** before bed.

10. The abbreviation "ac" stands for:
    - **a.** in between meals.
    - **b.** before meals.
    - **c.** after meals.
    - **d.** on an empty stomach.

Answers to the review questions can be found at the back of the book.

evolve Additional questions and activities can be found at *http://evolve.elsevier.com/asperheim/pharmacology*.

Administration of Medications

CHAPTER 5

Objectives

After completing this chapter, you should be able to do the following:

1 Differentiate between local and systemic effects, and give four examples of each.
2 Name the various methods of administering drugs for local and systemic effects.
3 Define the term *parenteral* and give examples of types of parenteral methods of administering drugs.
4 List advantages and disadvantages of giving drugs by the parenteral route.
5 List guidelines for safe administration of drugs.
6 Identify reasons for errors in medication administration.
7 Use common abbreviations with 100% accuracy.
8 Demonstrate beginning skill in pouring medications.
9 Calibrate the rate of flow of intravenous solutions.
10 Explain ways to properly dispose of tablets or capsules, liquid medications, and needles.

Key Terms

Calibration, p. 36
Dosage forms, p. 30
Inhaled administration, p. 32
Intra-arterial injection, p. 36
Intradermal injection, p. 33
Intramuscular (IM) injection, p. 33
Intravenous (IV) injection, p. 36
Local effect, p. 30
Oral administration, p. 31
Parenteral administration, p. 32
Subcutaneous injection, p. 33
Sublingual administration, p. 32
Systemic effects, p. 30

GUIDELINES FOR SAFETY IN DRUG ADMINISTRATION

Safety is the paramount concern in drug administration. Guidelines to be used in the promotion of safe medication administration include the following:

1. Know the policies of the hospital or agency.
2. Give only the medications for which the physician has written and signed the order.
3. Check with the head nurse or physician when in doubt about any medication.
4. Ensure that all data on the electronic medical record, medicine card, or Kardex corresponds exactly with the label on the patient's medicine.
5. Always have another person (e.g., the head nurse or pharmacist) check calculations.
6. Do not converse during drug administration unless seeking help. Attentiveness is the most important aspect of safety.
7. Keep the drug cart locked at all times when not in use.
8. Do not give keys to the drug cart to an unauthorized person.

See Box 5-1 for a summary of the "rights" of drug administration.

METHODS OF DRUG ADMINISTRATION

Drugs may have different effects on the body when they are administered by various routes. Certain drugs are suited to only one method of administration, whereas

Box 5-1 Six Rights for Correct Drug Administration

1. Right patient
2. Right time and frequency of administration
3. Right dose
4. Right route of administration
5. Right drug
6. Right documentation

others may be given in several ways, depending on the preparation used and the reason for which the medication is given. Generally, we are concerned with two types of drug administration: local (intended for an effect limited to the site of application) and systemic (intended for a general effect in which the drug is absorbed into the blood and carried to one or more tissues in the body).

The systems used to deliver drugs are called **dosage forms.** Drug companies package medications in certain ways to help with chemical stability and sometimes with bioavailability, which is the actual portion of the drug absorbed into the bloodstream and available for the desired effect.

Drug delivery systems may also serve a special purpose in specific patient populations. Patients with vomiting, seizures, asthma, or pain need quick relief. Nasal or pulmonary delivery via inhalers can achieve rapid blood levels of a required drug. Long-acting systems such as transdermal forms or extended-release oral or injectable forms help compliance because taking frequent doses is difficult for many patients.

New delivery systems being developed include bioadhesives that allow localization in mucosal routes of administration. Drug carriers that avoid removal of the drug by the liver, spleen, lung, and bone are also being developed.

ADMINISTRATION FOR LOCAL EFFECTS

A **local effect** is obtained when the drug is applied in the immediate area where its effect is desired. Occasionally, undesired absorption may be obtained from a local site, and an untoward or toxic effect may result. Boric acid, methyl salicylate, and hexachlorophene have been shown to exert harmful effects systemically, particularly when applied to large or denuded areas.

APPLICATION TO THE SKIN

Intact skin, with the exception of a newborn's skin, is generally impermeable to most agents. Ointments containing anti-inflammatory or antibiotic agents are useful for their local effects. Care should be taken not to apply topical agents to denuded areas without the physician's knowledge because undesired absorption may occur.

APPLICATION TO THE MUCOUS MEMBRANES

Drugs may be applied to the various mucous membranes of the body for local or systemic effects. The mucous membranes in the mouth, eye, nose, vagina, and rectum are constantly bathed in watery solutions and are generally more permeable than skin.

Suppositories

Suppositories may be inserted in the rectum for a local effect (e.g., bisacodyl [Dulcolax] for its local action to promote a laxative effect) or for the systemic effect they may produce after absorption through the mucous membrane (i.e., antinauseants, pain-relieving agents, or drugs such as aspirin for an antipyretic effect). Vaginal suppositories are generally used for treatment of local conditions, although some systemic absorption may occur.

Enemas

Enemas are most commonly used to promote a laxative effect; however, some oil-based retention enemas may contain drugs intended for systemic effects.

Intranasal Preparations

Intranasal preparations may be used to treat systemic conditions, such as asthma, or to exert a local effect in decreasing nasal congestion. Care should be taken that the nasal passages are free from exudate before administering a nasal preparation, and the tip of the spray bottle should be protected from contamination. Nasal spray nozzles should be cleaned after each use.

Ophthalmic Preparations

Care should be taken to protect eye preparations from contamination. The eyedropper bottle or ointment tube should never touch the membranes of the eye. These preparations generally have an expiration date to guarantee their sterility; this should be checked before using any ophthalmic preparation.

Ear Preparations

Absolute sterile technique is unnecessary for ear preparations. With the patient lying down, ear drops should be instilled into the ear canal after first gently pulling the external ear to straighten the ear canal. The patient should remain in a recumbent position for a few minutes after instillation of the drops to ensure their effect.

ADMINISTRATION FOR SYSTEMIC EFFECTS

To obtain **systemic effects** from a drug, it first must be absorbed into the blood and carried to the tissue or organ on which it acts. To produce these effects, drugs may be given orally, sublingually, rectally, parenterally, by inhalation, or in some cases by topical administration.

ORAL ADMINISTRATION

Although it is the most popular method from the standpoint of convenience and patient acceptance, **oral administration** (i.e., allowing the drug to be swallowed) has the disadvantage of being slower in onset of action than parenteral administration. This method should not be used if a rapid effect is desired. Some drugs, such as insulin, are ineffective when given orally because they are destroyed by the secretions in the gastrointestinal tract.

Drugs given orally may be available as tablets, capsules, or liquids. Taste is an important factor when using a liquid, particularly when giving a medication to a child. Many drugs that have disagreeable tastes may be disguised by giving them in a large amount of fluid, such as fruit juices or effervescent drinks, or in syrups or emulsions. Fluids that have an unpleasant taste should be given cold, often with ice, and followed by a drink of water.

Food can delay or reduce the absorption of many drugs, including aspirin and some forms of penicillin. Other drugs are better absorbed and less irritating to the stomach when taken with food. Examples of drugs better taken with food are iron products and some forms of erythromycin. Reduced absorption may occur if certain drugs are given with certain food products. Tetracycline used to be given with milk to reduce gastric irritation. It was later found that tetracycline was severely disabled and rendered much less effective because the calcium, magnesium, and mineral supplements in milk bound with the tetracycline, reducing the amount of the drug available to the body.

When taking oral medications, the patient should be advised as follows:

1. Read all directions, warnings, and interactions about the drug. These are generally clearly printed on the package insert that comes with the drug or the labels of over-the-counter (OTC) preparations. OTC preparations are drugs too and should not be ignored as a cause of possible side effects owing to interactions with prescription drugs.
2. Take medications with a full glass of water to enable the drugs to be dissolved and begin working faster.
3. Medications should never be combined with alcohol. Some cough syrups contain alcohol in sufficient amounts to be noted.
4. Do not mix medications in hot drinks. The hot temperature can destroy some drugs, and the tannic acid in hot tea can reduce the absorption of certain medications.
5. Do not mix medications in food unless specifically ordered.
6. Vitamin, mineral, and herbal supplements have substances that can interfere with drug absorption. Information about these supplements should be noted in the same way as for OTC drugs.

Procedure for Pouring and Administering Oral Medications

Observe the following guidelines when administering oral medications:

1. Wash your hands.
2. Identify the patient by checking his or her identification armband. If the armband is missing and there is any question as to the patient's ability to respond correctly to his or her name, ask a reliable staff member to identify the patient.
3. Compare the drug label with the patient's order when taking the container from its location, before pouring, and before returning the container to its location.
4. Pour tablets and capsules into the lid of the bottle before placing in a medicine cup. Avoid touching them with your fingers.
5. When pouring liquids, pour away from the label. Wipe the neck of the bottle with a damp paper towel or tissue before replacing the cap.
6. Hold a medicine cup or graduate (see Fig. 5-1) at eye level, and place a thumb on the glass at the desired volume.
7. When giving more than one medication to a patient, the following order should be used: Give tablets and capsules followed by water or other liquid; then give liquids diluted with water as required. Cough medicine is given undiluted and is not followed by liquids. Sublingual and buccal tablets are given last.
8. Remain with the patient until all medication has been swallowed.

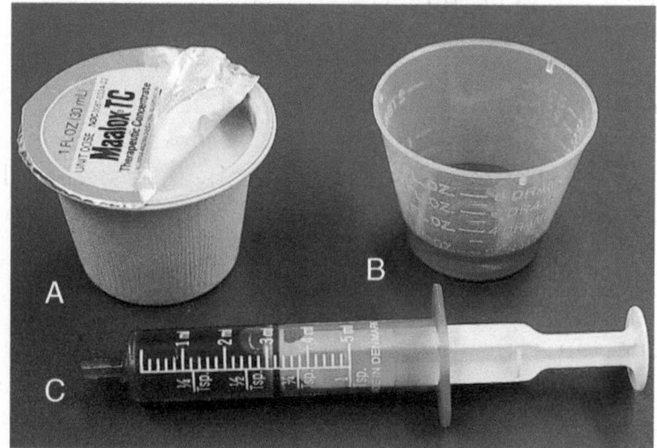

FIGURE 5-1 **A,** Liquid medication in a unit-dose package. **B,** Liquid measured into a medicine cup from a multidose container. **C,** Liquid medicine in an oral-dosing syringe. (From Lilley LL, et al: *Pharmacology and the nursing process*, ed 6, St. Louis, 2011, Mosby.)

9. Record on the electronic medical record, Kardex, or medicine sheet only after the medication has been given.
10. Report and record medication ordered but not given.

Many commonly used drugs are available in unit-dose packages. A unit-dose package contains the amount of drug for a single dose in the proper dosage form for administration by the prescribed route. Tablets, capsules, and liquids can be prepared in single-dose packages. All unit-dose packages are labeled with the generic name, trade name, packaging date, expiration date, and often a bar code.

Unit-dose packaging of drugs provides increased medication safety. Strip packages provide for ease of counting narcotics because all doses in the strip are numbered. This package also prevents contamination caused by pouring tablets into the hands when counting.

Liquid medications may be measured in a graduate glass or medicine cup, depending on the volume desired and the amount of accuracy required (see Fig. 5-1). Very small or exact volumes should not be measured in a medicine cup. A syringe should be used for the measurement of volumes less than 5 mL.

SUBLINGUAL ADMINISTRATION

The procedure for giving sublingual medications follows that for oral administration of drugs. However, with **sublingual administration,** the medication is not swallowed; it is placed under the patient's tongue, where it must be retained until it is dissolved or absorbed. The number of drugs that may be administered in this way is limited but includes nitroglycerin.

INHALED ADMINISTRATION

Certain drugs may be given by **inhaled administration.** The most common inhaled drugs are agents intended for direct use on the respiratory tract, as in the treatment of asthma, but an increasing number of agents for systemic use are becoming available in a form that is suitable for inhalation.

PARENTERAL ADMINISTRATION

The term *parenteral* refers to all the ways in which drugs are administered with a needle. **Parenteral administration** is the most efficient method of drug administration because it avoids all of the variables involved in topical and gastrointestinal absorption. However, it can also be the most hazardous; untoward effects may be rapid and even fatal.

Whenever the skin is punctured, it is possible for infections to develop; strict aseptic technique must be used. Injections may cause nerve damage if placed incorrectly, and the accidental penetration of blood vessels may cause hematoma formation or the incorrect placement of a drug intended for intramuscular use directly into a blood vessel.

Medications intended for use by injection are supplied in the form of ampules or vials (Fig. 5-2). Ampules are designed for one-time use, and the unused portion must be discarded. Vials with rubber

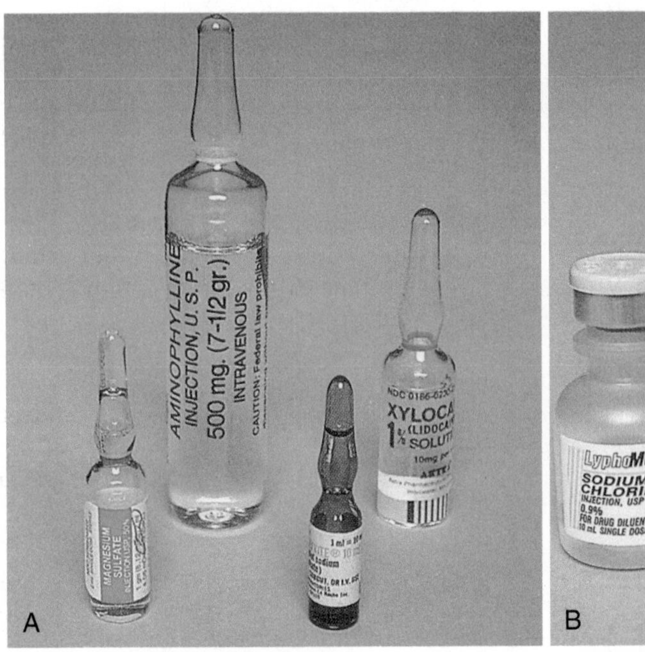

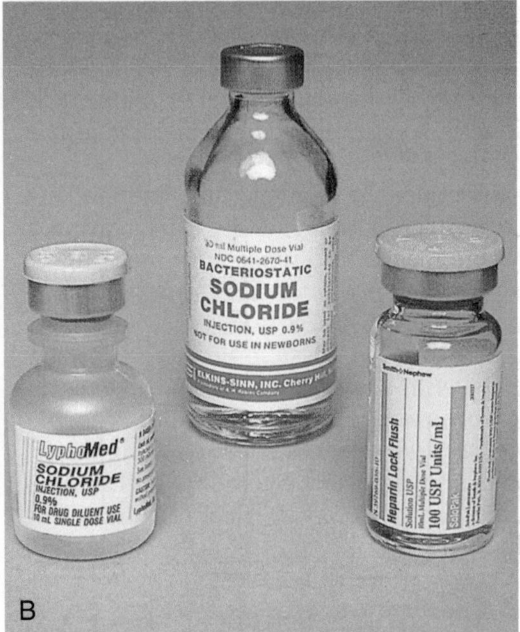

FIGURE 5-2 **A,** Medication in ampules. **B,** Medication in vials. Rubber top must be cleansed with alcohol when vial is opened or when it is reused. (From Potter PA, et al: *Basic nursing,* ed 7, St. Louis, 2011, Mosby.)

stoppers are used for single-dose amounts and for multiple withdrawals of drugs. The label should be examined carefully for the strength of the drug and the intended use of the particular vial. If any sign of precipitation, color change, or cloudiness develops within the vial, it should be discarded.

Some parenteral drugs are supplied within the ampule as a powder that first must be diluted by the nurse or pharmacist before administration. Directions for reconstitution are enclosed with the package literature, advising dilution with sterile saline or water, and should be strictly observed.

Prefilled disposable syringes for all medications to be given subcutaneously, intramuscularly, and intravenously are available (Fig. 5-3). Advantages of prefilled disposable syringes include the following:

1. Sterility is ensured.
2. Accuracy is ensured.
3. Trauma to tissue caused by blunt needles is avoided.
4. Drug doses are immediately available.

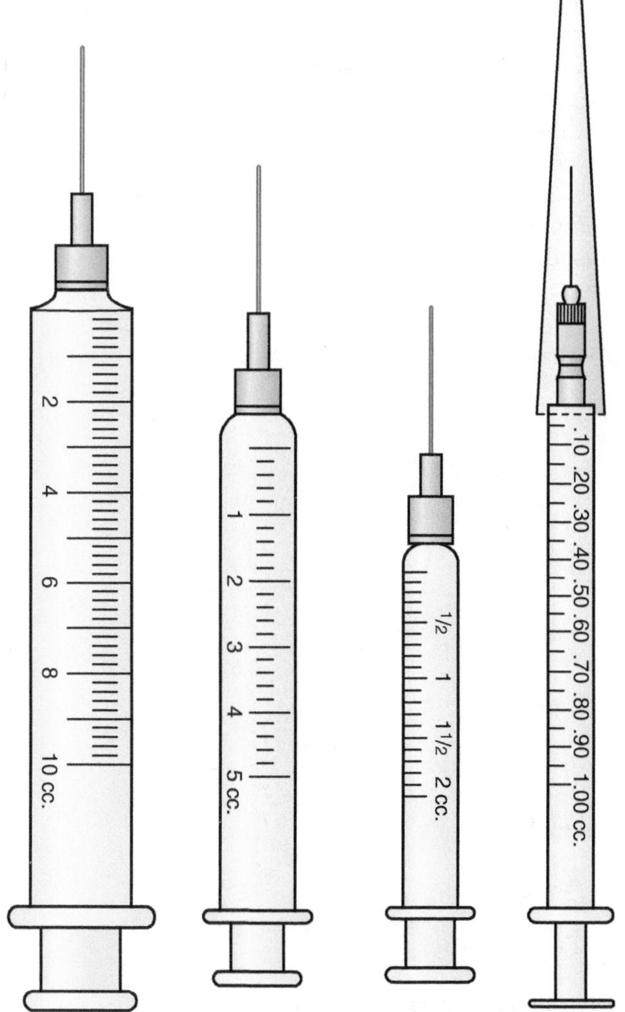

FIGURE 5-3 Prefilled disposable syringes.

These unit doses of disposable syringes are the most convenient but also the most costly forms of parenteral medications.

Intradermal Injection

To perform an **intradermal injection** (which is used exclusively for skin testing), the needle is inserted at an angle almost parallel to the skin surface, placing the drug within the dermis. When correctly placed, a small bubble is raised in the skin surface where the intradermal material is deposited. The inner surface of the arm or the back is generally chosen for skin testing (Fig. 5-4).

Subcutaneous Injection

In a **subcutaneous injection,** the solution is placed beneath the skin into the fat or connective tissue lying just under the dermis layer. A 25-gauge needle is generally used, with the length from ⅜ to ⅝ inch, depending on the thickness of the patient's subcutaneous tissue. A 45-degree angle is generally used, although with a short needle a 90-degree angle may also be used (see Fig. 5-4).

After careful cleansing with alcohol or another anti-infective, the skin is gently pinched and lifted away from the muscle. The needle is inserted, and the pinched-up skin is released. Before the medication is injected, the needle is aspirated to ensure a blood vessel has not been entered, and then the material is deposited. Generally, amounts injected subcutaneously are less than 2 mL.

Intramuscular Injection

For **intramuscular (IM) injection** (i.e., administration directly into a muscle), a 1- to 3-inch needle is used. The gauge of the needle generally is based on the viscosity of the material injected. A 21-gauge needle is often used for penicillin injections, but a smaller gauge is chosen for solutions of other drugs.

Several sites may be used for IM injections, including the deltoid muscle in the upper arm (Fig. 5-5), the vastus lateralis in the lateral thigh (Fig. 5-6), and the gluteus maximus in the buttocks (Fig. 5-7). Sites should be rotated if repeated administration of IM medications is ordered.

When giving IM injections to children, a smaller length needle is chosen. With infants, often a ½-inch needle is used. The vastus lateralis in the anterolateral thigh is the preferred site for infants and young children because the gluteal muscles are not well developed. The needle is inserted in an anteroposterior position after the muscle is firmly grasped and the child is firmly restrained (Figs. 5-8 and 5-9). Care should be taken to aspirate the syringe before the medication is delivered.

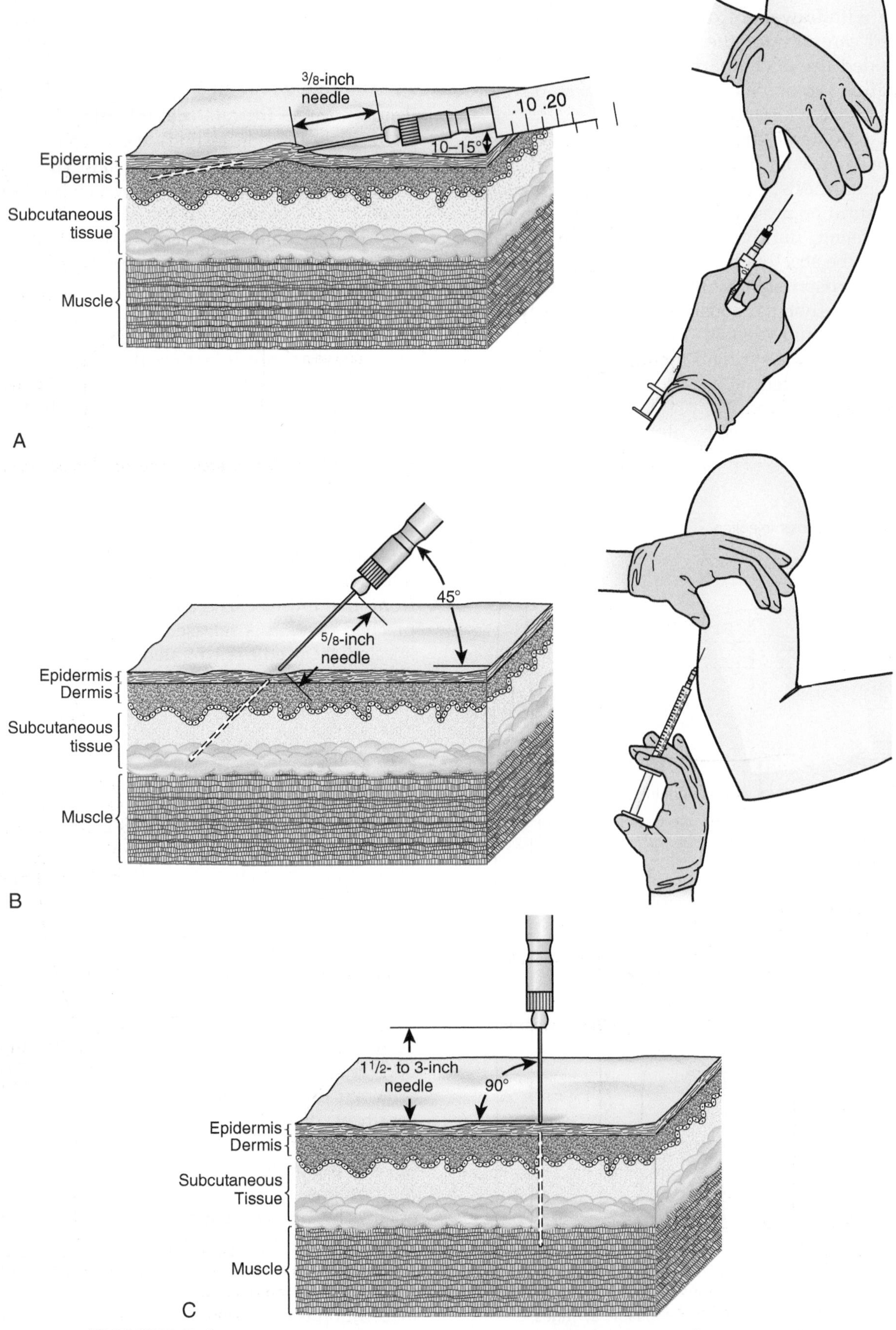

FIGURE 5-4 Three types of injections. **A,** Intradermal. **B,** Subcutaneous. **C,** Intramuscular (IM). (From Asperheim MK: *Pharmacologic basis of patient care,* ed 5, Philadelphia, 1985, Saunders.)

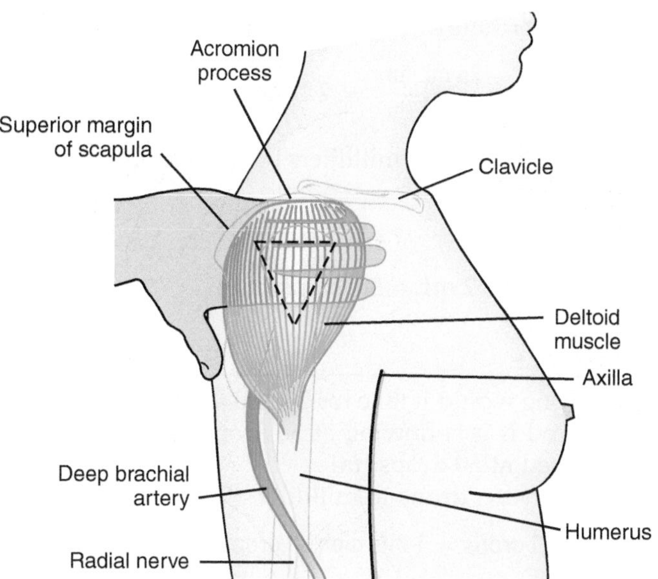

FIGURE 5-5 View of the deltoid site for IM injection. (From Asperheim MK: *Pharmacologic basis of patient care*, ed 5, Philadelphia, 1985, Saunders.)

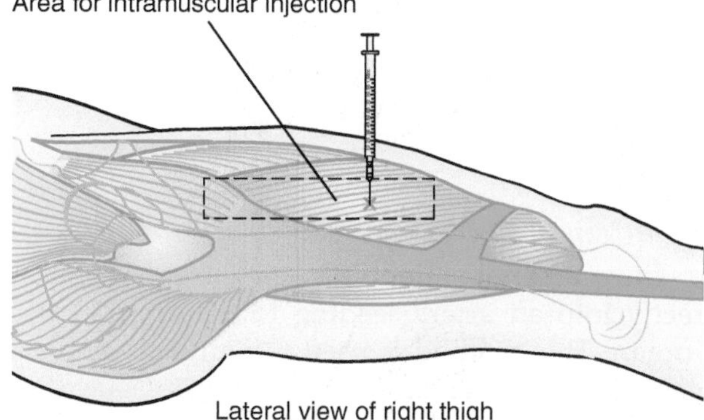

FIGURE 5-6 Vastus lateralis site for IM injection in adults. (From Asperheim MK: *Pharmacologic basis of patient care*, ed 5, Philadelphia, 1985, Saunders.)

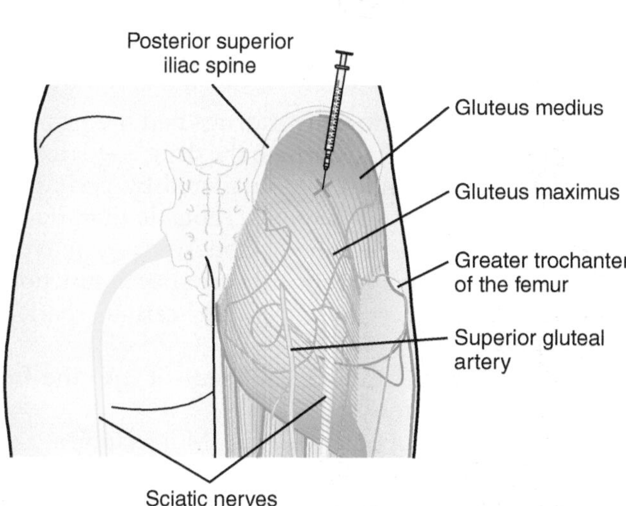

FIGURE 5-7 IM injection in the gluteal area. (From Asperheim MK: *Pharmacologic basis of patient care*, ed 5, Philadelphia, 1985, Saunders.)

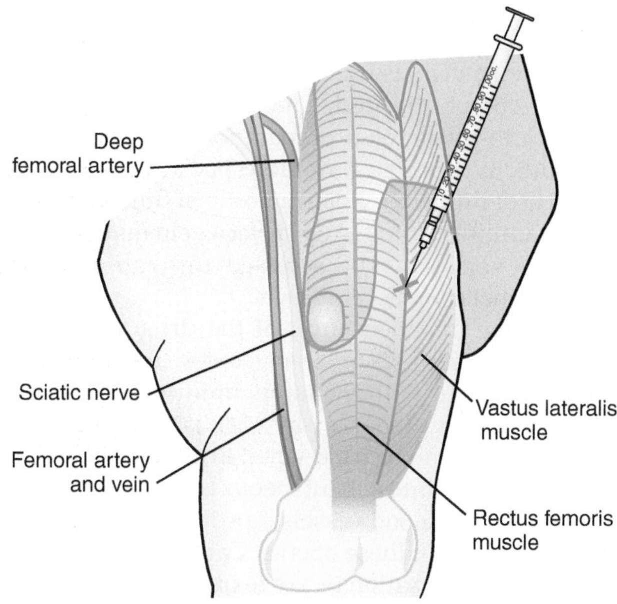

FIGURE 5-8 Vastus lateralis site for IM injection in children.

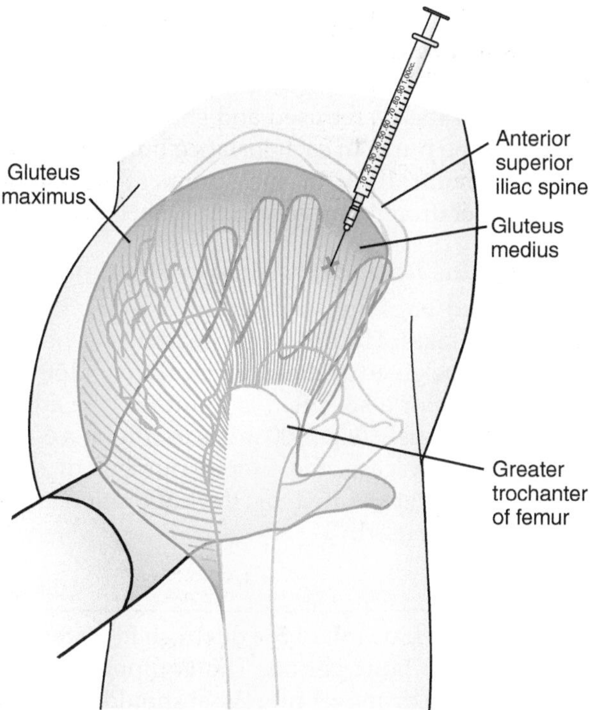

FIGURE 5-9 Ventrogluteal site. The injection is made between the index and middle fingers, which are spread apart as far as possible to form a "V." (From Asperheim MK: *Pharmacologic basis of patient care*, ed 5, Philadelphia, 1985, Saunders.)

Intravenous Administration

Intravenous (IV) injection, which places a drug directly into a vein, is used when the most rapid onset of drug action is desired. The medication is injected directly into a vein as a preparation, either administered directly from an ampule especially constituted for IV use or diluted in a bag or bottle of fluids for more gradual administration. Any surface vein may be used, or deeper veins may be accessed through a central venous catheter or via cutdown.

Just as the intended effect of the drug takes place within a few seconds in many cases, the untoward effects may occur with the same rapidity. For this reason, direct supervision by a physician is often necessary.

The IV route can be used when drugs are too irritating to be injected into subcutaneous or IM sites because the intima of the blood vessels is ordinarily quite resistant to the effect of these agents. Care should be taken to prevent extravasation (leakage of the substance into the surrounding tissues); sloughing of local tissues can result.

The IV route is also used to administer fluids, electrolytes, dextrose or other sugars, and proteins. Care should be taken to avoid incompatibilities when mixing drugs in various IV solutions. If cloudiness, discoloration, or precipitates occur when two drugs are mixed, the solution should not be used.

The rate of flow of the IV solution may be monitored by using a calibration pump to set the rate of administration. It may also be calculated by maintaining the proper number of drops per minute. The number of drops per minute varies with the caliber (diameter of the tubing) of the IV set used and should be carefully checked by the nurse in each instance if this method is used. The **calibration,** or measurement of solution delivered "per drop," may vary from 10 to 60 drops/mL.

Calibrating the Rate of Intravenous Solutions

IV bottles and bags are supplied in 250-mL, 500-mL, and 1000-mL sizes. The order may read that a specified solution is to be given at stated intervals (e.g., 150 mL/hr for 8 hours), or a specified amount may be administered continuously (e.g., 500 mL is to run for a 6-hour period). In every case, the proper number of drops per minute is determined by the calibration of the particular IV set used.

EXAMPLE

The order is for 1000 mL of 5% dextrose in water to be given over an 8-hour period. The equipment is calibrated so that 15 drops = 1 mL. What should be the rate of flow in drops per minute?

1. Determine the number of milliliters per hour.

$$\frac{1000 \text{ mL}}{8 \text{ hr}} = 125 \text{ mL/hr}$$

2. Determine the number of milliliters per minute.

$$\frac{125 \text{ mL/hr}}{60 \text{ min/hr}} = 2.1 \text{ (or 2 mL/min)}$$

3. Convert the milliliters per minute to the number of drops required.

$$1 \text{ mL} = 15 \text{ drops}$$

Therefore, 2 mL = 30 drops/min.

EXAMPLE

How long would it take for 250 mL of IV solution to be delivered if it is flowing at 30 drops/min? This set is calibrated at 60 drops/mL.

1. Convert drops to milliliters.

   If 60 drops = 1 mL, then 30 drops = 0.5 mL/min.

2. Determine how many minutes it would take for this amount of fluid to be infused.

$$\frac{250 \text{ mL}}{0.5 \text{ mL/min}} = 500 \text{ minutes}$$

3. Convert minutes to hours.

$$\frac{500 \text{ minutes}}{60 \text{ min/hr}} = 8.3 \text{ hr}$$

Intra-arterial Injection

For **intra-arterial injection,** the drug is injected directly into an artery leading to the affected tissue or organ. This method is used infrequently and most notably in the administration of antineoplastic agents. A special administration set is used for this purpose. Intra-arterial administration can deliver high doses of a drug to a restricted area of the body, eliminating some of the systemic side effects of the agent.

INNOVATIVE DRUG DELIVERY SYSTEMS

Historically, systems to deliver drugs had the primary purpose of allowing "no harm to the drug"—to deliver the drug to the intended site unaltered by body processes and defenses, so that an acceptable therapeutic blood level could be attained. Modern drug delivery systems are intended to perform very special functions with regard to certain drugs in certain patient populations.

New innovations in drug delivery fit into the following broad categories:

- Biocompatible subcutaneous or IM injectables
- Reticuloendothelial systems, drug carriers that avoid removal from the body by the liver, spleen, lung, and bone
- Bioadhesives that allow localization in mucosal routes of administration

- Systems for oral delivery of peptides and proteins, most of which are now destroyed on oral administration
- New polymers for tissue engineering
- New systems to solubilize new drugs (43% of new drugs are insoluble in water)
- Implantable polymer chips, which could replace many of the oral and injectable forms now in use. The paper-thin, dime-sized chip contains a series of tiny reservoirs. Each reservoir can store a single drug dose and is sealed with a membrane made from a second polymer. The membranes can be programmed to burst and release the contents of the reservoir at specific times. Microchips now developed have up to 36 reservoirs and release their drugs over 35 to 60 days. When the chip is empty, the biocompatible materials slowly degrade. The development of and research on polymer chips continues.

Research into tissue engineering is changing many aspects of medicine. Development in this field started with artificial skin; now other engineered artificial tissues, such as cartilage, are progressing toward U.S. Food and Drug Administration (FDA) approval. By designing polymers that do not fit the white blood cell receptors, it is possible to prevent white blood cells from attacking the polymers as they would foreign tissue. This research has implications in organ transplant, drug delivery, wound healing, and tissue engineering.

PROPER DISPOSAL OF UNWANTED MEDICINE

It is important to remember not to flush unwanted medications into a sink or toilet. This method of drug disposal is now discouraged since it was discovered that the drugs may leak into streams and groundwater, entering the freshwater system. Many drugs are not readily biodegradable.

Drugs should be disposed of in household trash, and they should be modified to discourage consumption. They should not be placed in recycling bags. Ways to modify drugs include the following:

1. Keep the drugs in their original container. For tablets or capsules, you may add water or alcohol to dissolve them partially. Tape the lids shut with packing or duct tape. After blacking out the label and name of the drug, place the bottle in a yogurt or margarine tub to avoid detection and place in the trash.
2. For liquid medicines, add enough table salt, chili powder, or mustard to make a pungent, unsightly mixture. Black out the label and conceal in another container as before, and place in the trash.
3. Liquid or solid drugs may be mixed with substances such as coffee grounds, cat litter, or sawdust. Place in a plastic bag and place in the garbage.
4. Take advantage of community take-back programs or hazardous waste collection events to dispose of medications. You can find out about these in your area by calling the household trash and recycling services in your city or county. Pharmacies occasionally advertise take-back days.
5. Needles should be placed in a sharps container. Less satisfactory containers would be empty bleach, detergent, or soda bottles. Some pharmacies or hospitals accept sharps containers for disposal. Alternatively, they should be disposed of with biohazardous waste.

REVIEW QUESTIONS

1. The most convenient systemic dosage form is:
   a. IV medication.
   b. subcutaneous injection.
   c. oral tablet.
   d. rectal suppository.

2. Which method of administration would have the most rapid systemic effect?
   a. Intravenous
   b. Subcutaneous
   c. Intramuscular
   d. Intradermal

3. An IV solution should generally *not* be used if it is:
   a. cloudy.
   b. discolored.
   c. noted to have "floaters."
   d. all of the above.

4. Parenteral administration refers to:
   a. local administration.
   b. administration into the parenchyma.
   c. administration by injection.
   d. topical administration.

5. Patient compliance may be increased with all of the following dosage forms *except:*
   a. transdermal patches.
   b. four-times-daily oral medication.
   c. extended-release tablets.
   d. long-acting injections.

6. Preparations generally applied for local effect are:
   a. ointments.
   b. subcutaneous injections.
   c. oral tablets.
   d. transdermal patches.

7. The main advantage of prefilled disposable syringes is:
   a. cost.
   b. fewer side effects.
   c. accuracy.
   d. less tissue trauma.

8. The hourly volume administered by an IV solution is calculated by:
   a. drops per minute.
   b. noting how long the IV bottle lasts.
   c. milliliters per second.
   d. urine volume of the patient.

9. Unused drugs should be disposed of by:
   a. flushing down the sink or toilet.
   b. storing in the medicine cabinet.
   c. placing in the garbage.
   d. giving to a neighbor.

10. Which of the following is *not* an example of an appropriate modification made to a drug for disposal?
    a. Flushing down the toilet
    b. Mixing solid tablets or capsules with water
    c. Mixing unpalatable ingredients in a liquid preparation
    d. Addition of coffee grounds or cat litter

Answers to the review questions can be found at the back of the book.

evolve Additional questions and activities can be found at *http://evolve.elsevier.com/asperheim/pharmacology*.

Vitamins, Minerals, and General Nutrition

CHAPTER 6

Objectives

After completing this chapter, you should be able to do the following:

1. List the characteristics of vitamins.
2. State the function of vitamins in the body.
3. State the function of minerals in the body.
4. Identify fat-soluble vitamins.
5. Identify water-soluble vitamins.
6. Give an example of a source of each vitamin.
7. Identify symptoms of specific vitamin deficiencies.
8. Identify symptoms of specific mineral deficiencies.
9. Identify the components of a healthy diet.
10. Understand the significance of MyPlate
11. Understand the role of antioxidants in nutrition.
12. Realize that nutrition can affect various bodily functions.

Key Terms

Anemia, p. 40
Antioxidants (ĂN-tĭ-ŎK-sĭ-dĕnts), p. 40
Avitaminosis, p. 39
Dietary Reference Intake (DRI), p. 40
Essential fatty acids, p. 40
Fiber, p. 40
Hypervitaminosis, p. 39
Minerals, p. 39
Recommended Daily Allowance (RDA), p. 40
Vitamins, p. 39

The old adage "you are what you eat" is true. Modern understanding of nutrition has shown us that the body needs a balance of nutrients—vitamins, minerals, protein, water, carbohydrates, fiber, and essential fatty acids—for optimal health. An improper diet has been related to increased incidences of death from heart disease, certain types of cancer, stroke, and diabetes. Nutrition can also affect various neurologic states, such as depression, insomnia, migraine headaches, and mood disorders.

At the lowest scale of life, primitive microorganisms are able to synthesize most of the nutrients they need and demand few ready-made raw materials from their environment. However, some of this ability to synthesize required nutrients is lost in higher plants and animals because they have many highly specialized cells and organs that depend entirely on other cells for their nourishment. Humans depend on other organisms to supply many vital constituents of their food; this is particularly true of one class of organic compounds that is required in minute amounts: **vitamins.**

It has been known for some time that vitamin deficiencies in the diet cause diseases. A condition that develops as a result of a lack of vitamins is referred to as **avitaminosis** (or hypovitaminosis). It was noticed by the British that sailors on long voyages, without sufficient supplies of fresh fruits and vegetables, developed a disease known as scurvy, which was characterized by loosening of the teeth, bleeding gums, irritability, and fatigue. It was found that if citrus fruits were part of the diet, this disease could be prevented. (Citrus fruits are notably rich in vitamin C.) One of the fruits frequently used was the lime—hence, the word "limey" was often applied to an English sailor. Unfavorable symptoms are also noted when an overdose of vitamins (especially fat-soluble vitamins) is consumed—a condition known as **hypervitaminosis.** Individuals may accidentally overdose on vitamins by taking excessive over-the-counter supplements.

Minerals are nonorganic materials found in the earth's crust. Some, such as calcium, zinc, and iron, are essential components of the human body. It is now understood that calcium consumed early in life plays an important part in preventing osteoporosis in later life. The mineral zinc and vitamins A and C may help to prevent macular degeneration in the eye by blocking free radical damage to retinal blood vessels. One cause of **anemia,** a condition in which the number of red blood cells or the amount of hemoglobin in cells is less than normal, is a deficiency of iron in the diet.

Essential fatty acids are molecules found within fats that are not produced by the body but that are necessary for proper functioning. Each fatty acid molecule is composed of carbon and hydrogen. Fatty acids that contain the maximum number of hydrogen atoms for each carbon atom are called *saturated fatty acids* and can be produced by the human body. *Monounsaturated fatty acids* contain one less hydrogen atom per carbon atom; *polyunsaturated fatty acids* contain several fewer hydrogen atoms than saturated fatty acids. Unsaturated fatty acids are found in plants and fish and cannot be produced by the human body. Excessive fat and cholesterol are harmful to the body, but the brain and nervous system need polyunsaturated fatty acids for proper nerve functioning. Strict limitation of all fats in infants and toddlers was found to delay maturation of the nervous system. Moderation is in order, but fats should not be strictly limited, especially in infants and young children.

Antioxidants are agents that inhibit oxidation, neutralizing the effects of free radicals and other substances believed to play a part in tissue damage and the aging process. The antioxidant power of certain foods, such as blueberries and foods containing vitamins C and E, is just now becoming apparent. It is thought that age-related memory impairment may be prevented or reversed by a diet rich in antioxidants. Vitamin C and other antioxidants such as lutein and zeaxanthin are being studied because they may help fight sunlight-induced damage to the retina and may help to prevent cataracts. Long-term vitamin C consumption has been shown to prevent or delay cataract formation.

Nutrition is also adversely affected by gastrointestinal conditions such as constipation, diarrhea, diverticulosis, irritable bowel syndrome, lactose intolerance, and malabsorption. **Fiber** is a food substance found only in plants that is not digested by gastrointestinal enzymes. A high-fiber diet rich in vegetables such as broccoli and cauliflower may help prevent colon cancer (Table 6-1). A diet rich in tomato products may help prevent prostate cancer because of a substance called lycopene that is present in tomatoes.

Table 6-1 Sources of Fiber

Source	Portion	Fiber Content (gm)
Apple	Small	2.8
Banana	Medium	2.0
Beans, green	½ cup	2.1
Beans, kidney	½ cup	5.5
Beans, lima	½ cup	4.4
Bread, whole wheat	Slice	2.0
Broccoli	¾ cup	5.0
Carrots	4 sticks	1.7
Peas	½ cup	3.0
Oat bran	½ cup	3.0
Orange	Small	3.0
Peach	Medium	2.0
Pear	Small	3.0
Potato	Small	4.2
Rice, brown	½ cup	5.5
Watermelon	Thick slice	2.8

To guide people in obtaining the nutrients necessary for good health, the Food and Nutrition Board of the National Academy of Sciences publishes the **Dietary Reference Intakes (DRIs)** for vitamins and minerals. The DRIs include four different values: Estimated Average Requirement (EAR), **Recommended Daily Allowance (RDA),** Adequate Intake (AI), and Tolerable Upper Intake Level (UL). The RDA value is the average daily dietary intake sufficient to meet the nutrition requirement of about 97% to 98% of healthy individuals. All values reported in this chapter are the RDAs for a man. In the case that there is no established RDA, the AI recommended for a man is given in its place. The recommendations for women and children and older adults in some instances may vary.

NOMENCLATURE OF VITAMINS

The duplication and confusion apparent in the naming of vitamins are understandable only in the historical context of the development of our knowledge of vitamins. Successive letters of the alphabet were assigned to new vitamins as they were characterized and isolated, but some letters were assigned out of order. Vitamin K refers to the Swedish word *Koagulation* because of the part this vitamin plays in the clotting mechanism of blood. Vitamin H refers to the German word *Haut,* which means skin.

It soon became evident that the original vitamin B was not a single vitamin but a group of vitamins, and subscript numbers were added, giving us vitamins B_1, B_2, and others. There are currently many numbers missing in the series because some of the subtypes that were identified during early research were later found to be identical.

CHARACTERISTICS OF VITAMINS

Vitamins are:
- Organic in nature
- Required in very small amounts
- Required preformed in the diet or synthesized by intestinal flora
- Necessary for normal growth and maintenance
- Sensitive to light, heat, and oxidation and so must be stored in a cool place in dark bottles
- Necessary for enzyme systems

Common symptoms of vitamin deficiency include tiredness, aches, pains, and a generalized "poor" feeling. The general populace has far too many symptoms of this type, however, to blame them exclusively on vitamin deficiencies. An adequate diet is the best answer for the prevention of vitamin deficiencies.

FAT-SOLUBLE VITAMINS

VITAMIN A

Source: Fish liver oils (especially cod liver), dairy products, and vegetables such as carrots and spinach

Deficiency symptoms: Night blindness, immune system deficiencies, skin lesions

RDA: 900 mcg

VITAMIN D

Source: Vitamin D_2 is digestible and is found in fish liver oils (especially cod, halibut, sardines, salmon, and oysters), dairy products, and enriched foods. Ultraviolet radiation (sunshine) produces vitamin D in the skin, which is known as cutaneous vitamin D or D_3. It is now known that the use of sunscreen interferes with cutaneous vitamin D formation. Some studies have shown that it is possible to absorb the full requirement of cutaneous vitamin D only when south of Latitude 32 and then only if there is full exposure of arms and legs or back without sunscreen for at least 1 hour a day between 10 A.M. and 3 P.M. on 3 days a week. The incidence of melanoma increases with excessive and unprotected sun exposure, so some balance is necessary. Dermatologists contend that there is no safe level of sun exposure that allows for satisfaction of the vitamin D requirement without increasing cancer risk. Dark-skinned persons and patients with gastrointestinal disorders, such as lactose intolerance or Crohn's disease, have additional difficulties meeting the requirements.

Substances that interfere with vitamin D absorption: Antacids, phenobarbital, phenytoin (Dilantin), primidone (Mysoline), valproic acid (Depakote), cholestyramine (Questran), colestipol (Colestid), rifampin, mineral oil, orlistat (Alli)

Deficiency symptoms: Major deficiency of vitamin D that occurs in childhood is known as *rickets*. Rickets is characterized by an abnormally large abdomen, soft skull, bowed legs, and deformed arms. Infants would often have the "rachitic rosary," a condition characterized by enlarged knoblike structures on the ribs from widening of the costochondral junctions. Later in life, vitamin D deficiency is known as *osteomalacia*, characterized by softening of the bones. Osteopenia and osteoporosis, traditionally believed to be just calcium deficiency particularly in older women, are now believed to be due to a vitamin D deficiency as well. There are escalating reports of widespread American vitamin D deficiency, with some reports citing adult deficits of 85% in the general population. Many studies show that infants also are subject to more deficiencies than previously considered.

Activity: All vitamin D, whether from a dietary or ultraviolet source, goes to the liver and kidneys, where it is converted to 25-hydroxyvitamin D, the main circulating form. The kidneys further convert it to 1,25-dihydroxyvitamin D, which is the effective vitamin D hormone. It then helps boost calcium levels in the intestines, it transforms calcium and phosphate in the blood into building blocks for bones, and regulates some aspects of cell growth. Because calcium depends on vitamin D to fulfill its role in bone development, having only one or the other leads to interference in the formation and maintenance of the skeletal system. In addition, much research is being done on the effect of vitamin D on the immune system and its role in the prevention of various types of cancer and other disorders. Parathyroid hormone is involved as well because it enhances the tubular absorption of calcium and stimulates the kidneys to produce more 1,25-dihydroxyvitamin D.

Overdose symptoms: Nausea, cardiac symptoms, confusion, and kidney stones. Overdose is highly unlikely from either oral or skin absorption.

RDA (surely to be revised upward):

Birth through 50 years: 200 international units

51 to 70 years: 400 international units

71 years and older: 600 international units

Practical recommended intake by many experts:

Breastfed infants: 400 international units supplement daily

Sun-deprived individuals, pregnant and lactating women, and adults older than 50 years: 1000 to 2000 international units daily

Seriously deprived individuals are often prescribed 50,000 international units weekly until corrected.

The best indication of vitamin D deficiency is the blood level of 25-hydroxyvitamin D. A deficiency would show a level of less than 20 ng/mL. It is now believed that an optimal value is 40 or more ng/mL.

VITAMIN K

Source: Spinach, broccoli; synthesized by intestinal flora
Deficiency symptoms: Hemorrhagic tendency
Activity: This vitamin is required for the formation of prothrombin in the liver, which is needed for blood to clot normally.
Adequate intake: 120 mcg/day

VITAMIN E (ALPHA-TOCOPHEROL)

Source: Wheat germ, vegetable oils, nuts, sunflower seeds
Deficiency symptoms: No deficiency states have been identified.
Activity: Vitamin E is an antioxidant. Antioxidants have been linked with decreased atherosclerosis in experimental studies. Studies have also suggested that it may boost the immune system and prevent cataracts. There is some evidence that vitamin E may have a protective effect against coronary events by reducing the oxidation of low-density lipoprotein (LDL), or "bad cholesterol," which can cause atherosclerosis. It is believed by some authors to have some activity in slowing down the progression of Alzheimer's disease. Further studies have not corroborated these claims, however.
Toxic effects: Vitamin E prolongs bleeding time, causing an increased tendency to hemorrhage. Patients with bleeding disorders and patients who take anticoagulants are generally advised not to take supplemental vitamin E.
RDA: 15 mg/day as alpha-tocopherol equivalents

WATER-SOLUBLE VITAMINS

Water-soluble vitamins may be subdivided into two groups: vitamins concerned with the release of energy from food (e.g., thiamine, riboflavin) and vitamins concerned with the formation of red blood cells (e.g., folic acid, vitamin B_{12}).

THIAMINE (VITAMIN B_1)

Source: Widely distributed in nature, especially in yeast, liver, and lean meat
Deficiency symptoms: Thiamine deficiency produces a condition known as beriberi, which is characterized by inflammation of the peripheral nerves, paralysis, mixed sensations of heat and cold, congestive heart failure, and edema.
RDA: 1.2 mg/day

RIBOFLAVIN (VITAMIN B_2)

Source: Liver, kidney, milk
Deficiency symptoms: Vascularization of the cornea followed by ulcerations, dermatitis, and lip lesions
RDA: 1.3 mg/day

NICOTINAMIDE (NIACINAMIDE) AND NICOTINIC ACID (NIACIN)

Source: Liver, tuna, peanuts
Deficiency symptoms: The condition produced by deficiency of niacin is known as pellagra ("raw skin"). Symptoms are insomnia, appetite loss, irritability, dizziness, and morbid fears, followed by lesions of the mucous membranes and dermatoses, especially on areas of the chest and neck exposed to the sun.
Activity: When prescribed in large doses, niacin has been shown to reduce severity of atherosclerosis and may be used as an adjunct in the treatment of hyperlipidemia.
Side effect: A facial flush occurs quite often when nicotinic acid is administered, but the flush is not commonly seen when nicotinamide is used.
RDA: 16 mg/day
Dose for atherosclerosis: 2 g daily.

PYRIDOXINE (VITAMIN B_6)

Source: Liver, yeast, milk, meats, molasses
Deficiency symptoms: Skin lesions, hypochromic anemia, and convulsions in some instances
RDA: 1.0 to 1.7 mg/day

PANTOTHENIC ACID (VITAMIN B_5)

Source: Meat, vegetables, cereals, legumes, eggs, milk
Deficiency symptoms: Symptoms as an isolated deficiency have not been described; occurs in overall deficiency states
Adequate intake: 5 mg/day

FOLIC ACID

Source: Green leafy vegetables, cantaloupe, breakfast cereals
Deficiency symptoms: Macrocytic anemia. Erythrocytes (red blood cells) do not mature properly and are larger than normal. This increased size reduces the amount of total surface area; consequently, less oxygen is transported to the tissues.
Neural tube defects: Intrauterine deformities of the neural tube have been reduced by incorporating folic acid in prenatal vitamins and fortified foods.

Memory loss: Although controversial, some studies have shown that a combination of high-dose folate and vitamin B_{12} was associated with protection against cognitive impairment. Cerefolin NAC is a commercial product that is being studied in older adults. One capsule daily contains 5.6 mg of L-methylfolate, 2 mg of methylcobalamin, and 600 mg of N-acetylcysteine. Research is ongoing with this product.

RDA: 0.4 mg/day

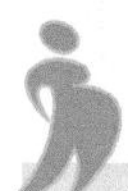

Considerations for Pregnant and Nursing Women

Folic Acid

Folic acid is particularly important for pregnant women. Evidence indicates that prophylactic therapy with folic acid initiated at least 1 month before pregnancy and continued through early pregnancy can reduce the incidence of neural tube defects, including spina bifida, anencephaly, and encephalocele. It is essential for DNA formation. Women of childbearing age should consume 0.4 mg of folic acid from fortified food or supplements in addition to folic acid available in a balanced diet.

VITAMIN B_{12} (CYANOCOBALAMIN)

Source: Animal tissue, especially liver

Deficiency symptoms: Pernicious anemia. Vitamin B_{12} is known as the extrinsic factor for the production of red blood cells. For effective use of this vitamin from the gastrointestinal system, the intrinsic factor must be present in the stomach of the individual. If it is not, the vitamin is not absorbed. In most cases of demonstrated deficiency of this vitamin, it is this intrinsic factor that is at fault because vitamin B_{12} is so widely distributed in nature that a dietary inadequacy in an individual would be unlikely. In a deficiency, vitamin B_{12} is ordinarily administered parenterally to circumvent the lack of this intrinsic factor needed for absorption from the oral route.

RDA: 2.4 mcg/day

VITAMIN C (ASCORBIC ACID OR CEVITAMIC ACID)

Source: Green vegetables, berries, citrus fruits, red bell peppers. Because this vitamin is rapidly destroyed by air, the fruits must be fresh. Canning and cooking destroy the vitamin.

Deficiency symptoms: Scurvy, characterized by gingivitis, loose teeth, slow healing of wounds, and petechial hemorrhages

Activity: Vitamin C is a potent antioxidant and is used as a popular daily supplement. Large doses of vitamin C—1000 mg or more daily—have been thought by some to prevent or lessen the severity of respiratory viral illnesses, although this is controversial. At these dose levels, severe abdominal cramps, nausea, vomiting, and diarrhea have occurred. Taking larger doses in the form of natural food sources is better than taking them in tablet form. A dose of 100 mg daily is generally recommended for a supplement. Increased vitamin C requirements may be associated with pregnancy, lactation, fever, stress, infection, smoking, and the use of certain drugs (e.g., estrogens, oral contraceptives, tetracyclines, barbiturates, and salicylates).

RDA: 90 mg/day

MULTIPLE VITAMIN PREPARATIONS

It is well recognized that when one vitamin deficiency exists, there is invariably a dietary deficiency in several other vitamins as well. A multiple vitamin supplement is commonly prescribed. Many multivitamin supplements are available. Multivitamins available over-the-counter generally have a lower vitamin content, particularly in the fat-soluble vitamins, than multivitamins available by prescription only.

MINERALS

Many minerals, or essential elements, are necessary for normal body functions. Most of these are required in trace amounts only and are found so freely in the environment—the soil, plants used for food, and seafood—that they rarely, if ever, need to be discussed in terms of a deficiency leading to ill health. Minerals known as trace elements are used by the body as components of enzymes and in some cases as catalysts necessary for proper enzymatic function. Copper, cobalt, fluorine, manganese, and zinc are a few of the trace elements known to be essential. Zinc is believed to help in the prevention of age-related retinal deterioration by slowing down the disease process. Other minerals perform a more dynamic function in the body and must be ingested regularly in some form because they either are excreted daily in urine or feces or are depleted in the process of forming or repairing body tissues.

IRON

Iron has long been known to be an essential component of blood hemoglobin. Blood is not a static tissue but is constantly being reformed as old red blood cells are trapped and destroyed by the spleen and other organs. Iron can be stored in the body, most notably in the bone marrow, but a dietary deficiency or a malabsorption problem in the intestinal tract soon manifests itself as an iron-deficiency anemia.

Iron-enriched infant formulas, such as Similac with Iron and Enfamil with Iron, have been designed to prevent this problem in very young children. Cow's milk is a very poor source of iron, and iron-deficiency anemia is a frequent finding in children 6 months to 3 years of age. The problem is compounded if an infant is allowed to stay on the bottle after 1 year of age and to satisfy most of his or her appetite with a bottle of milk between meals, coming to mealtime with a poor appetite for more nutritious meats and vegetables.

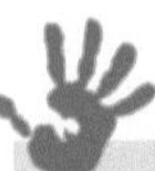

Considerations for Children

Iron

Iron deficiency is a very common cause of anemia in children, resulting in developmental delays and behavioral disturbances. Childhood anemia is generally nutritional, but it may also be caused by lead poisoning. Blood tests for persistent childhood anemia usually include serum lead levels.

The teenage years are another time in life when iron-deficiency anemias are common. This common incidence of iron-deficiency anemias is primarily due to a teenager's common pattern of fad diets and generally poor eating habits.

Menstruating women lose iron in the menstrual flow each month and are much more susceptible to deficiencies than men of the same age. Pregnancy is also a common time for anemia because the developing fetus takes what it needs for development and can cause alarmingly low hemoglobin values in women whose diets are nutritionally inadequate.

Sources: Meat, green vegetables, legumes, fortified cereals

RDA: 8 mg/day

COMMERCIAL PREPARATIONS OF IRON

ferrous sulfate, USP-NF, BP (Feosol). Ferrous sulfate is the most inexpensive and most commonly used form of iron supplement. It is available in tablet and liquid forms. Occasional abdominal cramping or discomfort is noted if it is taken on an empty stomach. The patient should be advised that all iron supplements turn the stool black.

Dosage: (Oral) 325 mg three times daily.

ferrous gluconate, USP-NF, BP (Fergon). Very little therapeutic difference is noted between the gluconate and sulfate salts of iron. Ferrous gluconate has the advantage of being slightly less irritating to the gastric mucosa but the disadvantage of being relatively more expensive.

Dosage: (Oral) 320 to 640 mg three to four times daily.

iron dextran injection, USP-NF, BP (INFeD). Designed for deep intramuscular injection or intravenous use, iron dextran injection is reserved for cases of severe iron-deficiency anemia and malabsorption problems. It should be administered with the Z-track technique in the upper outer quadrant of the buttock to minimize skin discoloration and irritation at the site of injection. The primary disadvantage of this, as of any parenteral iron preparation, is the ever-present danger of iron overdosage. Hemosiderosis, fever, urticaria, and headache are among the symptoms of iron overload.

Dosage: Calculated individually, based on the patient's hemoglobin level and weight. The dosage range is generally 50 to 100 mg/day given IM or IV.

CALCIUM AND PHOSPHORUS

Conditions arising from calcium and phosphorus deficiencies may be due to metabolic problems as well as nutritional deficits. These elements, under the control of the parathyroid glands, perform a very dynamic and complex function in the body. A constant balance is maintained between levels of these minerals in the blood and levels in calcified tissues of the body, primarily bone and teeth. Serum calcium levels should vary only slightly in healthy individuals. If calcium levels are too low, tetany occurs; if they are too high, cardiac irregularities are noted. Calcium is also required for muscle contraction, blood vessel expansion and contraction, secretion of hormones and enzymes, and transmitting impulses through the nervous system.

The kidneys are primarily responsible for the excretion of calcium, and severe or prolonged kidney damage can produce calcium deficiencies unrelated to the endocrine system. This condition is termed *renal rickets*. Vitamin D–deficient rickets, in which insufficient amounts of vitamin D limit proper calcium absorption, is uncommon in the United States but may still be noted in underdeveloped countries.

Osteoporosis is a condition in which there is thinning of the calcified portions of bones owing to deficient formation of bone matrix. It may be seen in postmenopausal women and in individuals with a severely protein-deficient diet. Osteoporosis in women may be alleviated by oral calcium supplements. It has been shown that the amount of calcium consumed in the first 3 decades of life can dramatically influence future risk for developing osteoporosis. Osteoporosis is also discussed in Chapter 24.

The adequate intake (AI) for elemental calcium is 1 gm for men and women 19 to 50 years of age. More calcium is needed in younger and older adults. One of the best sources of calcium is nonfat milk and other milk products such as yogurt and cheese. Besides providing calcium, milk is fortified with vitamin D, which helps the body absorb calcium.

The dosage for the treatment of calcium depletion can be up to 2 gm of elemental calcium daily. Certain salts of calcium contain a relatively small percentage of elemental calcium; calcium lactate contains only 84.5 mg of elemental calcium per 650 mg of the salt. Large doses of the salt are required to obtain the desired amount of elemental calcium.

Calcium salts are used intravenously in advanced cardiac life support during cardiopulmonary resuscitation. The dose may be repeated intravenously if necessary.

Dietary sources of calcium include dairy products such as milk, yogurt, and cheese. Nondairy sources include sardines and salmon with bones and vegetables such as Chinese cabbage, kale, turnip greens, and broccoli. Grains do not have high amounts of calcium naturally but may be fortified. Foods fortified with calcium include many fruit juices and drinks, tofu, breads, and cereals.

COMMERCIAL PREPARATIONS OF CALCIUM

calcium lactate, USP-NF, BP
Dosage: (Oral) 2 to 3 tablets daily (each 650-mg tablet has 84.5 mg of elemental calcium).

calcium gluconate, USP-NF, BP
Dosage: (Oral) 3 to 4 tablets daily (each 650-mg tablet has 58.5 mg of elemental calcium); (IV) 10 mL of 10% solution.

calcium chloride, USP-NF, BP
Dosage: (IV) 5 to 20 mL of a 10% solution.

calcium carbonate, USP-NF, BP (Tums)
Dosage: (Oral) 2 to 4 tablets daily (each 500-mg tablet has 200 mg of elemental calcium).

Calcium supplements should be taken with vitamin D, in combination with the calcium tablet or separately.

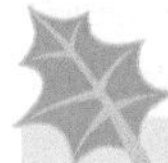

Considerations for Older Adults

Calcium

When taking calcium supplements for the prevention of osteoporosis, it is important to take vitamin D as well. New recommendations advise that 1000 international units of vitamin D should be taken daily along with the calcium. Many calcium tablets have combined vitamin D, and an additional amount may be taken in a vitamin and mineral supplement.

POTASSIUM

Potassium, similar to sodium and chloride, has a dynamic function in the maintenance of water and electrolyte concentrations within the body tissues and cells. In addition, potassium has a unique function in the transmission of nerve impulses and the control of cardiac rhythm.

Potassium depletion results from metabolic changes occurring in diabetic acidosis, in prolonged vomiting or diarrhea, and in the debilitation caused by surgery. It is often accidentally induced by prolonged administration of certain diuretics. Familial periodic paralysis is a hereditary disease characterized by bouts of muscular weakness and hypokalemia. The dose of potassium administered during medical treatment varies greatly based on the patient's state of depletion.

COMMERCIAL PREPARATIONS OF POTASSIUM

potassium chloride, USP-NF, BP
Dosage: (Oral) 40 to 80 mEq/day in divided doses; (IV) Based on potassium depletion. Maximum rate of administration would be 20 mEq/hr; usually 40 to 80 mEq is given in a 24-hour period. Maximum daily dose by IV infusion is 200 mEq/24 hr. *Caution:* This must be diluted before IV infusion; it may be fatal if given by IV push.

Slow-K. This coated tablet has 600 mg (8 mEq) of potassium chloride in a wax matrix to minimize gastrointestinal irritation.
Dosage: (Oral) 1 tablet up to three or four times daily.

TEN-K. Each tablet has 10 mEq of potassium chloride.
Dosage: (Oral) 1 tablet up to three times daily.

K-DUR 10. Each tablet has 10 mEq of potassium chloride.
Dosage: (Oral) 1 tablet up to three times daily.

COPPER

Copper is an essential component of many proteins and enzymes. It is necessary for the integrity of the red blood cell membrane, and as a component of ceruloplasmin it is necessary for the transport of ferrous iron in the body. Anemia, neutropenia, and thrombocytosis have been described in copper deficiency. It has been associated with poor balance, peripheral neuropathy, and leg spasticity and may lead to irreversible disability.

Deficiency states generally occur secondary to gastric surgery and may occur along with zinc deficiency. Copper deficiency often goes undiagnosed.

No minimum daily requirement has been described. Copper is a component of many multivitamin and mineral products.

FLUORIDE

Beginning in the 1950s, information that the addition of fluoride to the drinking water would be beneficial in reducing dental caries was publicized. After many years of controversy, the advantages of fluoride won the argument, and it is routinely administered to most municipal water supplies in a concentration of up to the allowed EPA limit of 4 mg/L. Most supplies are considerably lower than this limit, however.

Many food items such as juice drinks, soda pop, cranberry juice cocktails, ice pops, beef gravy, and canned crabmeat have notable levels of fluoride, probably added via the water used in processing. Higher levels get into grapes and raisins via pesticides, into processed chicken products via ground-up bone, and into tea leaves via absorption from soil and water.

It now seems that because of the unknown amounts of fluoride that may be ingested by children whose permanent teeth are still developing, an overdose condition known as *fluorosis* may occur, which causes a disruption in the development of the permanent teeth. The permanent teeth may be mottled or disfigured. There are no health risks with this condition, but the tooth marks are unattractive and are permanent. Masking treatments are available.

Excessive fluoride may also be deposited in the bone and may increase the risk of bone fracture by altering the crystalline structure of bone, especially in vulnerable populations such as older adults and diabetics. Fluoride may increase bone volume, but the strength of the bone apparently declines.

OMEGA-3 FATTY ACIDS

There is a great deal of information on the fat humans need to lose, but now there is heightened interest in the fat needed to live optimally. Part of a group known as the *essential fatty acids*, omega-3 is currently being touted as a preventive for heart disease, arthritis, skin problems, and mental health conditions, and the list keeps growing. Eicosapentaenoic acid (EPA) and dehydroepiandrosterone (DHA) are two of the components of omega-3, and aminolevulinic acid (ALA) is a precursor. The body cannot make omega-3; it must be ingested. Salmon, tuna, anchovies, herring, mackerel, and sardines are particularly rich sources. Walnuts, flaxseed oil, canola, olive oil, and soybean oil contain the precursor ALA. There is no minimum daily requirement, just an advisory to incorporate omega-3 sources in the diet.

CHANGES IN NUTRITIONAL INFORMATION

For many years, it was believed that proper nutrition could be achieved by eating the basic food groups: proteins (meat, fish, and eggs), breads and grains, fruits, vegetables, and dairy products. Increased information has become available with regard to overnutrition, particularly in the red meat and fat groups, with resulting elevation of cholesterol and increased incidence of vascular diseases, cerebrovascular accidents (or strokes), and heart attacks. It has become important to control and reduce the amount of these food items in the diet.

To coincide with the latest nutrition information, the U.S. Department of Agriculture developed MyPlate (Fig. 6-1) to replace MyPyramid. MyPlate emphasizes the fruit, vegetable, grains, protein, and dairy food groups and serves as a reminder to make healthier food choices. Individuals can visit *www.choosemyplate.gov* to access their own personalized plate and food plan.

Some nutritionists now recommend that fish or poultry be consumed only two or three times a week, with consumption of red meat being reduced to two or three times a month. It has been recommended that no more than 30% of the calories a person consumes come from fat.

Caloric requirements vary with age and activity. Children and active teenagers and men may need up to 2800 calories a day. Sedentary adults may require only 1600 calories.

When trying to select healthy foods, food labels can often be misleading. For instance:

- "Cholesterol free" does not mean fat free. Cholesterol comes only from animal sources. A food that does not contain animal products may still be fatty.
- "Made with vegetable oil" may or may not be a good sign. Good oil choices are canola, olive, corn, sunflower, and soybean oils. Saturated fats are present in coconut oil, palm kernel oil, or any hydrogenated oil. Whenever any oil is heated (i.e., for frying), it becomes a saturated oil and loses its advantage.

Look on the back of the package for the grams of fat or saturated fat per serving.

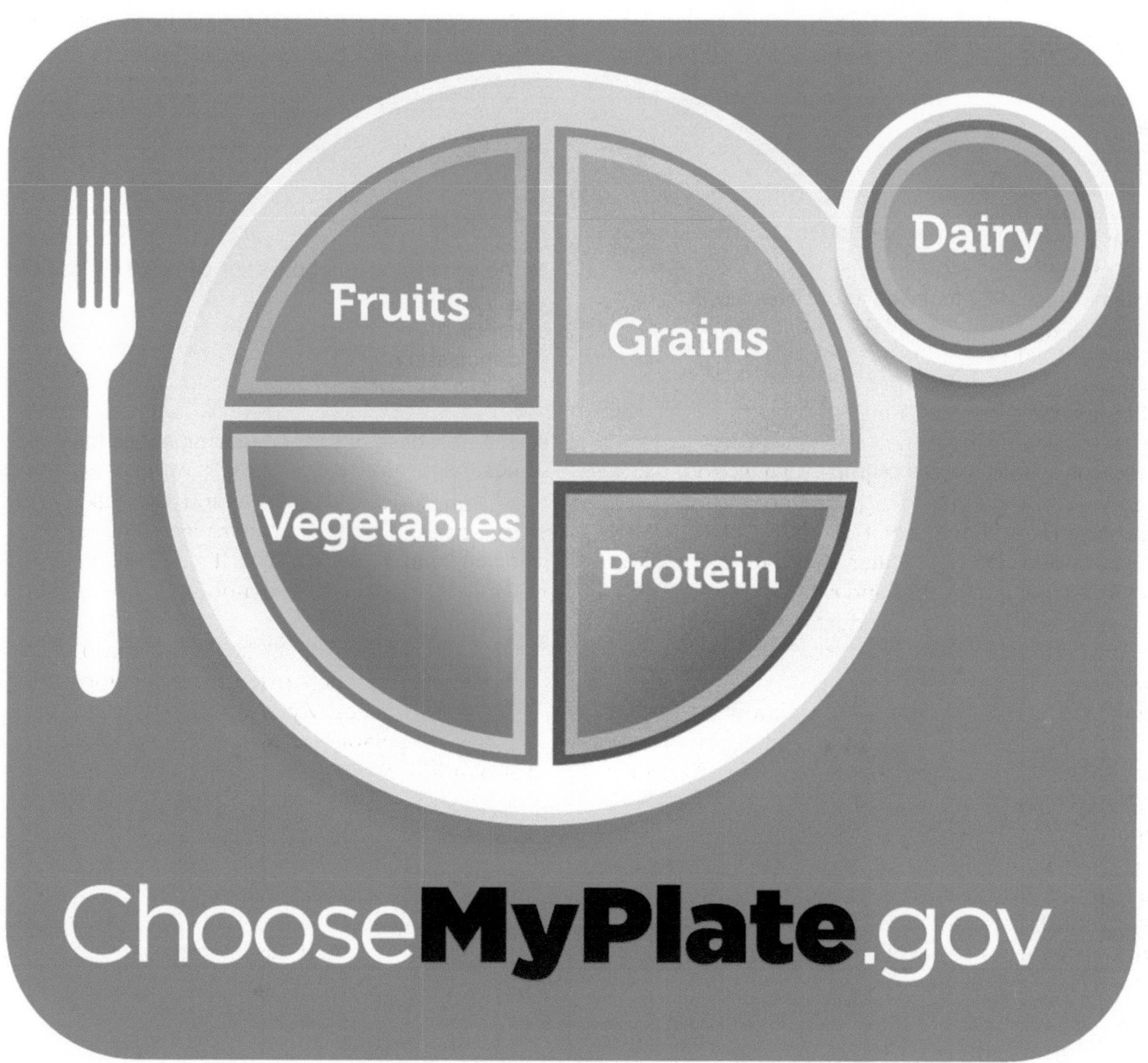

FIGURE 6-1 MyPlate guideline to make healthier food choices. (From U.S. Department of Agriculture, Center for Nutrition Policy and Promotion, June 2011; available at *www.choosemyplate.gov*.)

REVIEW QUESTIONS

1. The disease that develops because of an overdose of vitamins is:
   a. scurvy.
   b. beriberi.
   c. hypervitaminosis.
   d. avitaminosis.

2. A vitamin necessary for blood to clot normally is:
   a. vitamin A.
   b. thiamine.
   c. vitamin K.
   d. vitamin D.

3. Pernicious anemia may be caused by a deficiency of:
   a. vitamin B_1.
   b. vitamin B_2.
   c. vitamin B_6.
   d. vitamin B_{12}.

4. A mineral that is a component of blood hemoglobin is:
   a. zinc.
   b. iron.
   c. calcium.
   d. phosphorus.

5. Osteoporosis may result when the body is depleted of:
   a. vitamin C.
   b. vitamin A.
   c. calcium.
   d. iron.

6. A vitamin known to be an antioxidant is:
   a. vitamin A.
   b. vitamin B_1.
   c. vitamin D.
   d. vitamin E.

7. The administration of diuretics can cause a loss of:
   a. calcium.
   b. iron.
   c. potassium.
   d. zinc.

8. The daily dose of calcium recommended for a postmenopausal woman who is calcium depleted is:
   a. 1 gm.
   b. 2 gm.
   c. 300 mg.
   d. 5 gm.

9. A nonorganic material found in the earth's crust is a(n):
   a. vitamin.
   b. mineral.
   c. oxidant.
   d. antioxidant.

10. Rickets is a deficiency disorder caused by a lack of:
    a. vitamin A.
    b. vitamin C.
    c. vitamin D.
    d. vitamin E.

Answers to the review questions can be found at the back of the book.

evolve Additional questions and activities can be found at *http://evolve.elsevier.com/asperheim/pharmacology.*

Antibiotics and Antifungal, Antiviral, and Antiparasitic Agents

CHAPTER 7

Objectives

After completing this chapter, you should be able to do the following:

1. Identify the antibiotics, and give their general uses.
2. Identify serious side effects of antibiotics.
3. Distinguish between a broad-spectrum antibiotic and a narrow-spectrum antibiotic.
4. Distinguish among first-generation, second-generation, and third-generation cephalosporins.
5. Give examples of antibiotics that are used to treat specific conditions.
6. Identify common antiparasitic agents.
7. Identify antiviral agents and their general uses.
8. List current uses of sulfonamides.
9. List symptoms of toxic effects of sulfa drugs.

Key Terms

Antibiotics, p. 49
Broad-spectrum antibiotic, p. 49
Cephalosporins (SĔF-ĕ-lō-SPŎR-ĭns), p. 51
Fungus (*pl.* fungi), p. 57
Narrow-spectrum antibiotic, p. 49
Para-aminobenzoic acid (PABA), p. 55
Penicillin, p. 50
Quinolones (KWĬN-ĕ-lōns), p. 54
Sulfonamides ("sulfa drugs") (sĕl-FŌN-ĕ-mīds), p. 55
Tetracyclines (TĔT-rĕ-SĪ-klēns), p. 53
Virus, p. 58

ANTIBIOTICS

Antibiotics are substances that kill or inhibit the growth of microorganisms. They are either produced naturally, by living cells, or synthetically, as analogs of the natural substances. The first knowledge of antibiotics was provided by Fleming in 1928, when he discovered that a product of the *Penicillium* mold had the power to destroy many disease-producing microorganisms.

Currently, we obtain many antibiotics from molds, bacteria, and yeasts, but an increasing number are now manufactured synthetically. Often only a small change in the structure of a naturally produced antibiotic can result in significant changes in the action and effect of a drug.

Each antibiotic has its own characteristic "spectrum" of activity against various microorganisms. A **broad-spectrum antibiotic** is effective against many microorganisms; a **narrow-spectrum antibiotic** is effective against only a few.

Much has been discovered in recent years about the growing resistance of many microorganisms to the action of antibiotics. It is believed that the use of antibiotics to treat many trivial infections has allowed microorganisms to develop mutant forms that are resistant to these drugs. This is particularly likely if an antibiotic is taken for only a few days instead of the generally prescribed 10-day minimum for antibiotic use. When treatment time is shortened, the organisms that are more naturally resistant to the drug are allowed to increase and multiply, and only the weaker ones are killed.

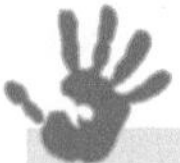

Considerations for Children

Unnecessary Antibiotics

Children do not need an antibiotic to treat every minor illness, and antibiotics are ineffective against viruses, which cause most colds and other minor illnesses. However, parents often feel uncomfortable leaving a child's illness untreated. Teach parents that overuse of antibiotics is producing antibiotic-resistant organisms, and reassure them when antibiotics are unnecessary.

Allergic reactions to various antibiotics are also common. With repeated exposure to a drug, various defensive mechanisms of the body begin to be sensitized, and allergic reactions result. Often these reactions are mild and may produce just a rash, which is easily treated. However, subsequent exposures to the drug may produce severe and fatal reactions.

PENICILLINS

A **penicillin** is any antibiotic derived from the *Penicillium* mold. Since its discovery as the first antibiotic, there have been many alterations in the structure of penicillin to increase its usefulness.

penicillin G, USP-NF; benzylpenicillin, BP. Used as either the sodium salt (intramuscular [IM] or intravenous [IV] administration) or the potassium salt (IM or IV administration) to increase its water solubility, this early form of penicillin is still the drug of choice for syphilis. It is also used for prophylaxis against group B streptococcus infections during pregnancy and against certain other susceptible organisms. Its main disadvantages are that it has a short duration of action in its crystalline form, and it must be injected because it is destroyed by stomach acids when taken orally. Before any form of penicillin is given, the patient must be carefully questioned concerning allergic reactions to the drug.

Dosage: Adults: (IV) 5 million to 20 million units daily in divided doses. Dosage is individualized.

Children: (IM, IV) 25,000 to 50,000 units/kg/day in divided doses four times daily. Dosage is individualized.

Neonates: (IM, IV) 25,000 units twice daily. Dosage is individualized.

penicillin V potassium, USP-NF, BP. By changing the structure of penicillin G, a form of penicillin was developed that can be absorbed better orally. It is used to treat respiratory infections, cutaneous anthrax, and gingivitis, and to prevent rheumatic fever recurrences.

Dosage: Adults: (Oral) 250 to 500 mg every 6 hours.

Children: (Oral) 25 to 50 mg/kg daily in four divided doses.

LONG-ACTING FORMS OF PENICILLIN G

Because of the short duration of the crystalline form of penicillin G, several long-acting forms have been developed. These agents have the advantage of IM administration so that a repository of the drug remains in the muscle tissue and can be absorbed slowly by the body.

These long-acting forms may be given *only* by IM route. They can produce fatal embolization if administered by IV route.

penicillin G procaine, USP-NF, BP (Wycillin). The addition of procaine to the penicillin molecule results in a product that provides good blood levels of penicillin for about 6 hours.

Dosage: Adults: (IM) 600,000 to 4 million units daily in divided doses every 6 hours.

Children: (IM) 300,000 to 1.2 million units daily in divided doses every 6 hours.

Neonates: This form is not recommended.

penicillin G benzathine, USP-NF, BP (Bicillin). By the addition of benzathine to the penicillin molecule, a very insoluble form of penicillin is formed. The drug is slowly leached from the repository in the muscle and may provide a prolonged low dose of penicillin for 1 month. This form is used in monthly injections to treat patients with syphilis, for prophylaxis in patients who have had rheumatic fever, and in other cases when prolonged action is desired.

Bicillin L-A. This drug is pure benzathine penicillin.

Dosage: Adults: (IM only) 1.2 million to 4.8 million units.

Children: (IM only) 600,000 to 1.2 million units.

Bicillin C-R. This drug combines equal parts of benzathine penicillin and procaine penicillin so that a therapeutic blood level is reached sooner. Dosage range is similar to that of Bicillin L-A.

SEMISYNTHETIC PENICILLINS

Considerable research and alteration of the penicillin molecule have resulted in new forms of penicillin that have a broader spectrum of activity than the parent molecule and greater effectiveness with oral administration. Table 7-1 presents an overview of this class of antibiotics.

GENERAL TOXICITY AND SIDE EFFECTS

Hypersensitivity to penicillins should always be considered. In some instances, individuals who are sensitive to penicillin G may be able to tolerate the altered forms of penicillin. When penicillin is prescribed orally, abdominal cramping or diarrhea may result. Overgrowth of nonsusceptible organisms such as *Monilia* may occur, with resultant diarrhea or vaginal or perineal infections.

Table 7-1 Semisynthetic Penicillins

Generic Name	Trade Name	General Uses	Dosage
amoxicillin, USP-NF, BP	Amoxil	Same as ampicillin	Adults: (Oral) 250-500 mg q8h Children: (Oral) 20-80 mg/kg/day in divided doses q8-12h
amoxicillin and clavulanic acid	Augmentin	Same as ampicillin but includes some ampicillin-resistant organisms	Adults: (Oral) 250-500 mg q8h Children: (Oral) 25-45 mg/kg/day in divided doses q8h
ampicillin, USP-NF, BP		Otitis media, respiratory tract infections, urinary tract infections, meningitis (in IV form)	Adults: (Oral, IM, IV) 1-2 gm/day in divided doses Children: (Oral) 50-400 mg/kg/day divided q6h
ampicillin sodium and sulbactam sodium	Unasyn	Severe skin, bone, abdominal infections	Adults and children >40 kg: (IM, IV) 1.5-3 gm q6h Children <40 kg: Not recommended
dicloxacillin sodium, USP-NF, BP		Staphylococcal infections	Adults: (Oral, IM, IV) 250-500 mg q6h Children: (Oral, IM, IV) 12.5-50 mg/kg/day in divided doses
nafcillin sodium, USP-NF, BP		Staphylococcal infections	Adults and children >40 kg: (IM, IV) 0.5-1 gm 4-6 times daily Children <40 kg: (IM, IV) 50-100 mg/kg/day in 4 divided doses
oxacillin sodium, USP-NF, BP		Staphylococcal infections	Adults and children >40 kg: (IM, IV) 250-500 mg q4–6h Children <40 kg: (IM, IV) 50 mg/kg/day in 4 divided doses
piperacillin and tazobactam sodium	Zosyn	Abdominal, skin, and respiratory tract infections	Adults: (IV) 3.375 gm q6h Children <12 yr: Not recommended
ticarcillin disodium and clavulanate potassium	Timentin	Urinary tract infections	Adults: (IM, IV) 3.1 gm q4-6h Children: (IM, IV) 200 mg/kg/day in divided doses

BETA-LACTAM ANTIBIOTICS: CEPHALOSPORINS

Also derived originally from a mold, **cephalosporins** are structurally related to penicillin. Similar to penicillin, these agents exert their activity against young dividing bacterial cells by interfering with the formation of cell walls.

Because of their similarity to the penicillin molecule, there is a considerable cross-sensitivity with penicillin. Although it is thought that the cross-allergic reaction occurs only about 25% of the time, all patients with a history of allergy to penicillin should be given these agents with caution. General toxic effects of these agents include gastrointestinal distress when they are administered orally and allergic skin rashes.

Cephalosporins are divided into four general groups on the basis of their spectrum of activity (Table 7-2). Because of the order in which they were developed, these groups are referred to as first, second, third, and fourth generations.

FIRST-GENERATION CEPHALOSPORINS

First-generation cephalosporins are effective against organisms such as streptococci and some strains of staphylococci. They are also effective against some organisms that invade the urinary tract.

SECOND-GENERATION CEPHALOSPORINS

In addition to activity against the same organisms as first-generation cephalosporins, second-generation agents are also effective against *Haemophilus influenzae,* an organism that commonly invades the middle ear and respiratory tract.

THIRD-GENERATION CEPHALOSPORINS

Third-generation cephalosporins are less effective against streptococci and pneumococci than earlier cephalosporins but are more effective against gram-negative organisms that invade the gastrointestinal and urinary tracts. They are generally reserved for serious infections that do not respond to other agents.

FOURTH-GENERATION CEPHALOSPORINS

Only one fourth-generation cephalosporin is available at the present time. Cefepime (Maxipime) is used to treat urinary tract infections, including infections associated with pyelonephritis, and severe infections of the skin, soft tissue, and abdomen.

Table 7-2 Cephalosporins and Other Beta-Lactam Antibiotics

Generic Name	Trade Name	Dosage
FIRST-GENERATION CEPHALOSPORINS		
cefadroxil, USP-NF, BP	Duricef	Adults: (Oral) 1-2 gm/day in 1-2 divided doses Children: (Oral) 10-15 mg/kg twice daily
cefazolin sodium, USP-NF, BP		Adults: (IM, IV) 250 mg–1.5 gm q6h Children: (IM, IV) 25-100 mg/kg/day in 3-4 divided doses
cephalexin, USP-NF, BP	Keflex	Adults: (Oral) 250-500 mg q6h Children: (Oral) 25-50 mg/kg/day in divided doses
SECOND-GENERATION CEPHALOSPORINS		
cefaclor, USP-NF, BP		Adults: (Oral) 250-500 mg q8h Children: (Oral) 20-40 mg/kg/day in divided doses q8h
cefoxitin sodium, USP-NF, BP	Mefoxin	Adults: (IM, IV) 1-2 gm q6-8h Children: (IM, IV) 80-160 mg/kg/day in 4-6 divided doses
cefprozil, USP-NF, BP	Cefzil	Adults: (Oral) 250-500 mg q12h Children 6 mo–12 yr: (Oral) 15 mg/kg/q12h
cefuroxime axetil, USP-NF	Ceftin	Adults: (Oral) 250-500 mg twice daily Children: (Oral) 125-250 mg twice daily
cefuroxime sodium, USP-NF	Zinacef	Adults: (IM, IV) 750 mg–1.5 gm q8h Children: (IM, IV) 50-100 mg/kg/day in divided doses
THIRD-GENERATION CEPHALOSPORINS		
cefdinir, USP-NF	Omnicef	Adults: (Oral) 600 mg daily, 1 dose or divided Children: (Oral) 14 mg/kg/day, 1 dose or divided
cefixime, USP-NF	Suprax	Adults: (Oral) 400 mg daily in 1 or 2 doses Children: (Oral) 8 mg/kg/day in 1 or 2 doses
cefditoren pivoxil	Spectracef	Adults and children >12 yr: (Oral) 200-400 mg twice daily
cefotaxime sodium, USP-NF, BP	Claforan	Adults: (IM, IV) 1-2 gm q6-8h Children: (IM, IV) 25-180 mg/kg/day in 4-6 divided doses
cefpodoxime proxetil	Vantin	Adults: (Oral) 100-400 mg q12h Children: (Oral) 10 mg/kg/day in 2 divided doses
ceftazidime sodium, USP-NF, BP	Fortaz	Adults: (IM, IV) 1-2 gm q8-12h Children: (IV) 30-50 mg/kg q8h
ceftibuten, USP-NF	Cedax	Adults: (Oral) 400 mg once daily Children: (Oral) 9 mg/kg once daily
ceftriaxone sodium, USP-NF, BP	Rocephin	Adults: (IM, IV) 1-2 gm/day in 1 or 2 divided doses Children: (IM, IV) 50-75 mg/kg/day in 2 divided doses
FOURTH-GENERATION CEPHALOSPORINS		
cefepime hydrochloride	Maxipime	Adults: (Deep IM or IV) 1-2 gm q12h Children: (IV) 50 mg/kg q12h
OTHER BETA-LACTAM ANTIBIOTICS		
aztreonam	Azactam	Adults: (IM, IV) 0.5-2 gm q8-12h Children: (IV) 30 mg/kg q8h
doripenem	Doribax	Adults: (IV) 500 mg q8h
ertapenem sodium	Invanz	Adults: (IM, IV) 1 gm once daily
imipenem and cilastatin sodium	Primaxin	Adults: (IM, IV) 250/250 up to 750/750 q6-12h
meropenem	Merrem	Adults and children >50 kg: (IV) 1 gm q8h Children <50 kg: (IV) 20 mg/kg q8h
CEPHAMYCINS		
cefotetan disodium		Adults: (IM, IV) 1-3 gm q12h Children >1 mo: (IM, IV) 40-80 mg/kg/day in 2 divided doses
cefoxitin sodium	Mefoxin	Adults: (IM, IV) 1-2 gm q6-8h Children >3 mo: (IM, IV) 80-160 mg/kg/day in 4-6 divided doses

TETRACYCLINES

Tetracyclines are broad-spectrum antibiotics that are effective against many organisms, particularly bacteria infecting the respiratory system and soft tissues. Although many agents can be given parenterally, they are well absorbed orally and are generally given by mouth. Tetracyclines are used principally in the treatment of infections caused by susceptible *Rickettsia, Chlamydia,* and *Mycoplasma* organisms and various gram-negative and gram-positive bacteria. Tetracyclines are the drug of choice for Rocky Mountain spotted fever and Lyme disease.

General adverse effects include gastrointestinal irritation; the overgrowth of nonsusceptible organisms such as yeasts, which may produce diarrhea; a perineal monilial rash; and vaginal infection. Tetracyclines are generally not given during pregnancy or to any child younger than 8 years of age because the drug concentrates in developing tooth enamel and produces a brown or yellow stain on the teeth. Doxycycline may be given to younger children when necessary, however, because it has less of an effect on tooth development. Tetracyclines are summarized in Table 7-3. All doses given are for adults and children older than 8 years of age.

Table 7-3 Tetracyclines

Generic Name	Trade Name	Dosage*
demeclocycline hydrochloride, USP-NF, BP	Declomycin	(Oral) 150 mg q6h
doxycycline hyclate, USP-NF, BP	Vibramycin	(Oral) 100 mg q12h initially, then 100 mg once daily
minocycline hydrochloride, USP-NF, BP	Minocin	(Oral, IV) 200 mg initially, then 100 mg q12h
tetracycline hydrochloride, USP-NF, BP	Sumycin	(Oral) 250-500 mg q6h
tigecycline	Tygacil	(IV) 100 mg initially, then 50 mg q12h

*All dosages are for adults and children older than 8 years of age.

MACROLIDE ANTIBIOTICS: ERYTHROMYCINS

Erythromycin is a macrolide antibiotic and this class of antibiotics, as it has become more diverse, has become known as the macrolides. Erythromycin itself is usually bacteriostatic only and exerts its effect only against multiplying organisms. It is a relatively narrow-spectrum antibiotic, effective generally against the same organisms that penicillin affects. It is often used in penicillin-sensitive patients. Although effective parenterally, it is generally used orally, primarily for upper and lower respiratory tract infections. Erythromycin is effective against gram-positive cocci, such as staphylococci and streptococci, and gram-positive bacilli, such as *Bacillus anthracis,* the causative agent of anthrax.

The synthetic agents in this class, such as azithromycin, clarithromycin, and dirithromycin, have expanded spectra of activity and generally are more potent than erythromycin itself. General untoward effects include pain and cramping after oral administration and skin reactions. Macrolide antibiotics are summarized in Table 7-4.

Table 7-4 Macrolide Antibiotics (Erythromycins)

Generic Name	Trade Name	Dosage
ERYTHROMYCINS		
erythromycin, USP-NF, BP	Eryc, Ery-Tab	Adults: (Oral) 250-500 mg q6h Children: (Oral) 20-50 mg/kg/day in 4 divided doses
erythromycin estolate, USP-NF, BP		Adults: (Oral) 250-500 mg q6h Children: (Oral) 30-50 mg/kg/day in 4 divided doses
erythromycin ethylsuccinate, USP-NF, BP	EES, Ery-Ped	Adults: (Oral) 400 mg twice daily Children: (Oral) 30-50 mg/kg/day in 2-4 divided doses
erythromycin lactobionate, USP-NF, BP	Erythrocin lactobionate	Adults and children: (IV) 15-20 mg/kg/day in 4 divided doses
erythromycin stearate		Adults: (Oral) 500 mg q12h Children: (Oral) 30-50 mg/kg/day in divided doses
SYNTHETIC MACROLIDES		
azithromycin, USP-NF, BP	Zithromax, Z-Pak	Adults: (Oral, IV) 250-500 mg once daily Children: (Oral) 30-50 mg/kg in divided doses over 3 days; single dose of 30 mg/kg for otitis media
clarithromycin, USP-NF, BP	Biaxin	Adults: (Oral) 250-500 mg q12h Children: Not recommended
telithromycin	Ketek	Adults only: (Oral) 800 mg once daily

Table 7-5 Quinolone Antimicrobials

Generic Name	Trade Name	General Uses	Dosage*
ciprofloxacin hydrochloride, USP-NF	Cipro	Respiratory tract, urinary tract, bone, and soft tissue infections	(Oral) 250-750 mg q12h
gemifloxacin mesylate	Factive	Respiratory tract	(Oral) 320 mg once daily
levofloxacin, USP-NF	Levaquin	Sinus, respiratory tract, and soft tissue infections	(Oral, IV) 250-500 mg q24h
moxifloxacin hydrochloride	Avelox	Respiratory tract infections	(Oral) 400 mg once daily
norfloxacin, USP-NF	Noroxin	Urinary tract infections and sexually transmitted diseases	(Oral) 400 mg q12h
ofloxacin		Respiratory tract, prostate, and urinary tract infections and sexually transmitted diseases	(Oral) 200-400 mg q12h

*All dosages are for adults only.

QUINOLONE ANTIMICROBIAL AGENTS

The **quinolones** are a class of orally effective antimicrobial agents that act by inhibiting the bacterial enzyme DNA gyrase. Quinolones are effective against pathogens of the respiratory, urinary, and gastrointestinal tracts and against some organisms that cause sexually transmitted diseases. They may be used in infections resistant to older antibiotics. These agents are analogs of nalidixic acid (see Chapter 19). They are entirely synthetic, and they act specifically to inhibit DNA synthesis by the microorganism, causing abnormalities that result in death of the microbe.

Quinolones exhibit concentration-dependent bacterial killing. That is, bactericidal activity is more pronounced as the serum drug concentration increases. They are well absorbed orally even in the presence of food. Their slow rate of elimination allows administration every 12 to 24 hours. Because of this slow elimination, doses may have to be adjusted for patients with renal or hepatic impairment.

Quinolone resistance has significant clinical impact. Mutations may occur rapidly during therapy and may be the most significant factor limiting the use of these antimicrobials. Side effects are mild with these agents and usually do not cause them to be discontinued. The most common reactions are gastrointestinal (i.e., nausea and vomiting). Rashes, insomnia, irritability, and arthralgia occur less commonly. Quinolones should be administered with caution in patients taking anticoagulants because in some cases they have prolonged the bleeding time. Quinolones are summarized in Table 7-5.

OTHER ANTIBIOTICS

Other antibiotics that are commonly used for various bacterial infections are presented in Table 7-6.

Table 7-6 Other Antibiotics

Generic Name	Trade Name	Uses	Toxic Effects	Dosage
amikacin sulfate, USP-NF	Amikin	Serious infections of bone and soft tissues	Auditory and kidney damage	Adults and children: (IM, IV) 15 mg/kg/day in divided doses
capreomycin sulfate	Capastat	Tuberculosis	Auditory and kidney damage	Adults: (IM, IV) 1 gm daily Children: (IM, IV) 15 mg/kg/day
chloramphenicol, USP-NF, BP	Chloromycetin	Meningitis, typhoid fever	Bone marrow depression	Adults: (Oral, IV) 12.5 mg/kg 4 times daily Children: (Oral, IV) 50-75 mg/kg/day in 4 divided doses
clindamycin hydrochloride, USP-NF, BP	Cleocin	Infections of respiratory tract and soft tissues	Leukopenia, vomiting, diarrhea, skin rash	Adults: (Oral) 150-300 mg q6h; (IM, IV) 600 mg twice daily Children: (Oral, IM, IV) 10-40 mg/kg/day in divided doses
colistimethate sodium, USP-NF, BP	Coly-Mycin M	Infections of urinary tract and soft tissues	Kidney damage	Adults: (Oral) 3-5 mg/kg/day in 2-4 divided doses
colistin sulfate, USP-NF, BP	Coly-Mycin S	Infections of urinary tract and soft tissues	Kidney damage	Adults and children: (IM, IV) 1.5-5 mg/kg/day in 2-4 divided doses
cycloserine	Seromycin	Tuberculosis	Disorientation, seizures	Adults only: (Oral) 250 mg q12h
dapsone		Leprosy	Hemolytic anemia	Adults: (Oral) 100 mg/day Children 10-14 years: (Oral) 50 mg/day
ethambutol hydrochloride, USP-NF, BP	Myambutol	Tuberculosis	Optic neuritis, rash, mental changes	Adults and children: (Oral) 15-25 mg/kg/day

Continued

Table 7-6 Other Antibiotics—cont'd

Generic Name	Trade Name	Uses	Toxic Effects	Dosage
ethionamide	Trecator	Tuberculosis	Abdominal pain, psychoses	Adults: (Oral) 15-20 mg/kg/day in divided doses Children: (Oral) 10-20 mg/kg/day in divided doses
gentamicin sulfate, USP-NF, BP	Garamycin	Serious infections of soft tissue, genitourinary tract, and respiratory tract	Auditory and kidney damage	Adults and children: (IM, IV) 1-2 mg/kg/day in 2-3 divided doses
isoniazid, USP-NF, BP	INH, Nydrazid	Tuberculosis	Neuritis, liver dysfunction	Adults: (Oral) 5 mg/kg once daily Children: (Oral) 10-20 mg/kg/day
kanamycin sulfate, USP-NF, BP	Kantrex	Infections of bone, genitourinary tract, respiratory tract, and soft tissues	Auditory damage	Adults: (Oral) 1 gm 3-4 times daily; (IM, IV) 7.5 mg/kg twice daily Children: (Oral) 12.5 mg/kg 4 times daily; (IM, IV) 3-7.5 mg/kg twice daily
metronidazole, USP-NF, BP	Flagyl	Trichomoniasis	Metallic taste, giardiasis, amebiasis, diarrhea, intolerance to alcohol, rash	Adults: (Oral) single dose of 2 gm or 250 mg 3 times daily for 7 days Children: (Oral) 15 mg/kg/day
neomycin sulfate	Neo-Fradin	Gastrointestinal infections	Hepatotoxicity	Adults only: (Oral) 4-12 gm daily in divided doses
polymyxin B sulfate, USP-NF, BP	Aerosporin	Serious infections of soft tissue or urinary tract	Neurologic and kidney damage	Adults and children: (IM) 40,000 units/kg/day in 4 divided doses; (IV) 40,000 units/kg/day in 2 divided doses; (Intrathecal) 20,000 units once daily
pyrazinamide, USP-NF, BP		Tuberculosis	Liver toxicity, rash	Adults: (Oral) 15-30 mg/kg/day Children: (Oral) 15-30 mg/kg/day
rifabutin	Mycobutin	Tuberculosis	Abdominal pain, neutropenia, rash	Adults only: (Oral) 300 mg once daily
rifampin, USP-NF, BP	Rifadin, Rifamate	Tuberculosis, carriers of meningitis organisms	Diarrhea, anemia, liver and kidney toxicity	Adults: (Oral) 600 mg/day Children: (Oral) 10-15 mg/kg/day
rifapentine	Priftin	Tuberculosis	Hepatic and hematologic side effects	Adults only: (Oral) 600 mg twice weekly
spectinomycin hydrochloride, USP-NF, BP	Trobicin	Gonorrhea	Chills, fever, nausea, dizziness, kidney damage	Adults only: (IM) 2-4 gm as a single injection
streptomycin sulfate, USP-NF, BP	Streptomycin	Tuberculosis	Auditory damage	Adults: (IM) 0.5-1 gm 4 times daily Children: (IM) 10 mg/kg 2-4 times daily
tobramycin sulfate, USP-NF, BP	Nebcin	Serious infections of bone, soft tissue, and respiratory tract	Auditory and kidney damage	Adults and children: (IM, IV) 1-2 mg/kg q8h
vancomycin hydrochloride, USP-NF, BP	Vancocin	Severe septicemia, meningitis	Nausea, thrombophlebitis at IV site, skin rashes	Adults: (IV) 0.5-2 gm/day in 3-4 divided doses Children: (IV) 10-15 mg/kg 2-3 times daily

Considerations for Children

Antibiotics and Ototoxicity (Auditory Damage)

Many antibiotics, but particularly the aminoglycosides such as gentamicin (Garamycin) and kanamycin (Kantrex), may produce auditory damage as a side effect. These agents are generally reserved for serious infections caused by gram-negative organisms, and the dosage must be carefully controlled. Hearing testing at an early age is beneficial when these agents have been used in the neonatal period.

SULFONAMIDE DRUGS

Sulfonamides ("sulfa drugs") combat infection in the body by checking the growth of bacteria and other microorganisms, enabling the body's own defenses to cope with the infection. These are synthetic drugs and are made to resemble **para-aminobenzoic acid (PABA)**, a substance that the microorganisms need for the synthesis of folic acid, an essential enzyme. The microorganism takes in the sulfa drug but cannot use it to make folic acid, and it is prevented from growing and multiplying.

Sulfa drugs are less effective in the presence of a large amount of PABA because the microorganisms prefer PABA to the drug. For this reason, the patient must not be taking medications containing PABA (e.g., Pabalate, an agent used for rheumatic conditions) when taking sulfa drugs. These drugs are usually administered by mouth, the method of choice from the standpoint of convenience and because they are well absorbed from the intestinal tract.

There has been concern over the increasing frequency of bacterial resistance to sulfonamides. In addition, the development of newer and more effective agents has sharply limited the usefulness of sulfonamides in many instances. The use of sulfonamides is recommended for the following conditions only:

- Chancroid
- Trachoma
- Inclusion conjunctivitis
- Nocardiosis
- Uncomplicated urinary tract infections caused by susceptible organisms
- Toxoplasmosis
- Malaria, as adjunctive therapy in some cases
- *Haemophilus influenzae* infections of the middle ear

Although sulfa drugs aid in controlling infections, they now have been largely replaced by the antibiotics, which have faster action and fewer side effects.

A patient who is taking sulfa drugs needs to maintain an adequate fluid intake. Sulfonamides have a tendency to crystallize in the urine and be deposited in the kidneys, resulting in a painful and dangerous condition. The chances of crystallization in the urine are minimized if the urine is kept dilute by high fluid intake.

Sulfa drugs used today produce fewer symptoms of toxicity than older compounds. However, toxic reactions may result from the use of any drugs that are absorbed and exert systemic effects. In this case, toxic reactions include nausea, vomiting, cyanosis, drug fever (often confused with a recurrent fever from the infection), rash, acidosis, jaundice, blood complications, and kidney damage. In a few cases, Stevens-Johnson syndrome, which may be fatal, has occurred. The general treatment of toxic symptoms includes discontinuing the drug and forcing fluids. The severity of symptoms determines whether the drug is permanently discontinued. The high incidence of toxicity associated with sulfonamides explains why they have been largely supplanted by the antibiotics.

Drug interactions have occurred with anticoagulants such as warfarin. The effect of warfarin may be potentiated. Sulfonamides may also potentiate the hypoglycemic effects of oral antidiabetic agents. Interference with the absorption and metabolism of digoxin and phenytoin has been described.

LONG-ACTING SULFONAMIDES

Because most sulfonamides are excreted rapidly, it has been necessary until more recently to give relatively high doses at short intervals to maintain an effective blood level of the drug. The use of long-acting sulfonamides permits lower doses to be given, because the drug remains in effective concentrations for a longer time in the blood. Often only one dose is needed daily to maintain effective blood levels. Because a lower dose may be used, side effects occur less frequently than with other sulfa drugs.

sulfasalazine, USP-NF, BP (Azulfidine). Sulfasalazine is used orally in the treatment of ulcerative colitis and Crohn's disease. It is often used in conjunction with corticosteroid therapy.

Dosage: Adults: (Oral) 2 to 4 gm daily in divided doses.

Children: (Oral) 40 to 60 mg/kg/day in three to six divided doses.

co-trimoxazole (trimethoprim and sulfamethoxazole), USP-NF, BP (Bactrim, Septra, Bactrim DS, Septra DS). This combination of agents blocks two successive steps in bacterial growth and has become one of the more successful antibacterial agents in the sulfonamide groups. The regular strength of the two brands of this combination contains 80 mg of trimethoprim and 400 mg of sulfamethoxazole. The "DS" form noted for both brands signifies the double strength of the tablet. The suspension contains 40 mg of trimethoprim and 200 mg of sulfamethoxazole per teaspoonful.

In addition to considerable effectiveness in the treatment of urinary tract infections, the combination of trimethoprim and sulfamethoxazole is now used successfully in the treatment of acute otitis media, particularly when routine antibiotic therapy has been ineffective. It should not be used in the treatment of streptococcal pharyngitis because it has been shown to have little effect.

Dosage: Adults: (Oral) Regular strength, 1 to 2 tablets every 12 hours; double strength, 1 tablet every 12 hours.

Children: (Oral) 8 mg/kg of trimethoprim and 40 mg/kg of sulfamethoxazole per 24 hours in two divided doses.

ALLERGIC REACTIONS TO SULFONAMIDES AND CROSS-REACTION ALLERGIES WITH OTHER MEDICATIONS

A particularly common allergic reaction to sulfonamides is an extensive bright red, pruritic rash, which may occur in 3% of patients prescribed sulfonamides. Also, there is an association between hypersensitivity reactions that may develop after taking a sulfonamide and a subsequent allergic reaction after

Box 7-1 Related Drugs That May Cross-React with Sulfonamides

acetazolamide	glipizide
acetohexamide	glyburide
bendroflumethiazide	hydrochlorothiazide
benzthiazide	hydroflumethiazide
bumetanide	indapamide
chlorothiazide	methyclothiazide
chlorpropamide	metolazone
chlorthalidone	piretanide
clopamide	polythiazide
cyclopenthiazide	probenecid
dapsone	quinethazone
diazoxide	sulfasalazine
dichlorphenamide	tolazamide
furosemide	tolbutamide
gliclazide	torsemide
glimepiride	

taking a drug with a similar sulfanilamide base. Cross-reaction with the related drugs is extremely common. Of particular note are the number of thiazide diuretics and antidiabetic agents that may react with sulfonamides (Box 7-1).

ANTIFUNGAL AGENTS

Fungi are eukaryotic organisms that contain no chlorophyll or vascular tissue. They are unable to eat or to manufacture their own food but rather survive by growing on and absorbing nutrients from the surrounding organic matter (e.g., a log or a piece of cheese). When the organic matter is the human body, fungi can cause disease. Fungal infections of humans include tinea pedis (athlete's foot), tinea corporis (fungal rashes on the skin), and thrush (a superficial infection of the mouth often seen in infants).

When the immune system is impaired, fungal infections can become overwhelming and life-threatening. Acquired immunodeficiency syndrome (AIDS) and AIDS-related complex are both caused by human immunodeficiency virus (HIV). Because of their severely compromised immune system, patients with these conditions are often subject to severe and life-threatening fungal infections. Cryptococcal meningitis, severe oropharyngeal candidiasis, and esophageal candidiasis can occur in these patients. IV forms of antifungal agents are generally used to treat these conditions (Table 7-7).

Table 7-7 Antifungal Agents

Generic Name	Trade Name	Uses	Dosage
amphotericin B, USP-NF, BP	Fungizone	Serious systemic fungal infections	Adults: (IV) 0.5-1 mg/kg in diluted infusion once daily Children: (IV) 0.25-1 mg/kg in diluted infusion once daily
anidulafungin	Eraxis	Candidiasis	Adults only: (IV) 100-200 mg/day
caspofungin acetate	Cancidas	Aspergillosis	Adults only: (IV) 50-70 mg/day
fluconazole	Diflucan	Vaginal candidiasis, systemic candidiasis	Adults: (Oral, IV) 200-400 mg/day Children: (Oral, IV) 3-12 mg/kg/day
flucytosine, USP-NF, BP	Ancobon	Serious systemic infections	Adults and children: (Oral) 50-150 mg/kg/day in 4 divided doses
griseofulvin, USP-NF, BP	Fulvicin, Grifulvin, Grisactin	Superficial fungal infections	Adults: (Oral) 500-1000 mg/day Children: (Oral) 10-20 mg/kg/day in 2 divided doses
itraconazole	Sporanox	Systemic fungal infection in immunocompromised patients	Adults: (Oral) 200-400 mg/day in 1-2 divided doses; (IV) 200 mg 1-2 times daily Children: Not established
ketoconazole USP-NF, BP	Nizoral	Serious systemic fungal infections	Adults: (Oral) 200-400 mg/day as a single dose Children: (Oral) 3.3-6.6 mg/kg/day as a single dose
micafungin sodium	Mycamine	Candidiasis	Adults only: (IV) 100-150 mg/day
miconazole, USP-NF, BP	Monistat	Vaginally and topically for yeast infections; systemically for major infections	Adults: (IV) 1.2-3.6 gm/day in divided doses; (Vaginal, topical) 2%-4% cream twice daily or one 200-mg insert once daily for 3 days Children: (IV) 20-40 mg/day in divided doses
nystatin, USP-NF, BP	Mycostatin	Orally for moniliasis; topically and vaginally for skin moniliasis	Adults: (Oral) 500,000-1,000,000 units 3 times daily; (Vaginal) 100,000-unit suppository 3 times daily Children: (Oral) 100,000-200,000 units 4 times daily
posaconazole	Noxafil	Aspergillosis, candidiasis	Adults only: (Oral) 200 mg 3 times daily
terbinafine hydrochloride, USP-NF	Lamisil	Orally for toenail and fingernail fungal infections	Adults: (Oral) 250 mg daily Children <12 years: Not recommended
voriconazole	VFEND	Aspergillosis	Adults and children: (IV) 6 mg/kg q12h for 1 day, then 4 mg/kg q12h

ANTIVIRAL AGENTS

A **virus** is a microscopic infectious agent that requires an intact living host cell for metabolism; when it enters this host cell, the virus is able to reproduce and mutate. Using the metabolic processes of the host cell, viruses can direct the synthesis of hundreds to thousands of progeny viruses (viral copies) during a single cycle of infection. When the discovery of antibiotics began a revolution in the ability to treat bacterial infections, it was anticipated that similarly effective antiviral agents would soon be identified as well; however, this has not proven to be the case. A major problem in the development of antiviral agents has been the more intimate relationship between viral and host metabolic activities. This relationship makes it nearly impossible to develop a drug to kill the virus effectively in a person's body without also causing great harm to the existing cells of the body. The search for selective inhibitors of viral activity that are not too toxic to the human host has been much more difficult than first appreciated.

The primary uses of the available antiviral agents are in the treatment of influenza, hepatitis, herpesvirus infections, and AIDS. Antiviral agents commonly used for these infections are discussed next; additional antiviral agents are listed in Table 7-8.

ANTIVIRALS USED IN THE TREATMENT OF INFLUENZA

When oseltamivir (Tamiflu) and zanamivir (Relenza) (see Table 7-8) are used to treat acute influenza, the duration of the symptoms of influenza is shortened, although only by a few days. Generally, older adults and very young children are at the greatest risk from serious complications of the flu; these agents may be considered for therapy in these groups especially. They have not been shown to have any prophylactic effects in preventing infection with the influenza virus.

Table 7-8 Antiviral Agents

Generic Name	Trade Name	Uses	Dosage
acyclovir sodium, USP-NF	Zovirax	Herpes simplex infections, oral or genital varicella-zoster (shingles), varicella (chickenpox) in immunocompromised patients	Adults: (Oral) 400 mg 5 times daily; (IV) 5 mg/kg q8h Children: (Oral) 15-20 mg/day in 3-5 divided doses; (IV) 5-10 mg/kg q8h
amantadine hydrochloride, USP-NF, BP	Symmetrel	Prevention and treatment of influenza A infections	Adults: (Oral) 100-200 mg/day Children: (Oral) 5 mg/kg/day in 1-2 divided doses
cidofovir, USP-NF	Vistide	Cytomegalovirus retinitis	Adults only: (Oral) 5 mg/kg weekly
famciclovir	Famvir	Varicella zoster, genital herpes	Adults only: (Oral) 500 mg 3 times daily
foscarnet sodium, USP-NF	Foscavir	Cytomegalovirus retinitis	Adults: (IV) 60 mg/kg q8h for 14-21 days
		Herpes simplex, varicella zoster	Adults: (IV) 40 mg/kg q8h
ganciclovir sodium, USP-NF	Cytovene	Cytomegalovirus retinitis in immunocompromised patients	Adults and children: (IV) 5 mg/kg q12h
oseltamivir	Tamiflu	Influenza A and B	Adults: (Oral) 75 mg twice daily Children 1-12 years: (Oral) 30 mg twice daily
palivizumab	Synagis	Respiratory syncytial virus	Children: (IM) 15 mg/kg once a month
ribavirin, USP-NF	Rebetol, Virazole	Respiratory syncytial virus infections, adenovirus pneumonia, chronic hepatitis C	Adults and children: (Oral) 600 mg twice daily; (Nasal) 20 mg/mL for 12-18 hr/day for 3-7 days
rimantadine hydrochloride, USP-NF	Flumadine	Influenza A prophylaxis	Adults: (Oral) 100 mg twice daily for up to 6 wk Children <10 years: (Oral) 5 mg/kg/day up to 150 mg/day maximum
trifluridine, USP-NF	Viroptic	Herpes simplex conjunctivitis, keratitis of eye	Adults and children: (Topical) 1% solution applied to eye 1 drop every 2 hr up to 9 drops/day for 7-14 days
valacyclovir hydrochloride	Valtrex	Varicella zoster, genital herpes	Adults only: (Oral) 1 gm twice daily
vidarabine, USP-NF, BP	Vira-A	Topically to eyes for herpes simplex keratitis	Adults and children: (Topical) 3% ointment applied 5 times a day
zanamivir	Relenza	Influenza A and B	Adults and children >5 yr: (Oral inhalation) 2 inhalations (10 mg) twice daily

ANTIVIRALS USED IN THE TREATMENT OF HEPATITIS AND HERPESVIRUSES

HEPATITIS VIRUSES

Hepatitis A

Hepatitis A virus is generally a short-lived virus and is not treated with antiviral agents. It is contracted orally from contaminated food or water.

Hepatitis B

Hepatitis B virus affects 5% of the worldwide population and may lead to cirrhosis and hepatocellular carcinoma. It was formerly called serum hepatitis and is contracted from blood or bodily fluids. Most infected persons do not progress to the chronic form.

Hepatitis C

Hepatitis C virus is believed to be the most common cause of end-stage liver disease. Nearly 85% of individuals who contract this virus develop the chronic form. It is contracted from infected blood or body fluids.

Other forms of hepatitis virus have been identified to at least hepatitis G. Generally, they are spread by infected blood and body fluids as well.

entecavir. Entecavir is active against hepatitis B virus. Resistance can develop slowly during long-term therapy.
Dosage: Adults only: (Oral) 0.5 mg once daily at least 2 hours before a meal.

interferon alfa-2b (Intron A). Interferon alfa, a synthetic version of the naturally occurring interferon-alpha, is composed of a family of proteins that possess antiviral, antineoplastic, and immunomodulating properties. It is used to treat hepatitis B, C, and D and West Nile virus infections. Infrequently, thyroid abnormalities occur during treatment; thyroid function should be evaluated before the start of therapy.
Dosage: Adults: (Subcut or IM) 5 million units per day.

lamivudine (Epivir, Epivir-HBV). Lamivudine is a synthetic nucleoside analog that has activity against hepatitis B virus and HIV. Clinical exacerbations of hepatitis B have occurred after the drug is discontinued, as shown by an increased level of alanine aminotransferase.
Dosage: Adults: (Oral) 100 mg once daily.
Children 2 to 17 years: (Oral) 3 mg/kg once daily.

peginterferon (PEG-Intron). Peginterferon is a conjugate of recombinant alfa-2b interferon. It binds to cell receptors and initiates intracellular events such as induction of certain enzymes and suppression of cell proliferation.
Dosage: Adults: (Subcut) 1.5 mcg/kg once weekly.

ribavirin (Rebetol, Virazole). Ribavirin is ineffective for the treatment of hepatitis C when used alone, but it is a useful adjunct when used with peginterferon.
Dosage: Adults: (Oral) 600 mg twice daily.

ribavirin plus interferon alfa-2b (Rebetron). This is a combination therapy product containing ribavirin capsules and interferon alfa-2b injection. The dosages are as noted for the two separate drugs (ribavirin and interferon alfa-2b).

HERPESVIRUSES

Herpesviruses are DNA viruses that can lie dormant in sensory neurons after an initial infection and then reactivate and cause disease. Viruses in this family are herpes simplex virus (HSV) and varicella-zoster virus (VZV).

Agents used to treat these viruses may be oral or topical. Oral agents are the following (see Table 7-8):

- acyclovir (Zovirax)
- famciclovir (Famvir)
- valacyclovir (Valtrex)

The available topical agents are:

acyclovir (Zovirax). This 5% cream or ointment can be applied topically to herpes lesions of the lips and to genital herpes lesions.
Dosage: Adults: (Topical) Apply six times daily for 7 days.

penciclovir (Denavir). For orolabial herpes.
Dosage: Adults and children over 12 years: (Topical) Apply every 2 hours while awake for 4 days. Safety in children younger than 12 years has not been established.

ANTIVIRALS USED IN THE TREATMENT OF ACQUIRED IMMUNODEFICIENCY SYNDROME

Since its identification in the early 1970s, acquired immunodeficiency syndrome (AIDS) has generated much research into antivirals that are effective against this disease. AIDS is caused by human immunodeficiency virus (HIV), a virus of the family Retroviridae. It is a ribonucleic acid (RNA) virus and has two strands of RNA as its genetic material. It is called a retrovirus because it converts genetic information "backward" from RNA to DNA. (Information generally goes from DNA to RNA; the twisted strand of DNA "unzips" itself to allow the RNA within to be copied.)

HIV fuses with the membrane of a host cell and enters the cytoplasm of the cell. Packaged within HIV is a DNA polymerase called reverse transcriptase, which transcribes single-stranded viral RNA into numerous copies of single strands of viral DNA and then combines these into double-stranded viral DNA. The viral DNA is transcribed in the normal way to form viral RNA. Some of these RNA copies are used to make new HIV, which is assembled near the surface of the host cell in a process that involves the action of the enzyme protease.

Drug development for treatment of AIDS has concentrated on drugs that interfere with the activity of the viral RNA, primarily at the point of fusion with the host cell, during the process of reverse transcription, or at the point of action of protease on the new virus. These drugs are usually given to patients in combinations because of the high likelihood that the virus will develop resistance to any one of them. Resistance occurs because HIV reverse transcriptase is prone to making errors during transcription of viral RNA into viral DNA, which can allow HIV to mutate to a drug-resistant form.

Two mechanisms determine the progression of AIDS and the need to treat or to change drugs if the treatment is becoming less effective:

1. *Viral load.* This is directly measured at the HIV RNA level in units indicating the number of viral copies per microliter. At a viral count of greater than 30,000/mcL, therapy is recommended. The goal is an undetectable viral load, or at least a viral load less than 5000 copies/mcL.
2. *CD4 cell count.* CD4 cells are the subpopulation of lymphocytes referred to as the helper T cells (T4 cells). The severity of the CD4 count reduction corresponds to the severity of AIDS disease progression. The CD4 cell count in unaffected individuals should be significantly greater than 400 cells/mL. At the present time, treatment is recommended when the CD4 count is less than 350 cells/mL.

Three major categories of antiviral drugs are used to treat AIDS: nucleoside reverse transcriptase inhibitors (NRTIs), non-nucleoside reverse transcriptase inhibitors (NNRTIs), and protease inhibitors. A fourth category, fusion inhibitors, is used less often. Dosages given are for adults only.

NUCLEOSIDE REVERSE TRANSCRIPTASE INHIBITORS

Nucleoside reverse transcriptase inhibitors (NRTIs) exert their antiviral activity by intracellular conversion of the drug to a triphosphate metabolite. These triphosphate metabolites are analogs of one of the four essential components of the DNA molecule (adenine, thymine, guanine, or cytosine) and can fit into a DNA molecule that is being assembled. The analog slips into the viral DNA molecule during its construction and interferes with the viral RNA–directed DNA polymerase (i.e., reverse transcriptase) activity, causing the assembly of the viral DNA molecule to stop prematurely.

abacavir (Ziagen)

Dosage: Adults: (Oral) 300 mg twice daily.
Children: (Oral) 8 mg/kg twice daily.

didanosine (Videx). Didanosine triphosphate competes with adenosine triphosphate for incorporation into the viral DNA. Antacids increase the bioavailability of this drug by preventing its breakdown in the acid pH of the stomach. Didanosine has been associated with fatal pancreatitis; the patient must be observed for abdominal symptoms. Patients need frequent eye examinations to assess for optic neuritis or retinal changes. This drug also has been associated with peripheral neuropathy and renal impairment.
Dosage: Adults: (Oral) 400 mg once daily.
Children: (Oral) 100 mg/m^2 twice daily.

emtricitabine (Emtriva)

Dosage: Adults and children: (Oral) 200 mg once daily.

lamivudine (Epivir)

Dosage: Adults: (Oral) 300 mg once daily.

stavudine (Zerit)

Dosage: Adults: (Oral) 40 mg every 12 hours.

zidovudine (Retrovir). Zidovudine triphosphate competes with thymidine triphosphate for incorporation into the viral DNA. DNA synthesis is prematurely terminated. Side effects include nausea and vomiting; generally there are no hematologic effects.
Dosage: Adults: (Oral) 600 mg daily in two to three divided doses.

NON-NUCLEOSIDE REVERSE TRANSCRIPTASE INHIBITORS

Non-nucleoside reverse transcriptase inhibitors (NNRTIs) interfere with HIV by binding directly to the viral reverse transcriptase and act as specific reverse transcriptase inhibitors. In contrast to NRTIs, they do not require conversion to a metabolite.

delavirdine mesylate (Rescriptor). Although delavirdine is active against HIV type 1, as with nevirapine, resistance develops quickly, so it should be used with other agents to diminish resistance. Delavirdine is ineffective against HIV type 2. It should be taken with an acidic beverage (e.g., orange juice) to enhance absorption. Rash is the major side effect.
Dosage: Adults: (Oral) 400 mg every 8 hours.

efavirenz (Sustiva). Efavirenz is also effective only against HIV type 1 and should be used with other agents to diminish resistance. Side effects include central nervous system effects, abnormal dreams, vertigo, delusions, rash, nausea, and liver toxicity.
Dosage: Adults and children older than 3 years and weighing more than 40 kg: (Oral) 600 mg once daily.

etravirene (Intelence). Etravirene is administered orally and should always be taken after a meal. It should always be combined with other antiviral agents.
Dosage: Adults only: (Oral) 200 mg twice daily.

nevirapine (Viramune). Nevirapine is active against HIV type 1 but not HIV type 2. Resistance develops quickly unless it is used with other antiviral agents. Side effects include severe skin reactions (Stevens-Johnson syndrome type of bullous lesions) and hepatotoxicity.
Dosage: Adults: (Oral) 200 mg twice daily.

PROTEASE INHIBITORS

Protease inhibitors directly interfere with viral protease, which plays an essential role in the replication cycle of HIV and the formation of infectious virus. These agents act at a different stage of the HIV replication cycle than NRTIs or NNRTIs and may be used alone or in combination with other agents. Cross-resistance forms between drugs within this class.

atanazir sulfate (Reyataz). This agent is often used in conjunction with other drugs to treat HIV.
Dosage: Adults: (Oral) 100 to 400 mg once daily with food.

darunavir (Prezista). This agent is administered along with 100 mg of ritonavir.
Dosage: Adults: (Oral) 800 mg once daily.

fosamprenavir calcium (Lexiva). This agent should not be used alone and is generally given with two or three other antiviral agents.
Dosage: Adults: (Oral) 700 mg daily.
Children: (Oral) 30 mg/kg twice daily.

indinavir sulfate (Crixivan). Indinavir works against HIV type 1 and HIV type 2. Side effects include nausea, vomiting, hyperbilirubinemia, skin rash, and anaphylaxis.
Dosage: Adults: (Oral) 800 mg every 8 hours.

lopinavir and ritonavir (Kaletra). This fixed combination is administered orally. Ritonavir enhances the effectiveness of lopinavir.
Dosage: Adults: (Oral) 800 mg lopinavir and 200 mg ritonavir daily.
Children older than 6 months: (Oral) 12 mg/kg lopinavir and 3 mg/kg ritonavir twice daily.
Infants younger than 6 months: (Oral) 300 mg/m^2 lopinavir and 75 mg/m^2 ritonavir twice daily.

nelfinavir mesylate (Viracept). Nelfinavir is active against HIV type 1 and HIV type 2. Side effects include diarrhea, skin rashes, and new-onset diabetes.
Dosage: Adults: (Oral) 750 mg three times daily.

ritonavir (Norvir). Ritonavir works against HIV type 1 and HIV type 2. Side effects include nausea, vomiting, diarrhea, taste perversion, and peripheral paresthesias.
Dosage: Adults: (Oral) 600 mg every 12 hours.

saquinavir (Invirase). Saquinavir is active against HIV type 1 and HIV type 2. Absorption of this agent is greatly enhanced by the presence of food in the gastrointestinal tract, so it should be taken 2 hours after meals. It should not be used alone because of resistance. Side effects include nausea, diarrhea, and hepatotoxicity.
Dosage: Adults: (Oral) 1000 mg twice daily given with ritonavir (100 mg twice daily).

tipranavir (Aptivus). This agent should be used in combination with other antiviral agents such as ritonavir.
Dosage: Adults: (Oral) 500 mg twice daily.
Children older than 2 years: (Oral) 14 mg/kg twice daily.

FUSION INHIBITORS

The fusion inhibitor class of antiretroviral drugs is mainly used when the available combination antiretroviral regimens are no longer effective because of the development of viral resistance. These agents prevent the fusion of the HIV type 1 transmembrane glycoprotein with the CD4 receptor of the host cell. Fusion inhibitors can work synergistically with other classes of AIDS drugs. Only one agent in this class is approved for use.

enfuvirtide (Fuzeon). Enfuvirtide is useful when the patient has become resistant to the more standard combinations of AIDS drugs. It must be administered subcutaneously.
Dosage: Adults: (Subcut) 90 mg twice daily.
Children 6 to 16 years: (Subcut) 2 mg/kg twice daily.

maraviroc (Selzentry). This agent is used in conjunction with other antiviral drugs.
Dosage: Adults only: (Oral) 300 mg twice daily.

ANTIPARASITIC AGENTS

Numerous parasites, including the helminths (worms), are able to invade the human body. Tropical parasites are not discussed here.

ANTHELMINTIC DRUGS

Worm infestations appear throughout the world but are particularly prominent in warmer climates. Cultural hygienic practices are important in the prevention of worm infestations because in every case they are spread by a feces-to-mouth route. Day care centers where the diaper changer is also the food handler have been important sources for the spread of worms and other parasites.

Herb Alert
Goldenseal

Goldenseal has shown some clinical effectiveness in the treatment of bacterial infections, notably infections with *Salmonella, Shigella,* and *Klebsiella* species, and in vitro activity against intestinal parasites, such as *Giardia lamblia, Trichomonas,* and *Entamoeba histolytica.* It has been used in the past to treat eye infections, notably trachoma. Prolonged use can cause digestive disorders including constipation, irritation of mucous membranes, and occasionally hallucinations. Goldenseal reduces the anticoagulant activity of heparin and enhances the effectiveness of antihypertensives and sedatives. Avoid the use of goldenseal in patients with glucose-6-phosphate dehydrogenase (G-6-PD) deficiency. See Chapter 28 for more information on goldenseal.

albendazole, USP-NF (Albenza). Albendazole is used to treat active central nervous system lesions caused by the larval form of *Taenia solium* (pork tapeworm), generally in combination with corticosteroids. In addition, it is used for cystic hydatid disease involving lesions in the lung, liver, and peritoneum caused by the larval form of the dog tapeworm.
Dosage: Adults: (Oral) 400 mg twice daily for 8 to 30 days.
Children: (Oral) 15 mg/kg divided in two doses for 8 to 30 days.

ivermectin (Stromectol). Ivermectin is effective against hookworms and ascaris and may be used orally as an adjunct in the treatment of pediculosis and scabies.
Dosage: Adults and children: (Oral) 150 to 400 mcg/kg as a single dose.

mebendazole, USP-NF, BP (Vermox). Mebendazole is used to treat roundworms, hookworms, threadworms, pinworms, and many tropical parasites.
Dosage: Adults and children: (Oral) One 100-mg tablet twice daily for 3 days. For pinworms, one dose of 100 mg is usually sufficient.

praziquantel (Biltricide). Praziquantel has been shown to be active against many tapeworms pathogenic to humans, including fish tapeworms, dog and cat tapeworms, and beef and pork tapeworms. It is also active against all *Schistosoma* species. Generally treatment is for 1 day only.
Dosage: Adults and children: (Oral) 60 to 75 mg/kg/day in three divided doses.

thiabendazole, USP-NF, BP (Mintezol). This agent is used for cutaneous larva migrans (creeping eruption) and threadworm infestations.
Dosage: Adults and children: (Oral) 25 mg/kg twice daily for 2 days. A 10% suspension of the drug may be applied topically to cutaneous larva migrans as well.

MEDICATION FOR LICE AND SCABIES

Lice and scabies occur indiscriminately among all socioeconomic groups. Outbreaks of head lice in school systems create a public health challenge, particularly in the fall. It is often impossible to see the lice themselves, but the infestation is characterized by pruritus and the presence of nits, which are the small, silver eggs attached to the hair shaft.

Scabies is caused by a mite that burrows under the skin and causes intense body pruritus. It is often spread by shaking hands because the thin skin between the fingers is a typical spot for infestation.

crotamiton (Eurax). Crotamiton is applied in a 10% solution for the treatment of scabies.
Dosage: Adults and children: (Topical) Apply to all skin surfaces once daily for 2 days.

lindane, USP-NF, BP (Kwell). Lindane may be used as a shampoo for head lice or as an application to the entire body for scabies. Because of the possibility of neurotoxic effects, this prescription product should not be used unless over-the-counter (OTC) agents have failed.
Dosage: Adults and children: (Topical) 1% solution applied to the body and/or scalp once. Treatment may be repeated one more time in a week, if necessary.

malathion (Ovide). Malathion is used to treat head and pubic lice.
Dosage: Adults and children: (Topical) 0.5% lotion is applied to hair. The hair is allowed to dry naturally. Shampoo after 8 to 12 hours. Dosage may be repeated after 7 days if necessary.

permethrin (Nix Creme Rinse). This product is recommended as a single-dose treatment for head lice.
Dosage: Adults and children: (Topical) After hair has been washed, rinsed, and towel dried, the cream rinse is applied and left on hair for 10 minutes.

permethrin topical cream (Acticin, Elimite). When applied as a skin cream, this agent is effective against scabies. It should be applied evenly to all skin surfaces and left on for 8 to 14 hours, then washed off thoroughly.
Dosage: Adults and children: (Topical) One application of the cream; may be repeated in 2 weeks if necessary.

pyrethrins with piperonyl butoxide (Tisit Liquid, Licide). When used in combination, these agents are very effective as a topical treatment for head lice and pubic lice. They are supplied as a solution, shampoo, or gel containing 0.17% to 0.33% pyrethrins.
Dosage: Adults and children: (Topical) Apply to affected body surface once. Wash agent off after 10 minutes. Application may be repeated in 7 to 10 days if necessary.

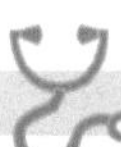

Clinical Implications

1. All injectable antibiotics should be carefully checked for the expiration date before administration.
2. The patient should be carefully questioned concerning previous allergic reactions to antibiotics.
3. After administration, the patient should be checked for possible untoward effects, such as a skin rash, respiratory distress, or other allergic responses.
4. Become familiar with the special tags placed on patients' charts noting drug allergies.
5. Remember to check for a MedicAlert tag that an unresponsive patient may be wearing.
6. The health care professional should be aware of cross-sensitivity reactions of antibiotics, such as reactions between penicillin and cephalosporins.
7. Patients should be carefully instructed to take their entire supply of antibiotics to prevent the development of resistant strains of bacteria.
8. Old antibiotic prescriptions should be discarded if they are not finished because antibiotics quickly become outdated.
9. Aseptic technique is still the most effective way to prevent infection. Antibiotics must not be relied on to remedy infections caused by disregard for asepsis.
10. Many antibiotics are irritating when given by injection. IM injections should be given deeply in large muscles.
11. Resolution of fever is a sign used to check the early effectiveness of an antibiotic against an infection.
12. The student should be aware of possible side effects of antibiotic agents.
13. Superinfection by organisms not susceptible to antibiotics is a common sequela to antibiotic therapy. Superinfections may occur as a rash, commonly *Monilia* in the oral or genital region, or as diarrhea.
14. Good nutrition, adequate rest, and general cleanliness are important to the overall well-being of a patient recovering from an infection.
15. Instruct patients in the importance of hygiene in preventing the spread of parasites. Short fingernails that are kept very clean, good handwashing techniques, and the avoidance of nail biting and "mouthing" of objects such as pencils should be stressed.
16. Become familiar with steps used to prevent head lice cross-infection. Combs, brushes, and other toilet articles should not be shared. Outer garments hung in cloakrooms can spread an infestation from garment to garment.
17. Stools should be inspected for the presence of worms. Transmission of infestations by toilet seats and bedpans should be considered and avoided.
18. Superinfections with fungal and bacterial agents are common in immunocompromised patients. These patients should be observed carefully and instructed to report changes in skin, mucous membranes, or bowel habits.
19. Infections such as chickenpox and common colds can have life-threatening implications for immunocompromised patients. An immunocompromised patient and family members should be instructed to avoid infected persons.
20. The urine should remain acid for optimal effectiveness of sulfonamides. Prunes and cranberries in any form promote an acidic urine. The patient should be encouraged to drink plenty of fluids while taking sulfonamides.
21. Sulfonamides produce frequent allergic reactions, most notably a pruritic, bright red skin rash and occasionally a drug fever.
22. Patients should be carefully questioned about former drug allergic reactions whenever they begin taking a new drug. Agents that commonly cross-react with sulfa drugs include thiazide diuretics and antidiabetic agents.

CRITICAL THINKING QUESTIONS

1. A patient was referred by his family physician to a local ear, nose, and throat specialist for his hearing deficit. The physician took the following case history: The patient had been well until age 35 years, when he had had a severe case of lobar pneumonia that did not resolve on appropriate penicillin therapy. Further studies showed that he had tuberculosis, and he was treated effectively. What further inquiries might be made as to the cause of his deafness?
2. A patient was treated for recurrent and persistent sinusitis with tetracycline and the decongestant Ornade. On the 8th day of medication, her condition improved, but she presented with complaints of diarrhea and gripping abdominal discomfort. What recommendations should be made?
3. A mother brought her 2-month-old infant in for a routine well-baby examination. The infant's length and weight had increased normally. The infant appeared healthy except for a yellowish white plaque that covered most of her tongue and a few spots that were noted on the buccal mucous membranes. What is this? How is it treated? Is it serious?
4. A 3-year-old boy was placed on ampicillin 3 days ago for otitis media. Today his mother called to report that she noted a pale pink flat rash on his chest when she bathed him. The rash did not appear to itch. She also reported that his fever was gone now, and he did not complain of his earache anymore. Should the medication be discontinued? What precautions should be taken?
5. A 76-year-old woman presented with a new pruritic rash. She had formerly been in good health but recently had begun taking verapamil and hydrochlorothiazide for hypertension. What questions may be included in the evaluation?

REVIEW QUESTIONS

1. The term used for an antibiotic that is effective against many different types of bacteria is:
   a. broad spectrum.
   b. narrow spectrum.
   c. fungicide.
   d. anthelmintic.

2. Penicillin may be used prophylactically (without evidence of an acute infection) in the management of:
   a. sinusitis.
   b. allergies to penicillin.
   c. rheumatic fever.
   d. tuberculosis.

3. Amoxicillin is superior to oral penicillin V in every respect *except:*
   a. it has increased absorption after oral administration.
   b. it is less likely to be broken down in the stomach.
   c. it needs to be taken more frequently during the day.
   d. it has a broader spectrum of activity.

4. Cross-sensitivity may occur between penicillin and:
   a. tetracycline.
   b. erythromycin.
   c. cephalexin.
   d. zidovudine.

5. Another name for macrolide antibiotics is:
   a. penicillins.
   b. tetracyclines.
   c. fungicides.
   d. erythromycins.

6. Viruses differ from other microorganisms in that they:
   a. are less likely to cause severe illnesses.
   b. are more easily treated.
   c. require an intact cell to replicate.
   d. reproduce slowly.

7. Interferon alfa is used to treat:
   a. the common cold.
   b. hepatitis A.
   c. hepatitis B.
   d. AIDS.

8. An agent often used in the treatment of AIDS is:
   a. zidovudine.
   b. Zithromax.
   c. Zelnorm.
   d. Xanax.

9. A common use for sulfonamides is for:
   a. drug allergies.
   b. urinary tract infections.
   c. streptococcal sore throat.
   d. respiratory tract infections.

10. Drugs that may cross-react with a sulfonamide to cause an allergic reaction include all of the following *except:*
    a. hydrochlorothiazide.
    b. tolazamide.
    c. dapsone.
    d. penicillin.

Answers to the review questions can be found at the back of the book.

evolve Additional questions and activities can be found at *http://evolve.elsevier.com/asperheim/pharmacology*.

Antihistamines

CHAPTER

8

Objectives

After completing this chapter, you should be able to do the following:

1. Identify the symptoms of an allergic reaction.
2. Understand the role of histamines in allergic reactions.
3. Understand the antigen-antibody reaction and how it may cause allergic reactions.
4. Help detect the various environmental causes of allergic reactions.
5. Discuss information the health care professional should give to a patient taking antihistamines.
6. Describe the symptoms of anaphylaxis.
7. Understand drug allergies and their importance in drug therapy.

Key Terms

Allergen, p. 65
Allergy, p. 65
Anaphylaxis (ĂN-ĕ-fĭ-LĂK-sĭs), p. 65
Antibody, p. 65
Antigen, p. 65
Antihistamines (ĂN-tĭ-HĬS-ta-mēns), p. 67
Drug allergies, p. 66
Histamine (HĬS-tă-mēn), p. 65
Immunotherapy (IM-yĕ-nō-THĔR-ĕ-pē), p. 69

Early in the 20th century, it was discovered that the release of histamine from body tissues was largely responsible for symptoms that occurred after certain viral infections or on the introduction of sensitizing foreign substances. Examples of these substances are pollen, dust mites, and animal dander, all of which can cause allergic reactions in the body. **Histamine** is a chemical released from body tissues in response to an allergic reaction. It is found in many plant and animal tissues. Under normal circumstances, it is probably bound to an intracellular protein. Histamine evokes the allergic reaction, which may be manifested by symptoms of red watery eyes, urticaria, sneezing, coryza, rash, and bronchiolar constriction of asthma.

ALLERGIC REACTIONS

When an **antigen** (the general term for a foreign substance capable of inducing sensitivity and causing an allergic reaction) is introduced into the body, it evokes a tissue response in the form of a substance called an **antibody,** which is synthesized specifically to combat the particular antigen. When the tissue response is a hypersensitive reaction, known as an **allergy,** the antigen is referred to as an **allergen.** It is believed that the complex reactions and interactions that follow cause the release of histamine.

Anaphylaxis is a severe, life-threatening allergic reaction, marked by an extreme decline in blood pressure and body temperature, a decrease in the circulating blood volume, and cardiac abnormalities. If emergency measures are not taken immediately (e.g., administration of epinephrine or corticosteroids and rapid administration of intravenous [IV] fluids), death may occur.

The emotional component of allergic reactions is not as well understood. It is a well-established fact that certain individuals can experience urticaria, or hives, after severe emotional stress. It has likewise been observed that asthmatic children and occasionally adults develop severe and life-threatening attacks of asthma in times of emotional upheaval and stress, when no precipitating antigen can be shown.

Allergic rhinitis is characterized by nasal itching, sneezing, watery rhinorrhea, and nasal congestion. It also may cause various non-nasal physical symptoms including headache; sore throat; postnasal drip; plugged or itchy ears; chronic cough; and ocular symptoms such as itching, tearing, and swelling. It has been estimated that allergic rhinitis may affect 30% of adults and at least 40% of children. The symptoms may exert a significant negative impact on the quality of life.

A wide variety of complications may affect patients with chronic congestion caused by allergic rhinitis, including sinusitis, halitosis, sleep disturbances (including apnea and frequent arousals), allergic "shiners" (dark coloring under the eyes from venous congestion), and exacerbations of asthma. Up to 38% of patients with rhinitis have also received a diagnosis of asthma. In many cases, the diagnosis of allergic rhinitis precedes a diagnosis of asthma, but the two disorders may manifest simultaneously as well.

The prevalence of allergic rhinitis over the past 4 decades has increased dramatically. This is believed to be due to the increasing concentrations of airborne pollutants, growing dust mite populations, and poor ventilation in buildings.

DETERMINING THE CAUSE OF ALLERGIES

In some cases, the source of an allergy can be determined by a little investigation or attention to circumstances prevailing when allergic symptoms appear. Individuals who are allergic to certain animal dander often determine this fact for themselves, noting that symptoms arise shortly after contact with dogs, cats, or other animals. Likewise, an individual who sneezes uncontrollably after contact with a certain flower is likely to remember the circumstances and avoid the allergen in the future.

Food allergies can be more difficult to determine, but if suspected, they can often be discovered by keeping a careful record of all food consumed. Allergic reactions to a food may occur quickly or any time within a 3-day period after the offending food is eaten; all food that was eaten during this time span should be investigated. Fish, chocolate, wheat, milk, eggs, and nuts are common offenders, but any food may be involved. Peanut allergies are common and often severe enough to be life-threatening.

Skin tests may be used to determine an offending allergen, but these are often disappointing. It is impossible to prepare testing solutions of every existing antigen. It is also rare to have one or even two allergens defined as the offending substance, even under optimal conditions. Many persons react to multiple allergens. If a patient is allergic to a given substance, wheals or areas of swelling and induration occur when the allergen is injected during skin testing. At best, a probable diagnosis can be obtained, and some improvement in severe allergic reactions can be achieved following regular injection of desensitizing vaccines.

ADVERSE DRUG REACTIONS AND DRUG ALLERGIES

Adverse drug reactions are common and often mislabeled as **drug allergies.** Identifying a true drug allergy is often difficult. Overdiagnosis of drug allergies is common because they can be confused with a viral rash or other unusual or unwanted symptom that may have appeared as part of an illness or as a nonallergic side effect of a drug. In addition, very few laboratory tests are available for drug allergies, and the diagnosis depends on clinical findings.

Drug reactions can be classified into immunologic, or immune-mediated, and nonimmunologic causes. *Idiosyncratic reactions* are abnormal reactions not related to the known pharmacologic action of the drug and occur in only a small percentage of the population. An example of an idiosyncratic reaction is the hemolysis that occurs when a person with glucose-6-phosphate dehydrogenase deficiency takes a drug such as a sulfonamide. *Drug intolerance* would be defined as a lower threshold to the normal action of a drug, such as experiencing tinnitus after a single tablet of aspirin or abdominal pain after a single dose of erythromycin.

In some cases, an adverse effect may be tolerated if it is minimal and not too disruptive. The signs of a generalized allergic reaction are more alarming. Warning signs of impending cardiovascular collapse include urticaria, laryngeal or upper airway edema, wheezing, and hypotension. Fever, mucous membrane lesions, lymphadenopathy, joint tenderness or swelling, and a generalized skin rash are also suggestive of more serious reactions.

The most common therapeutic intervention is to discontinue the suspected drug. In most patients, the symptoms resolve within 2 weeks. Antihistamines and corticosteroids may be given to lessen symptoms and hasten recovery.

General criteria for drug hypersensitivity reactions are as follows:

1. The patient's symptoms are consistent with a drug reaction.
2. The patient was administered a drug known to cause such symptoms.
3. The timing of the appearance of symptoms is consistent with a drug reaction.
4. Other causes of the symptoms are excluded.

TREATMENT OF ALLERGIES

Environmental controls should not be overlooked in the management of allergies. Measures that may be effective in minimizing exposure to allergens include encasing mattresses and pillows in plastic covers, replacing woolen blankets with cotton ones, replacing carpeting with hardwood flooring, replacing fabric curtains with plastic or wooden blinds, vacuuming with a system that filters through water, avoiding humidifiers, and freezing soft toys in a plastic bag for 24 hours.

When it is necessary to use drug therapy, **antihistamines** (drugs that combat the symptoms generated by histamine in an allergic reaction) are the mainstay of treatment for allergic reactions. The first-generation antihistamines, although effective in treating the symptoms of allergic symptoms, have been implicated in worsening quality of life by causing drowsiness and exacerbating fatigue and depression. First-generation antihistamines should not be taken when working around machinery, when driving, or at any other time when drowsiness could be hazardous. The sedative effect of these agents is greatly increased when combined with other depressants such as alcohol, tranquilizers, sleeping pills, and some antihypertensive agents; the combination of these agents should be avoided. These agents are also associated with anticholinergic effects such as dry mouth, dry eyes, and urinary retention.

The U.S. Food and Drug Administration (FDA) advised more recently that use of all over-the-counter (OTC) cough and cold medications be avoided in children younger than 2 years. Serious and potentially life-threatening adverse effects may occur as a result. The FDA is reviewing use of OTC cold preparations in children older than 2 years and recommends that these products be used with caution.

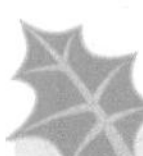

Considerations for Older Adults
Antihistamines

Older adults are much more susceptible to the sedating effects of antihistamines than younger people. Before administering antihistamines, ask about other prescriptions for sedating drugs such as sedatives, hypnotics, tranquilizers, and beta blocker antihypertensive agents.

TRADITIONAL (SEDATING) ANTIHISTAMINES

brompheniramine maleate, USP-NF, BP (Lodrane). Brompheniramine maleate is very similar in action and uses to chlorpheniramine. It is available in tablets and delayed-action dosage forms.

Dosage: Adults: (Oral) One 4-mg tablet every 4 to 6 hours. Delayed-action form is 8 to 12 mg every 8 hours.

chlorpheniramine maleate, USP-NF, BP (Chlor-Trimeton, Teldrin). Chlorpheniramine maleate is available in both tablet form and delayed-action preparations, which allow effective release of the antihistamine for up to 8 hours. Drowsiness generally is more troublesome in the delayed-release forms.

Dosage: Adults: (Oral) 4 mg every 4 to 6 hours. Delayed-release form is 8 to 12 mg every 12 hours. The 24-hour dosage should not exceed 24 mg.

Children 6 to 12 years: (Oral) 2 mg every 4 to 6 hours. Delayed-release form is 8 mg at bedtime. The 24-hour dosage should not exceed 12 mg.

cyproheptadine hydrochloride, USP-NF (Periactin). Cyproheptadine hydrochloride is generally used for skin reactions such as urticaria or the pruritus of varicella eruptions (chickenpox). This agent is one of the more effective antihistamines for the treatment of dermatologic disorders.

Dosage: Adults: (Oral) 4 mg three times daily.

Children older than 2 years: (Oral) 2 mg three times daily.

dimenhydrinate, USP-NF, BP (Dramamine). Dimenhydrinate is used primarily for the relief of motion sickness and is quite successful in this respect if taken a half-hour before air or ground travel. It may be administered parenterally as well for nonspecific nausea and vomiting.

Dosage: Adults: (Oral) 50 mg two to four times daily; (IM) 50 mg as necessary.

Children 6 to 12 years: (Oral) 25 to 50 mg every 6 to 8 hours to a maximum of 150 mg; (IM) 1.25 mg/kg four times daily.

Children 2 to 5 years: (Oral) 12.5 to 25 mg every 6 to 8 hours to a maximum of 75 mg; (IM) 1.25 mg/kg four times daily.

diphenhydramine hydrochloride, USP-NF, BP (Benadryl). Diphenhydramine hydrochloride is useful when given as oral, IV, or IM dosages to control moderately severe allergic reactions such as those occurring in serum sickness, urticaria, and drug reactions. In addition, diphenhydramine hydrochloride is often used as a mild sedative and hypnotic.

Dosage: Adults: (Oral) 25 to 50 mg three to four times daily; (IM, IV) 10 to 50 mg three times daily. Oral dosage should not exceed 300 mg in 24 hours. IM, IV dosage should not exceed 400 mg in 24 hours.

Children 12 years and older: (Oral) 25 to 50 mg every 4 to 6 hours to a maximum of 300 mg/day.

Children 6 to 12 years: (Oral) 12.5 to 25 mg every 4 to 6 hours to a maximum of 150 mg/day.

Children 2 to 6 years: (Oral) 6.25 mg every 4 to 6 hours to a maximum of 37.5 mg/day.

meclizine hydrochloride, USP-NF, BP (Bonine, Antivert). Meclizine hydrochloride has long been used to control nausea and vomiting in pregnancy. It is also effective in the prevention of motion sickness.
Dosage: Adults: (Oral) 12.5 to 50 mg one to three times daily.

Children: Not recommended.

promethazine hydrochloride, USP-NF, BP (Phenergan). The drowsiness and antisecretory effects caused by promethazine hydrochloride make it particularly useful in preoperative patients. If this drug is administered parenterally with a narcotic agent, the sedative effect is increased. Oral forms and rectal suppositories are available as well.
Dosage: Adults: (Oral) 25 mg three to four times daily; (IM, IV) 25 to 50 mg as necessary.

Children older than 2 years: (Oral) 6.25 to 12.5 mg three to four times daily; (IM) 0.25 to 1 mg/kg every 6 to 8 hours.

trimethobenzamide hydrochloride, USP-NF, BP (Tigan). Trimethobenzamide hydrochloride is used in the form of capsules, rectal suppositories, and IM injections to control nausea and vomiting in children and adults. It is not recommended for use in pregnant women. Side effects have been infrequent, but occasional hypersensitivity reactions have occurred. Hypotension, coma, disorientation, dizziness, headaches, blurred vision, and opisthotonos have been reported. Because the suppositories contain benzocaine, they should not be administered to individuals known to be sensitive to local anesthetics.
Dosage: Adults: (Oral) 300 mg three to four times daily; (Rectal Suppository) 200 mg three to four times daily; (IM) 200 mg three to four times daily.

Children weighing more than 30 lb: (Oral) 100 mg three to four times daily; (Rectal Suppository) 50 to 200 mg three to four times daily. The injectable form should not be used in children.

NONSEDATING ANTIHISTAMINES

cetirizine hydrochloride (Zyrtec). Cetirizine hydrochloride is a long-acting antihistamine used to provide relief of seasonal allergic rhinitis and chronic urticaria.
Dosage: Adults and children older than 5 years: (Oral) 5 to 10 mg once daily.

Children 2 to 5 years: (Oral) 2.5 mg once daily.

desloratadine (Clarinex). Desloratadine is a long-acting antihistamine used for once-daily treatment of allergic symptoms in individuals older than 12 years.
Dosage: Adults and children older than 12 years: (Oral) 5 mg once daily.

fexofenadine hydrochloride (Allegra). Fexofenadine hydrochloride is a selective antihistamine that exhibits an antihistamine effect within 1 hour and is effective in allergic rhinitis.
Dosage: Adults and children older than 12 years: (Oral) 60 mg twice daily or 180 mg once daily.

fexofenadine plus pseudoephedrine (Allegra-D). This combination contains 60 mg of fexofenadine hydrochloride and 120 mg of pseudoephedrine. It is useful in controlling nasal congestion and exerts an antihistamine effect.
Dosage: Adults and children older than 12 years: (Oral) One tablet twice daily.

loratadine (Claritin). Loratadine is a long-acting antihistamine that is used for symptomatic improvement of rhinitis and urticaria in adults and children older than 6 years.
Dosage: Adults and children older than 6 years: (Oral) 10 mg once daily.

loratadine plus pseudoephedrine (Claritin-D). This combination of 5 mg of loratadine and 120 mg of pseudoephedrine is formulated in a 12-hour extended-release tablet. It provides decongestant activity and an antihistamine effect.
Dosage: Adults and children older than 12 years: (Oral) One tablet every 12 hours.

INTRANASAL ANTIHISTAMINE

azelastine hydrochloride (Astelin). Azelastine hydrochloride is formulated to be administered intranasally to treat seasonal allergic rhinitis in adults and children older than 5 years. Each spray delivers 137 mcg of azelastine hydrochloride.
Dosage: Adults and children older than 12 years: (Intranasal) One to two sprays in each nostril twice daily.

Children 5 to 12 years: (Intranasal) One spray in each nostril twice daily.

ANTIHISTAMINE COMBINATIONS

Antihistamine combinations vary greatly in composition. The proprietary "cold capsules" generally contain a small dose of antihistamine in combination with a decongestant and often aspirin, acetaminophen, or another pain reliever. Examples are Allerest, Contac, Coricidin D, Dristan, and Sinutab. Other combinations are available by prescription only and generally have higher doses of the respective drugs. The FDA has recommended that cough and cold medications should not be administered to children younger than 2 years of age.

acrivastine (Semprex-D). This fixed-combination preparation containing 8 mg of acrivastine and 60 mg of pseudoephedrine hydrochloride is used to provide symptomatic relief of seasonal allergic rhinitis.
Dosage: Adults and children older than 12 years: (Oral) 8 mg four times daily.

carbinoxamine maleate (Palgic). Also combined with pseudoephedrine hydrochloride (Rondec, Cardec), carbinoxamine maleate may be used for adults and children older than 6 years for control of allergic symptoms.
Dosage: Adults and children older than 6 years: (Oral) 4 mg four times daily.

clemastine fumarate (Tavist). This combination of clemastine with pseudoephedrine can be used in adults and young children with seasonal allergies.
Dosage: Adults and children older than 12 years: (Oral) 1.34 mg every 12 hours.

Children 6 to 12 years: (Oral) 0.67 to 1.34 mg every 12 hours.

ROLE OF IMMUNOTHERAPY

Many studies show that **immunotherapy,** the systematic repeated exposure to small amounts of an allergen, reduces symptoms of allergic rhinitis in certain patients. It is particularly useful in patients who are unable or unwilling to avoid the allergen, patients who experience inadequate relief or intolerable side effects from pharmacologic therapy, and patients with comorbid conditions such as asthma. Initially, very low concentrations of the allergen are used. The strength of the solution is gradually increased until the symptoms are relieved or a maximum tolerable dose is reached. Immunotherapy requires careful monitoring because of the possibility of acute allergic reactions to the allergens used in treatment. Continuous treatment lasting 3 to 5 years is generally required. The therapy then may be discontinued in some cases.

A home remedy that some authorities believe is helpful is to take 1 to 2 tablespoons of local honey daily. The small amounts of antigen from local grasses and flowers are believed by some authorities to become gradually effective as a treatment for respiratory allergies.

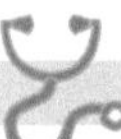

Clinical Implications

1. Allergic conditions are best managed by avoidance of the suspected allergen. Animals should be removed from the home if possible, as should items that collect dust, such as curtains, carpets, and collectibles, particularly in the bedroom.
2. Foam pillows should be used, and feather pillows should be avoided. All pillows and mattresses should be encased in dust mite–proof covers.
3. Become familiar with MedicAlert tags, and remember to check them for potential drug allergies.
4. Common symptoms of mild allergic reactions include rhinitis, coryza, conjunctival injection, and skin rashes.
5. Anaphylaxis is an acute emergency and is manifested by itching, urticaria, and respiratory distress with wheezing and bronchospasm, progressing to edema of the face and extremities, hypotension, and death.
6. The primary side effect of antihistamines is drowsiness. The patient should be instructed not to work around machinery or to drive long distances after taking antihistamines.
7. The sleepiness produced by antihistamines is an individual variation; certain people become rapidly resistant to the drowsiness induced by these agents and can take them routinely without drowsiness.
8. Bed rails and assistance with ambulation may be indicated when an individual, particularly an older adult, has received an antihistamine.
9. The antihistamines potentiate the central nervous system depression caused by many other agents such as alcohol, tranquilizers, sedatives, and hypnotics.
10. Certain antihistamines are useful in the prevention of motion sickness and should be given 30 minutes before entering the vehicle for optimal effect.
11. Most drugs have adverse effects and the ability to produce allergic reactions.
12. A patient who develops an unusual or unwanted symptom while taking a drug should be questioned about previous drug allergies. The drug should be discontinued until full evaluation of a potential allergic reaction can be made.

CRITICAL THINKING QUESTIONS

1. A patient has been miserable since his daughter bought a cat. He has coryza, excessive sneezing, and rhinitis. Because his daughter insists on keeping the cat, he wants to control his allergies with antihistamines. What health teaching is indicated here?
2. You have a part-time job in a drugstore as a drug clerk. A pregnant woman comes in and asks your advice as to which OTC antihistamine she can safely take for her spring allergies. How would you respond to this woman?
3. A patient stepped in a nest of fire ants and has a severe local reaction over both lower legs. It is 10 o'clock in the morning, and you detect a strong odor of alcohol on his breath. The physician decides to prescribe Benadryl, 50 mg four times a day, and the man reports that he has to go back to work. What suggestions might be made?
4. A patient has been taking Bactrim, a sulfonamide, for 5 days to treat a urinary tract infection. She wants to know which lotion she should buy for a bright red rash on her face and arms. How should you respond?

REVIEW QUESTIONS

1. Symptoms of an allergic reaction may include all of the following symptoms *except:*
   a. red, watery eyes.
   b. runny nose.
   c. asthma.
   d. thirst.
2. A severe and life-threatening allergic reaction is known as:
   a. epileptic equivalent.
   b. anaphylaxis.
   c. coryza.
   d. urticaria.
3. A drug that may be given orally to treat an allergic reaction is:
   a. loratadine.
   b. epinephrine.
   c. azelastine hydrochloride.
   d. weekly immunotherapy.
4. An example of an intranasal antihistamine is:
   a. desloratadine.
   b. trimethobenzamide.
   c. promethazine.
   d. azelastine hydrochloride.
5. Immunotherapy consists of:
   a. giving increasing doses of antihistamines.
   b. treating asthma aggressively with high doses of drugs.
   c. repeated administration of small amounts of antigen.
   d. introducing allergens in inhalants daily.
6. The primary side effect of diphenhydramine (Benadryl) is:
   a. drowsiness.
   b. jitteriness.
   c. skin rash.
   d. watery eyes.
7. The advantage loratadine has over diphenhydramine is that it:
   a. is less sedating.
   b. is more sedating.
   c. causes fewer skin rashes.
   d. is less expensive.
8. The best first step in the treatment of allergies is to:
   a. begin allergy immunotherapy immediately.
   b. avoid the allergen.
   c. expose the patient to the allergen frequently.
   d. give antihistamines.
9. An agent that may be potentiated or have an increased effect when given with antihistamines is:
   a. penicillin.
   b. rifampin.
   c. alcoholic beverages.
   d. tetracycline.
10. An example of a nonsedating antihistamine is:
    a. trimethobenzamide.
    b. brompheniramine.
    c. cyproheptadine
    d. fexofenadine.

Answers to the review questions can be found at the back of the book.

evolve Additional questions and activities can be found at *http://evolve.elsevier.com/asperheim/pharmacology.*

Drugs That Affect the Skin and Mucous Membranes

CHAPTER 9

Objectives

After completing this chapter, you should be able to do the following:

1. Describe the functions of the skin.
2. Describe the effects of emollients, demulcents, and keratolytics on the skin.
3. Understand the uses of the various acne preparations.
4. Describe the action of astringents.
5. Give examples of local anesthetics and the purpose for which each one is used.
6. Identify agents used to treat *Candida* infections.
7. Identify agents used to treat fungal infections.
8. Identify local anti-infectives.
9. Explain how sun-induced skin damage can occur, and become familiar with sunscreens and their action.
10. Recognize drugs that are photosensitizers.

Key Terms

Acne (ĂC-nē), p. 76
Anesthetics (ăn-ĕs-THĔ-tĭks), p. 72
Astringents (ĕ-STRĬN-jĕnts), p. 72
Candida albicans (KĂN-dĭ-dĕ ĂL-bĕ-kănz), p. 73
Candidiasis (KĂN-dĭ-DĪ-ĕ-sĭs), p. 73
Demulcents (dĭ-MŬL-sĕnts), p. 71
Emollients (ĭ-MŌL-yĕnts), p. 71
Moniliasis (MŌ-nĕ-LĪ-ĕ-sĭs), p. 73
Photosensitizer (FŌ-tō-SĔN-sĭ-TĪZ-ĕr), p. 76

The skin is a complex structure that serves many functions. Chief among these are regulation of body temperature; maintenance of electrolyte and water balance; protection; excretion of waste substances; and some metabolic activity, such as formation of vitamin D (the "sunshine vitamin").

Drugs applied to the skin likewise may serve many functions and may be intended for either a local effect or a systemic effect after absorption through the skin. These drugs may be divided into several classes.

SOOTHING SUBSTANCES

Agents classified as soothing substances are applied to irritated and abraded areas to protect them and alleviate itching.

EMOLLIENTS

Emollients are fatty or oily substances applied to soothe the skin or mucous membranes. Irritants, air, and airborne bacteria are excluded by the oily layer, and the skin is rendered softer and more pliable by penetration of the emollient into the surface layers. Emollient substances are used chiefly as vehicles for fat-soluble drugs and as protective agents. Some commonly used emollients are the following:

- Petrolatum
- Rosewater ointment
- Hydrous wool fat (lanolin)

DEMULCENTS

Demulcents are protective agents used primarily to alleviate irritation, particularly of mucous membranes and abraded tissue. They are generally applied to the surface in sticky preparations that rapidly cover the area. Demulcents may be incorporated in lozenges to soothe the oral and throat mucosae and are swallowed in liquid form as an antidote for corrosive poisons.

Various substances possess demulcent properties; some common demulcents are the following:

- Gums and mucilages (e.g., acacia and tragacanth)
- Starch
- Cream, milk
- Egg white

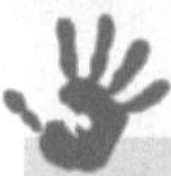

Considerations for Children

Hexachlorophene

The skin of infants and children is particularly susceptible to absorption of drugs, such as hexachlorophene. Do not routinely use hexachlorophene to bathe infants. Symptoms of neurotoxicity, including seizures, have been observed after systemic absorption of hexachlorophene from the skin. Also, do not apply it to the mucous membranes or abraded skin of patients of any age.

ASTRINGENTS

Astringents precipitate protein but ordinarily do not penetrate beyond cell surfaces, so the cell remains viable. This action is accompanied by contraction and blanching of skin, and mucus and other secretions may be reduced so that the affected area becomes drier. These agents are used to arrest minor hemorrhage, check perspiration, reduce inflammation, promote healing, and toughen skin. The principal astringents are the following:

- Salts of aluminum, zinc, and other heavy metals
- Tannins (e.g., tannic acid in alcohol, witch hazel)
- Alcohols, phenols

IRRITANTS

Irritants produce irritation, the degree of which is determined by the concentration and the duration of action. There are three types of irritants, as follows:

Counterirritants: Used to irritate unbroken skin to relieve deep pain in muscles, joints, bursae, and other areas

Rubefacients: Produce local vasodilation, redness, and a feeling of warmth

Vesicants: Cause a strong irritation; blisters may be produced if used in high concentrations or for a prolonged time

The following agents may be counterirritants, rubefacients, or vesicants, depending on the concentration used and the length of time of application:

- Camphor, menthol, chloroform
- Mustard, as in a mustard plaster
- Oil of wintergreen

KERATOLYTICS

Keratolytics cause sloughing of hardened epithelium. They are used to cauterize ulcers and to destroy excess tissue such as calluses and warts. Common keratolytics are the following:

- Benzoic and salicylic acids
- Resorcinol
- Lactic acid

LOCAL ANESTHETICS

Anesthetics are substances that cause a loss of sensation. They may have systemic effects, or the effects may be localized. Many ointments contain local anesthetics and are applied topically for minor conditions such as sunburn and insect bites and for more serious dermatoses, burns, hemorrhoids, and other conditions. These agents may be either applied directly to the skin or injected. A few local anesthetics are described.

benzocaine, USP-NF, BP. Benzocaine is used in throat lozenges and topical preparations. Examples are the following:

- Medicone rectal ointment
- Unguentine ointment
- Surfacaine ointment

cocaine, USP-NF, BP. Cocaine is used especially in topical solutions and nasal preparations. It is quite addictive and comes under the restrictions of the Controlled Substances Act.

dibucaine, USP-NF, BP (Nupercainal). Dibucaine is applied topically in ointments.

procaine, USP-NF, BP (Novocain). Procaine is used in dentistry and before minor surgery. Because it is not effective topically, it must be injected.

ANTIFUNGAL AGENTS

Fungal infections of the skin are a common problem in warm and temperate climates. They particularly affect areas of the skin that tend to remain warm and moist, such as the feet, the underarms, under the breasts, and the perineal area *(intertrigo)*. Topical therapy is often sufficient in uncomplicated infections, but systemic therapy, such as oral griseofulvin, may be necessary to treat long-standing infections.

ciclopirox olamine, USP-NF, BP (Loprox). Ciclopirox olamine may be applied topically for the treatment of various fungal and yeast infections. It has a low toxicity, but some burning may be felt at the site of application.

Dosage: 1% cream or lotion applied topically twice daily for up to 4 weeks.

ciclopirox solution (Penlac Nail Lacquer). Ciclopirox solution may be applied topically directly to the fingernails and toenails in immunocompromised patients for the treatment of fungal infections.
Dosage: 8% topical solution applied to nails daily for 4 weeks.

clioquinol (formerly iodochlorhydroxyquin), USP-NF, BP (Vioform). The antibacterial and antifungal properties of clioquinol make it extremely useful in nonspecific or mixed infections. It is also available in combination with hydrocortisone to suppress local inflammatory reactions. Topical application is helpful in some cases of eczema, athlete's foot, or intertriginous rashes.
Dosage: 3% clioquinol applied topically twice daily for 2 to 4 weeks. The combination forms contain 0.5% or 1% hydrocortisone.

clotrimazole, USP-NF, BP (Lotrimin). Clotrimazole has a broad spectrum of activity against fungi and yeasts. It is available in the form of a solution or cream for topical application. Erythema, blistering, peeling, pruritus, and general skin irritation have been observed in sensitive individuals; application of clotrimazole should be discontinued if these symptoms occur.
Dosage: 1% clotrimazole in solution or cream applied topically twice daily for 2 to 4 weeks.

econazole nitrate (Spectazole). A once-daily application of econazole nitrate cures many topical tinea infections (Fig. 9-1). *Candida* (monilial) infections require twice-daily application.
Dosage: 1% in ointment once or twice daily for 2 weeks.

ketoconazole, USP-NF, BP (Nizoral). Ketoconazole is used topically to treat fungal and yeast infections. It is also effective for seborrheic dermatitis. Local application is generally well tolerated, but there may be some local irritation at the site of application.
Dosage: 2% topical cream applied once daily for up to 6 weeks.

tolnaftate, USP-NF, BP (Tinactin). When applied twice daily to topical fungal infections, tolnaftate is effective against ringworm, athlete's foot, and similar conditions. To prevent recurrences, care must be taken to continue the use of this preparation for 2 weeks after all visible signs of the infection have cleared. Sensitivity reactions are rare.
Dosage: 1% cream, solution, powder, or aerosol applied twice daily. Continue use for 2 weeks after disappearance of visible signs of infection.

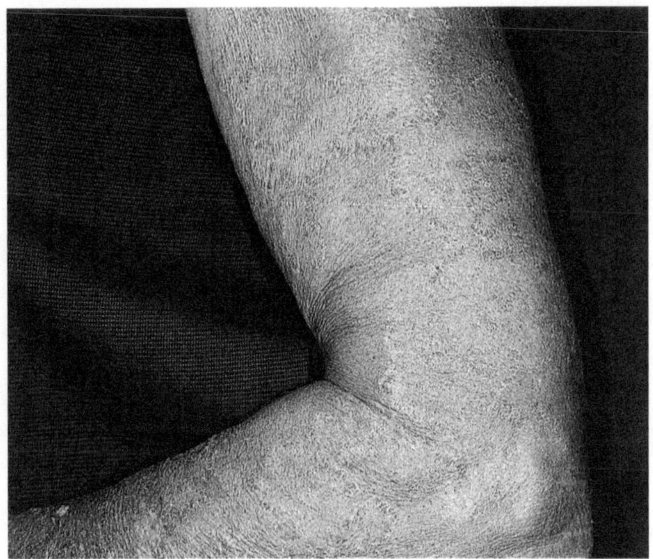

FIGURE 9-1 Tinea corporis. Widespread lesions in an immunosuppressed patient. (From Callen JP, et al: *Color atlas of dermatology*, ed 2, Philadelphia, 2000, Saunders.)

zinc undecylenate ointment, USP-NF, BP (Desenex). Zinc undecylenate was one of the first topical antifungal agents and continues to be a popular over-the-counter (OTC) preparation for the treatment and prevention of athlete's foot. It has been surpassed in effectiveness by tolnaftate and other preparations, however.
Dosage: 20% ointment applied topically twice daily (often in combination with varying amounts of undecylenic acid) for 2 to 4 weeks.

Other antifungal agents are listed in Table 9-1.

ANTIMONILIAL PREPARATIONS

Moniliasis (or **candidiasis**) is an infection caused by ***Candida albicans***—a yeastlike organism that infects the skin and mucous membranes. Similar to fungal

Table 9-1 Other Antifungal Agents

Name	Use	How Supplied
butenafine hydrochloride (Mentax)	Tinea pedis, corporis, cruris; tinea versicolor	1% cream
ketoconazole (Nizoral)	Tinea pedis, corporis, cruris	2% cream or shampoo
miconazole nitrate tincture (Fungoid)	Tinea pedis, corporis, cruris	2% solution
oxiconazole nitrate (Oxistat)	Antifungal and antimonilial; tinea pedis, corporis, cruris	1% lotion or cream
terbinafine (Lamisil)	Tinea pedis, corporis, cruris	1% lotion or cream

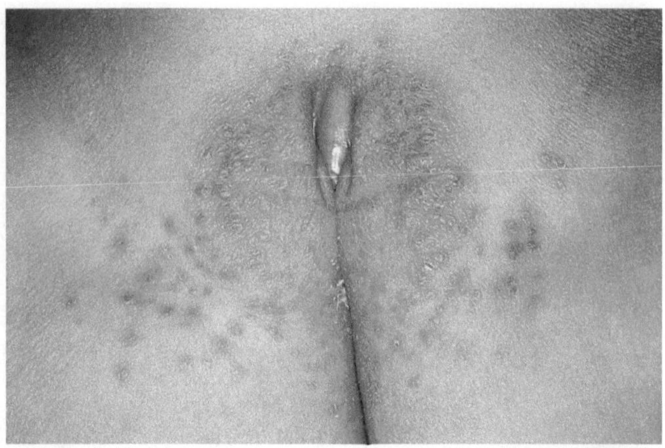

FIGURE 9-2 Vulvovaginal perirectal candidiasis. (From Lebwohl MG, et al: *Treatment of skin disease*, ed 2, St. Louis, 2002, Saunders.)

infections, topical monilial infections tend to occur in warm, macerated areas. Monilial diaper rash is common in infants, particularly after antibiotic therapy, which can disturb the normal intestinal flora. Monilial vaginitis and perineal and intertriginous *Candida* infections tend to occur with increased frequency in diabetic patients and obese individuals (Fig. 9-2).

clotrimazole, USP-NF, BP (Lotrimin, Gyne-Lotrimin). Clotrimazole is used intravaginally for monilial infections.
Dosage: (Vaginal) One applicator of the 1% cream inserted daily for 7 days or 1 200-mg tablet inserted daily for 3 days.

miconazole nitrate vaginal cream (Monistat). Miconazole nitrate is a water-miscible cream that is indicated for vaginal use in the treatment of vulvovaginal *Candida* infections. Vaginal burning, pelvic cramps, hives, skin rash, and headache are very rarely observed.
Dosage: (Vaginal) One applicator of the 2% cream inserted daily for 7 days.

Mycolog Cream and Ointment. This commercial preparation consists of a combination of nystatin, neomycin, gramicidin, and triamcinolone acetate. The topical antibiotics and corticosteroid included in this product have been shown to be highly effective in all forms of topical *Candida* infections and aid in clearing secondary infections caused by local irritation and scratching of the areas. When applied two to three times daily, noticeable improvement is seen within 1 week in most cases. Topical sensitivity reactions have been noted but are rare.

Dosage: 100,000 units nystatin, 2.5 mg neomycin, 0.25 mg gramicidin, and mg triamcinolone acetate per gram of cream or ointment two to three times daily for 1 week or longer.

nystatin vaginal tablets, USP-NF, BP (Mycostatin). Vulvovaginal *Candida* infections may be treated topically with the use of vaginal tablets. Irritation or sensitization to this agent may occur very rarely.
Dosage: (Vaginal) One tablet containing 100,000 units inserted daily for 2 weeks.

terconazole (Terazol). Terconazole is used for the treatment of vulvovaginal monilial infections.
Dosage: (Vaginal) One applicator of 0.4% cream inserted daily for 7 days or one suppository inserted daily for 3 days.

GENERAL ANTI-INFECTIVE AGENTS

benzalkonium chloride, USP-NF, BP (Zephiran Chloride). A rapid-acting, nonirritating antibacterial agent, benzalkonium chloride may be used safely on skin and mucous membranes in concentrations of 1:1000 to 1:10,000. One precaution to be observed, however, is that all soap or detergent must be completely removed before application of benzalkonium chloride because it is inactivated by anionic agents.

ethyl alcohol, USP-NF, BP (alcohol). The alcohol most frequently used as an anti-infective is ethyl alcohol; the optimal antiseptic activity is obtained from a 70% solution. Higher concentrations have a decreased antiseptic action. In addition to its antiseptic activity, alcohol has an astringent effect when applied topically and is frequently used in the treatment of decubitus ulcers; it is commonly used to cleanse the skin before giving hypodermic injections and while dressing wounds.

gentian violet, USP-NF, BP. Gentian violet is an antiseptic dye that may be applied to surface areas for many infectious conditions. In strengths of 1:1000 to 1:100, it is used to treat impetigo, thrush, fungal infections, cystitis, urethritis, and similar conditions.

hexachlorophene, USP-NF, BP (incorporated in Gamophen and Dial soaps, Septisol, and pHisoHex). Preparations containing hexachlorophene in 3% concentrations are used widely as antiseptic scrubs. When it is used regularly, a residual layer of the antiseptic forms on the skin and reduces the normal bacterial flora. Its activity is lessened by the presence of serum and organic materials. Because hexachlorophene has been found to be systemically absorbed from skin surfaces, it is no longer recommended for the routine bathing of infants. It should be used in its more concentrated forms (e.g., pHisoHex) only on the advice of a physician.

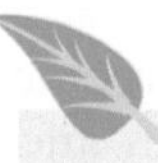

Herb Alert
Aloe

Aloe is commonly rubbed on the skin to soothe minor burns, treat infections, and moisturize dry patches. It has been taken internally as a cathartic but is not generally recommended for this use because it may produce cardiac arrhythmias, edema, and nephropathies when taken orally. It also enhances potassium loss in patients taking diuretics. See Chapter 28 for more information on aloe.

hydrogen peroxide solution, USP-NF, BP. The antiseptic activity of hydrogen peroxide solution results from the liberation of oxygen, which destroys many anaerobic bacteria and produces an effervescent action that cleans wounds of dead tissue and pus. It deteriorates on standing, however, and should be stored in a cool, dark place. The 3% solution is most frequently used.

iodine tincture, USP-NF, BP. One of the oldest and most effective of the germicides and fungicides, iodine tincture is used in 2% solution for application to wounds and abrasions. It is not safe for application to large wounds. The agent of choice for application to mucous membranes is a 2% solution of iodine in glycerin.

isopropyl alcohol. Isopropyl alcohol is approximately twice as germicidal as ethyl alcohol and is much less corrosive to instruments. Isopropyl alcohol is more toxic, however. It is used in full strength.

povidone-iodine solution, USP-NF, BP (Betadine). The iodine content of this preparation furnishes its germicidal activity. The iodine is released more slowly than from the tincture, but the prolongation of action largely compensates for this. It is used in 1% to 1.5% solutions and has various applications in aerosol, douche, vaginal gel, shampoo, and topical forms.

saponated cresol solution, USP-NF, BP (Lysol, Creolin). In strengths of approximately 2%, this solution is used for disinfection of contaminated bedpans, basins, and linens. The presence of organic material does not interfere with its action. It may be used for vaginal douches in very weak dilutions.

WOUND CARE PRODUCTS

Wounds such as pressure ulcers, venous stasis ulcers, and burns need special care. Various products can aid in their treatment. The goal of treatment is to remove any dead tissue *(débridement)*, control the level of bacterial growth (cleansing), and provide a moist wound environment while keeping the surrounding intact skin dry.

mafenide acetate cream, USP-NF (Sulfamylon Cream). Mafenide acetate cream is a nonstaining white cream that can be applied topically on second and third-degree burns.
Dosage: 85 mg mafenide per 1 gm cream applied topically one to two times daily until healing has occurred.

mupirocin calcium (Bactroban). Mupirocin calcium is a topical antibiotic ointment that is used to treat local infections, such as impetigo. Few adverse effects occur; burning or local irritation is an indication for discontinuing the drug.
Dosage: 2% ointment applied three times daily for 2 to 4 weeks. OTC antibiotic ointments are readily available and may be used as well.

silver sulfadiazine, USP-NF (Silvadene Cream). Silver sulfadiazine has a broad spectrum of anti-infective activity. It is used topically to prevent wound infection in patients with second and third-degree burns.
Dosage: 1% cream applied topically one to two times daily until healing has occurred.

SUN DAMAGE TO SKIN

Knowledge of sun-induced skin disorders has expanded tremendously in recent decades. The radiant energy from the sun produces a thermal burn, giving light-skinned persons a coveted tan for a short time; over the years, however, sun damage produces premature aging and leathery skin and greatly increases the chances of skin cancer. The potential for sun damage may be increasing with the loss of the ozone layer. It is now believed that even one significant sunburn in early life measurably increases the risk of skin cancer later. Effects of sun exposure are cumulative, and preventing sun exposure at any age is beneficial.

Many commercial sunscreen products are available. They are labeled with a sun protection factor (SPF) number. Higher numbers indicate greater levels of sun protection. For significant protection, the SPF number should be 15 or higher. Many individuals have become sensitized or allergic to many components of sunscreen. Some individuals may be para-aminobenzoic acid (PABA)–sensitive, and some are allergic to the replacements for PABA, such as the cinnamic acid derivatives.

In addition, the potential for sun damage to the skin may be enhanced by certain drugs. Many chemicals and foods act as **photosensitizers,** meaning that they make the skin more susceptible to burning and sun damage. It is impossible to give a complete list, but photosensitizers include the following:

- Cosmetics (lipsticks, many perfumes)
- Pigments and dyes in clothes and tattoos
- Plants (buttercup, carrots, celery, dill, fennel, figs, limes, mustard, parsley, parsnip)
- Some soap deodorants containing hexachlorophene or bithionol or both

Drugs that act as photosensitizers are listed in Box 9-1.

Box 9-1 Drugs Containing Photosensitizers

acetazolamide	hydrochlorothiazide
acetohexamide	ibuprofen
amantadine	imipramine
amiloride	indomethacin
amitriptyline	ketoconazole
astemizole	methyldopa
azathioprine	nalidixic acid
barbiturates	naproxen
captopril	nifedipine
carbamazepine	nitrofurantoin
cephalosporin	nonsteroidal anti-inflammatory drugs
chlordiazepoxide	nortriptyline
chloroquine	ofloxacin
chlorothiazide	para-aminobenzoic acid (PABA)
chlorpromazine	phenothiazine
chlorthalidone	phenylbutazone
contraceptives, oral	promazine
coumarin	promethazine
desipramine	quinidine
diflunisal	retinoic acid
diltiazem	sulfa drugs
diphenhydramine	tetracycline
doxycycline	tolazamide
fluorescein	tolbutamide
fluorouracil	trazodone
furosemide	triamterene
glyburide	trimethoprim
griseofulvin	vinblastine
haloperidol	warfarin

ACNE PREPARATIONS

Acne, an inflammatory eruption of the skin, occurs in most adolescents and many adults and can cause physical and emotional scars when severe. Many new preparations are available to treat this disorder.

Various factors can aggravate acne. Young women should be counseled to avoid oily cosmetics and creams and to choose makeup that is hypoallergenic and water-based. The hair should be kept clean and worn in a style off the face. The use of styling gels, creams, or sprays may clog pores. Dietary theories regarding the relationship of foods to acne come and go. According to some theories, seafood contributes iodine, an irritant, to the perspiration and may enhance folliculitis. There may also be an individual intolerance to chocolate or acid fruits when eaten in excessive amounts.

CLEANSING AGENTS

It is recommended that the patient cleanse the face twice daily with a mild, nonirritating soap, such as Dove or Neutrogena or a product containing triethanolamine. Astringent drying lotions (Stri-Dex Pads, Clearasil Medicated Astringent) help accelerate the resolution of lesions. They may be used for prolonged periods if necessary.

DRUGS USED TO TREAT ACNE

adapalene solution (Differin). Adapalene solution is applied topically to treat acne. Adverse effects such as pruritus, burning, scaling, and erythema may occur in 30% to 60% of patients.
Dosage: 0.1% topical solution applied daily for 2 to 4 weeks.

benzoyl peroxide, USP-NF, BP (Brevoxyl). Also a peeling agent, benzoyl peroxide is usually applied to the face in the morning after washing. Some irritation or inflammation is common; if these become severe, the product should be discontinued. It takes 6 to 8 weeks to determine whether treatment is effective.
Dosage: Applied locally in strengths of 4% or 8% in various vehicles.

benzoyl peroxide plus clindamycin (Benzaclin, Duac). These topical products combine 5% benzoyl peroxide with 1% clindamycin phosphate to treat acne.
Dosage: Applied twice-daily to lesions.

clindamycin phosphate, USP-NF, BP (Cleocin-T, Clindagel). Clindamycin is a topical antibiotic applied directly to acneiform lesions and has been shown to be effective against *Propionibacterium acnes,* one of the agents contributing to acne. Some systemic absorption occurs, and the side effects of diarrhea and colitis can require discontinuation of the product.
Dosage: Solution form equivalent to 10 mg of clindamycin per milliliter applied twice daily or as a 1% gel.

erythromycin topical gel (Emgel, Erygel). Erythromycin topical gel is an antibiotic solution that should be applied twice daily for local treatment of acne. Peeling occurs. Severe dryness and irritation necessitate discontinuing the product.
Dosage: 2% topical gel applied twice daily.

isotretinoin, USP-NF, BP (Accutane). The principal effect of isotretinoin seems to be the regulation of cell proliferation, in addition to exhibiting anti-inflammatory and antineoplastic activities. It is used in nodular acne to reduce the size of sebaceous glands and inhibit sebum production. It inhibits the adhesion of epithelial cells and permits them to be sloughed more easily. Side effects include conjunctivitis, thinning of the hair, photosensitivity, and hyperlipidemia. It is teratogenic to a developing fetus and must not be taken by a woman who is either pregnant or planning to become pregnant.
Dosage: Adults and children older than 12 years: (Oral) 0.5 to 1 mg/kg/day in two divided doses.

tretinoin (Retinoic Acid, Retin-A). Tretinoin seems to act as a follicular irritant, preventing cells from sticking together. A mild inflammatory reaction is produced, with peeling and extrusion of the comedo. Topical tretinoin has been shown to enhance repair of skin that has been damaged by ultraviolet radiation. It is used cosmetically for this effect to reduce the wrinkling of aging, sun-damaged skin.
Dosage: Adults and children older than 12 years: (Topical) Applied once-daily at bedtime in the form of a cream, gel, or solution. Strengths of 0.025% to 0.1% are prescribed.

AGENTS USED IN THE TREATMENT OF ATOPIC DERMATITIS (ECZEMA)

Atopic dermatitis is a common skin condition, seen especially in children (Fig. 9-3). Topical steroids may be used in treatment, but they have side effects, as discussed subsequently. A few nonsteroidal products are available for this condition.

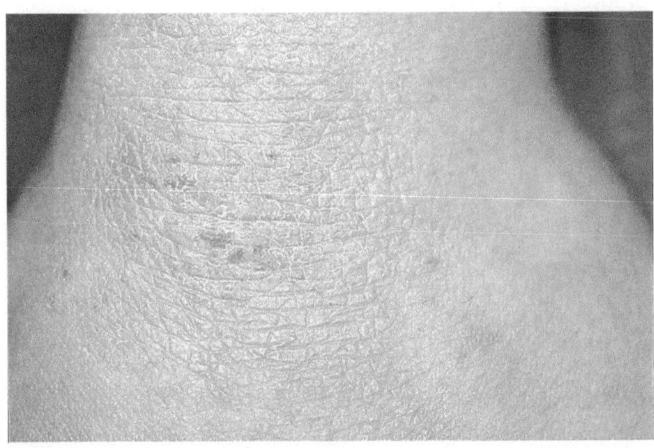

FIGURE 9-3 Lichenified eczematous plaque. A patch of lichenified skin with increased skin markings on the dorsum of the hand is evident in this girl with atopic eczema. (From Lawrence CM, Cox NH: *Physical signs in dermatology,* ed 2, London, 2002, Mosby.)

pimecrolimus (Elidel). The exact mechanism of action of pimecrolimus is unknown. It has been shown to be an effective topical treatment for atopic dermatitis in nonimmunocompromised patients.
Dosage: 1% cream applied topically twice daily for as long as symptoms persist.

tacrolimus (Protopic). Tacrolimus is an immunosuppressant and is used in other applications to prevent organ rejection. When used for atopic dermatitis, topical tacrolimus has been shown to bind to specific receptors on the T cells, which causes a series of reactions that act to reduce the inflammatory response of the skin. The most common side effect is a burning of the skin after application.
Dosage: 0.03% or 0.1% ointment applied topically twice daily until symptoms have resolved for 1 week.

AGENTS USED IN THE TREATMENT OF WARTS

imiquimod cream 5% (Aldara). Imiquimod is an immune response modifier. It is used primarily in the treatment of external genital and perirectal warts (Fig. 9-4), but it may also be used to treat basal cell carcinoma, actinic keratoses, and condylomata acuminata. Side effects include redness, swelling, skin peeling, itching, and changes in skin color.
Dosage: Adults and children older than 12 years: (Topical) Apply a thin layer of cream to the affected area; rub in well. Do not cover the area with a bandage. Leave on for 6 to 10 hours, and then wash off with soap and water. Use 3 days a week until the lesions are gone, or up to 16 weeks.

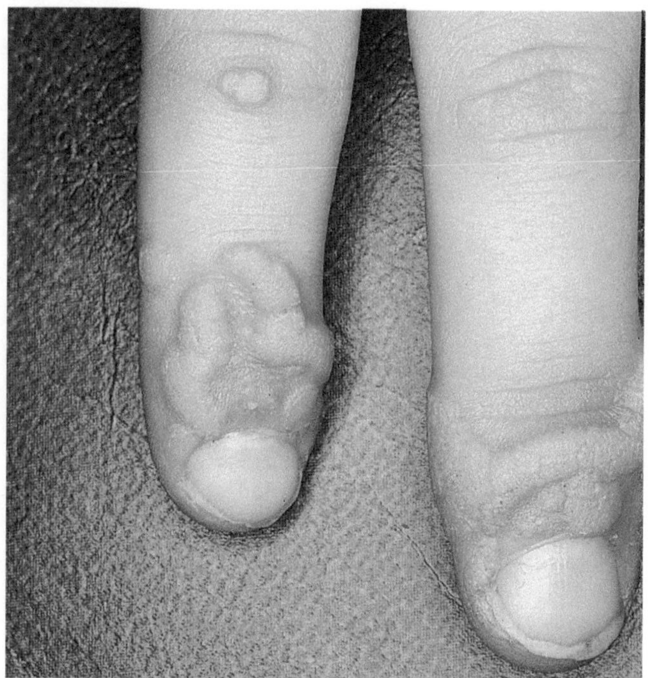

FIGURE 9-4 Verruca vulgaris or common viral warts. These papules often have verrucous surface changes. (From Callen JP, et al: *Color atlas of dermatology*, ed 2, Philadelphia, 2000, Saunders.)

Applying duct tape to topical skin warts (not to the genital or perirectal variety) is a nonprescription treatment method. The duct tape is applied directly, left on for a few days, then changed. A substance in the adhesive is apparently inhibitory to the virus causing the warts.

TOPICAL CORTICOSTEROIDS

Topical corticosteroids have anti-inflammatory, antipruritic, and vasoconstrictive properties. They can be absorbed from intact, healthy skin. Occlusion and disease processes enhance the absorption. The potency of the commercially available products varies greatly (Table 9-2).

Generally, a lower potency corticosteroid should be used when possible, and the corticosteroid should be discontinued when the desired effect is produced. Predictably, adverse effects—which include skin atrophy, depigmentation of dark skin, and dermatologic absorption of the steroid with possible adrenal suppression—increase with duration of use and with application of higher potency steroid preparations.

Table 9-2 Corticosteroids

Generic Name	Trade Name	How Supplied
HIGHEST POTENCY		
betamethasone dipropionate, augmented	Diprolene	0.05% gel, ointment, lotion
clobetasol propionate	Temovate, Temovate E, Olux, Olux-E	0.05% cream, gel, ointment, foam
diflorasone diacetate	Psorcon E	0.05% ointment, cream
halobetasol propionate	Ultravate	0.05% cream, ointment
HIGH POTENCY		
amcinonide	Cyclocort	0.1% cream, ointment, lotion
desoximetasone	Topicort, Topicort LP	0.25%, 0.05% cream, ointment
fluocinonide	Lidex, Lidex-E	0.05% cream, gel, ointment
mometasone furoate	Elocon	0.1% lotion, cream, ointment
INTERMEDIATE POTENCY		
betamethasone valerate	Luxiq	0.12% foam
fluticasone propionate	Cutivate	0.005% ointment, 0.05% cream
hydrocortisone butyrate	Locoid	0.1% cream, ointment
hydrocortisone valerate	Westcort	0.2% cream, ointment
LOW POTENCY		
alclometasone dipropionate	Aclovate	0.05% cream, ointment
desonide	DesOwen	0.05% cream, ointment, lotion
hydrocortisone	Hytone	1% cream, ointment, lotion

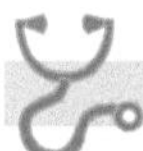

Clinical Implications

1. For the desired effect when topical application of medications is ordered, the skin should be cleansed before application.
2. The site of application should be observed for edema and inflammation. The physician should be informed if the patient complains of discomfort during or after the application of topical medications.
3. Signs of healing in skin lesions are the development of a healthy, pink color and the appearance of granulation tissue.
4. Orders should be followed carefully regarding the application of dressings after administration of topical medications. In some cases, adverse effects can occur as a result of bandaging the area after application.
5. To prevent cross-contamination, a different container of a topical medication should be used for each patient.
6. Aerosol containers should be stored in a cool, dry place. The aerosol container should be held at least 6 inches from the skin at the time of application. Care should be taken that the aerosol does not spray into the eyes.
7. If improper hygiene contributed to the formation of skin lesions, the patient should be carefully instructed in proper hygiene.
8. Gloves should be worn when applying topical medications to infected areas.
9. The health care professional should be aware of the psychological effects of severe and disfiguring skin disorders. Counseling may be advisable in some patients.
10. Many skin disorders are worsened by self-treatment by the patient. If improper application of proprietary medications has occurred, the patient should be counseled against self-treatment.
11. The health care professional should become familiar with ways to improve acne through the proper use of cosmetics and hygienic aids.
12. Topical acne agents sometimes can have severe side effects. The health care professional should take time to read the product literature on all preparations.
13. Many prescription drugs cause photosensitization. The patient should be advised to avoid prolonged sun exposure and to wear sunscreens.
14. The prolonged use of potent topical corticosteroids should be avoided. The health care professional should look for signs of skin atrophy or depigmentation if the product has been used for a long time.

CRITICAL THINKING QUESTIONS

1. A patient came home from college with a severe case of athlete's foot. What products could be recommended to her? Is there any further advice she could be given?
2. An older patient complains of dry, itchy skin. She states that she is a very clean person because she takes a hot bath daily and always uses plenty of soap. What health teaching is indicated?
3. Your roommate returned from the dentist after a tooth extraction. She stated that the dentist gave her a "lot of Novocain." Later in the day her face was markedly swollen. She had difficulty talking and appeared very nervous. On the basis of your knowledge of pharmacology, what do you think might have been the cause of the problem? Is it necessary to call the dentist?
4. A patient comes into the clinic with a fiery red rash over her face and arms. She said the rash developed after she played golf yesterday, and she thinks she might be allergic to her medication. Her health is generally good. She has a urinary tract infection and is nearly finished with her 14-day supply of trimethoprim-sulfamethoxazole (Bactrim). Do you think it is an allergic reaction? What else could it be?

REVIEW QUESTIONS

1. A use for a counterirritant such as camphor may be to:
   - **a.** relieve allergic symptoms.
   - **b.** treat irritated skin or mucous membranes.
   - **c.** promote healing.
   - **d.** relieve deep muscle pain.

2. Cocaine is an effective local anesthetic for:
   - **a.** nasal mucous membranes.
   - **b.** the gastrointestinal tract.
   - **c.** deep muscle pain.
   - **d.** weeping eczema.

3. Which of the following is *not* an antifungal agent?
   - **a.** tolnaftate
   - **b.** zinc sulfate
   - **c.** zinc undecylenate
   - **d.** clioquinol

4. Tretinoin (Retin-A) is used in the treatment of:
   - **a.** urticaria.
   - **b.** weeping eczema.
   - **c.** cellulitis.
   - **d.** acne.

5. An agent effective in the topical treatment of monilial infections is:
   - **a.** Chlor-Trimeton.
   - **b.** clotrimazole.
   - **c.** Chloromycetin.
   - **d.** clonidine.

6. A topical agent useful in the treatment of burns is:
   - **a.** miconazole.
   - **b.** Mycolog.
   - **c.** mafenide acetate.
   - **d.** Motrin.

7. Topical corticosteroids have all of the following properties *except:*
   - **a.** enhanced wound healing.
   - **b.** anti-inflammatory.
   - **c.** antipruritic.
   - **d.** vasoconstriction.

8. An example of the highest potency topical corticosteroid is:
   - **a.** hydrocortisone.
   - **b.** desonide.
   - **c.** diflorasone.
   - **d.** alclometasone.

9. An agent used in the treatment of atopic dermatitis is:
   - **a.** camphor.
   - **b.** lactic acid.
   - **c.** econazole.
   - **d.** pimecrolimus.

10. An indication of the effectiveness of a sunscreen would be the:
    - **a.** PABA content.
    - **b.** emollient ingredients.
    - **c.** SPF number.
    - **d.** photosensitizer ingredients.

Answers to the review questions can be found at the back of the book.

evolve Additional questions and activities can be found at *http://evolve.elsevier.com/asperheim/pharmacology.*

Drugs That Affect the Respiratory System

CHAPTER 10

Objectives

After completing this chapter, you should be able to do the following:

1. Understand the function of the respiratory system.
2. Identify important drug groups that produce respiratory depression.
3. Define *expectorant* and give three examples.
4. Become familiar with environmental changes that may reduce the need for asthma medications.
5. Discuss the action of bronchodilators and give three examples.
6. Identify side effects produced by bronchodilators.
7. Recognize which asthma medications are more effective when administered by inhalation.
8. Discuss nursing measures related to assisting patients with respiratory tract disorders.

Key Terms

Asthma (ĂS-mĕ), p. 83
Bronchoconstriction (brŏng-kō-kŏn-STRĬK-shŭn), p. 83
Bronchodilators (brŏng-kō-DĪ-lā-tĕrs), p. 83
Inflammation (ĬN-flĕ-MĀ-shŭn), p. 81
Respiration (RĔS-pĕ-RĀ-shŭn), p. 81

Respiration is the process of exchanging oxygen and carbon dioxide and is accomplished via the respiratory system. The respiratory system in humans includes the nasal cavity, larynx, pharynx, trachea, bronchi, lungs, muscles of the larynx, intercostal muscles, diaphragm, and respiratory center in the medulla (Figs. 10-1 through 10-3).

The chief functions of respiration are to supply oxygen to the tissues and remove carbon dioxide and to aid in the evaporation of water from the respiratory passages, a function that helps to regulate body temperature. Disruptions to the system can occur when the medulla signals the lungs to breathe too much or too little; when the bronchioles constrict (tighten or narrow), reducing gas exchange; and when inflammation occurs within the lungs. **Inflammation** is a pathologic reaction by the body in response to an injury or abnormal stimulation by a physical, chemical, or biologic agent. When inflammation occurs within the lungs or bronchioles, wheezing, breathlessness, and other symptoms can result.

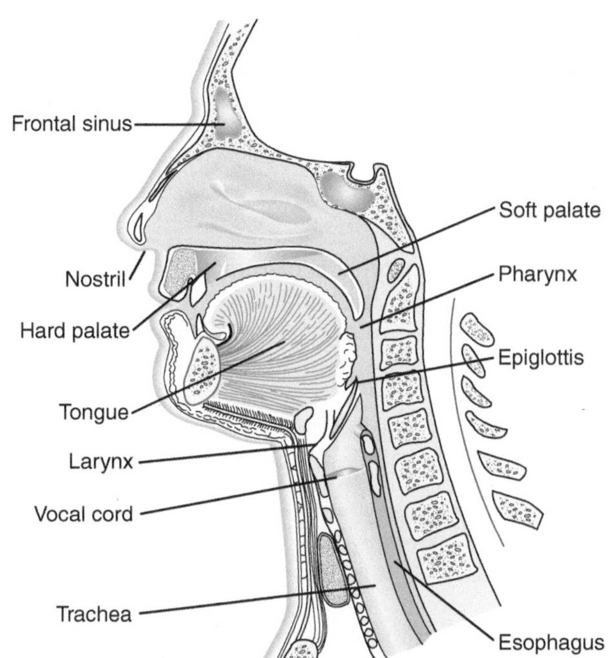

FIGURE 10-1 The upper respiratory organs.

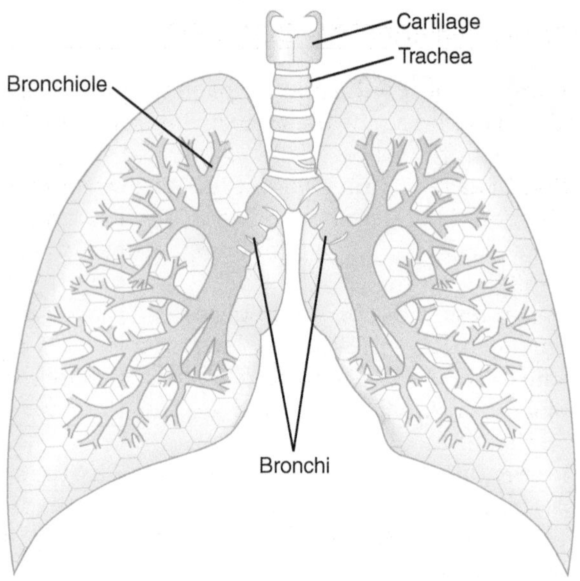

FIGURE 10-2 The lungs.

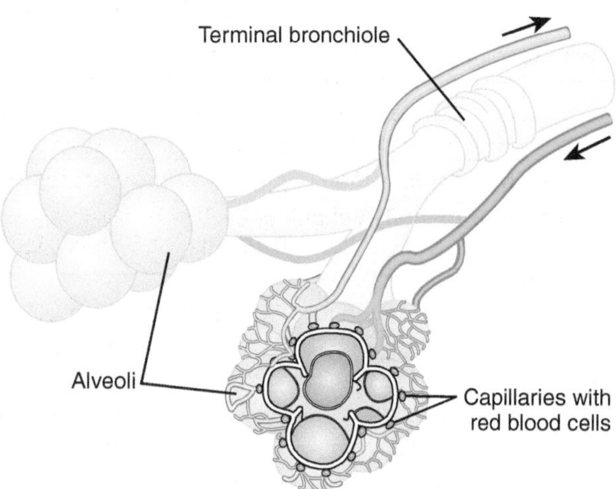

FIGURE 10-3 The terminal respiratory unit.

Drugs that act on the respiratory system may be classified as agents that do the following:

1. Act on the respiratory center in the brain
2. Affect the mucous membrane lining of the respiratory tract
3. Affect the size of the bronchioles
4. Act to decrease inflammation in the lungs

DRUGS THAT ACT ON THE RESPIRATORY CENTER IN THE BRAIN

RESPIRATORY STIMULANTS

carbon dioxide, USP-NF, BP. Carbon dioxide is used, in combination with oxygen, to stimulate deep breathing. It is the natural respiratory stimulant; the increase in carbon dioxide in the blood influences the respiratory center in the brain to cause the individual to take a breath. The lack of oxygen in the tissues does not stimulate respiration. During strenuous exercise, more carbon dioxide is produced, the respiratory center is stimulated, and breathing becomes deeper and more frequent.

RESPIRATORY DEPRESSANTS

The most important respiratory depressants are the central depressants of the opium group (e.g., morphine, codeine) and the barbiturate group (e.g., phenobarbital, secobarbital). Respiratory depression is an undesirable side effect of these drugs, however. They are not given therapeutically to produce respiratory depression.

DRUGS THAT AFFECT THE MUCOUS MEMBRANE LINING OF THE RESPIRATORY TRACT

Agents that affect the mucous membrane lining of the respiratory tract are used chiefly to relieve or enable effective coughing. A cough is a reflex action produced by irritation in the upper portion of the respiratory tract. This irritation can be due to a foreign body (e.g., a particle of food accidentally inhaled), excessive mucus, or a malignant growth. Treatment of the cough is secondary to treatment of the underlying cause of the cough.

Expectorants are drugs that liquefy the mucus in the bronchi and facilitate the expulsion of sputum. They are used for coughs resulting from the common cold, bronchitis, and pneumonia. Numerous over-the-counter (OTC) cough and cold remedies are available, many with the addition of antihistamines or decongestants.

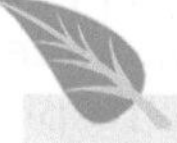

Herb Alert

Red Clover

Red clover is taken internally to treat coughs and respiratory conditions. Externally, it is used for the treatment of chronic skin conditions, such as psoriasis and eczema. Red clover exerts a coumarinlike anticoagulant effect; it should be used with caution in patients with bleeding disorders and in patients taking warfarin, other anticoagulants, or nonsteroidal anti-inflammatory drugs. See Chapter 28 for more information on red clover.

Many remedies used to treat coughing contain codeine or codeine and morphine derivatives to depress the cough reflex. Suppressing the cough reflex by these agents is desirable in certain circumstances, such as a persistent and irritating nonproductive cough.

ASTHMA AND ALLERGIC DISORDERS

Allergic disorders that involve the respiratory tract range from occasional allergic rhinitis to life-threatening asthma. Chronic obstructive pulmonary disease (COPD) may be a result of long-standing asthma or the result of smoking or contact with other pollutants. Many of the same agents are used for this spectrum of disorders.

Asthma is a disorder that affects the airways of the lungs. It is estimated that about 7% of the U.S. population is affected, and it is the most common chronic illness in childhood. Asthma is characterized by airway hyperresponsiveness to allergens and variable airflow obstruction. Episodic, recurrent coughing, wheezing, and shortness of breath are the hallmark symptoms of asthma. Asthma is now understood to be an inflammatory condition rather than a simple constriction of the smooth muscles of the bronchial tree. Numerous cells and cellular mediators are involved, including mast cells, eosinophils, and T lymphocytes.

Asthma attacks can be triggered by allergens, physical exertion, foods, and environmental changes. Reactive airways disease is a condition common in childhood in which a child wheezes only with infections and has no demonstrable known allergies.

Herb Alert

Ephedra (Ma Huang)

The herbal preparation ephedra (not to be confused with the drug ephedrine sulfate) is used to treat colds, asthma, and other respiratory conditions. However, this herb can produce toxic psychosis, life-threatening seizures, tachycardia, hypertension, and heart failure. Life-threatening poisonings occur with very high dosages. It reduces the effects of antihypertensives and phenothiazines and enhances the effects of theophylline, epinephrine, caffeine, decongestants, and stimulants. Ephedra should be avoided in patients with hypertension, diabetes, psychiatric disorders, and cardiac arrhythmias and in patients taking monoamine oxidase inhibitors. Its use is currently restricted. See Chapter 28 for more information on ephedra.

Pathophysiologic features in the lungs associated with asthma include the following:

- Variable airflow obstruction
- Bronchoconstriction
- Edema
- Airway hyperreactivity
- Airway inflammation
- Mucus hypersecretion
- Impaired mucus clearance
- Smooth muscle hypertrophy or hyperplasia
- Subendothelial matrix protein deposits
- Collagen deposits

ENVIRONMENTAL CONTROL

It is important to educate the patient and his or her family to minimize the presence of environmental triggers of asthma. Allergens bind to mast cells, which release histamine and other allergic and inflammatory mediators. Allergens and noxious agents can cause **bronchoconstriction,** a tightening or narrowing of the lung bronchioles. Control of the environment assists in lessening these influences.

- Smoke from personal smoking and second-hand smoke should be eliminated as well as smoke from wood-burning fireplaces and gas from fuel-burning appliances.
- Pet dander is a common allergen. It is best that animals not be present in the home of an asthma patient.
- Dust harbors the dust mite, which is a culprit in triggering asthma.
- Cockroaches should be controlled as much as possible.
- Air filtration and air conditioning should be used to minimize seasonal pollen and mold.
- Seasonal factors should be evaluated, including grass, ragweed, and other plants.
- Occupational concerns must be evaluated. Farmers are around molds and mites in hay and fungal agents in silage. Asbestos, dust, and chemical allergens are implicated as asthma triggers. Latex allergies may develop in health care workers and in patients.
- Sports should be chosen that do not involve dusty environments.
- Foods that provoke asthma include dairy products, peanuts, tree nuts, eggs, soy, chocolate, wheat, corn, fish, and citrus fruits. Tartrazine (yellow dye No. 5), used in many foods including cereals and soft drinks, is believed to be a trigger. Foods with sulfites such as beer, dried foods, shrimp, and wine, also may trigger symptoms.
- Foods that may lessen asthma symptoms include foods rich in natural anti-inflammatories such as omega-3 (tuna, sardines, salmon) and vitamin C. The spice turmeric and the plant flavanoid quercitin found in apples and onions also are anti-inflammatories.

DRUGS THAT AFFECT THE SIZE OF THE BRONCHIOLES

Bronchodilators are agents that dilate, or widen, the bronchioles of the lung by relaxing the smooth muscle of the bronchioles, allowing better air exchange.

ephedrine sulfate, USP-NF, BP. Although not as potent as epinephrine, ephedrine sulfate has the added advantages of being active when taken orally and having a longer duration of action. Nervousness and central nervous system stimulation may occur.

Dosage: Adults: (Oral) 25 mg three to four times daily.

Children: (Oral) 2 to 3 mg/kg/day in four to six divided doses.

epinephrine injection, USP-NF, BP (Adrenalin). The rapid action of epinephrine makes it best for an acute attack. It has a short duration of action, however, so it is not suitable for long-term therapy. Epinephrine must be given by subcutaneous or intravenous (IV) injection. A rapid heart rate and an acute increase in blood pressure may be observed after administration; caution must be used when administering this agent.
Dosage: Adults: (Subcut, IV) 0.3 mg, often repeated three times at 20-minute intervals.

Children: (Subcut) 0.01 mg/kg, often repeated three times at 20-minute intervals.

Considerations for Older Adults
Epinephrine

Older adults often have underlying disorders such as atherosclerosis or hypertension, that may make them particularly sensitive to the side effects of epinephrine. Tachycardia, premature ventricular contractions, a severe increase in blood pressure, and palpitations may occur after administration of epinephrine. Cerebrovascular hemorrhage (i.e., stroke or brain attack) may occur as a result of a marked increase in blood pressure related to the administration of epinephrine. Administer this drug with extreme caution in older adults.

terbutaline sulfate, USP-NF, BP (Brethine). Terbutaline has a dilating effect on the smooth muscles of the bronchioles and may be administered to treat acute asthma attacks or COPD. Side effects include an increase in blood pressure and heart rate.
Dosage: Adults and children older than 12 years: (Oral) 2.5 mg three to four times daily; (Subcut) 0.25 mg with a second dose in 15 to 30 minutes. Other agents should be used if two doses are ineffective.

theophylline, theophylline ethylenediamine (aminophylline), USP-NF, BP (Theo-24, Theolair, Uniphyl). Various forms of pure theophylline are available commercially. Most of these preparations are designed to prolong theophylline levels in the blood. Although a very effective bronchodilator, this agent has largely been replaced in the treatment of asthma because of the availability of more effective treatments. Current therapy is usually directed toward treating the inflammatory aspects of asthma.

The primary side effect of theophylline is central nervous system stimulation, which may be exhibited as nervousness, excitation, or tachycardia. Gastric distress may be produced by oral administration. Many drugs have interactions with theophylline. It increases the secretion of lithium and may decrease its effectiveness. It may enhance the effects of anticoagulants, cardiac glycosides, ephedrine, and similar sympathomimetic agents.

The dose of theophylline is most accurately controlled by measuring the serum level of the drug. Although texts state that 10 to 20 mcg/mL is generally a safe dose, toxic effects have been noted at levels greater than 15 mcg/mL.
Dosage: Adults: (Oral) 300 to 600 mg two to three times daily; (IV) 500 mg over a 20-minute period; (Rectal) 0.25 to 0.5 gm two to three times daily.

Children: (Oral, IV) Initial dose: 5 to 7.5 mg/kg. Subsequent administration is 20 to 24 mg/kg/day in divided doses.

ADMINISTRATION OF DRUGS BY INHALATION

Various drugs may be administered by inhalation directly to the respiratory tract to exert local bronchodilator or anti-inflammatory effects. These agents may be used to treat allergic rhinitis, asthma, or COPD including emphysema.

The availability of metered-dose oral aerosols has simplified the dosing of oral inhalants. The inhaled dose is generally given in terms of the commercially available aerosols. If greater depth within the respiratory tract is desired, the drugs may be administered under pressure by means of an intermittent positive-pressure breathing machine. Respiratory therapists generally monitor the use of these machines. The settings may be varied to obtain the desired pressure (usually 15 to 20 cm H_2O). The patient should breathe slowly and must be observed for side effects of the drugs such as nausea, vomiting, dizziness, and tachycardia. Hand-held nebulizers are useful as well.

Current guidelines emphasize using severity to guide initial therapy and making adjustments to therapy as the disease progresses. Inhaled corticosteroids are the preferred first-line medication for long-term control in patients with persistent asthma. All patients should have an inhaled, short-acting bronchodilator available for quick relief of symptoms. When using long-acting bronchodilators, it is thought that they should be used for the shortest duration possible and preferably should be combined with an inhaled corticosteroid. The goal of therapy is the maintenance of normal or near-normal lung function to improve the quality of life and prevent asthma-related complications.

albuterol, USP-NF, BP (Proventil HFA, Ventolin HFA, ProAir HFA, Accuneb). Albuterol is the classic short-acting agent that is used for acute asthma attacks. It is a sympathomimetic agent and causes rapid bronchodilation. The onset of action occurs within 15 minutes by oral inhalation. Duration of action is 3 to 4 hours.
Dosage: Adults and children older than 12 years: (Inhalation) One to two inhalations (90 mcg/spray) every 4 to 6 hours.

arformoterol tartrate (Brovana). Arformoterol tartrate is used as a bronchodilator for long-term symptomatic treatment of bronchospasm associated with COPD.
Dosage: Adults: (Inhalation) 15 mcg twice daily via nebulizer.

azelastine hydrochloride (Astelin). Azelastine hydrochloride is a histamine receptor antagonist that is used as a nasal spray to provide symptomatic relief of seasonal allergic rhinitis.
Dosage: Adults and children older than 12 years: (Intranasal Spray) Two sprays (274 mcg) in each nostril twice daily.

beclomethasone dipropionate, USP-NF, BP (Beclovent). Beclomethasone dipropionate is a corticosteroid that is used as a nasal spray for symptomatic treatment of seasonal rhinitis.
Dosage: Adults and children older than 12 years: (Intranasal Spray) One or two sprays (42 mcg or 84 mcg) in each nostril twice daily.

budesonide (Rhinocort). Budesonide is a corticosteroid spray used for intranasal treatment of seasonal or allergic rhinitis.
Dosage: Adults and children older than 6 years: (Intranasal Spray) One or two sprays (32 to 64 mcg) in each nostril once daily.

ciclesonide (Alvesco). Ciclesonide is a synthetic corticosteroid that is recommended as a step-down drug after a patient has been controlled on a combination long-acting beta agonist and corticosteroid combination (i.e., Advair).
Dosage: Adults and children older than 12 years: (Inhalation) Two sprays (80 to 160 mcg) once daily.

flunisolide nasal solution, USP-NF, BP (Aerobid, Nasalide). Intended for use as a spray to the nasal mucosa, flunisolide is an anti-inflammatory corticosteroid that reduces the symptoms of rhinitis and swollen nasal mucous membranes resulting from allergic rhinitis. Although relief is generally apparent after a few days of therapy, it may take 2 weeks before a full therapeutic effect is obtained.
Dosage: Adults: (Nasal) Two sprays (250 mcg/spray) in each nostril two times daily.

Children older than 6 years: (Nasal) One spray in each nostril three times daily.

fluticasone propionate (Flonase). Fluticasone propionate is a synthetic corticosteroid that is used as a nasal spray to treat seasonal or allergic rhinitis.
Dosage: Adults and children older than 12 years: (Nasal) Two sprays (100 mcg) in each nostril once daily.

fluticasone propionate and salmeterol (Advair Diskus). This combination corticosteroid-bronchodilator is used twice daily for prevention of asthma. It is not intended to be used for the relief of an acute attack. The commercial Diskus inhaler comes in three sizes: the fluticasone dosage is 100 mcg, 250 mcg, and 500 mcg per Diskus, whereas the salmeterol dosage is 50 mcg in all three sizes: 100/50, 250/50, 500/50.
Dosage: Adults and children older than 12 years: (Inhalation) One inhalation twice daily.

formoterol fumarate (Foradil). Formoterol fumarate is a long-acting bronchodilator that generally produces maximum improvement in 1 to 3 hours, with improvement noted to last for 12 hours. It should not be used to treat acute asthma symptoms; it is used twice daily for maintenance treatment of asthma and to prevent exercise-induced asthma. The drug is supplied in the form of a dry powder, intended for use only with its supplied inhaler.
Dosage: Adults and children older than 5 years: (Inhalation) One dosage unit (the contents of one 12-mcg capsule) every 12 hours.

levalbuterol inhalation solution (Xopenex). Levalbuterol is indicated for the treatment or prevention of bronchospasm. It is supplied in individual vials of solution. The vials come in different strengths and contain 0.31 mg, 0.63 mg, and 1.25 mg of levalbuterol. This agent is administered by a nebulizer.
Dosage: Adults and children older than 12 years: (Inhalation) 0.63 to 1.25 mg three times daily.

Children older than 6 years: (Inhalation) 0.31 mg three times daily.

salmeterol (Serevent Diskus). This form of salmeterol provides the drug in a patented delivery system. The drug is provided in powder form, and each blister on the package contains a dose of the drug.
Dosage: Adults and children older than 4 years: (Inhalation) One dosage unit (50 mcg) twice daily.

tiotropium bromide (Spiriva). Tiotropium bromide is intended for the long-term, once-daily maintenance of bronchospasm associated with chronic pulmonary disease, including chronic bronchitis and emphysema. The drug is supplied in a capsule form and comes with its own HandiHaler.
Dosage: Adults only: (Inhalation) Contents of one capsule (18 mcg) inhaled daily.

triamcinolone acetonide (Azmacort). Triamcinolone acetonide is indicated for the maintenance treatment of asthma in patients who require systemic corticosteroid medication. Adding this inhaler may reduce the need for systemic corticosteroids.
Dosage: Adults: (Inhalation) Two inhalations (200 mcg) three to four times daily.

Children younger than 12 years: (Inhalation) One inhalation three to four times daily.

OTHER AGENTS USED IN THE TREATMENT OF ASTHMA

Various agents may be given orally or by injection to aid in the treatment of asthma.

montelukast sodium (Singulair). Montelukast sodium is indicated for the prevention of asthma. It should not be used for the reversal of bronchospasm during attacks. It should be taken daily even when the patient is asymptomatic. The patient must be advised to have appropriate rescue medications available for an attack.
Dosage: Adults: (Oral) 10 mg daily in the evening.
Children 6 to 12 years: (Oral) 5 mg daily in the evening.
Children 2 to 5 years: (Oral) 4 mg daily in the evening.

omalizumab (Xolair). Omalizumab is a monoclonal antibody that is used for the management of moderate to severe persistent asthma in patients who have a positive skin test to an allergen and whose asthma is not adequately controlled with corticosteroids.
Dosage: Adults and children older than 12 years: (Subcut) 150 to 375 mg every 2 to 4 weeks.

zafirlukast (Accolate). Zafirlukast is used for the prevention of asthma; it may be used daily and in some cases may be considered an alternative to daily inhaled corticosteroids or cromolyn. The patient should be advised that zafirlukast does not provide immediate relief from bronchospasm, but it should be continued during an attack along with other rescue medications.
Dosage: Adults: (Oral) 20 mg twice daily.
Children 5 to 11 years: (Oral) 10 mg twice daily.

OTHER AGENTS THAT ACT ON THE RESPIRATORY TRACT

acetylcysteine, USP-NF, BP (Mucomyst). A derivative of the amino acid cysteine, acetylcysteine is effective by inhalation when the liquefaction of mucus and purulent material is desired. It loosens pulmonary secretions and aids in their removal by postural drainage.
Dosage: Adults and children: (Inhalation) 3 to 5 mL of a 10% to 20% solution three to four times daily.

cromolyn sodium, USP-NF, BP (Aarane, Intal). Although ineffective in the treatment of acute asthma, cromolyn sodium is useful in the prevention of asthma attacks. It is believed to stabilize the membranes of the mast cells that are responsible for liberating histamine and initiating the allergic reaction.
Dosage: Adults and children: (Inhalation) 20 mg four times daily.

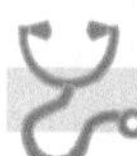

Clinical Implications

1. Adequate fluid intake is necessary during treatment of respiratory infections or wheezing to liquefy mucus and aid in its expulsion.
2. Coughing is beneficial in some cases to clear secretions from the respiratory tract. Antitussives are often prescribed if coughing is excessive or nonproductive.
3. Because coughing is often increased when the patient is lying flat, greater comfort is attained if the patient is placed in a sitting position.
4. Cough preparations, particularly preparations with codeine or similar drugs, cause drowsiness. The patient should be cautioned against combining cough preparations with self-prescribed antihistamines because increased central nervous system sedation may result.
5. In patients with severe chronic respiratory conditions such as emphysema or late forms of cystic fibrosis, respiration is stimulated by high blood carbon dioxide levels. High levels of oxygen administered suddenly to these patients may result in respiratory arrest and death.
6. Arterial blood gases are useful in monitoring the severity of an acute asthma attack and are often used as a guideline in adjusting the oxygen and the drug dosage necessary for the treatment of asthma.
7. Cyanosis, particularly on the lips and perioral area, is a sign of decreased blood oxygen level. A decrease in cyanosis and in respiratory distress can be used to assess quickly improvement in a patient's condition.
8. Corticosteroids, when administered for asthma, have many side effects related to the endocrine system.
9. Prevention of asthma by avoiding or minimizing contact with allergens is always advisable.
10. Health care measures should be directed toward relief of anxiety in patients with respiratory conditions.
11. The patient should be instructed carefully in the use of her or his asthma medications and should be counseled to be compliant with the dosing schedule.

CRITICAL THINKING QUESTIONS

1. A 6-year-old patient is brought to the physician's office after his mother noticed he had some trouble breathing following a strenuous soccer game in the backyard. He has had wheezing a few times after playing outside but has never been brought to the physician for this. What drugs do you think may be prescribed? What may be his problem?

2. A patient reports that she had one of her asthmatic spells last night and spent most of the night in a chair. In the office today, she has only scattered and minimal wheezing. Her activities yesterday included vigorous spring housecleaning and grooming her three cats for a show. What medications or other advice may be helpful for this patient?

REVIEW QUESTIONS

1. The chief function of the respiratory system is to:
   - **a.** guard against infections.
   - **b.** supply oxygen to tissues and remove carbon dioxide.
   - **c.** supply carbon dioxide to tissues and remove oxygen.
   - **d.** relax the lung bronchioles.

2. Agents that are known to be respiratory depressants include all of the following *except:*
   - **a.** phenobarbital.
   - **b.** alcohol.
   - **c.** morphine.
   - **d.** carbon dioxide.

3. Asthma may include all of the following symptoms *except:*
   - **a.** bronchoconstriction.
   - **b.** bronchodilation.
   - **c.** edema.
   - **d.** airway inflammation.

4. A drug that widens the bronchioles of the lung is:
   - **a.** carbon dioxide.
   - **b.** oxygen.
   - **c.** montelukast.
   - **d.** epinephrine.

5. A side effect of drugs administered by inhalation may be:
   - **a.** dizziness.
   - **b.** sweating.
   - **c.** bradycardia.
   - **d.** inflammatory response.

6. A long-acting bronchodilator used in the treatment of asthma is:
   - **a.** epinephrine.
   - **b.** zafirlukast.
   - **c.** theophylline.
   - **d.** salmeterol.

7. Advair Diskus contains a combination of:
   - **a.** salmeterol and fluticasone.
   - **b.** salmeterol and epinephrine.
   - **c.** acetylcysteine and fluticasone.
   - **d.** cromolyn and salmeterol.

8. A drug that is used to liquefy thick mucus in the lungs is:
   - **a.** salmeterol.
   - **b.** triamcinolone.
   - **c.** acetylcysteine.
   - **d.** cromolyn.

9. Cyanosis, when observed in an asthma patient, may be a sign of:
   - **a.** increased response to the asthma medication.
   - **b.** increased blood oxygen level.
   - **c.** hypotension.
   - **d.** decreased blood oxygen level.

10. Respiratory stimulants act on receptors in the:
    - **a.** lining of the lungs.
    - **b.** alveoli.
    - **c.** bronchial tree.
    - **d.** brain.

Answers to the review questions can be found at the back of the book.

evolve Additional questions and activities can be found at *http://evolve.elsevier.com/asperheim/pharmacology*.

CHAPTER 11

Drugs That Affect the Circulatory System

Objectives

After completing this chapter, you should be able to do the following:

1. Discuss the ways drugs may affect the heart.
2. Identify drugs used to treat heart failure.
3. Identify drugs used to treat hypertension.
4. Explain the action of antiarrhythmic agents.
5. Explain the action of vasoconstrictors.
6. Explain the action of vasodilators.
7. Identify drugs used to hasten the process of coagulation.
8. Discuss the uses of anticoagulants.
9. Identify the specific antidote for an overdose of sodium heparin.
10. Identify the specific antidote for an overdose of warfarin sodium.
11. Identify the classes of antihypertensive drugs and their general mechanisms of action.
12. Become familiar with side effects of antihypertensive drugs.
13. Understand the role of platelets in blood clotting and cardiovascular disease.
14. Identify drugs used in antiplatelet therapy.
15. Identify drugs used as thrombolytic agents.
16. Identify drugs used in antilipemic therapy.

Key Terms

ACE inhibitors, p. 90
Anticoagulants (ăn-tĭ-kō-ĂG-ū-lănts), p. 97
Antidote (ĂN-tĭ-dōt), p. 90
Antilipidemic (ăñ-tĭ-LĬP-DĒ-mik) **drugs,** p. 101
Antiplatelet (ăn-tĭ-PLĂT-lĭt) **agents,** p. 100
Beta blockers, p. 91
Coagulants (kō-ĂG-ū-lănts), p. 97
Congestive heart failure, p. 90
Diuretics (dĭ-ū-RĔT-ĭks), p. 89
Inotropic (ĬN-ō-TRŎP-ĭk) **drug,** p. 89
Thrombolytic (THRŎM-bō-LĬT-ĭk) **therapy,** p. 99
Vasoconstrictors (văs-ō-kŏn-STRĬK-tŏrs), p. 94
Vasodilators (văs-ō-DĪ-lā-tŏrs), p. 94

The circulatory system includes the heart and all the blood vessels (Fig. 11-1). The heart is a hollow, muscular organ that is roughly cone-shaped; it is situated near the center of the thoracic cavity, in close relation to the lungs. It is divided by partitions (septa) into four chambers: the right and left atria and the right and left ventricles. The left ventricular wall is about twice the thickness of the right ventricular wall because the work the left ventricle must perform is much greater than the work performed by the right ventricle.

In normal circulation of blood throughout the body, the oxygenated blood comes into the left atrium from the lungs and passes into the left ventricle on contraction of the atrium. The ventricle contracts shortly after the atrium, and the blood is forced into the aorta, which branches into other major arteries. The blood is carried to the gastrointestinal tract, liver, and capillary beds in the systemic circuit. In this capillary region, the objectives of circulation are fulfilled: oxygen and nutritive materials are carried to the tissues, and carbon dioxide and waste products are carried away.

The venous capillaries merge to form larger veins; the blood returns to the heart via the vena cava and enters the right atrium. Contraction of the atrium forces blood into the right ventricle; the subsequent

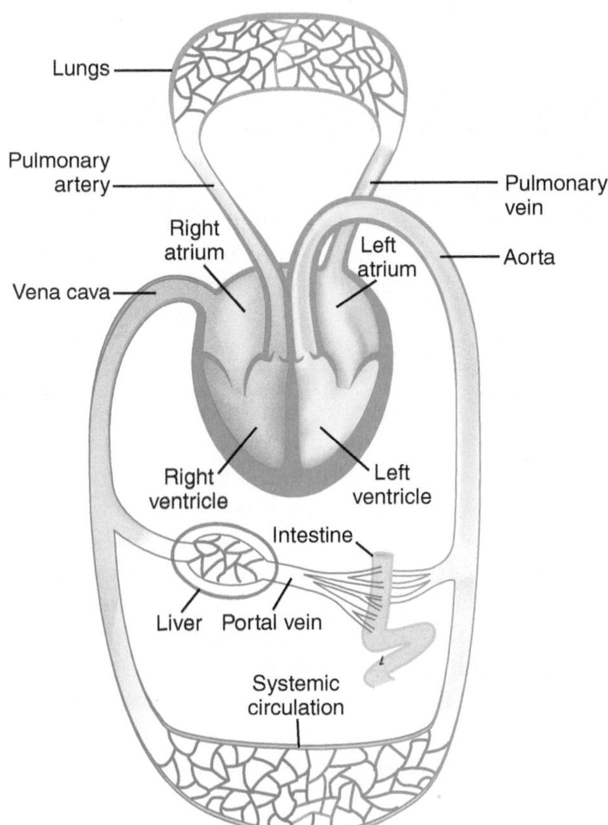

FIGURE 11-1 The circulatory system.

contraction of the ventricle forces the blood to the lungs where it is oxygenated and then returned again to the left atrium to begin the cycle anew.

DRUGS THAT AFFECT THE HEART

Cardiac drugs may affect (1) the heart rate, (2) the rhythm of the heartbeat, (3) the amount of output of blood, (4) the strength of contraction, or (5) the intracellular energy production of the heart muscle. Generally, there are three main conditions for which cardiac drugs are used: heart failure, myocardial infarction, and arrhythmias.

HEART FAILURE

Heart failure means that the heart is not circulating blood at a satisfactory rate to meet the body's demands. When a person is in good health, the heart accomplishes the circulation of blood without faltering. It does not allow an abnormal amount of blood to accumulate in the veins of the body, in the chambers of the heart, or in the lungs. The rate of flow is sufficient to provide a normal pressure in the systemic arteries and the veins in the vascular bed of the lungs.

A diseased heart may have such a handicap that it is unable to move the blood efficiently. If this defect is moderate, it may occur only during physical exertion (e.g., running or climbing stairs), or it may be noticeable when lying flat in bed. The increased venous return when lying down may cause shortness of breath. Heart failure should be suspected when a patient must elevate the upper body on two or three pillows to breathe comfortably in bed.

The following changes may occur during heart failure:

- The capillaries and all veins contain more than the normal amount of blood.
- The hydrostatic pressure is greater than normal in these areas, forcing fluid into the lungs and body tissues.
- The blood in the periphery retains more carbon dioxide and waste products.
- The blood has less oxygen combined with hemoglobin.
- Respiration in the lungs may be so reduced that the blood pumped into the aorta may contain more carbon dioxide and less oxygen than it should.
- Cyanosis, or bluish discoloration of the skin and mucous membranes, may be present.
- Edema, or swelling caused by abnormal accumulation of fluid in tissues, may occur.

Several classes of drugs are used in the treatment of heart failure. They are often used in combination. An **inotropic drug** (a drug that increases the contractility of the heart), such as digoxin, may be combined with an angiotensin-converting enzyme (ACE) inhibitor, a beta blocker, or a diuretic.

DIURETICS

Diuretics (drugs that promote the formation and excretion of urine) are used in the treatment of heart failure and in the treatment of hypertension to reduce fluid overload. The symptoms of orthopnea and dyspnea are reduced with treatment. Recording of daily weight changes also is helpful to monitor fluid retention. Diuretics are most helpful in combination with other agents. Furosemide (Lasix) at a dosage of 50 to 200 mg daily, metolazone (Zaroxolyn) at a dosage of 2.5 mg daily, chlorthalidone (Thalitone) at a dosage of 12.5 to 25 mg daily, or hydrochlorothiazide (HydroDIURIL) at a dosage of 25 to 50 mg daily may be used. The dosages are subsequently adjusted as the condition improves.

INOTROPIC DRUGS

All inotropic drugs increase the contractility of the myocardium. Digitalis was the first inotropic drug identified and used. The crude digitalis leaf is no longer used because of problems with its standardization.

The synthetic form, digoxin, is used exclusively at the present time in oral, intramuscular (IM), and intravenous (IV) formulations.

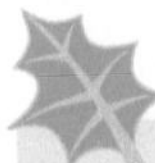

Considerations for Older Adults

Digitalis Preparations

Calcium salts, such as calcium carbonate (Os-Cal) and calcium citrate (Citracal), should be used cautiously, if at all, by patients receiving cardiac glycosides (digitalis preparations). The inotropic and toxic effects of cardiac glycosides and calcium are synergistic, and arrhythmias may occur if these drugs are given together. Also, avoid IV administration of calcium in these patients.

digoxin, USP-NF, BP (Digitek, Lanoxin). The most important action of digoxin on the heart is the strengthening of the heart musculature. The digitalized fibers contract more vigorously and enable the heart to empty more completely. The result is an increase in the amount of blood propelled with any contraction of the ventricles.

The efficiency of the heart is also improved by the slowing of the rate of contraction. This is a desired effect of digoxin, but in overdose the excessive slowing of the heart becomes an untoward effect. The dosage of digoxin should be adjusted so that the pulse remains in the normal range of 60 to 80 beats/min. Excessive doses of digitalis depress the heart rate still further; the pulse must always be taken before administering a dose. If the pulse is less than 60 beats/min, the medication should not be given.

Early side effects that warn of overdose of digoxin are nausea, vomiting, and visual disturbances (objects appear brighter than they actually are; green objects may appear almost white). At this point, the digoxin dosage is usually decreased, or the drug is discontinued for a few days. A lethal dose of digoxin causes death by stopping the heart. The **antidote** (i.e., the substance that neutralizes the effects of a toxin) to digoxin is digoxin immune Fab.

Dosage: Adults: (Oral, IM, IV) Initial loading dose, 0.6 to 1 mg; maintenance: 0.125 to 0.25 mg/day.

Children: (Oral, IM, IV) Initial loading dose: 20 to 35 mcg/kg/day; maintenance: 20% to 30% of the digitalizing dosage.

digoxin immune Fab (Digibind). This agent is the antidote to life-threatening digoxin poisoning. It is composed of antigen-binding fragments (Fab) derived from antidigoxin antibodies produced in sheep serum.

Dosage: Adults and children: (IV) Highly variable, based on the number of tablets ingested and the serum level of digoxin. Tables for dosage calculation are available with the drug literature.

milrinone lactate (Primacor). Milrinone lactate is administered intravenously for the short-term management of acute congestive heart failure. It should be given only when the patient and the electrocardiogram (ECG) can be closely monitored, with equipment available to treat untoward effects such as ventricular arrhythmias.

Dosage: Adults only: (IV) Given as a slow initial IV injection of 50 mcg/kg over 10 minutes, followed by maintenance IV infusion of 0.375 to 0.75 mcg/kg/min.

ACE INHIBITORS

Agents that inhibit angiotensin-converting enzyme (ACE) have become more important in the treatment of **congestive heart failure,** a condition in which the heart is unable to circulate blood satisfactorily. The benefits provided by these agents for patients with congestive heart failure have been shown for all levels of left ventricular dysfunction. **ACE inhibitors** are the agents of choice for congestive heart failure and are used in combination with other agents such as diuretics, thrombolytic agents, aspirin, beta blockers, nitrates, angiotensin II receptor blockers, and digoxin. Their exact mode of action in the treatment of congestive heart failure is still being debated. ACE inhibitors, beta blockers, and angiotensin II blockers appear to work within the metabolic pathways that generate cellular energy for the cardiac muscle.

ACE inhibitors are also used to treat hypertension. ACE is important in the development of hypertension because it enables angiotensin I (a precursor) to be converted to angiotensin II. Angiotensin II is a vasoconstrictor, meaning that it causes narrowing of the blood vessels, which increases blood pressure. Inhibiting the production of angiotensin II reduces vasoconstriction and assists in the treatment of hypertension.

The annoying side effect of a chronic nonproductive cough occurs in a significant percentage of patients. If cough is not severe, it may be simply tolerated for the beneficial effects that the drug has on the heart and blood vessels. When cough is severe, it is necessary to discontinue the drug. Cough can persist for 4 weeks after the drug is discontinued. The other notable side effect of ACE inhibitors, angioedema, is a serious, although infrequent, side effect and is always a reason for discontinuing these agents.

benazepril (Lotensin)

Dosage: Adults: (Oral) 10 to 80 mg in one or two divided doses daily.

captopril (Capoten)

Dosage for heart failure: Adults: (Oral) 6.25 mg three times a day to 25 to 75 mg.

Dosage for hypertension: Adults only: (Oral) 12.5 to 150 mg three times daily.

enalapril (Vasotec)
Dosage for heart failure: Adults: (Oral) 5 mg daily, increased to 10 to 20 mg twice a day.
Dosage for hypertension: Adults only: (Oral) 5 to 40 mg daily in one or two divided doses.

fosinopril sodium (Monopril)
Dosage: Adults: (Oral) 10 to 80 mg once daily.

lisinopril (Prinivil, Zestril)
Dosage for heart failure: Adults: (Oral) 2.5 mg initially, increased to 10 to 30 mg/day.
Dosage for hypertension: Adults only: (Oral) 10 to 40 mg daily in one dose.

moexipril hydrochloride (Univasc)
Dosage: Adults only: (Oral) 7.5 to 30 mg once daily.

perindopril erbumine (Aceon)
Dosage: Adults only: (Oral) 4 to 16 mg once daily.

quinapril (Accupril)
Dosage: Adults only: (Oral) 10 to 80 mg daily in one or two divided doses.

ramipril (Altace)
Dosage: Adults only: (Oral) 2.5 to 20 mg once daily.

trandolapril (Mavik)
Dosage: Adults only: (Oral) 1 to 4 mg once daily.

BETA BLOCKERS

Beta blockers are so named because they block the beta-adrenergic receptors in the sympathetic nervous system. They have been shown to be beneficial for patients who have had myocardial infarctions. The benefit is greatest in patients with reduced ejection fractions. Increased survival rates and decreased hospitalizations have long been noted when beta blockers are used in treatment. They are also used alone or in combination with other agents to treat hypertension.

atenolol (Tenormin)
Dosage for acute myocardial infarction: Adults: (IV) 5 mg over 5 minutes, followed by another 5-mg injection 5 minutes later.
Dosage for hypertension: Adults only: (Oral) 50 to 200 mg once daily.

betaxolol (Kerlone)
Dosage: Adults: (Oral) 10 to 20 mg once daily.

bisoprolol fumarate (Zebeta, ingredient in Ziac)
Dosage: Adults: (Oral) 2.5 to 5 mg once daily; may increase to 20 mg daily.

carvedilol (Coreg)
Dosage for myocardial infarction or hypertension: Adults: (Oral) 6.25 mg twice a day; may increase to 25 mg twice daily.

esmolol (Brevibloc)
Dosage for atrial flutter or fibrillation: Adults: (IV) Infusion containing 10 mg/mL adjusted by response.

labetalol (Normodyne, Trandate)
Dosage for hypertension: Adults: (Oral) 100 to 400 mg in one or two divided doses.

metoprolol (Toprol, Toprol-XL)
Dosage for myocardial infarction: Adults: (IV) 2.5 to 5 mg every 5 minutes up to 15 mg.
Dosage for hypertension: Adults: (Oral) 200 to 800 mg in one or two divided doses.

nadolol (Corgard)
Dosage for hypertension or angina pectoris: Adults: (Oral) 40 to 240 mg once daily.

nebivolol (Bystolic)
Dosage for hypertension: Adults: (Oral) 5 to 40 mg once daily.

pindolol (Visken)
Dosage for hypertension or angina: Adults: (Oral) 10 to 60 mg daily in divided doses.

propranolol hydrochloride (Inderal)
Dosage for myocardial infarction or arrhythmias: Adults: (Oral) 10 to 30 mg three times a day; (IV) 1 mg/min with monitoring.
Dosage for hypertension: Adults: (Oral) Dosages are highly individualized and range from 40 to 160 mg/day. Maximum allowable dosage is 640 mg/day. Long-acting tablets facilitate once-daily dosing.

Children: (Oral only) 2 to 4 mg/kg/day in two divided doses.

sotalol (Betapace)
Dosage for ventricular arrhythmias: Adults: (Oral) 80 mg twice daily, increased to 320 mg daily as required to a maximum of 640 mg/day.

timolol maleate (Blocadren)
Dosage: Adults only: (Oral) 10 mg one to two times daily to a maximum daily dose of 60 mg.

ANGIOTENSIN II RECEPTOR BLOCKERS

Angiotensin II receptor blockers are used after myocardial infarction or heart failure, primarily in patients who cannot tolerate ACE inhibitors. They also reduce left ventricular dilation or dysfunction after a myocardial infarction but do so less effectively than ACE inhibitors. As the name implies, these agents inhibit the effect of angiotensin II by blocking the receptors for the enzyme. They can be used alone or in combination with a diuretic to treat hypertension.

There is a low incidence of side effects to these agents. The side effects include skin rash, facial edema, insomnia, and myalgia.

candesartan cilexetil (Atacand)
Dosage: Adults: (Oral) 8 to 32 mg daily.

eprosartan mesylate (Teveten)
Dosage: Adults: (Oral) 600 to 800 mg daily in one to two divided doses.

irbesartan (Avapro)
Dosage: Adults: (Oral) 150 mg daily.

losartan (Cozaar, ingredient of Hyzaar)
Dosage: Adults: (Oral) 25 to 50 mg daily.

olmesartan (Benicar)
Dosage: Adults: (Oral) 20 to 40 mg daily.

telmisartan (Micardis)
Dosage: Adults: (Oral) 40 to 80 mg once daily.

valsartan (Diovan)
Dosage for hypertension: Adults: (Oral) 80 to 120 mg once daily.
Dosage for heart failure: Adults: (Oral) 40 mg twice daily.

ALDOSTERONE INHIBITORS

Although aldosterone inhibitors are helpful in the treatment of congestive heart failure when the preceding two classes of drugs are not tolerated, they cannot be used if the patient has hyperkalemia or reduced renal function. This class can also be used to treat hypertension.

eplerenone (Inspra)
Dosage: Adults only: (Oral) 25 to 50 mg/day.

spironolactone (Aldactone)
Dosage: Adults only: (Oral) 25 mg/day.

RENIN INHIBITORS

Renin inhibitors act directly on the kidneys to improve the management of hypertension. These agents are generally used with angiotensin II receptor antagonists or diuretics. There does not seem to be a similar additive effect when they are used with beta blockers or ACE inhibitors.

aliskiren hemifumarate (Tekturna)
Dosage for hypertension: Adults only: (Oral) 150 to 300 mg daily.

aliskiren and valsartan (Valturna). This combination agent has been shown to offer good blood pressure control. It is available as 150 mg/160 mg or 300 mg/320 mg of the aliskiren/valsartan combination.
Dosage for hypertension: Adults only: (Oral) One tablet daily of the combination.

CARDIAC ARRHYTHMIAS

The rate and rhythm of the heart are controlled by the sinoatrial (SA) node, known as the "pacemaker" in the right atrium. The SA node generates tiny electrical impulses to the adjacent muscle of the atria, causing the atria to contract and pump blood into the ventricles. The impulses sent out by the SA node are received by the atrioventricular (AV) node, travel down the bundle of His, and are transported to the ventricular muscles by a network of nerves. The ventricles contract shortly after the atria. Both the SA node and the AV node receive autonomic innervation that, to a certain extent, controls the heart rate.

Any deviation from this normal orderly sequence is a disturbance of the rhythm and is called an *arrhythmia*. Sometimes an area of muscle in one of the atria becomes more excitable than the SA node and fires more rapid impulses. The rest of the heart responds to this new pacemaker, and the resulting arrhythmia is known as atrial tachycardia.

Such a new focus may discharge impulses at extremely rapid rates of 180 to 250 impulses per minute. The atria, instead of beating in unison, are swept by wave on wave of contraction and relaxation known as atrial fibrillation. When fibrillation occurs, the AV node is literally bombarded with impulses and is unable to let them all through. The result is that the ventricles, which are the more important chambers, are irregularly stimulated and, consequently, beat less efficiently.

DRUGS USED TO TREAT ARRHYTHMIAS

amiodarone hydrochloride (Pacerone, Cordarone). Amiodarone is used to treat supraventricular and ventricular arrhythmias. It may also be used for this purpose during cardiopulmonary resuscitation. Side effects include bradycardia, heart block, and hypothyroidism.
Dosage: Adults: (IV) Bolus 150 mg over 10 minutes, then 60 mg/hr for 6 hours, followed by 30 mg/hr for up to 18 hours; (Oral) 200 to 400 mg/day in one to two divided doses.

disopyramide phosphate, USP-NF, BP (Norpace). The antiarrhythmic activity of this agent is similar to that of quinidine and procainamide in the treatment of arrhythmias. Side effects include bradycardia.
Dosage: Adults only: (Oral) 100 to 150 mg every 6 hours.

dofetilide (Tikosyn). Dofetilide is used to maintain normal sinus rhythm in patients with atrial fibrillation and atrial flutter. The dose should be modified in the presence of renal impairment. Side effects include bradycardia.
Dosage: Adults: (Oral) 125 to 500 mcg twice daily without regard to meals.

dronedarone hydrochloride (Multaq). This agent is used to control paroxysmal supraventricular tachycardia or for atrial flutter or atrial fibrillation.
Dosage: Adults: (Oral) 400 mcg twice daily with monitoring of the ECG to adjust as necessary.

ibutilide fumarate (Corvert). Ibutilide fumarate is used for the rapid conversion of atrial fibrillation to sinus rhythm. The dose should be adjusted if there is renal or hepatic impairment.
Dosage: Adults: (IV) Injection containing 0.1 mg/mL may be administered undiluted. Injection may be repeated in 10 minutes.

lidocaine hydrochloride, USP-NF, BP (Xylocaine). When administered intravenously, lidocaine hydrochloride has been shown to be extremely effective in controlling and preventing ventricular fibrillation. The drug must be administered by a physician and must be monitored carefully with ECG tracings. Lidocaine is often used in cardiac intensive care units for the prevention of arrhythmias, particularly in patients who have recently had a severe myocardial infarction. Side effects of lidocaine primarily affect the central nervous system and include drowsiness, disorientation, confusion, visual disturbances, and, very rarely, convulsions or coma.
Dosage: Adults: (IV) 50 to 100 mg at a rate of 25 to 50 mg/min. Maximum dosage per hour is 300 mg. Prophylactic IV infusions are administered to deliver a dosage of 1 to 4 mg/min.

nadolol, USP-NF, BP (Corgard). This beta blocking agent has a mechanism of action similar to propranolol. It is used to prevent arrhythmias and to treat hypertension. Side effects include bradycardia.
Dosage: Adults only: (Oral) 40 to 80 mg daily increased to 320 mg daily.

procainamide hydrochloride, USP-NF, BP (Pronestyl). Although also effective in atrial fibrillation, procainamide hydrochloride is used more commonly in ventricular arrhythmias in which premature contractions occur. It is usually administered orally or intravenously. Side effects include bone marrow depression, abdominal pain, and dizziness.
Dosage: Adults: (Oral) 50 mg/kg/day in divided doses every 3 hours; (IM) 50 mg/kg/day in divided doses every 3 to 6 hours; (IV) 50 to 100 mg every 5 minutes, or a loading dose of 500 to 600 mg may be given.
Children: (Oral) 15 to 50 mg/kg/day in divided doses; (IV) 2 to 5 mg/kg, repeat in 10 to 30 minutes; (IV) Bolus 3 to 6 mg/kg; maintenance infusions: 10 to 50 mcg/kg/min.

propranolol hydrochloride, USP-NF, BP (Inderal). Propranolol is an antiarrhythmic agent that exerts its influence by blocking the effect of circulating norepinephrine on the myocardium of the heart. It is used for the treatment of life-threatening arrhythmias, generally in an intensive care unit. By blocking the receptor sites for norepinephrine, this agent reduces cardiac irritability. It is used to treat and prevent atrial flutter and fibrillation and to control extrasystoles. Side effects include nausea, vomiting, diarrhea, skin rash, hallucinations, and blood disorders.
Dosage: Adults: (Oral) 10 to 30 mg three times daily; (IV) For life-threatening arrhythmias, 1 to 3 mg administered slowly at a rate not more than 1 mg/min.
Children: Dosage has not been established.

quinidine sulfate, USP-NF, BP. This drug is used to decrease the number of times the atrial muscle can contract in a given period. It is administered orally or intravenously to treat atrial or ventricular tachycardia.
Dosage: Adults only: (Oral, IV) 200 to 400 mg three to four times daily for 1 to 3 days.

DRUGS THAT AFFECT THE BLOOD VESSELS

Abnormal conditions that affect the arteries, arterioles, capillaries, and veins are many in number and variety. Drugs may be used to increase or decrease the size of the blood vessels and affect the flow of blood through them.

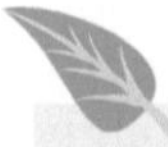

Herb Alert

Horse Chestnut

The seeds and leaves of the horse chestnut tree have been used to treat lower extremity edema caused by venous insufficiency. However, this herb enhances the effect of coumarin and must be used cautiously in patients with bleeding disorders, patients taking warfarin or other anticoagulants, and patients taking nonsteroidal anti-inflammatory drugs. Also, long-term use may cause liver and kidney damage. See Chapter 28 for more information on horse chestnut.

VASOCONSTRICTORS

Vasoconstrictors bring about constriction of the muscle fibers in the walls of the blood vessels, either by direct action on the vessels or by stimulation of the vasomotor center in the medulla. They may be used to (1) stop superficial hemorrhage, (2) relieve nasal congestion, (3) increase the blood pressure, or (4) increase the force of heart action.

epinephrine injection, USP-NF, BP; epinephrine solution, USP-NF (Adrenalin). The chief use of epinephrine is to constrict peripheral blood vessels by local application. It is commonly used in the eye for this purpose. Although used to control bleeding from capillaries or small arteries, it does not stop bleeding from a larger vessel.

Given parenterally, epinephrine produces powerful vasoconstriction, which causes a marked increase in blood pressure. The heart is stimulated as well, which also contributes to the increase in blood pressure. The peak of this elevation is rarely sustained for more than a few minutes, and the blood pressure returns to normal usually within ½ hour after the dose has been given. Because of this transitory action, epinephrine is not the agent of choice when a gradual, sustained elevation of blood pressure is desired. It is quite effective in emergency situations, however. When used with local anesthetics, the vasoconstricting properties prolong the action of the anesthetic.
Dosage: Adults: (Subcut) 0.3 mg.
Children: (Subcut) 0.01 mg/kg.

midodrine hydrochloride (ProAmatine). Midodrine is indicated for the treatment of symptomatic orthostatic hypotension. Because it can cause elevation of supine blood pressure, its use should be restricted to the most severely affected patients. It is contraindicated in severe organic heart disease, acute renal disease, urinary retention, or thyrotoxicosis.
Dosage: Adults only: (Oral) 10 mg three times daily.

VASODILATORS

Vasodilators cause the blood vessels to relax or increase in diameter and have a role in the treatment of peripheral vascular diseases, heart conditions, and hypertension. Many vasodilators are currently in use.

NITRATES AND NITRITES

Nitrates and nitrites cause relaxation of the muscle fibers in the walls of the blood vessels. The relaxation increases the width of the vessels and reduces the pressure of the blood flow through the mucous membranes of the mouth, stomach, or lungs. Tablets often are prescribed to be dissolved under the tongue rather than swallowed. One of the chief uses of nitrates is in the treatment of angina pectoris (chest pain caused by ischemia of the heart muscle). Nitrates are also used to treat hypertension and to relax the smooth muscle spasm in bronchial asthma.

amyl nitrite. Amyl nitrite acts in a similar fashion to nitroglycerin and has been used for relief of angina pectoris. It is administered by nasal inhalation.
Dosage: Adults only: (Inhalation) 0.18 to 0.3 mL as required.

glyceryl trinitrate, USP-NF (nitroglycerin) (Nitrostat). This drug is used in the form of small soluble tablets that are dissolved under the tongue to prevent or relieve attacks.
Dosage: Adults: (Sublingual) 0.2 to 0.6 mg as necessary.
Children: Dosage has not been established.

ranolazine (Ranexa). Ranolazine is used in combination with amlodipine besylate, beta blockers, or nitrates in the management of angina pectoris.
Dosage: Adults only: (Oral) 500 mg to 1 gm twice daily.

topical nitroglycerin (transdermal systems) (Minitran, Transderm-Nitro, Nitro-Dur, Nitrodisc). These transdermal patches should be applied daily to hairless portions of the upper body. The system is designed to last 24 hours.
Dosage: Adults only: (Transdermal) Ranges from 0.1 to 0.8 mg/hr.

ANTIHYPERTENSIVE AGENTS

As previously noted, many agents that are used in the management of congestive heart failure and myocardial infarction are also used to treat hypertension. There are several categories of drugs used to treat hypertension, and some have already been reviewed with the cardiac drugs. The remaining classes are discussed here. When hypertension is not well controlled, it is often better to choose an additional drug from another class rather than increase the dose of the first drug. The classes of antihypertensive agents are as follows:

- ACE inhibitors
- Aldosterone inhibitors
- Alpha blockers
- Angiotensin II antagonists (also called angiotensin II receptor blockers)
- Beta blockers
- Calcium channel blockers
- Central alpha agonists
- Diuretics
- Renin inhibitors

Effective treatment of hypertension can reduce the incidence of stroke, myocardial infarction, heart failure, kidney failure, and overall cardiovascular disease. Nearly one-third of patients with hypertension do not take their medication properly, and many stop the medication altogether because of unpleasant side effects. In addition, hypertensive patients, particularly in the early stages of the disease, feel well; they tend to take their medication irregularly or not at all. From the patient's point of view, the treatment often seems worse than the illness.

Herb Alert

Garlic

Garlic has been widely promoted for treatment of high cholesterol and high blood pressure. Although it has shown some effectiveness in lowering cholesterol and triglyceride levels and raising high-density lipoprotein ("good" cholesterol) levels, studies have not shown any impact on lowering blood pressure. Garlic interferes with platelet adhesiveness and enhances the antiplatelet effects of nonsteroidal anti-inflammatory drugs and warfarin. It also reduces blood glucose levels. See Chapter 28 for more information on garlic.

Lifestyle changes such as weight reduction, increased exercise, and limiting alcohol and sodium intake, are usually the first treatment options that physicians give their patients. If lifestyle changes do not work, single-drug therapy is used, beginning with a low dose and gradually titrating upward. Combination drug therapy often is used to reach the target blood pressure, generally in the range of no higher than 120/80 mm Hg.

Although diastolic blood pressure was formerly thought to be the important number to consider when treating the patient, systolic blood pressure is emerging as a more important criterion for diagnosis and decision making, particularly in middle-aged or older adults who have hypertension. Of hypertensive patients older than 60 years, 65% have isolated systolic hypertension, defined as a systolic blood pressure greater than 140 mm Hg with a diastolic pressure less than 90 mm Hg. It is now recommended that these patients be treated until the target systolic pressure of 120 mm Hg is attained. The old-fashioned rule of thumb that an appropriate systolic pressure is "100 plus your age" is incorrect.

Most patients have "essential" hypertension; that is, no cause is identified. Organic causes of hypertension include renal artery stenosis or other renal abnormalities, pregnancy, use of oral contraceptives, and estrogen replacement therapy.

Several classes of drugs used to treat hypertension are also used to treat cardiovascular disease and were previously discussed. Following are some agents that are used only in the treatment of hypertension.

CENTRAL ALPHA-AGONISTS

Central alpha-agonist agents generally stimulate central alpha-adrenergic receptors in the brain, resulting in a decreased sympathetic outflow from the brain to the circulatory system, causing less vaso constriction.

clonidine (Catapres TTS). This transdermal delivery system consists of patches of clonidine that may be applied and are effective for 1 week of therapy. The patches deliver 0.1 mg, 0.2 mg, or 0.3 mg daily transdermally.

clonidine hydrochloride, USP-NF, BP (Catapres). Clonidine hydrochloride has a rapid onset of activity, with lowering of blood pressure within 30 to 60 minutes after an oral dose. Dry mouth and drowsiness are the most common side effects. In addition to its use as an antihypertensive agent, this drug has been found helpful in controlling impulsivity in hyperactive children or in children with attention-deficit/hyperactivity disorder. It has been used in cases when methylphenidate (Ritalin) has not been helpful. In contrast to methylphenidate, clonidine does not seem to improve school performance and may need to be combined with methylphenidate in some cases. This indication is still under study.

Dosage: Adults: (Oral) 0.1 to 0.3 mg every 12 hours.

Children: (Oral) 5 to 10 mcg/kg/day in two to three divided doses to a maximum of 0.9 mcg/kg/day.

methyldopa hydrochloride, USP-NF, BP (Aldomet). The actions of methyldopa hydrochloride are primarily due to its effect on the central nervous system. The hypotensive effect is attributed to a decrease in peripheral vascular resistance with little change in heart rate. Side effects include drowsiness, impotence, and gynecomastia.

Dosage: Adults: (Oral) 250 to 1000 mg in two divided doses; (IV) 250 to 1000 mg every 6 to 8 hours.

Children: (Oral, IV) 10 to 40 mg/kg/day in divided doses.

ALPHA BLOCKERS

The agents in this group are believed to work by blocking alpha-adrenergic receptors. Alpha blockers cause a vasodilator effect and a lowering of peripheral resistance, which is not usually accompanied by an increased heart rate. Alpha blockers are given to adults only; no dosages have been established for children.

doxazosin mesylate (Cardura). Doxazosin is well tolerated and has few side effects. It has a first-dose effect of occasionally lowering the blood pressure significantly. The first dose should be taken at bedtime.
Dosage: Adults only: (Oral) 1 to 16 mg daily in one dose.

prazosin hydrochloride (Minipress). Prazosin hydrochloride is generally well tolerated and effective orally, with few systemic side effects after treatment is established. The most notable problem is the first-dose effect, a sudden, severe postural hypotension and a sudden syncopal episode, or "drop attack." This problem occurs in a very small percentage of patients and is generally avoided by stressing that the first dose should be taken after the patient has gotten into bed for the night. The drug is generally begun with a lower dose and titrated upward.
Dosage: Adults only: (Oral) 1 to 5 mg three times daily to a maximum of 20 mg/day.
Children: (Oral) 5 mcg/kg every 6 hours, gradually increased to 25 mcg/kg every 6 hours.

terazosin hydrochloride (Hytrin). Action and effects of terazosin hydrochloride are similar to those of prazosin, including the first-dose effect of postural hypotension. The drug is initiated with a low dose and slowly titrated upward.
Dosage: Adults only: (Oral) 1 mg once daily initially to a maximum dosage of 20 mg daily.

CALCIUM CHANNEL BLOCKERS

The class of antihypertensive agents known as calcium channel blockers acts by blocking the entry of extracellular calcium ions into myocardial and vascular smooth muscle cells; this leads to reduced cardiac output and reduced total peripheral resistance, with a subsequent reduction in blood pressure. Calcium channel blockers are also effective for angina pectoris, supraventricular arrhythmias, and cardiomyopathy.

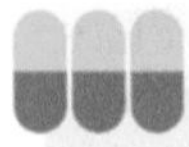

Special Considerations
Calcium Channel Blockers

Calcium channel blockers should not be taken with grapefruit juice, which increases the effects of these medications, sometimes resulting in symptoms of overdose. The interaction apparently occurs because of an inhibition of the cytochrome P-450 enzyme system by some constituent in the juice. Other juices, such as orange juice, do not have this effect.

amlodipine besylate (Norvasc, ingredient of Lotrel). Amlodipine besylate may be used alone or in combination with other agents to treat hypertension. Its side effects are similar to other agents in this class, with dizziness and bradycardia being the most common.
Dosage: Adults only: (Oral) 2.5 to 5 mg once daily.

clevidipine butyrate (Cleviprex). This agent is administered intravenously for the control of hypertension when oral therapy is undesirable.
Dosage: Adults only: (IV) 1 to 2 mg/hr in IV infusion. Dosage may be increased slowly to a maximum of 32 mg/hr.

diltiazem hydrochloride, USP-NF, BP (Cardizem). This agent is used to treat hypertension and angina pectoris. Nausea, dizziness, and bradycardia are side effects.
Dosage: Adults only: (Oral) 90 to 480 mg/day in three to four divided doses.

felodipine (Plendil). Felodipine is generally used in combination with other antihypertensives and seems to be most effective when combined with enalapril.
Dosage: Adults only: (Oral) 5 to 10 mg once daily.

nicardipine (Cardene). Nicardipine is useful for managing hypertension in patients with underlying cardiovascular disease or diabetes. Side effects include pedal edema, headache, and nausea.
Dosage: Adults only: (Oral, IV) 30 to 60 mg twice daily.

nifedipine, USP-NF, BP (Procardia, Adalat). This agent is particularly effective in managing hypertension in patients with coexisting angina or peripheral vascular disease. Hypotension, dizziness, and nausea are side effects.
Dosage: Adults only: (Oral) 10 mg three times daily; as extended-release capsules: 30 to 60 mg once daily.

nimodipine (Nimotop). Nimodipine is used to improve neurologic outcome in patients with ruptured cerebral aneurysms and strokes. It has been found to be useful in the treatment of migraine headaches. Thrombocytopenia and rashes have been reported as side effects.
Dosage: Adults only: (Oral) 20 to 90 mg daily.

nisoldipine (Sular). Nisoldipine is an effective antihypertensive whether used alone or with other agents. Nausea and skin rashes have been reported.
Dosage: Adults only: (Oral) 10 to 40 mg once daily.

verapamil hydrochloride, USP-NF, BP (Calan, Isoptin, Verelan). This agent is used for hypertension, angina, and tachyarrhythmias. Bradycardia, heart block, and constipation are side effects.
Dosage: Adults: (Oral) 120 to 240 mg daily to a maximum dosage of 480 mg/day; (IV) 0.075 to 0.2 mg/kg, repeated once in 30 minutes.

Children: (IV) 0.1 to 0.3 mg/kg, repeated in 30 minutes.

DRUGS THAT AFFECT THE BLOOD

COAGULANTS

Coagulants hasten the process of blood coagulation, or clotting.

CALCIUM SALTS

Calcium salts are needed for the reactions in blood coagulation and may be given orally just before surgery to prevent excessive bleeding. Calcium salts may also be given intravenously by slow IV push or diluted in an infusion to treat tetanic convulsions.

calcium gluconate, calcium chloride, calcium lactate
Dosage: Adults: (Oral, IV) 1 gm as necessary.

VITAMIN K

Vitamin K is a fat-soluble vitamin that is needed for normal blood coagulation. Bile salts must be present in the gastrointestinal tract for absorption of natural vitamin K; in the event of a bile obstruction, an oral preparation of natural vitamin K would be of no use.

phytonadione injection, USP-NF, BP (AquaMEPHYTON). This colloidal solution of vitamin K has smaller particles that permit this preparation to be given by the IM, subcutaneous, and IV routes. It can be used to treat overdoses of coumarin.
Dosage: Adults: (IM, Subcut) 1 to 10 mg once daily. Adults only: (IV) After being diluted with 5% dextrose in 0.9% saline solution, it should be administered at a rate not exceeding 1 mg/min.

Newborns: (IM, Subcut) 0.5 to 1 mg administered immediately after birth to prevent hemorrhagic disease of the newborn.

ANTICOAGULANTS

Anticoagulants increase the time it takes for blood to coagulate by interfering with thrombin production and the subsequent formation of fibrin from fibrinogen. They are used to treat thromboembolic disorders.

Laboratory tests are used to determine the correct dosage of anticoagulants. The prothrombin time (PT), which is sensitive to plasma concentrations of functional blood coagulation factors, has long been used to evaluate the effectiveness of an anticoagulant and to guard against overdose. Valid PT determinations can be made if the blood samples are drawn at least 4 to 6 hours after an IV dose or 12 to 24 hours after a subcutaneous dose of heparin. The generally accepted therapeutic value of the PT ratio is 1.5 to 2.5 times the control value in seconds.

A system of standardizing PT values through determination of an international normalized ratio (INR) has been introduced. It is derived from calibrations of commercial thromboplastin reagents against an international reference preparation. An INR of 2.5 to 3.5 corresponds to a PT ratio of 1.4 to 1.6 and is now used as the optimal value for determining the effectiveness of anticoagulation therapy.

HEPARIN

sodium heparin injection, USP-NF, BP. Heparin is not active orally and must be given parenterally. The preferred method of administration is by IV infusion. In addition, it may be administered by deep subcutaneous (intrafat) injection. It may not be administered by the IM route because of problems with local reactions and the development of hematomas.

Heparin is used for the prevention and treatment of venous thrombosis and, by extension, for prevention and treatment of pulmonary embolism, prevention and treatment of arterial emboli, and treatment of consumption coagulopathies (e.g., disseminated intravascular coagulation). Heparin is the anticoagulant of choice when an immediate effect is desired. An oral anticoagulant (coumarin derivative) is generally started at the same time that heparin is started. After allowing several days for the oral anticoagulant to reach its full effect, heparin can be discontinued. The effect of heparin is generally monitored by PT, although other clotting factors such as the clotting time and activated partial thromboplastin time are also affected.

Heparin-induced thrombocytopenia (HIT) is a significant side effect of heparin therapy in which the heparin induces formation of platelet antibodies. When HIT occurs, another agent must be used. Platelet

counts should be ordered when the patient is receiving heparin, and the drug should be discontinued if the platelets decrease to 100,000/mm^3. Newer low-molecular-weight heparins have less effect on platelets than heparin.
Dosage: Adults: (IV) 5000 units initially, then 20,000 to 40,000 units as a slow infusion over 24 hours.

protamine sulfate. Protamine sulfate is the antidote for heparin overdose.
Dosage: Adults: (IV) 1 to 1.5 mg; recheck PT/INR in 15 minutes. Administration of 1 mg of protamine neutralizes about 100 units of heparin.

LOW-MOLECULAR-WEIGHT HEPARINS

Low-molecular-weight forms of heparin are made by peroxide fragmentation of the heparin molecule, with a resulting molecular weight approximately one-half that of heparin. Similar to older unfractionated heparin, these agents are used to prevent and treat thromboembolic disorders (disorders in which a blood clot is carried away from its site of origin and blocks a blood vessel). They are administered by deep subcutaneous injection; they are not intended for IM or IV injection.

Compared with unfractionated heparins, low-molecular-weight heparins have a few advantages. They may be given by subcutaneous injection rather than intravenously, they have greater bioavailability after subcutaneous injection, and they have a longer half-life and may be administered less frequently. There is a lower incidence of antiplatelet antibody formation and HIT after these heparin forms are administered.

ardeparin sodium injection (Normiflo)
Dosage: Adults only: (Deep subcut) 50 units/kg twice daily.

dalteparin sodium injection (Fragmin)
Dosage: Adults only: (Deep subcut) 2500 to 5000 units daily.

enoxaparin sodium injection (Lovenox)
Dosage: Adults only: (Deep subcut) 30 mg twice daily.

tinzaparin sodium injection (Innohep)
Dosage: Adults only: (Deep subcut) 175 units/kg once daily.

DIRECT INHIBITORS OF THROMBIN

Direct inhibitors of thrombin are used to prevent and treat HIT.

argatroban. Argatroban is administered by continuous IV infusion. Before administering this agent, all parenteral anticoagulants must be discontinued.
Dosage: Adults only: (IV) 2 mcg/kg/min by continuous infusion.

bivalirudin (Angiomax). Bivalirudin is used with aspirin to reduce the risk of ischemia in patients with unstable angina. It is administered intravenously only.
Dosage: Adults only: (IV) 0.75 mg/kg by direct IV injection followed by a continuous infusion of 1.75 mg/kg/hr.

lepirudin (Refludan). Lepirudin, or recombinant DNA for injection, is a highly specific direct inhibitor of thrombin. The natural hirudin was initially extracted from the saliva of the medicinal leech. Although it is structurally and chemically unrelated to heparin, it produces a similar pharmacologic effect through direct interaction with thrombin. It is used for anticoagulation in patients with HIT, to prevent further embolic complications. As with all agents of this class, side effects are primarily associated with hemorrhagic events.
Dosage: Adults only: (IV) 0.4 mg/kg by infusion over 15 to 20 seconds, followed by 0.15 mg/kg/hr as a slow infusion.

COUMARIN ANTICOAGULANTS

Similar to heparin, coumarin anticoagulants are used in the prevention and treatment of thromboembolic disorders. Their main advantage is that they may be taken orally. Their main disadvantage is that they do not take effect for 2 to 7 days. Heparin must be given for initial treatment while coumarin is being started. Neither administration of large loading doses nor administration by the IM or IV route hastens the onset of antithrombotic action. The anticoagulant effect lasts for several days after the drug is discontinued.

Coumarin anticoagulants function by altering the synthesis of blood coagulation factors. Coumarin does nothing to hasten the clearance of existing factors from the blood; the anticoagulant effect does not occur until depletion of the factors occurs.

The dose of coumarin anticoagulants may be adjusted by using the PT/INR, a standardized format for reporting thromboplastin values. A therapeutic PT ratio of 1.3 to 2 times the control PT is equivalent to an INR of 2 to 4. Blood tests should be done weekly until the patient is stabilized and continually monitored every 3 to 4 weeks as long as the patient is receiving coumarin.

The antidote for a coumarin overdose is vitamin K. Phytonadione in the amount of 1 to 10 mg is administered intravenously. Subsequent doses are administered as needed. Many drugs have interactions with the coumarins (Box 11-1).

Box 11-1 Drugs That Interact with Coumarin*

DRUGS THAT MAY INCREASE RESPONSE TO COUMARIN	
acetaminophen	streptokinase
allopurinol	sulfonamides
amiodarone	sulindac
azithromycin	tamoxifen
chloramphenicol	tetracyclines
cimetidine	thiazide diuretics
clofibrate	thyroid drugs
diazoxide	tricyclic antidepressants
diflunisal	vitamin E
disulfiram	
erythromycin	**DRUGS THAT MAY DECREASE RESPONSE TO COUMARIN**
ethacrynic acid	barbiturates
fenoprofen calcium	corticosteroids
fluoxetine	ethchlorvynol
glucagon	glutethimide
lovastatin	griseofulvin
mefenamic acid	mercaptopurine
metronidazole	nafcillin
nalidixic acid	oral contraceptives
nonsteroidal anti-inflammatory drugs	rifampin
quinolone antibiotics	spironolactone
salicylates	sucralfate
	trazodone
	vitamin K

*This list is not absolute; check the most up-to-date drug reference before administering any unfamiliar drug.

warfarin sodium, USP-NF, BP (Coumadin). Warfarin sodium may be absorbed orally and is used to prevent clot formation and extension. Warfarin takes 12 to 18 hours for onset of action. When immediate action is desired, heparin is given intravenously, followed by orally administered warfarin for prolonged anticoagulant therapy. Several herbs and medications can have a cumulative effect with this drug. Patients should always report other medications they are taking and should not take any herbal preparations without permission of their physician.
Dosage: Adults: (Oral, IV) 2 to 5 mg daily initially, followed by daily dosage adjustments based on PT/INR. Most patients are satisfactorily maintained on 2 to 10 mg once daily.

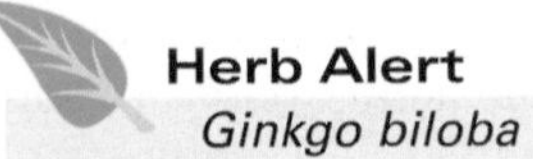

Herb Alert
Ginkgo biloba

Ginkgo biloba has been used to relieve the symptoms of intermittent claudication (leg pain caused by arterial insufficiency) and to treat Alzheimer's disease. Prolonged use has been associated with increased bleeding times and subdural hematomas. This herb also enhances the antiplatelet effects of warfarin and nonsteroidal anti-inflammatory drugs. It should not be used by patients taking tricyclic antidepressants. See Chapter 28 for more information on *Ginkgo biloba*.

THROMBOLYTIC THERAPY FOR MYOCARDIAL INFARCTION

Myocardial infarction, the death of heart muscle resulting from prolonged ischemia, is a life-threatening condition. It is usually caused by obstruction of a coronary artery by a blood clot, probably because of rupture of an atherosclerotic plaque. Advances have been made in aggressive treatment aimed at dissolving the blood clot and minimizing damage to the myocardium. **Thrombolytic therapy,** in which blood clots are dissolved, has been shown to rescue myocardium, reduce mortality in patients with acute myocardial infarction, and improve left ventricular function.

Thrombolytic therapy is also used for acute stroke; the disabling effects of stroke may be reversed if the therapy is given quickly enough. The ideal window is 4.5 hours after the onset of a stroke—there is not a moment to lose after the patient presents with myocardial infarction or stroke symptoms.

alteplase, t-PA, rt-PA (Activase). This biosynthetic form of the human enzyme tissue-type plasminogen activator (t-PA) is a thrombolytic agent. Alteplase is a relatively fibrin-selective plasminogen activator. For maximum effectiveness, it should be administered within 3 to 5 hours after myocardial infarction or stroke. The most frequent complication is hemorrhage.
Dosage: Adults: (IV) 100 mg in a small amount of diluent over a 3-hour period and a subsequent maintenance infusion of 0.25 mg/kg/hr for the next 2 hours.

urokinase. Urokinase may be used intravenously for lysis of acute massive pulmonary emboli. It is most effective in recently formed thrombi. In addition, it is used to treat coronary artery thrombosis, to treat occlusions in peripheral vessels, and occasionally to restore the patency of occluded IV catheters.
Dosage: Adults only: (IV) Loading dose of 4400 units/kg diluted and administered over 10 minutes. At the end of the infusion, heparin may be administered by continuous IV infusion.

ANTIPLATELET THERAPY IN CARDIOVASCULAR DISEASE

Blood platelets are small, granular bodies that number about 250,000 to 350,000 per milliliter of blood. They have three functions:

1. Platelets stick to the inner surfaces of damaged blood vessels, plug up leaks, and cement over injured tissues.

2. When they rupture, platelets release thromboplastin, a substance that begins a series of reactions that forms a blood clot.
3. Once a clot is formed, platelets make it shrink or retract, during which the clot changes from a soft mass to a firm one. This helps stop bleeding from damaged vessels.

Platelet activity and blood clot formation are important functions in the body. However, when a patient has atherosclerosis and the linings of many of the blood vessels are ragged with plaques of cholesterol, the formation of clots is unwanted. **Antiplatelet agents** interfere with platelet aggregation on the surface of atherosclerotic plaques, preventing the formation of thrombi and emboli that block blood vessels.

abciximab (ReoPro). Abciximab may be used with low-molecular-weight heparin or clopidogrel to prevent ischemic complications of cardiac procedures. The most severe side effect is bleeding.
Dosage: Adults: (IV) 2 mg/mL solution; 0.25 mg/kg administered by direct IV injection. The condition should be followed for further doses.

aspirin, USP-NF, BP. By inhibiting enzymes within the platelet, aspirin prevents platelet aggregation. When given daily to patients after a myocardial infarction, there is a reduction in the incidence of recurrent myocardial infarction and cardiovascular death. It may be used daily in low doses to prevent cardiovascular disease. After a transient ischemic attack (TIA), aspirin may be used to prevent further clotting. Aspirin should not be taken when the patient is taking warfarin or other anticoagulants because potentiation of the anticoagulant effect occurs.
Dosage for antiplatelet effect: Adults: (Oral) 65 to 325 mg daily. Higher dosages are not more effective than lower dosages.

aspirin and extended-release dipyridamole (Aggrenox). With the addition of dipyridamole, which is a coronary vasodilator and an inhibitor of platelet aggregation, the effect of aspirin is increased. This combination agent is used to reduce the risk of stroke in patients who have had TIAs. Each capsule contains 25 mg of aspirin and 200 mg of extended-release dipyridamole.
Dosage: Adults only: (Oral) One capsule twice daily.

cilostazol (Pletal). Cilostazol is used as a platelet aggregation inhibitor, mainly in the treatment of intermittent claudication. Grapefruit juice is contraindicated while taking this drug.
Dosage: Adults only: (Oral) 100 mg twice a day.

clopidogrel bisulfate (Plavix). This inhibitor of platelet aggregation is used to reduce atherosclerotic events such as myocardial infarction, stroke, and vascular death in patients with atherosclerosis.
Dosage: Adults only: (Oral) 75 mg once daily.

eptifibatide (Integrilin). Eptifibatide is used to reduce the risk of cardiac ischemic events in patients with unstable angina or myocardial infarction. The risk of bleeding is the main side effect.
Dosage: Adults: (IV) Loading dose of 90 to 250 mcg/kg followed by slower infusions.

prasugrel hydrochloride (Effient). Prasugrel hydrochloride is used to reduce the risk of thrombotic cardiovascular events in patients undergoing percutaneous cardiac intervention procedures. This agent helps in the management of unstable angina, and it is advised that it be used in combination with aspirin therapy.
Dosage: Adults only: (Oral) Initial loading dose of 60 mg followed by 10 mg once daily.

ticlopidine hydrochloride (Ticlid). This agent is used to reduce the risk of thrombotic stroke in patients who have previously had a thrombotic stroke or its precursor, a TIA.
Dosage: Adults only: (Oral) 250 mg twice a day.

tirofiban (Aggrastat). Tirofiban is a selective platelet aggregation inhibitor. It is used to reduce the risk of acute cardiac ischemic events in patients with unstable angina. It may be given concomitantly with heparin in the same IV line.
Dosage: Adults only: (IV) 0.4 mcg/kg/min for 30 minutes.

Considerations for Older Adults

Antiplatelet Agents and Proton Pump Inhibitors

Antiplatelet agents should not be used with proton pump inhibitors such as omeprazole, esomeprazole, rabeprazole, lansoprazole, or pantoprazole, because they reduce the effectiveness of the antiplatelet agents. Non–proton pump inhibitors such as ranitidine and cimetidine do not have this effect and may be used.

ANTILIPIDEMIC DRUGS

The measuring of cholesterol and the definition of "good," or high-density lipoprotein (HDL), and "bad," or low-density lipoprotein (LDL), cholesterol have become a matter of public and personal concern in recent years. As the understanding of the relationship between blood cholesterol levels and atherosclerotic diseases of the blood vessels became known, the "optimal" cholesterol level was decreased farther and farther. Most recent studies have shown that a total cholesterol level of 160 mg/dL is optimal for vascular health. LDL should ideally be less than 70 mg/dL. These numbers may be unattainable for many older individuals even with the use of antilipidemic drugs, but they represent a goal.

After dietary restrictions have been tried, drug therapy is used to attain acceptable cholesterol levels. Many **antilipidemic drugs** have been used and continue to be developed. All drugs in this category are contraindicated in pregnant and nursing women. When a woman of childbearing age is a candidate for these agents, a careful history must be taken with regard to childbearing potential. Blood screening should be done at least every 6 months when patients are receiving these agents. If an elevation of liver enzymes is noted, the drug should be withdrawn until the values return to normal. Another antilipidemic agent may be used with continued monitoring. Elevation of serum creatine kinase may indicate myopathy or skeletal muscle damage. If not soon resolved, these are indications for withdrawal of the drug.

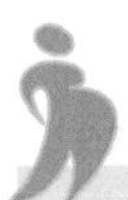

Considerations for Pregnant and Nursing Women

Antilipidemic Drugs

All antilipidemic agents are contraindicated for pregnant and nursing women.

atorvastatin calcium (Lipitor). Atorvastatin calcium is used along with dietary control to reduce serum cholesterol. It may be taken without regard to meals or the time of day.
Dosage: Adults only: (Oral) 10 to 80 mg once daily.

cholestyramine for oral suspension, USP-NF, BP (Questran). Cholestyramine is used orally to bind with bile acids in the intestine, forming an insoluble complex that is excreted in the feces. Cholesterol is the precursor of bile acids; when bile acid loss is accelerated, this stimulates cholesterol to form bile acids, resulting in a net loss of cholesterol from the bloodstream. Cholestyramine is ineffective and contraindicated in patients with bile duct obstruction. The most common adverse effect is constipation. Abdominal pain and flatulence may also be noted. Constipation may be treated with conventional laxative therapy.
Dosage: Adults only: (Oral) 15 gm (one packet or one scoopful) two to four times daily.

colestipol granules (Colestid). Similar to cholestyramine, colestipol acts to remove bile acids from the gastrointestinal tract, causing more cholesterol to be converted to bile acids and lowering the serum cholesterol level. Constipation is the most common side effect.
Dosage: Adults only: (Oral) 5 to 30 gm daily in divided doses. It should always be mixed with fluids.

ezetimibe (Zetia). This agent may be used as monotherapy or in combination with another agent to reduce serum cholesterol.
Dosage: Adults only: (Oral) 10 mg once daily.

ezetimibe with simvastatin (Vytorin). This combination has been shown to be an effective treatment for the reduction of serum cholesterol. It comes in combinations of 10 mg/10 mg, 10 mg/20 mg, 10 mg/40 mg, and 10 mg/80 mg of ezetimibe and simvastatin.
Dosage: Adults only: (Oral) One capsule at bedtime beginning with the 10 mg/10 mg combination and increasing as necessary.

fenofibrate (Tricor). Fenofibrate may be used as monotherapy or with other agents to reduce cholesterol. It is used to reduce hypertriglyceridemia as well.
Dosage: Adults only: (Oral) 130 to 200 mg daily.

fenofibric acid (Trilipix). This delayed-release capsule used in combination with a statin reduces triglycerides and increases HDL cholesterol.
Dosage: Adults only: (Oral) 45 to 135 mg once daily.

gemfibrozil (Lopid). This lipid-lowering agent reduces serum levels of triglycerides and very-low-density cholesterol. Renal and liver abnormalities have occurred with prolonged treatment; the patient should be monitored frequently.
Dosage: Adults only: (Oral) 1200 mg daily in two divided doses.

lovastatin (Mevacor). This agent was isolated from a strain of *Aspergillus terreus*, a fungus. Through complex enzyme activation, it interferes with the biosynthesis of cholesterol. It can cause liver dysfunction.
Dosage: Adults only: (Oral) 20 to 80 mg daily in single or divided doses.

niacin (Advicor, Niacor, Niaspan). Niacin is a B vitamin that is useful as an adjunct to dietary therapy to assist in the management of hypercholesteremia. It may be used along with cholestyramine if other agents are discontinued because of untoward effects. The most common side effects are flushing, nausea, and diarrhea.
Dosage: Adults only: (Oral) 500 to 2000 mg at bedtime daily.

pravastatin sodium (Pravachol). Through a complex mechanism of action involving enzymes and membrane transport complexes, pravastatin sodium acts to clear the serum of cholesterol and triglycerides. The most significant side effect is alteration of liver function; liver enzymes should be tested before therapy and every 6 weeks.
Dosage: Adults only: (Oral) 10 to 80 mg daily at bedtime for 3 to 6 months.

rosuvastatin (Crestor). This agent is used in the management of primary hypercholesterolemia and mixed dyslipidemia.
Dosage: Adults only: (Oral) 5 to 40 mg daily.

simvastatin (Zocor). Also derived from *Aspergillus*, simvastatin reduces cholesterol by interfering with its biosynthesis. Hepatic, renal, and cardiac complications may occur with prolonged use.
Dosage: Adults only: (Oral) 5 to 80 mg daily in the evening.

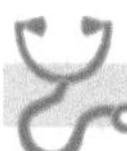

Clinical Implications

1. Care should be taken to monitor the pulse of a patient with cardiac disease before each dose of medication. If the pulse is less than 60 beats/min, digoxin should be withheld, and the physician should be notified.
2. Blood levels of digoxin provide an accurate method of determining the digoxin dose for an individual patient.
3. An increase in urine output is generally seen as an early sign of improvement in a patient being treated for congestive heart failure.
4. A decrease in visible edema from fluid retention is generally noted as a sign of improvement in patients with congestive heart failure.
5. Patients with congestive heart failure are generally more comfortable in a sitting position and should be placed in this position to minimize dyspnea.
6. Patients with cardiac disease are generally prescribed a low-sodium diet to minimize fluid retention. Patients should be carefully instructed about the importance of the diet.
7. Alterations in the serum calcium and potassium levels affect the performance of digoxin. Severe changes in the serum concentration of these electrolytes may be responsible for toxic effects from digoxin.
8. Patients should be monitored for any change in cardiac rhythm during administration of cardiac drugs. An irregular pulse rate should be reported to the physician.
9. Patients should be instructed to take cardiac medications exactly as prescribed. They should be told to report any weight gain, shortness of breath, or edema to the physician.
10. The prothrombin time (PT) may be used as a measure of the effectiveness of anticoagulation. PT is generally believed to be optimal for a patient receiving anticoagulants if it is double the control PT. When the value is more than double the control value, there is a danger of bleeding.
11. Hypertensive agents may have severe side effects. All untoward symptoms should be reported to the physician.
12. Many drugs and herbal remedies have interactions with warfarin. A patient receiving anticoagulants may not take herbal supplements.
13. A patient receiving anticoagulants should be instructed to report prolonged bleeding time from cuts and bloody or black bowel movements. Bleeding gums and petechiae (tiny, nonraised red spots caused by intradermal or submucous hemorrhage) may also be signs of elevated anticoagulant activity.

CRITICAL THINKING QUESTIONS

1. A patient is admitted to the emergency room with shortness of breath; cold, clammy skin; a heart rate of 100 beats/min; and cough producing pink, frothy sputum. A probable diagnosis of heart failure and pulmonary edema has been established. What nursing procedures might be taken immediately to make the patient more comfortable? What drugs are likely to be needed?
2. A patient comes into the emergency room in a state of extreme anxiety, expressing a fear that he is dying. His pulse is thready, rapid, and irregular with a rate of 150 beats/min. A probable diagnosis of atrial fibrillation is established. What drugs are likely to be needed? What other techniques are known to be useful in stopping an attack such as this?
3. A patient appears chronically ill. He has recurrent chest pain and reports shortness of breath. The probable diagnosis is angina. What drugs are likely to be useful in managing his condition?
4. After a heart attack, a patient was prescribed warfarin (Coumadin), 10 mg/day. He has returned to work and feels well. However, he is annoyed that he has to have periodic blood tests and checkups. How can you help him understand the need for these tests?
5. The patient comes to the office to have his rash checked. He fears he may be allergic to warfarin (Coumadin). You see that he has large, deep red spots on his forearms, some measuring 10 cm in diameter. What is the cause of the rash? What should be done?

REVIEW QUESTIONS

1. Heart failure means that the heart:
   a. has stopped beating.
   b. has stopped circulating blood.
   c. has stopped circulating blood efficiently.
   d. has lower hydrostatic pressure than normal.

2. A drug commonly used to increase the contractility of the heart is:
   a. digoxin.
   b. disopyramide.
   c. lidocaine.
   d. nitroglycerin.

3. Which of the following is used to treat angina pectoris?
   a. midodrine.
   b. digitalis.
   c. nitroglycerin.
   d. felodipine.

4. An agent that may be given intravenously to control hemorrhage is:
   a. phytonadione.
   b. felodipine.
   c. glyceryl trinitrate.
   d. perindopril.

5. An example of an ACE inhibitor is:
   a. amiodarone.
   b. olmesartan.
   c. isradipine.
   d. enalapril.

6. An antiplatelet drug may be used in the treatment or prevention of:
   a. hemophilia.
   b. hypertension.
   c. hemorrhage.
   d. transient ischemic attacks.

7. An advantage of low-molecular-weight heparins over traditional heparin is:
   a. shorter half-life.
   b. less bioavailability.
   c. subcutaneous injection rather than IV injection.
   d. IV injection only.

8. Coumarin is used for:
   a. coagulation.
   b. anticoagulation.
   c. hypertension.
   d. antidote for heparin overdose.

9. Gemfibrozil may be used to treat:
   a. hypertension.
   b. hypotension.
   c. constipation.
   d. hyperlipidemia.

10. A common problem when treating hypertensive patients is:
    a. increase in the cholesterol level in the blood.
    b. compliance with taking the medications.
    c. rapid decrease of the blood pressure.
    d. congestive heart failure.

Answers to the review questions can be found at the back of the book.

evolve Additional questions and activities can be found at *http://evolve.elsevier.com/asperheim/pharmacology*.

CHAPTER 12

Drugs That Affect the Central Nervous System

Objectives

After completing this chapter, you should be able to do the following:

1. Classify and give examples of drugs that affect the central nervous system.
2. Differentiate between narcotic and non-narcotic analgesics.
3. Identify narcotic analgesics.
4. State precautions to be observed when narcotic analgesics are administered.
5. List the symptoms of drug dependence.
6. Explain the action of general anesthetic agents.
7. Identify drugs used to prevent and treat migraine headaches.
8. Become familiar with the different types of epilepsy and the drugs used to treat each type.
9. Identify drugs used to treat attention-deficit/hyperactivity disorder.
10. Identify drugs used to treat Parkinson's disease.
11. Identify drugs used to treat fibromyalgia.

Key Terms

Addiction, p. 108
Analgesia (aň-ăl-JĒ-zē-ă), p. 109
Anesthesia (ăn-ĕs-THĒ-zē-ă), p. 106
Anticonvulsants (ăn-tī-kŏn-VŬL-sănts), p. 113
Barbiturates (băr-BĬCH-ū-rătes), p. 107
Narcotic (năr-KŎT-ĭk), p. 109
Opiates, p. 109
Opioids (Ō-pē-oids), p. 109
Tolerance, p. 108

The nervous system, including the peripheral nerves, constitutes the body's equipment for rapid coordination of many of its activities. These activities often must be set into motion and coordinated to the body's needs in a fraction of a second. An example is the very rapid closing of the eyelids when the eyes are unexpectedly touched (e.g., by a grain of sand). We move ourselves at will by sending electrical signals from the central nervous system (CNS) through the peripheral nervous system to the skeletal muscles.

The CNS comprises the brain and spinal cord; together, they coordinate many functions such as blood pressure, heart rate, the flow of saliva and gastric juices, skin temperature, and sensations such as pain. In addition, the brain serves to store knowledge and to cause conscious and unconscious reactions to stimuli and conditions on the basis of past experience. Our awareness of our environment and our satisfaction or dissatisfaction with it and happiness, love, and all emotions or moods are seated in the brain.

It has long been known that the brain can be both depressed and stimulated. The use of alcoholic beverages and plants with depressant effects has its origin in antiquity. The discovery of anesthesia made the performance of lifesaving surgical procedures possible.

In the 20th century, drugs that are effective in treating mentally ill patients were developed. After centuries of study, the first important steps have been taken in unraveling the mysteries of mental illness. Chapter 14 is devoted exclusively to drugs used in the management and treatment of mental illness; however, some of the agents discussed in this chapter have also been used therapeutically in this area.

CENTRAL NERVOUS SYSTEM STIMULANTS

CNS stimulants are drugs that increase the activity of the brain and spinal cord. CNS stimulants are commonly used to treat attention-deficit/hyperactivity disorder (ADHD). ADHD is recognized more frequently in children but is known to last into adulthood in many individuals. If unmedicated, children with this disorder may have cumulative effects of a lifetime of ADHD-associated behaviors. Distractibility, talkativeness, and inappropriate impulsive behavior make life difficult for the child and his or her associates.

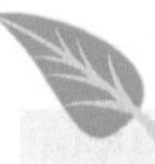

Herb Alert

Ginseng

Ginseng has been used as a stimulant, as a tonic, and to treat menopausal hot flashes. It is claimed to enhance cognitive function, but this has not been substantiated. Ginseng should not be used with warfarin or nonsteroidal anti-inflammatory drugs because it enhances the anticoagulant effect of these agents. Ginseng enhances the effects of phenelzine and should not be used by patients with diabetes or patients taking monoamine oxidase inhibitors. See Chapter 28 for more information on ginseng.

The diagnosis of ADHD is made clinically. In addition to drug treatment for ADHD, educational adjustments can be helpful in addressing the learning disabilities that are often associated with the condition.

amphetamine salts (Adderall). This mixture of the salts of amphetamine is used to treat ADHD and narcolepsy. Peripheral effects of this agent include elevation of blood pressure and a weak bronchodilator action. Heart palpitations, restlessness, dizziness, insomnia, anorexia, and weight loss may occur as adverse effects.
Dosage: Adults and children older than 12 years: (Oral) 5 to 60 mg daily in one to three divided doses.

Children 6 to 12 years: (Oral) 5 to 40 mg daily, dosage adjusted as necessary.

armodafinil (Nuvigil). Armodafinil is used to treat patients with excessive sleepiness associated with sleep disorders, such as shift work disruptions, narcolepsy and obstructive sleep apnea. It is the longer lasting isomer of modafinil.
Dosage: Adults only: (Oral) 150 to 250 mg once daily in the morning.

atomoxetine hydrochloride (Strattera). Atomoxetine hydrochloride is used in the treatment of attention-deficit disorder (ADD) and ADHD, as are the previously listed drugs, but is different in that it is *not* strictly a CNS stimulant and is *not* a controlled substance. Growth should be monitored in a child taking this agent because it has been shown to decrease the appetite. In addition, headache, nausea, abdominal pain, and increases in blood pressure and heart rate have been reported with use.
Dosage: Adults: (Oral) 40 to 100 mg once daily.

Children: (Oral) 0.5 mg/kg initially, increased to 1.2 mg/kg/day.

dextroamphetamine sulfate (Dexedrine). Dextroamphetamine may be used instead of amphetamine because its increased potency permits the use of a lower dosage. The side effects are similar to amphetamine.
Dosage: Adults: (Oral) 5 mg two to four times daily.

Children older than 5 years: (Oral) 5 to 20 mg/day in one to three divided doses to a maximum of 40 mg/day.

Children 3 to 5 years: (Oral) 0.1 to 0.5 mg/kg/day up to 40 mg daily in one to three divided doses.

doxapram hydrochloride, USP-NF, BP (Dopram). This CNS stimulant acts on the CNS at all levels but is used primarily as a respiratory stimulant to hasten arousal in individuals who have taken depressants or after anesthesia. There is a narrow margin of safety with this agent, and hypertension, tachycardia, and seizures have occurred with its use.
Dosage: Adults: (IV) 0.5 to 1 mg/kg for the first two doses at 5-minute intervals and then repeated as necessary at 1- to 2-hour intervals, diluted with IV fluids.

lisdexamfetamine dimesylate (Vyvanse) . Lisdexamfetamine dimesylate is used to treat ADD. It may be used in children 6 years old and is used in adults.
Dosage: Adults: (Oral) 30 mg daily to a maximum of 70 mg daily.

Children 6 to 12 years: (Oral) 20 to 30 mg daily, increased as necessary to a maximum of 70 mg daily.

methylphenidate hydrochloride, USP-NF, BP (Ritalin). The primary use of methylphenidate hydrochloride is in the treatment of ADHD, ADD, and other syndromes. Although the drug is a CNS stimulant, it causes a kinetic slowing of a hyperactive individual and increases the ability to concentrate. It is occasionally used in the treatment of narcolepsy and mild depressive states. The drug is short-acting, generally taking effect within ½ hour and lasting 4 hours. A mid-day dose is necessary to sustain the effect during the school day. Side effects, when they occur, are generally mild and include nervousness, headache, and insomnia; they can generally be controlled by alteration of the dosage.
Dosage: Adults and children: (Oral) 5 to 20 mg two to three times daily.

methylphenidate hydrochloride, extended-release tablets (Concerta). This extended-release form of methylphenidate eliminates the need for a mid-day dose for a school-age child and avoids the perceived stigma of taking the drug at school. The tablet must be taken whole, not crushed.
Dosage: Adults: (Oral) 36 mg once daily in the morning, up to a maximum of 72 mg daily.

Children: (Oral) 18 mg once daily in the morning. Dosage may be individually adjusted.

methylphenidate transdermal system (Daytrana). This patch is a transdermal system that allows once-daily dosing of methylphenidate. The patch should be worn for 9 hours daily, applied generally to the buttocks below the waistline and alternating locations daily. It may be used to treat narcolepsy and ADD, and the dose necessary for the expected effect is generally less than the required oral dose. Side effects are those of methylphenidate generally and some skin irritation at the site of the application.
Dosage: Adults and children: (Transdermal) Patches release 10 mg, 15 mg, 20 mg, or 30 mg per 9-hour period.

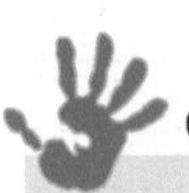

Considerations for Children

Methylphenidate (Ritalin)

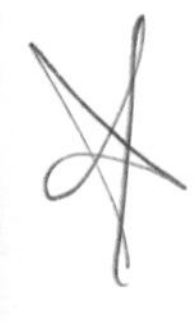

Methylphenidate (Ritalin) should be used with caution in children with a history of seizures or an abnormal electroencephalogram (EEG). There is some evidence that the seizure threshold is lowered in patients receiving methylphenidate.

modafinil (Provigil). Modafinil is indicated to improve wakefulness in patients with sleepiness associated with narcolepsy, sleep apnea, and shift work sleep disorder. Side effects include headache, nausea, nervousness, diarrhea, and back pain.
Dosage: Adults only: (Oral) 200 mg once daily.

phentermine (Adipex-P, Ionamin). Phentermine is used as an adjunct to diet and exercise for weight loss. It should be used for short-term management of a few weeks.

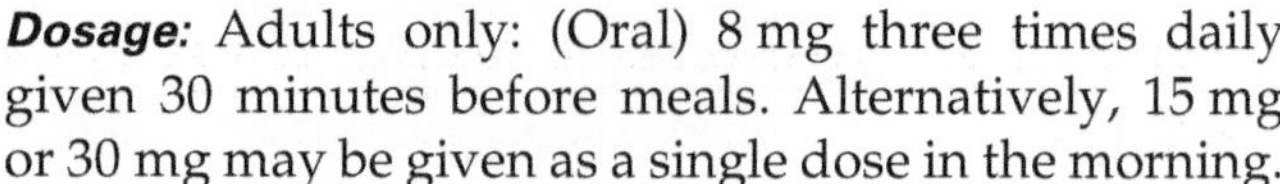

Dosage: Adults only: (Oral) 8 mg three times daily given 30 minutes before meals. Alternatively, 15 mg or 30 mg may be given as a single dose in the morning.

sibutramine hydrochloride (Meridia). Sibutramine hydrochloride is a CNS stimulant that is used as an appetite suppressant. Its side effects are increased blood pressure and heart rate and impaired mentation. This drug should be used with caution if there is a history of seizures.
Dosage: Adults only: (Oral) 5 to 15 mg once daily.

CENTRAL NERVOUS SYSTEM DEPRESSANTS

The action of CNS depressants may be general, depressing the CNS more or less as a whole, or they may act in a more specific way on one or more centers of the brain. **Anesthesia,** a pharmacologic CNS depressant, produces a loss of sensation, which also may be general, systemic, or localized.

GENERAL ANESTHETICS

General anesthetics produce a loss of sensation throughout the body by cutting off all sensory impulses to the brain, causing unconsciousness. General anesthetics are most commonly administered by inhalation, although a few, such as sodium pentothal, are administered intravenously (Tables 12-1 and 12-2).

STAGES OF ANESTHESIA

The stages of anesthesia provide guidelines regarding the level or depth of anesthesia. The anesthetist controls the depth of anesthesia for various procedures by observing the stages. All stages of anesthesia are passed through during induction; the order is then reversed during the recovery period.

I—Analgesia. This stage begins when the anesthetic is administered and lasts until loss of consciousness. It is characterized by analgesia, euphoria, perceptual distortions, and amnesia.

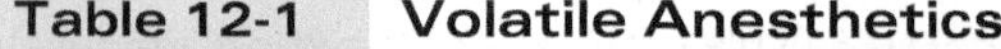

Table 12-1 Volatile Anesthetics

Generic Name	Trade Name	Uses	Concentration (vol %)
enflurane, USP-NF, BP	Ethrane	General use	1.5-4
ether, USP-NF, BP	—	Major surgical procedures	10-15
halothane, USP-NF, BP	Fluothane	Major procedures, particularly when vasoconstriction is desired	1-3
methoxyflurane, USP-NF, BP	Penthrane	Obstetrics, short procedures	2-3
nitrous oxide, USP-NF, BP	—	Short procedures	80
vinyl ether, USP-NF, BP	Vinethene	Major procedures	2-4

Table 12-2 General Anesthetics Administered Intravenously

Generic Name	Trade Name	Uses	Dosage or Concentration
diazepam, USP-NF, BP	Valium	Anticonvulsant, induction aid, preoperative medication	Adults: (IV) 2-10 mg slow IV push Children: (IV) 1-10 mg slow IV push
ketamine hydrochloride, USP-NF, BP	Ketalar	Obstetrics, short procedures	Adults: (IV) 1-4.5 mg/kg Children: (IV) 0.5-2 mg/kg
midazolam hydrochloride	Versed	Sedation anesthetic for short procedures	Adults: (IV) 10-50 mcg/kg initially, then 20-100 mcg/kg/hr Children: (IV) 100-150 mcg/kg initially, then as necessary
thiopental sodium, USP-NF, BP	Pentothal	Short procedures or to facilitate induction with volatile anesthetics	Adults and children >12 yr: (IV) 3-5 mg/kg Children 1-12 yr: (IV) 5-6 mg/kg

II—Delirium. This stage begins with loss of consciousness and extends to the beginning of surgical anesthesia. There may be excitement and involuntary muscular activity. Skeletal muscle tone increases, breathing is irregular, and hypertension and tachycardia may occur.

III—Surgical anesthesia. This stage lasts until spontaneous respiration ceases. It is divided further into four planes based on respiration, the size of the pupils, reflex characteristics, and eyeball movements.

IV—Medullary depression. This stage begins with cessation of respiration and ends with circulatory collapse. The pupils are fixed and dilated, and there are no lid or corneal reflexes.

LOCAL ANESTHETICS

Local anesthetics are presented in this section for completeness and clarity, but they are not CNS depressants. Local anesthetics interfere with nerve conduction from an area of the body to the CNS. In this way, they interfere with pain perception by the CNS. Table 12-3 presents a summary of the local anesthetics.

HYPNOTICS AND SEDATIVES

Hypnotic and sedative agents generally may be used in small doses for daytime sedation and in larger doses for the induction of sleep at bedtime. Patients who are taking these agents must be cautioned not to take other CNS depressants, such as alcohol. Antihistamines, with their side effect of drowsiness, can also produce adverse effects when administered concurrently with these agents. In some cases when these agents are used for their hypnotic effect, a morning "hangover" or sedative effect may be experienced. In many cases, this effect can be minimized by using a shorter acting hypnotic or reducing the dose.

BARBITURATES

Barbiturates produce sedation of the CNS. **Barbiturates** are derivatives of barbituric acid and act by depressing the CNS, respiratory rate, blood pressure, and temperature. The response to barbiturates may be mild sedation, hypnosis, or general anesthesia, depending on the dose and the method of administration. Barbiturates are not analgesics, however, and cannot be depended on to produce sleep when insomnia is caused by pain.

Table 12-3 Local Anesthetics

Generic Name	Trade Name	Uses	Concentration
bupivacaine hydrochloride, USP-NF, BP	Marcaine	Epidural or caudal block, local nerve block	0.25-0.5% subcut solution
chloroprocaine hydrochloride, USP-NF, BP	Nesacaine	Epidural, caudal, or local nerve block	1-2% subcut solution
cocaine hydrochloride, USP-NF, BP	—	Mucous membranes of the nose and throat	1-20% topical application
etidocaine hydrochloride	Duranest	Epidural or peripheral nerve block	1% subcut solution
lidocaine hydrochloride, USP-NF, BP	Xylocaine	Local nerve block	1-2% subcut solution
mepivacaine hydrochloride, USP-NF, BP	Carbocaine	Dental and local block	1% subcut solution
prilocaine hydrochloride	Citanest	Peripheral nerve block	4% subcut solution
procaine hydrochloride, USP-NF, BP	Novocain	Local nerve block	0.25-2% subcut solution
tetracaine hydrochloride, USP-NF, BP	Pontocaine	Spinal anesthesia	1% subarachnoid solution

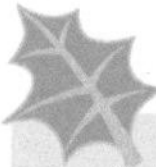

Considerations for Older Adults

Hypnotics and Sedatives

Sedative and hypnotic dosages may need to be reduced for older adults. The metabolism of these drugs is often impaired in older adults, and their excretion may be slower in older adults than it is in younger people. Symptoms of overdose may occur at or below standard doses.

Herb Alert

Valerian

Valerian is used as a sedative to treat insomnia. It enhances the effects of sedatives, hypnotics, antihistamines, and benzodiazepines. Use of valerian should be avoided during pregnancy and lactation. See Chapter 28 for more information on valerian.

These drugs are definitely habit-forming and produce **tolerance**—a condition where larger and larger doses are needed to produce the desired effect. They may lead to **addiction** (habitual dependence on a substance that is beyond voluntary control) if large doses are taken over a long time. The symptoms of barbiturate poisoning are similar to the symptoms of chronic alcoholism. There is impairment of mental efficiency, confusion, belligerence, blurred speech, and tremors. The skin is clammy and cyanotic, the temperature decreases, and respiratory depression continues, causing death.

Severe poisoning results at 5 to 10 times the hypnotic dose, and death results at 15 to 20 times the hypnotic dose. Barbiturate poisoning is treated with dialysis. The patient's blood is passed through an artificial kidney in which the barbiturate is diffused out of the blood.

There are many commonly used barbiturates. They differ in onset of action, duration of action, and method of administration, but for all practical purposes the pharmacologic effects on the body are the same.

mephobarbital, USP-NF, BP (Mebaral)

Dosage: Adults: (Oral) 30 to 100 mg three to four times daily.

pentobarbital, USP-NF, BP

Dosage: Adults: (IM) 150 to 200 mg; (IV) Begin with 10 to 15 mg/kg over 1 to 2 hours, then administer 1 to 2 mg/kg/hr.

phenobarbital, USP-NF, BP (Luminal)

Dosage: Adults: (Oral, IM, IV) 30 mg four times daily.

secobarbital, USP-NF, BP (Seconal)

Dosage: Adults: (Oral) 100 to 200 mg at bedtime.

NONBARBITURATE SEDATIVE-HYPNOTIC AGENTS

chloral hydrate, USP-NF, BP. Sleep is produced in a relatively short time after administration of chloral hydrate and lasts 5 to 8 hours. The sleep greatly resembles natural sleep, and the patient can be awakened without difficulty. There is no analgesic effect from this drug, so it is not used when restlessness or insomnia is due to pain.

Dosage: Adults: (Oral) 500 to 1000 mg at bedtime.
Children: (Oral) 50 mg/kg at bedtime.

flurazepam hydrochloride, USP-NF, BP (Dalmane). Flurazepam is used to treat all types of insomnia and is a hypnotic of moderate activity.

Dosage: Adults only: (Oral) 15 to 30 mg at bedtime.

ramelteon (Rozerem). This insomnia medication has not been shown to have a potential for habit formation or abuse. The most common adverse effects are somnolence, dizziness, and fatigue.

Dosage: Adults only: (Oral) 8 mg at bedtime.

zolpidem tartrate (Ambien). Zolpidem tartrate is used to treat insomnia, is administered orally at bedtime, and has a rapid onset of action. Amnesia, anxiety, and abnormal dreams have been reported as side effects.

Dosage: Adults only: (Oral) 5 to 10 mg at bedtime; (Long-acting Form) 6.25 to 12.5 mg at bedtime.

DOPAMINE RECEPTOR AGONISTS TO TREAT RESTLESS LEGS SYNDROME

Restless legs syndrome (RLS) is a sensorimotor disorder caused by a distressing urge to move the legs while at rest, especially in the evening and at night. The agents used to treat RLS are dopamine receptor agonists, not CNS depressants.

pramipexole dihydrochloride (Mirapex). In addition to being used to treat RLS, pramipexole has some effectiveness in the treatment of parkinsonism. Drowsiness and hallucinations have been reported with use of this agent.

Dosage: Adults only: (Oral) 0.125 to 0.5 mg 2 to 3 hours before bedtime.

ropinirole hydrochloride (Requip). Ropinirole hydrochloride has been found to be effective against RLS and may be used to treat parkinsonism. It may cause somnolence, with the possibility of falling asleep while engaged in daily activities.

Dosage: Adults only: (Oral) 0.25 to 4 mg 1 to 3 hours before bedtime.

OPIATES AND OPIOID ANALGESICS

In ancient times, the opium poppy was discovered to produce **analgesia** (the relief of pain). Opium is described in Chinese literature written long before the time of Christ. It is obtained from the hardened, dried juice of the unripened seeds of the species of poppy grown in Asia Minor. Three alkaloids derived from opium are in use today: morphine, codeine, and papaverine. Any drug derived from opium, or its synthetic analogs, is termed a **narcotic.** Drugs derived from opium are known as **opiates,** whereas drugs with actions similar to those of opium but not derived from opium are called **opioids.**

Although undoubtedly the most powerful and effective pain relievers known to humans, these agents are also the most addictive. After repeated doses, the dose must be continually increased to obtain relief of pain. In the case of narcotic addicts, the desired euphoria is also subject to dose tolerance, and the dosage levels must be continually increased to obtain the desired effect.

Addiction to opiates or opioids is characterized by tolerance, physical dependence, and habituation. Repeated doses of these drugs lead not only to marked tolerance but also to a very strong desire for the drug that the victim seems powerless to resist. The results vary in individuals, but long-term use may lead to depression and weakness not only of the body but also of the mind and morals. The patient has a loss of appetite and various other digestive disturbances and may become thin and anemic. An addict resorts to almost any method to obtain the drug. Ill health, crime, and low standards of living are the result not of the effects of morphine itself but of the sacrifices of money, social position, food, and self-respect made to obtain the daily dose of the drug.

OPIATES

All opiates are controlled substances. The class of controlled substance depends on the potency and potential for addiction and abuse. Generally, opiates that are combined with other substances are in a lower class than preparations of the pure drug.

morphine sulfate, USP-NF, BP (MS Contin, MSIR, Oramorph, Roxanol). Morphine depresses the cerebral cortex; sensation and perception are dulled. Anxiety and apprehension disappear, and euphoria may occur. When administered for painful situations, such as after surgery, the drug is most effective if administered before the pain becomes severe. As long as time intervals are strictly observed and the drug dose is reduced as the pain becomes less severe, addiction is not a frequent problem in short-term indications for this agent. Other effects of morphine include the following:

- The respiratory center is depressed, which is seen as the most dangerous effect of drug overdose.
- The pupils contract and become "pinpoint" in size.
- The emptying time of the stomach is delayed.
- Peristalsis is decreased (this and the previous effect explain why patients often experience abdominal pain, distention, and constipation when given morphine for pain).
- The cough center is depressed, and coughing is lessened.
- The patient may experience interference with motor coordination. He or she may have difficulty handling a glass of water, may misjudge distances when attempting to pick up articles, and may stagger when walking.

Uses of opium and its derivatives are as follows:

- The chief use, as stated before, is as a potent pain reliever.
- As a preliminary medication before general anesthesia, morphine is usually given with atropine. Atropine is used mainly to prevent excessive salivation and respiratory tract secretion, but it also antagonizes the depressant action of morphine on the respiratory center and tends to increase the heart rate. This combination promotes a relaxed state, which favors a more satisfactory induction of anesthesia and decreases the amount of general anesthetic needed for the induction.
- Opium derivatives are frequently used in cough preparations. These syrups or expectorants usually contain codeine, hydrocodone, or hydromorphone, but paregoric has been found useful as well.
- To treat diarrhea, paregoric (camphorated opium tincture) may be used alone or in combination with an absorbent. Laudanum (opium tincture) and synthetic derivatives of opium (Lomotil) have also been used.
- Because of the relaxant effect of morphine on the smooth muscles, opium derivatives may be used as antispasmodics.

Poisoning caused by opium or morphine results from overdoses that have been taken with a therapeutic or suicidal intent. Death usually results from asphyxia brought on by respiratory failure. The pupils are constricted at first and later become dilated as asphyxia deepens. The patient perspires freely and increasingly as poisoning advances. Body temperature decreases, and the skin feels cold and clammy and appears cyanotic or gray. In the treatment of opiate poisoning, attention must be especially focused on maintaining respiration. Naloxone is the treatment of choice for overdoses.

The toxic dose of morphine is 60 mg in a normal individual, and the fatal dose is about 240 mg. Addicts and patients needing control of chronic pain become tolerant of the drug, however, and need much higher doses to exert the desired action. Tolerance develops to the drug, and both the effectiveness and the potential for toxic effects wane over time.

Dosage: Adults: (Subcut, IM, IV) 10 mg, repeated up to six times daily.

Children: (Subcut, IM, IV) 0.1 mg/kg up to six times daily.

Doses may be much higher if tolerance develops.

codeine phosphate, USP-NF, BP; codeine sulfate, USP-NF, BP. Codeine, similar to morphine, is a narcotic regulated under the Controlled Substances Act. It is a mild analgesic, but its potential for abuse and the respiratory depression caused by overdose require that the usual precautions for narcotic analgesic therapy be taken. It is often prescribed in a combination form with aspirin, acetaminophen, or other analgesic agents. Its antitussive activity is well known, and it is included in many cough preparations.

Dosage: Adults: (Oral, Subcut) 15 to 120 mg four to six times daily.

Children: (Oral, Subcut) 3 mg/kg/day in four to six divided doses.

OPIATE ANTIDOTE

naloxone (Narcan). Naloxone is a competitive narcotic antagonist used in the management and reversal of overdoses of morphine and synthetic opioids. It antagonizes all the effects of morphine. When administered after a morphine overdose, naloxone assists in the reversal of the respiratory and CNS depression.

Dosage: Adults: (IV) 0.4 to 2 mg. Doses may be repeated every 2 to 3 minutes, up to 10 mg if needed.

Children: (IV) 0.01 mg/kg every 2 to 3 minutes, up to 0.2 mg.

OPIOIDS

Opioids are synthetic agents that exert a similar pharmacologic effect as the derivatives of the opium poppy, morphine, and codeine. They all are controlled substances and are placed in the various drug schedules based on their activity and their potential for abuse and addiction.

butorphanol tartrate (Stadol). Butorphanol is a synthetic agent that is structurally related to morphine. It is used for moderate to severe pain associated with cancer, burns, renal colic, and migraine headaches.

Dosage: Adults: (IM, IV) 1 to 2 mg every 3 to 4 hours; (Nasal) Metered pump, 1 mg per spray.

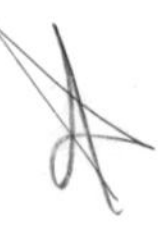

fentanyl transdermal system (Duragesic). This transdermal delivery system consists of patches that are applied to the skin and provide a continuous systemic delivery of fentanyl, a potent opioid narcotic. All the different sizes of patches have the same concentration of drug per area of patch. Increased doses are obtained by using larger patches for greater surface area of delivery. The patches may be used for acute and chronic pain conditions such as cancer and Paget's disease of bone. After removal of the patch, serum concentrations of fentanyl decline gradually and reach an approximate 50% reduction 17 hours after removal. The patch should be applied to a nonirritated area of skin on a flat surface or to the upper torso. Each patch is worn for 72 hours. Side effects are similar to side effects associated with opioids, along with the potential for addiction.

Dosage: Adults: (Topical) Patches deliver 25 mcg/hr, 50 mcg/hr, 75 mcg/hr, or 100 mcg/hr. A patch is applied every 72 hours; (Oral) 2.5 to 7.5 mg four times daily.

hydrocodone bitartrate (ingredient in Hycodan, Hydrocet, Lortab, Tussend, Vicodin). Hydrocodone is generally combined with other non-narcotic analgesics and is used for its analgesic and antitussive effect.

Dosage: Adults only: (Oral) 2.5 to 5 mg four times daily.

hydromorphone hydrochloride (Dilaudid). Hydromorphone hydrochloride is a strong analgesic and is used to relieve moderate to severe pain. It should be used in the smallest effective dose.

Dosage: Adults only: (Oral, Subcut, IM) 1 to 2 mg every 4 to 6 hours.

meperidine hydrochloride, USP-NF, BP (Demerol). Meperidine hydrochloride is a synthetic substitute for morphine. It can cause addiction, but tolerance develops at a slower rate, and the withdrawal symptoms are not as severe as those of morphine. In contrast to morphine, it does not produce sleep, but it is an effective analgesic agent. Because the respiratory depression produced is less than the respiratory depression caused by morphine, it is preferred to morphine in obstetrics.

Dosage: Adults: (Oral, Subcut, IM) 50 to 100 mg every 3 to 4 hours; (IV) 15 to 35 mg/hr.

Children: (Oral, Subcut, IM) 1 mg/kg four to six times daily.

methadone (Dolophine). Methadone was previously largely restricted to use as a withdrawal agent for narcotic addiction, but it is now used as an analgesic in its own right. Although it shares the toxic potential of the other opioids, its potential for addiction is diminished. The euphoria experienced when methadone is taken is less than that of other agents.

Dosage: Adults: (Oral, IM, IV) 2.5 to 10 mg every 8 to 12 hours.

Children: (Oral, IM, IV) 0.1 mg/kg every 6 to 12 hours.

oxycodone (OxyContin, OxyFAST, OxyIR, Roxicodone). This opioid is used orally to relieve mild to moderate pain. It is available in many combinations with acetaminophen or aspirin and in extended-release forms that facilitate pain control.
Dosage: Adults: (Oral) 5 mg every 6 hours.
Children 12 years and older: (Oral) 2.5 mg every 6 hours.
Children 6 to 12 years: (Oral) 1.25 mg every 6 hours.

oxymorphone hydrochloride (Numorphan). Also an opioid, oxymorphone may be given rectally, subcutaneously, intramuscularly, or intravenously. The onset of action is within 5 to 10 minutes after IV administration.
Dosage: Adults and children older than 12 years: (IM, Subcut) 1 to 1.5 mg every 4 to 6 hours; (IV) 0.5 mg every 4 to 6 hours; (Rectal) 5 mg every 4 to 6 hours.

sufentanil citrate (Sufenta). Sufentanil is primarily administered intravenously but also may be given intramuscularly. It is used alone for general anesthesia in some cases but generally is administered along with another anesthetic.
Dosage: Adults: (IV) 10 to 30 mcg/kg.
Children: (IV) 10 to 15 mcg/kg.

NON-NARCOTIC ANALGESICS

Although some can be habit-forming, non-narcotic analgesics generally do not have the addictive properties of narcotic analgesics. They also are not as effective as narcotic agents in analgesic activity.

acetaminophen, USP-NF, BP (Tempra, Tylenol). Acetaminophen has been shown to be an effective and safe analgesic and antipyretic. In contrast to aspirin, however, it has no antirheumatic or anti-inflammatory activity, and it is of limited benefit in the treatment of pain arising from joint disorders. It is not as irritating to the gastric mucosa as aspirin, so it is useful in patients who do not tolerate aspirin well. Acetaminophen has been found to be of great benefit in the treatment of fevers in infants and young children. It is not associated with Reye's syndrome, which has been noted in young children who have received aspirin products.

Sensitivity reactions are rare, and acetaminophen is usually well tolerated by patients sensitive to aspirin. The dosage limits should be carefully observed with acetaminophen. Overdoses lead to serious hepatotoxicity.
Dosage: Adults: (Oral) 325 mg every 4 hours as necessary.
Children: (Oral) 60 to 120 mg four times daily.

nalbuphine hydrochloride (Nubain). Although it is believed to be equivalent to morphine on a milligram-to-milligram basis for analgesia, nalbuphine does not produce euphoria.
Dosage: Adults only: (Subcut, IM, IV) 10 mg every 3 to 6 hours.

pentazocine hydrochloride, USP-NF, BP (Talwin). Pentazocine is a very effective non-narcotic analgesic that may be used for moderate to severe pain. It is effective orally and parenterally. It should not be stopped suddenly after prolonged use because some withdrawal effects may occur. The oral preparations of this drug are combinations, as follows:
- pentazocine with aspirin (Talwin Compound)
- pentazocine with naloxone hydrochloride (Talwin NX)
- pentazocine with acetaminophen (Talacen)

Dosage: Adults: (Subcut, IM, IV) 30 mg every 3 to 4 hours; (Oral): 50 mg every 3 to 4 hours.

tramadol hydrochloride (Ultram). Tramadol hydrochloride is used as an analgesic for mild to moderate pain.
Dosage: Adults and children older than 16 years: (Oral) 50 to 100 mg every 4 to 6 hours.

ANTIMIGRAINE AGENTS

A migraine headache is characterized by severe pain on one or both sides of the head, with aching around the temples or behind one eye. It is caused by a combination of enlarged blood vessels and the release of chemicals from nerve fibers that are adjacent to blood vessels. There may be an aura where the patient reports spots or flashes of light before or during an episode. Nausea and vomiting may occur. A migraine can last 2 to 48 hours and sometimes up to 72 hours. Triggers of migraine include stress, red wine, hard or aged cheese, spices such as monosodium glutamate (MSG), coffee or tea, chocolate, perfumes, bright lights and loud noises, and lack of sleep.

The agents that treat these headaches, also known as triptans, function as analgesics in the treatment of migraine headaches. They are not related to other analgesics, but are selective serotonin agonists. Many headaches are not vascular in origin, and the effective use of these agents is limited to "true" vascular headache.

almotriptan malate (Axert). Almotriptan is given orally to treat acute migraine headaches. It is contraindicated in the presence of ischemic heart disease. Increases in blood pressure and cerebral hemorrhage have been reported.
Dosage: Adults only: (Oral) 6.25 to 12.5 mg as one dose; may be repeated in 2 hours.

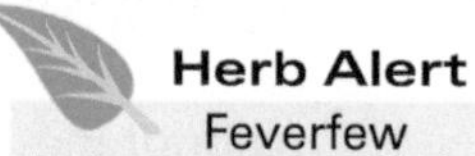

Herb Alert

Feverfew

Feverfew is used to prevent migraine headaches, and some new studies seem to confirm its effectiveness. Its effectiveness as a digestive aid and as a local anesthetic and for the treatment of intestinal parasites, arthritis, and menstrual cramps has not been confirmed. Feverfew enhances the antiplatelet action of nonsteroidal anti-inflammatory drugs and warfarin. Its use should be avoided during pregnancy and lactation. See Chapter 28 for more information on feverfew.

rizatriptan benzoate (Maxalt). This second-generation triptan binds to the 5-hydroxytryptamine (5-HT) receptors found on blood vessels and on sensory nerves. It crosses the blood-brain barrier and has enhanced activity at the 5-HT receptors within the CNS. It has better bioavailability and is successful with more patients than sumatriptan. This agent may be effective in patients who have had a previous drug failure with sumatriptan. Nausea, dizziness, and insomnia are the usual side effects. It may increase blood pressure and should be avoided in hypertensive patients. It should not be given to patients with a history of heart disease because of its vasoconstrictive effects.
Dosage: Adults only: (Oral) 5 to 10 mg at the onset of a migraine headache. A repeat dose may be taken in 2 hours. No more than 30 mg should be taken in 24 hours.

sumatriptan succinate (Imitrex). Sumatriptan succinate acts by binding to 5-HT receptors. It apparently constricts blood vessels in the carotid vascular bed and blocks nerve fibers that conduct pain. The agent is administered by self-injection or taken orally for the treatment of vascular or migraine headaches.

At first hailed as the most effective drug in migraine therapy, sumatriptan has proved disappointing in many cases, probably because many so-called migraines are not vascular headaches at all but are tension, cluster, or muscular contraction types of headaches instead. The drug may work well for some headaches but not all headaches that the patient may have. A positive response, defined as being pain-free 2 hours after the drug is administered, ranges from 50% to 60%. It effectively causes vasospasm, relieving vascular headache, but its side effects also relate to vasospasm: angina pectoris, hypertension, and Raynaud's phenomenon have been reported. It should be avoided in pregnancy. When sumatriptan fails to give the desired relief from migraine headaches, one of the other triptans may still provide a beneficial effect.
Dosage: Adults only: (Oral) 25 mg initially. If necessary, a second dose of up to 100 mg may be given after 2 hours. Maximum daily oral dosage is 200 mg; (Subcut) 6 mg, self-administered. A second dose may be given in 1 hour, but no more than 12 mg may be given in 24 hours.

sumatriptan/naproxen sodium (Treximet). The combination of sumatriptan with the nonsteroidal anti-inflammatory drug naproxen has been shown to be effective. Each tablet contains 85 mg sumatriptan and 500 mg naproxen.
Dosage: Adults only: (Oral) One tablet; may repeat after 1 hour to a maximum of 2 tablets in 24 hours.

zolmitriptan (Zomig). Also a second-generation triptan, zolmitriptan has enhanced bioavailability and crosses the blood-brain barrier to act on the 5-HT receptors in the brain. It is used to treat migraine headaches and may be effective when other triptans have not treated the migraine headaches satisfactorily. The side effects are similar to those of rizatriptan.
Dosage: Adults only: (Oral) 2.5 to 5 mg at the onset of a migraine headache. Dose may be repeated after 2 hours, not to exceed 10 mg in 24 hours.

Other similar agents for migraine headaches include the following.

eletriptan hydrobromide (Relpax)
Dosage: Adults only: (Oral) 20 to 40 mg, repeated in 2 hours.

frovatriptan succinate (Frova)
Dosage: Adults only: (Oral) 2.5 mg, repeated in 2 hours.

naratriptan hydrochloride (Amerge)
Dosage: Adults only: (Oral) 1 to 2.5 mg, repeated in 2 hours.

ALCOHOL

Alcoholic beverages have been prepared and used by humans as both beverages and medicinal agents since ancient times. At one time, alcohol was thought to be a remedy for practically all diseases. During the past century, therapeutic usefulness has diminished greatly because of the availability of more effective and efficient agents, but the abuse of alcohol as a beverage has continued to be a medical and a social problem.

Ethyl alcohol (grain alcohol) is obtained by fermentation. It is formed by the growth of yeast in fruit and vegetable juices containing sugar or starch. Undistilled beverages such as wines and beers contain less than 14% alcohol; distilled liquors such as whiskey, brandy, rum, and gin contain about 50% alcohol.

When consumed, alcohol depresses the cells of the cerebral cortex. In large quantities, its depressant action extends to the cerebellum, the spinal cord, and the respiratory center of the medulla. Alcohol kills by paralyzing the respiratory center, which controls breathing. One effect of alcohol on the cerebral cortex is depression of inhibitory behavior. Small amounts often produce a feeling of well-being, talkativeness, greater vivacity, and increased confidence in one's abilities. Large quantities may cause excitement and impulsive speech and behavior. The special senses become dulled; the person cannot hear normally and speaks in a louder voice. This sense of freedom from inhibitions has given alcohol a false reputation as a stimulant. Because the opposite is true, however, a sedative should not be given to an individual under the influence of alcohol because it would add to CNS depression.

Therapeutic uses of alcohol include the following:

- Dilation of peripheral blood vessels in vascular disease
- Improvement of appetite and digestion
- Hypnotic effect in some individuals
- Local antiseptic and astringent
- Analgesic when injected in or around the sensory nerve trunks for pain relief

EPILEPSY

Epilepsy is as old as the written pages of the history of humankind. It was the "royal illness" of Egyptian pharaohs. Descriptions of the convulsive seizure, the sinister cry, and the loss of consciousness can be traced back to the earliest medical records. Paracelsus described epilepsy as the "disease of lightning" for the individual was struck down as if by a bolt from the sky. Actually, the disease is characterized by an increase in electrical discharges from the brain, producing an irregular pattern. It is a chronic disorder caused by a brain dysfunction, associated with some alteration of consciousness and variable movement. The brain wave patterns obtained by taking an EEG permit diagnosis of the disease.

TYPES OF SEIZURES

TONIC-CLONIC SEIZURES (GRAND MAL SEIZURES)

Seizures are often preceded by an aura and are characterized by a cry, loss of consciousness, and tonic-clonic movements. There is often loss of bladder and bowel control. The attack lasts 2 to 5 minutes and may be followed by deep sleep.

ABSENCE SEIZURES (PETIT MAL SEIZURES)

A quick loss of consciousness for only 1 to 30 seconds may not be noticeable by others. The patient may not even realize the extent or number of seizures he or she has during the day.

COMPLEX PARTIAL SEIZURES

Complex partial seizure is characterized by a brief loss of contact with the environment or by repetitive motions. The patient is generally confused for a minute or two after the attack.

EPILEPTIC EQUIVALENTS

Episodes that resemble seizures may be caused by hypoglycemia, tetanus, poisoning, fluid overload, anaphylaxis, tremors, or drug withdrawal.

ANTICONVULSANTS AND OTHER DRUGS USED TO TREAT EPILEPSY

The first step taken to control epilepsy was in 1857, when Locock gave large doses of bromides to 14 epileptic patients. In nearly all of his cases, the frequency and severity of the seizures were diminished. Bromides produced many toxic effects when given over an extended time, however, which caused their use to be restricted.

In 1912 phenobarbital was found to be more effective than bromides in producing depression of the motor cortex and reducing the number of seizures. Phenobarbital has the disadvantage of depressing the sensory areas of the brain along with the motor areas.

The next advance was made in 1921, when one compound related to the barbiturates was found to depress the motor cortex only and not the sensory areas of the brain. This compound was diphenylhydantoin (now called phenytoin). Since that time, other analogs of this drug have been made and have brought epilepsy under excellent control. There is no cure for epilepsy, but the disease may be controlled through the use of **anticonvulsants.**

carbamazepine, USP-NF, BP (Tegretol). Carbamazepine is used to manage major motor seizures and complex partial seizures. It is ineffective in petit mal seizures. In addition, it may be useful in controlling the pain of trigeminal neuralgia and other forms of neuritis. The side effects of this agent may be dangerous and include aplastic anemia, liver toxicity, congestive heart failure, acute urinary retention, nausea, vomiting, and gastric distress. It should not be used for the control of seizures that respond to other, less toxic agents.

Dosage: Adults: (Oral) 200 to 400 mg four times daily.

Children: (Oral) 10 to 20 mg/kg/day in two to four divided doses.

clonazepam, USP-NF, BP (Klonopin). Clonazepam is used to manage absence attacks and complex partial seizures. The most frequent side effects are drowsiness, ataxia, and behavioral disturbances. Tolerance to this drug may occur.

Dosage: Adults: (Oral) 1.5 to 20 mg daily in three divided doses.

Children: (Oral) 0.01 to 0.03 mg/kg/day.

diazepam, USP-NF, BP (Valium). The injectable form of diazepam has been used intravenously with remarkable success for control of seizures from various causes. It may be administered to halt status epilepticus, seizures secondary to brain damage, or tetany. Valium is of little value in long-term control of epilepsy, however. Respiratory arrest may occur with IV infusion; resuscitation equipment should be available. Its oral use as a tranquilizer is discussed in Chapter 14.
Dosage: Adults: (IV) 2 to 10 mg administered slowly.
Children older than 5 years: (IV) 5 to 10 mg.
Children younger than 5 years: (IV) 1 to 5 mg.

ethosuximide, USP-NF, BP (Zarontin). Ethosuximide is used in the management of absence attacks. The most common side effects are nausea, vomiting, gastric distress, anorexia, drowsiness, ataxia, and irritability. Very rarely, blood disturbances, including aplastic anemia, have occurred.
Dosage: Adults: (Oral) 20 mg/kg/day in a single dose. Dose should not exceed 1.5 gm daily.

ethotoin (Peganone). Ethotoin is used to manage major motor and complex partial seizures. It is both less effective and less toxic than phenytoin. It is often combined with other agents for more effective seizure control. Reported side effects include blood dyscrasias, vomiting, diarrhea, chest pain, and nystagmus.
Dosage: Adults: (Oral) 1 to 3 gm daily.
Children: (Oral) 500 mg to 1 gm daily.

felbamate (Felbatol). Felbamate is believed to raise the seizure threshold and reduce seizure spread. It is used primarily in complex partial seizures.
Dosage: Adults and children older than 14 years: (Oral) Up to 3.6 gm/day in three to four divided doses.
Children younger than 14 years: (Oral) 15 mg/kg/day in three to four divided doses.

fosphenytoin sodium (Cerebyx). This synthetic agent is intended for parenteral administration only. Its active metabolite is phenytoin, and the therapeutic effect is that of phenytoin. Similar to phenytoin, it is used for the treatment of major motor epilepsy.

Each vial contains 75 mg of fosphenytoin, which is equivalent to 50 mg of phenytoin. The dose of this drug is expressed as phenytoin equivalents (PE) to avoid the need to calculate the equivalent dose of phenytoin each time this drug is used. It is used for short-term parenteral administration when other means of phenytoin administration are unacceptable. It is used to control status epilepticus and to prevent and treat seizures during neurosurgery. It may be administered at a faster rate than phenytoin.
Dosage: Adults: (IM, IV) 10 to 20 mg PE/kg. It may be administered at up to 150 mg/min.

gabapentin (Neurontin). Gabapentin is generally used in combination with other agents to control complex partial seizures. It is also used to treat many peripheral neuropathies and postherpetic neuralgia.
Dosage: Adults and children older than 12 years: (Oral) 900 mg to 1.8 gm daily in three divided doses.
Children 2 to 12 years: (Oral) 0.3 mg/kg/day in one to two divided doses.

lamotrigine (Lamictal). Lamotrigine is structurally different from most anticonvulsants. It is believed to act by stabilizing neuronal membranes. It is used primarily to manage complex partial seizures.
Dosage: Adults and children older than 12 years: (Oral) 25 mg daily; may be increased to 400 mg daily.
Children younger than 12 years: (Oral) 0.15 mg/kg/day.

levetiracetam (Keppra). Levetiracetam is generally used along with other agents to control partial seizures in adults.
Dosage: Adults only: (Oral) 500 mg twice daily.

magnesium sulfate. When administered by the IM or IV route, magnesium sulfate is a powerful anticonvulsant. It is used in toxemia of pregnancy and for management of seizures associated with encephalopathy, particularly in association with childhood acute nephritis.
Dosage: Adults: (IM, IV) Solution containing 200 mg/mL given at a rate not to exceed 150 mg/min. Dose is highly variable; 4 to 6 gm may be given initially, then adjusted.
Children: (IM, IV) Solution given at the adult dosage. Up to 2 gm may be administered over 10 to 20 minutes, then adjusted.

oxcarbazepine (Trileptal). Oxcarbazepine is used to treat partial seizures in adults and children older than 4 years. It is used in monotherapy or in combination with other agents.
Dosage: Adults and children older than 16 years: (Oral) 600 mg daily in two divided doses, up to a maximum of 2400 mg daily.
Children older than 4 years: (oral) 8 to 10 mg/kg daily in two divided doses. The dose may be increased in increments of 5 mg/kg/day every third day.

phenobarbital, USP-NF, BP. Its long duration of effect after oral administration makes phenobarbital useful in a once-daily dosage for management of all forms of epilepsy except absence attacks. It may be given to prevent febrile seizures and to treat acute seizure states. It has a relatively slow onset of action, however, even when administered intravenously. It is often combined with other agents for control of seizures.

The primary side effect is drowsiness; this is often minimized by a once-daily dosage administered at bedtime. There is some evidence that the sedation or even lowering of intelligence may be cumulative and progressive when this agent is used for a long time; however, this seems to be reversible if phenobarbital is discontinued.

Dosage: Adults: (Oral) 50 to 100 mg two to three times daily; (IV) For status epilepticus, 200 to 300 mg administered slowly.

Children: (Oral) 3 to 5 mg/kg/day one to two times daily; (IV) 10 to 20 mg/kg over 10 to 15 minutes.

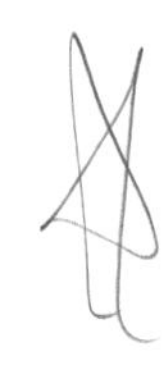

phenytoin, USP-NF, BP (Dilantin). Phenytoin causes depression of the motor cortex without depression of the sensory areas of the brain. It is used to a great extent for major motor epilepsy and often is combined with phenobarbital for more effective therapy.

The principal adverse reactions to phenytoin are dizziness, muscular incoordination, gastric distress, weight loss, and skin rashes. None of these symptoms is severe, however, and they may be overcome by temporarily decreasing the dosage or stopping the drug for a short time.

Plasma concentrations of phenytoin are used to regulate the dosage of this drug. Therapeutic concentrations are 7.5 to 20 mcg/mL. The steady-state serum level may not be achieved until about 1 week of therapy.

There are two types of phenytoin capsules:

1. *Phenytoin prompt*—rapidly absorbed and gives a peak activity in 1 to 3 hours
2. *Phenytoin extended*—formulated to be more slowly absorbed and produce peak concentrations in 4 to 12 hours; only this type of phenytoin may be used for once-daily dosing

Dosage: Adults: (Oral) 100 mg three to four times daily (prompt) or 300 mg once daily (extended); (IV) Rate of administration should not exceed 50 mg/min.

Children: (Oral) 5 mg/kg/day in two divided doses.

pregabalin (Lyrica). Pregabalin is used in combination with other agents to treat partial seizures. In addition, pregabalin has been used to treat postherpetic neuralgia, diabetic neuropathy, and fibromyalgia. When discontinued, it should be stopped gradually.

Dosage: Adults only: (Oral) 150 to 600 mg daily in divided doses.

primidone, USP-NF, BP (Mysoline). Primidone is used primarily in the treatment of complex partial seizures, but it has been used in major motor seizures as well. Mild toxic effects such as drowsiness, nausea, vomiting, ataxia, and dizziness are reported. Serious toxic effects are rare.

Dosage: Adults: (Oral) 250 mg to 2 gm/day in two to four divided doses.

Children: (Oral) 125 to 750 mg/day in divided doses.

tiagabine hydrochloride (Gabitril). This anticonvulsant is used primarily in combination with other agents to control complex partial seizures.

Dosage: Adults and children older than 12 years: (Oral) 4 to 8 mg/day in divided doses.

topiramate (Topamax). Topiramate is generally used in combination with other agents to manage complex partial seizures in children and adults.

Dosage: Adults: (Oral) 200 to 400 mg/day.

Children: (Oral) 5 to 9 mg/kg/day.

trimethadione, USP-NF, BP (Tridione). Trimethadione is used to manage absence attacks refractory to ethosuximide and may be combined with other agents for treatment of combined forms of epilepsy. It has been associated with severe blood disorders, but these are rare. Skin rashes, drowsiness, visual disturbances, and alopecia have been reported.

Dosage: Adults: (Oral) 300 mg three times daily. It may be increased to 2.4 gm daily in divided doses.

Children: (Oral) 25 to 50 mg/kg/day in three to four divided doses.

valproic acid, USP-NF, BP (Depakene). Valproic acid has been shown to be extremely useful in managing epilepsy. It may be used alone or with other agents to manage absence attacks, and it may be used with other agents to control multiple seizure types. The most frequent side effects are nausea, vomiting, and increased appetite with weight gain. Drowsiness, skin rashes, and decreased platelet counts have been observed.

Dosage: Adults: (Oral) 15 mg/kg/day to a maximum dosage of 30 mg/kg/day given once daily or in divided doses.

ANTIPARKINSONIAN AGENTS

Parkinson's disease is a clinical syndrome characterized by lesions of the basal ganglia in the brain. The lesions cause abnormalities in motor activities. About 1% of adults older than 65, or about 1 million people, in the United States are believed to have Parkinson's disease.

Parkinson's disease has no known cause, but it seems to be related to depletion of dopamine in the brain. The disease causes alterations in muscle tone, disturbances in postural stability, and abnormal involuntary movements. A resting tremor, described as a pill-rolling motion of the fingers, is characteristic of the condition. *Secondary parkinsonism* may be caused by drugs such as the phenothiazines and lithium, by toxins such as methanol or carbon monoxide poisoning, and by degenerative diseases such as Alzheimer's disease. Secondary parkinsonism is treated with the same agents. Treatment is generally individualized and may be delayed in the early stages of the disease, when physical therapy may provide enough assistance.

DOPAMINERGIC AGENTS

The following agents are used only in adults:

carbidopa (Lodosyn). Although available as a single agent, carbidopa is usually used in combination with levodopa because it inhibits the metabolic breakdown of levodopa and prolongs its activity in the body.
Dosage: Adults only: (Oral) 25 mg three times daily.

levodopa (Dopar, Larodopa). Levodopa is an isomer of dihydroxyphenylalanine and is the metabolic precursor of dopamine. It is converted to dopamine in the basal ganglia. It is used to treat Parkinson's disease and to control the symptoms of parkinsonism. Levodopa should be used with caution in patients who have a history of myocardial infarction or ventricular arrhythmias. In addition, gastrointestinal hemorrhage, psychiatric disorders, and bronchospasm have been reported as adverse effects of this drug.
Dosage: Adults only: (Oral) 500 mg to 1 gm/day in divided doses.

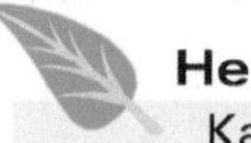

Herb Alert
Kava Kava

Kava kava is used to relieve anxiety and stress and to promote sleep. It reduces the effects of levodopa and other antiparkinsonian drugs. It enhances the effects of sedatives, hypnotics, antihistamines, alcohol, and alprazolam. Its use should be avoided in patients with depressive disorders and during pregnancy and lactation. See Chapter 28 for more information on kava kava.

levodopa plus carbidopa (Atamet, Sinemet). These combinations generally have either a 1:4 or a 1:10 ratio of carbidopa to levodopa. The combinations work well in many cases to reduce the number of medications that have to be taken each day.
Dosage: Adults: (Oral) 25 mg carbidopa/100 mg levodopa three times a day.

rotigotine transdermal patch (Neupro). This transdermal patch may be applied every 24 hours. The patch contains 2 mg, 4 mg, or 6 mg of drug. Side effects include sudden onset of sleepiness, postural hypotension, dizziness, and headache.
Dosage: Adults only: (Transdermal) One patch daily beginning with the 2-mg size.

OTHER AGENTS USED TO TREAT PARKINSON'S DISEASE

Other drugs used in the treatment of Parkinson's disease are listed in Table 12-4.

AGENTS USED TO TREAT FIBROMYALGIA

Fibromyalgia has many subjective and diverse symptoms and classically has been difficult to diagnose and to treat. It is characterized by widespread musculoskeletal pain and a generalized reduced threshold to pain. Depressive symptoms, cognitive disturbances, sleep disturbances, and other symptoms often accompany it. A few agents are now showing some effectiveness with this condition.

milnacipran (Savella). After treatment with milnacipran, patients generally reported a reduced pain level and overall global improvement in symptoms. Patient perception of cognitive function was improved as well. Reported side effects included nausea, dizziness, dry mouth, palpitations, and diarrhea.
Dosage: Adults only: (Oral) 100 to 200 mg daily.

pregabalin (Lyrica). Included with the medications for seizure disorders, pregabalin also has shown effectiveness in treating the symptoms of fibromyalgia. Dizziness, somnolence, and ataxia have been reported with continued use.
Dosage: Adults only: (Oral) 300 to 600 mg daily in divided doses.

Table 12-4 Other Agents for Treatment of Parkinson's Disease

Generic Name	Trade Name	Adult Dosage (Oral)
benztropine mesylate	Cogentin	1-4 mg/day, divided
bromocriptine mesylate	Parlodel	30-100 mg/day, divided
pergolide mesylate	Permax	0.05-3 mg/day, divided
pramipexole dihydrochloride	Mirapex	0.125-1.5 mg 3 times daily
procyclidine hydrochloride	Kemadrin	2.5-5 mg 3 times daily
ropinirole hydrochloride	Requip	0.25-6 mg 3 times daily
tolcapone	Tasmar	100-200 mg 3 times daily
trihexyphenidyl hydrochloride	Artane	1-6 mg 3 times daily

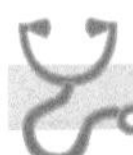

Clinical Implications

1. Central nervous system (CNS) stimulants are generally given early in the day because they may interfere with the patient's sleep pattern.
2. CNS stimulants may aggravate other medical conditions such as hypertension, cardiovascular disease, and hyperthyroidism.
3. Opioid analgesics are the most effective for pain relief.
4. All patients should have a full understanding of the addictive potential of opioid analgesics and should be cautioned not to overuse the drugs.
5. CNS stimulants such as methylphenidate (Ritalin) have a calming effect on individuals with attention-deficit/hyperactivity disorder.
6. Preanesthetic agents to promote sedation aid in the successful induction of general anesthesia. Efforts should be made to maintain the patient in a calm mental condition before surgery.
7. The health care professional should be available to explain the actions of the preanesthetic medication and to answer any questions the patient may have about anesthetic induction.
8. Local anesthetics may have CNS stimulation and irritability as a side effect. In some cases, stimulation may be severe enough to produce seizures.
9. Hypnotics are often given to produce restful sleep in unfamiliar surroundings such as hospitals. Nursing measures such as a back rub and the maintenance of a quiet environment also may be used to promote restful surroundings.
10. "Hangovers," or continued sedation, the day after a hypnotic medication is administered should be noted. Older adults are particularly susceptible to sedation from these agents and may need shorter acting hypnotics.
11. Guardrails are often used to prevent accidental injuries when a patient has been prescribed a sedative or hypnotic. The patient should be instructed not to get out of bed without assistance after administration of these agents.
12. When analgesics are prescribed, the health care professional should give the medication within the prescribed time frame but ideally before the patient experiences severe recurrence of pain. Small, frequent doses are sometimes more effective than longer spacing of larger doses.
13. Addiction is generally not a problem when narcotics are prescribed for relief of a temporary painful situation, such as postoperatively.
14. A patient with epilepsy should be cautioned against driving until seizures are controlled for 1 year and should be cautioned against working around machinery. These individuals should not swim unattended.
15. Parkinson's disease is a degenerative disease of the CNS. A similar condition, parkinsonism, may be due to the side effects of certain drugs.

CRITICAL THINKING QUESTIONS

1. On the second postoperative day, a patient was observed to have slow, shallow respirations and "pinpoint" pupils. His hand shook when he reached for a magazine on his overbed table, and he seemed to be less alert than before surgery. What medications do you think he had received for pain? What steps should be taken to handle this situation? Should the physician be called?
2. A patient is brought to the pediatrician's office with a temperature of 104° F and a draining left ear. The mother states that she did not have any acetaminophen (Tylenol) to give the child to control the fever. The child had a generalized seizure during the examination. What do you think caused the temperature elevation? What caused the seizure? Are there any other measures that the mother could have taken to reduce the fever? Does the child need medication for seizures?
3. A woman was brought to the emergency room after taking an overdose of phenobarbital. She is unconscious. What is the most important consideration in this emergency situation?
4. It has been reported that a patient in your unit has not been swallowing her sleeping pills; instead, she is hoarding them in her drawer. She has been very depressed lately. What is the responsibility of the health care professional when administering any medication? Does the health care professional have other responsibilities for this patient? What would you do in this situation?

REVIEW QUESTIONS

1. A major difference between opioid and nonopioid analgesics is:
   a. their potential for addiction.
   b. there is no difference.
   c. their effect on the blood pressure.
   d. their effect on the heart.

2. A symptom of long-term opioid use or abuse is:
   a. dilated pupils.
   b. agitation.
   c. diarrhea.
   d. constricted pupils.

3. Codeine is the opioid most often used in:
   a. IV pain relief.
   b. preoperative medication.
   c. postoperative medication.
   d. cough preparations.

4. A medication that is effective when administered in a transdermal patch is:
   a. codeine.
   b. morphine.
   c. fentanyl.
   d. meperidine.

5. An example of a non-narcotic analgesic is:
   a. codeine.
   b. oxycodone.
   c. morphine.
   d. acetaminophen.

6. An agent often used in the treatment of tonic-clonic seizures is:
   a. phenytoin.
   b. methylphenidate.
   c. levodopa.
   d. cocaine.

7. An absence attack is another name for:
   a. an episode in which a person has amnesia for a whole day.
   b. a convulsive seizure.
   c. absent blood pressure.
   d. loss of consciousness for less than 1 minute.

8. An agent that is used in the treatment of Parkinson's disease is:
   a. phenobarbital.
   b. phenytoin.
   c. diazepam.
   d. levodopa.

9. Which agent may be used to treat an overdose of morphine?
   a. naloxone
   b. nadolol
   c. codeine
   d. meperidine

10. Which of the following is *not* used to treat attention-deficit/hyperactivity disorder?
    a. methylphenidate
    b. dextroamphetamine
    c. ethotoin
    d. atomoxetine

Answers to the review questions can be found at the back of the book.

evolve Additional questions and activities can be found at *http://evolve.elsevier.com/asperheim/pharmacology.*

Pain Medications

CHAPTER 13

Objectives

After completing this chapter, you should be able to do the following:

1. Take a careful history of a patient's pain.
2. Understand the sources of chronic pain and the different types of treatment available.
3. Realize that it is the patient's assessment of pain that is most important.
4. Recognize that negative responses on the part of health care providers are inappropriate when assisting patients with chronic pain.
5. Understand that approaches to pain management may use drugs of varying potency.
6. Understand that tolerance to opioids may occur if the patient is treated over a long period, and that this is accepted.
7. Become aware of the methods used to prevent illegal use of narcotic medications.

Key Terms

Coanalgesic (KŌ-ăn-ăl-JĒ-sĭk), p. 124
Physical dependence, p. 123
Pseudoaddiction (SŪ-dō-ăd-DĬK-shŭn), p. 123
Withdrawal, p. 123

The relief of pain and suffering has always been an important goal in patient care. Pain is a problem for many people with many medical conditions, and it is the most feared symptom of any medical problem. Pain makes a person lose his or her appetite and become irritable, and it interferes with the quality of life.

The medical care system is designed to focus on acute care, but many patients with incurable and disabling illnesses that progressively worsen over time need management. Chronic pain is one of the most common complaints in primary care facilities; many patients complain that their pain has persisted for more than 5 years, either as a constant discomfort or as frequent flare-ups. Frequently, depression accompanies painful syndromes; depression may require separate medication and attention for the pain management to be effective.

Despite new and effective medications and new treatment procedures, pain is often undertreated. There are many reasons for this, including the following:

- Opioids have a well-known potential for abuse and addiction.
- Drug seekers go to extreme lengths to obtain narcotic medications that they do not need for any medical conditions. Some drug seekers are not truthful.
- Some abusers obtain medications from multiple physicians and clinics.
- Some pain medications are diverted to other persons.
- Some practitioners refuse to write prescription refills for all of these reasons. Meanwhile, truly painful conditions are undertreated.

In a patient with a terminal illness who is expected to live only a short time, tolerance and addiction to the pain medication must be of no concern, and the medications should be dispensed according to increasing need, to provide as much comfort as possible. For a patient with a painful condition who does not have a terminal disease, the goals are different. Some issues to be considered in pain management for these patients include the following:

- A realistic goal for therapy. Total freedom from pain is rarely an achievable goal. Instead, the patient should be questioned as to his or her needs and expectations. For example, one patient may wish to do simple housework and care for her children without excessive pain. Another patient may want to remain alert enough to drive his car and may accept some pain. A condition that has progressed to a more severe level may require more pain relief at night so that the patient can get a good night's sleep to be more alert during the day. It is important to discuss and think through the goals of therapy and use them to assess progress.

- A means of evaluating and describing pain. Because pain is subjective (determined by the patient's perception), a method of measuring and communicating issues related to pain must be found that is meaningful to both the patient and the health care professional. A pain intensity scale ranging from 0 to 10 is often used. On this scale, 10 represents the most pain that could be experienced while conscious, and 0 represents no pain.
- The progression of analgesia. Analgesic therapy should start with the agents that have lower potency and addiction potential and progress to more potent agents.
- Agreements with regard to the responsibility of the patient for the pain medication and the responsibility of the physician to prescribe the medication. These are often in the form of a written contract, which is discussed in more detail later in this chapter.

ETIOLOGY OF PAIN

Visceral pain from internal organs is generally poorly localized and can be due to an underlying condition such as cancer. Chronic pain that is not caused by cancer is generally of two types: *somatic pain,* which arises by activation of the pain receptors in the skin and musculoskeletal tissue, and *neuropathic pain,* which is caused by a disease or injury to the peripheral nerves or their ganglia (groupings of nerve junctions) in the central nervous system.

Back problems and degenerative joint disease are common causes of somatic pain. Osteoporosis in elderly adults is often associated with collapsed vertebrae and stress fractures, which are acutely painful. Degenerative joint disease is readily apparent in many instances because of signs of local inflammation. More troublesome is diagnosis of fibromyalgia, a musculoskeletal disorder that has no clear diagnostic markers. Examples of neuropathic pain include pain resulting from a herpes eruption or diabetic complications and pain resulting from many other conditions that cause inflammation or degeneration of nerves.

INVESTIGATION OF CAUSES OF PAIN

A careful history of pain is crucial. This should include the history of the condition that is causing the pain, a record of all previous diagnostic procedures, the names of all previous treating practitioners, a determination of the level of the pain, and an understanding of how the pain interferes with the patient's quality of life. Pain is subjective. The physical examination is extremely important in making the diagnosis, but it cannot be relied on to determine the amount of pain that the patient is experiencing.

Chronic pain causes both physical and psychological limitations in the patient's ability to manage his or her daily activities. A careful psychological history should be taken, investigating for signs of depression; if these are found, the depression should also be treated. Although it is important to diagnose and treat the underlying cause of the pain, in many cases it is equally important to treat the pain itself even when the diagnosis remains in doubt. Early and aggressive treatment of pain reduces the patient's risk of developing a chronic pain syndrome.

ASSESSMENT OF PAIN

Pain needs to be assessed before a plan can be made for management. Considerable effort must be made to gather information on the type, location, and severity of the pain and its impact on the patient's ability to function and on the quality of life. Psychological, spiritual, social, and family histories are important in the assessment.

Because pain is subjective, the patient's assessment of the severity and quality of pain should be accepted. Family members tend to overestimate the pain of their loved ones, and health care providers tend to underestimate it. Nevertheless, insight is gained by including all parties in the evaluation. The observation of grimacing, wincing, limping, profuse sweating, hypertension, pallor, or tachycardia is useful but not diagnostic. In the end, the clinician must accept the patient's report of pain—pain is what the patient says it is.

Pain should be assessed for severity, for factors that ease the pain or make it worse, and for the timing and characteristics of the pain. The history should include any previous painful situations or diagnoses of painful conditions, recent attempts at cure, issues and concerns of substance abuse, and previous response to various methods of pain control. The patient's beliefs about the origin of the pain should be assessed and included in the history.

Other issues involve how the pain affects the patient and how the patient responds to pain. What makes the pain worse, and what improves it? Does it interfere with sleep? It is extremely important to assess the ways in which the pain interferes with activities of daily living, work, hobbies, and social roles. The relationship between high levels of pain and psychological illness should not be ignored in the assessment of the pain. Depression and anxiety can magnify the expression of pain. Quality-of-life assessment tools are useful in addressing physical well-being and underlying problems. Fatigue is almost universal as a symptom in pain patients.

Particular care should be taken when assessing patients unable to communicate well, including young infants and children, older adults, mentally incompetent patients, emotionally disturbed patients, and individuals who speak only a foreign language. Children may be reluctant to report pain for fear of undergoing further painful diagnostic procedures. Often agitation, fear, and other unusual symptoms are the only way these patients can express their pain. In some cases, agitated patients are given sedatives when their pain should be addressed instead.

Patients may fear becoming addicted to controlled substances, and many health care professionals reinforce that fear. A patient may fear being labeled a "problem patient" and so may not complain to his or her physician about pain or inadequate pain relief. Negative responses by health care providers may cause patients to describe their pain as less severe than what they actually feel.

Effective communication with the patient is crucial. The most common reason for unrelieved pain in the U.S. health care system is the failure of staff to assess pain and pain relief routinely and accurately. Many patients tolerate unrelieved pain silently, especially if they are not specifically asked about it. The key to delivering high-quality pain management is effective communication. All team members must consistently communicate changes in patient status and become aware of treatment plans. Patients and family members value effective communication and an individualized approach to pain management and palliative care. Even patients with severe pain report greater satisfaction with their pain management if they have had good communication with their physician and can experience a reduction, if not total relief, of pain.

PROGRESSIVE LEVELS OF PAIN RELIEF

The approach to treatment of pain may be considered in three steps: treatments for (1) mild, (2) moderate, and (3) severe pain. In some cases, topical therapies may be tried before oral medication. A heating pad or a warm bath in the morning may alleviate arthritic stiffness. A topical therapy such as Aspercreme, Ben-Gay, or a cream containing capsaicin, the compound made from chili peppers, may be applied locally. These substances, known as *counterirritants,* may sting locally when applied, but they can relieve some painful stimuli from musculoskeletal and arthritic conditions.

A general rule is that when pain increases, a sustained-release form of a narcotic may be administered by mouth, and a shorter acting "rescue drug" may be given for breakthrough pain between doses. Frequent use of the rescue drug should be noted; if it is necessary for the patient to take the rescue drug more than three or four times a day, a larger dose of the baseline sustained-action drug should be given. The usual dose of the short-acting drug should be equivalent to 5% to 15% of the 24-hour dose of the long-acting drug.

Patients should be told the name of the medication, and they should clearly understand how it is to be taken. If there are restrictions with regard to food or water or combining the pain reliever with other medications, these should be clearly explained. The side effects should be mentioned, and any concerns of the patient should be addressed. The patient should be encouraged to ask questions and to participate in his or her own care.

Adult dosages are provided for all drugs listed in this chapter. Pediatric dosages may be obtained in the respective chapters where the drugs are covered in more detail. All are oral doses unless otherwise specified.

MILD PAIN

Mild pain generally can be treated with acetaminophen, aspirin, a nonsteroidal anti-inflammatory drug (NSAID), or a nonopioid analgesic. Unless contraindicated, any regimen should include one of these mild analgesics for baseline analgesia, even when pain is severe enough to require the addition of an opioid. Parenteral and rectal forms of some of these agents are available if the patient is unable to take oral medications.

The potential for gastric ulcer formation needs to be considered with the NSAIDs. The addition of misoprostol or a proton pump inhibitor may be considered. Aspirin may cause bleeding tendencies.

DRUGS FOR MILD PAIN

acetaminophen (Tylenol)

Dosage: (Oral, Rectal) Up to 3 to 4 gm/day in divided doses.

aspirin

Dosage: (Oral, Rectal) Up to 3 or 4 gm/day in divided doses.

celecoxib (Celebrex)

Dosage: (Oral) Up to 400 mg/day.

diflunisal (Dolobid)
Dosage: (Oral) Up to 1500 mg/day in divided doses.

etodolac (Lodine)
Dosage: (Oral) Up to 1000 mg/day.

ibuprofen (Advil, Motrin)
Dosage: (Oral) Up to 2400 mg/day.

indomethacin (Indocin)
Dosage: (Oral) Up to 200 mg/day.

ketorolac tromethamine (Toradol)
Dosage: (Oral, IM, IV) Up to 120 mg/day. Limit treatment to 5 days.

naproxen sodium (Anaprox, Naprosyn)
Dosage: (Oral) Up to 1650 mg/day.

sulindac (Clinoril)
Dosage: (Oral) Up to 400 mg/day.

MODERATE PAIN

Short-acting agents for relief of moderate pain may be administered alone or in combination with a nonopioid analgesic as pain increases. Agents in this class are also used when breakthrough pain occurs, or the patient may need step-up therapy using all stronger analgesics. Starting dosages are given in most instances, which may be increased.

DRUGS FOR MODERATE PAIN

codeine sulfate, combined
Dosage: (Oral) 30 to 200 mg every 3 to 4 hours.

hydrocodone bitartrate, combined (Lorcet Plus, Vicodin). Vicodin contains 5 mg/500 mg hydrocodone and acetaminophen. Lorcet Plus has 7.5 mg/650 mg hydrocodone and acetaminophen.
Dosage: (Oral) One to two tablets every 3 to 4 hours.

hydrocodone bitartrate and ibuprofen (Vicoprofen). This combination tablet contains 7.5 mg hydrocodone and 200 mg ibuprofen.
Dosage: (Oral) One tablet every 4 to 6 hours. Maximum 5 tablets a day.

oxycodone hydrochloride, combined (Percocet, Percodan). Percodan has 4.8 mg/324 mg oxycodone and aspirin. Percocet is available in 2.5 mg/325 mg, 5 mg/325 mg, 7.5 mg/325 mg, 7.5 mg/500 mg, 10 mg/325 mg, and 10 mg/650 mg oxycodone and acetaminophen.
Dosage: (Oral) 5 mg every 3 to 4 hours.

pentazocine (Talwin)
Dosage: (Oral, IM) 50 mg every 4 hours.

tapentadol (Nucynta)
Dosage: (Oral) 50 to 100 mg every 4 to 6 hours.

tramadol hydrochloride (Ultram)
Dosage: (Oral) 50 to 100 mg every 4 to 6 hours up to 400 mg/day.

SEVERE PAIN

Some agents for severe pain may need to be administered parenterally. Dosages are given for the beginning range used when these medications become necessary. Tolerance may bring the dosages well above the levels listed if the medications are used for a prolonged period. Milder analgesics are often continued with these drugs, and the use of shorter acting moderate pain drugs for breakthrough pain is often necessary as well.

DRUGS FOR SEVERE PAIN

butorphanol (Stadol)
Dosage: (IV) 1 to 2 mg; (IM) 2 to 4 mg; (Nasal Spray) 1 mg delivered per spray.

fentanyl citrate (Actiq, Duragesic)
Dosage: (Topical patch) 25 to 100 mcg/hr, patch applied every 72 hours; (IM, Slow IV) 50 to 100 mcg every 3 to 4 hours; (Oral) Lozenge, 0.2 to 1.6 mg; (Intranasal Spray) 50 to 200 mcg per spray every 48 hours.

hydromorphone hydrochloride (Dilaudid)
Dosage: (Oral) 7.5 mg every 3 to 4 hours; (Parenteral) 1.5 mg every 3 hours.

levorphanol tartrate (Levo-Dromoran)
Dosage: (Oral) 4 mg four times daily; (Parenteral) 2 mg every 6 hours.

meperidine hydrochloride (Demerol)
Dosage: (Oral) 100 to 150 mg every 3 to 4 hours; limit use to 1 to 2 days; (IV) 50 to 75 mg every 3 to 4 hours.

methadone hydrochloride (Dolophine)
Dosage: (Oral, Parenteral) 10 to 20 mg every 6 hours.

morphine sulfate
Dosage: (Oral) 30 to 60 mg every 3 to 4 hours; (IV) 2 to 10 mg every 4 to 6 hours.

morphine sulfate controlled-release (Kadian, MS Contin, Oramorph SR)
Dosage: (Oral) 30 to 60 mg every 12 hours.

morphine sulfate and naltrexone (Embeda). Three extended-release strengths are available: 20 mg/0.8 mg, 30 mg/1.2 mg, and 50 mg/2.6 mg morphine extended-release and naltrexone.
Dosage: (Oral) Individualize dose every 12 to 24 hours.

nalbuphine (Nubain)
Dosage: (IM, IV, Subcut) 10 mg every 4 hours.

oxycodone (OxyContin, OxyFAST, OxyIR)
Dosage: (Oral) 2.5 to 20 mg every 12 hours; dosage may be increased greatly according to needs.

oxymorphone hydrochloride (Numorphan)
Dosage: (Parenteral) 0.5 mg every 3 to 4 hours.

OPIATES AND OPIOIDS

As discussed in Chapter 12, an opioid is a synthetic drug made to imitate opium derivatives; examples include meperidine, hydromorphone, and oxycodone. Morphine, codeine, and papaverine are opium derivatives and correctly termed *opiates*. However, most narcotics currently in use are synthetic in part or whole, so for convenience we use the term *opioids* to discuss the narcotic drugs. Unless stated otherwise, it should be assumed that the opiate characteristics are identical to the characteristics discussed for opioids.

EQUIVALENT DOSES OF OPIOIDS

For comparison purposes, the oral doses of opioids that are equivalent to a dose of 10 mg of morphine administered by the IM route are shown in Table 13-1.

Table 13-1 Doses of Various Opioids That Are Equivalent to Morphine 10 mg Intramuscularly

Drug	Equivalent Dose
ORAL ANALGESICS	
morphine	60 mg
codeine	200 mg
hydrocodone	40 mg
hydromorphone	7.5 mg
levorphanol	4 mg
meperidine	300 mg
methadone	20 mg
oxycodone	30 mg
TRANSDERMAL EQUIVALENT	
fentanyl	25-mcg patch equivalent to 45-135 mg/day of oral morphine

LONG-TERM EFFECTS OF OPIOIDS

Early in the process of analgesia, severe pain seems to counteract the sedative effects of opioids. Tolerance develops to the sedating effects of opioids, but the mechanism for developing dose-related tolerance when these agents are used for analgesia is more poorly understood. The need for dosage increases develops more slowly when the drugs are given for true pain relief than when they are taken by addicts for the euphoria effect. There is no true ceiling or maximum dose for opioids. Extremely large doses may be necessary to relieve severe pain.

Physical dependence is a condition in which the patient requires continued use of a drug for proper functioning and would experience withdrawal symptoms if it were discontinued. It is a physiologic phenomenon that occurs following regular use of opioids for more than 2 weeks and should be expected. Physical dependence also occurs after administration of steroids or of beta blockers and other antihypertensive drugs for an extended period. This condition is not to be considered the same as drug addiction, which is generally driven by a desire for the euphoria associated with the drug and may involve criminal behavior.

The fear of opioid addiction should not be a primary concern when implementing appropriate therapy for acute pain and cancer pain. However, individuals attempt to obtain opioids for illegal use by trying to pass themselves off as patients with legitimate need. The use of drug screens, looking for appropriate levels of the prescribed drug and for other illegal agents, may assist in identifying these individuals.

Pseudoaddiction is a term that has been used to describe the drug-seeking behaviors that may occur when a patient's pain is undertreated. Patients may "clock watch," may become focused on obtaining medication, and may otherwise seem to be inappropriately "drug seeking." This behavior resolves when the pain is adequately treated.

Many patients with acute pain are anxious but are calmed when the pain is relieved with analgesics. Antianxiety agents may be necessary as adjunctive medication.

Withdrawal (a syndrome that occurs when a drug-dependent person discontinues the drug suddenly) must be prevented and can be avoided if drugs are tapered gradually. The time course of the withdrawal symptoms is a function of the half-life of the opioid. With drugs with a short half-life, such as morphine and hydromorphone, the symptoms may appear in 6 to 12 hours and peak at 24 to 72 hours. With drugs with a longer half-life, such as methadone and levorphanol, symptoms may be delayed for several days and are generally less severe. A clonidine patch may decrease symptoms of withdrawal. The dose is 0.1 to 0.3 mg/24 hours, and the patch is applied once every 7 days.

SIDE EFFECTS OF OPIOIDS

Respiratory depression is an adverse effect of opioids, particularly with higher doses. Precautions should be taken against combining opioids with other sedating drugs or alcohol.

Opioids may cause constipation, sleepiness, dry mouth, nausea, and vomiting. To manage constipation, the patient should be instructed to drink several 8-oz glasses of fluid per day and eat foods high in fiber, such as beans, lentils, and dried or fresh fruits. A stool softener should be given routinely when the patient requires daily opioids. Senna tablets or other laxatives may become necessary and should be taken as needed. Antihistamines, such as over-the-counter cold preparations, are additives for the sleepiness and dry mouth side effects and should be avoided if possible. Alternatively, the side effects should be anticipated and managed. Except in unusual cases, the nausea and vomiting associated with opioid therapy generally go away within a short time.

NEUROPATHIC PAIN

Neuropathic pain is burning or shooting pain that is usually caused by nerve injury or dysfunction from disease or trauma. Causes of neuropathic pain include diabetes, postherpetic neuralgia, phantom limb pain after limb amputation, trigeminal neuralgia, and spinal cord injury pain, but neuropathic pain can occur as a progressive condition in older adults without diabetes or other known causes of the neuropathy. Some drugs, when taken for long periods, have been implicated in causing neuropathic pain.

Neuropathic pain often begins with pain in lower extremities, the pain ascends, and then the extremities become numb. Individuals may lose proprioception (the unconscious perception of bodily movement and spatial orientation) without realizing it at first and then have difficulty walking on narrow platforms such as steps, docks, or boats; they may fall because of missteps. Individuals with neuropathic pain may have trouble driving because of decreased ability to distinguish the gas pedal from the brake pedal. In treating this type of pain, any analgesic agent may be used, but the following are particularly effective.

gabapentin (Neurontin)

Dosage: Adults: (Oral) 100 to 300 mg every 4 to 6 hours to a maximum of 3600 mg/day.

lidocaine patches 5% (Lidoderm)

Dosage: Adults: (Topical) Up to three patches applied to the painful area for up to 12 hours in a 24-hour period.

pregabalin (Lyrica)

Dosage: Adults: (Oral) 50 mg three times daily to a maximum of 600 mg/day.

DEPRESSION AND PAIN

There is a strong association between chronic pain and depression. Serotonin and norepinephrine, the neurotransmitters associated with depression, play key roles in the modulation of pain. Depressive symptoms have been shown to coincide with the development of chronic musculoskeletal pain. Somatic symptoms of depression in patients with chronic pain include change in appetite, change in weight, loss of energy, motor retardation, and sleep disturbance. Predictors of depression in patients with chronic pain may be the frequency that severe pain is experienced, functional disability, the number of painful areas in the body, and poor coping ability and problem solving.

Tricyclic antidepressants seem to be most effective when combined with pain medications. Selective serotonin reuptake inhibitors (i.e., fluoxetine, paroxetine, citalopram) are much less effective.

COANALGESICS

A **coanalgesic** is any of a group of drugs that may be used to enhance pain relief. Numerous other classes of drugs may be used to increase the effects of opioids or NSAIDs, and some may have independent analgesic properties as well.

ANTICONVULSANT DRUGS

Examples: carbamazepine, gabapentin, lamotrigine, oxcarbazepine, phenytoin, sodium valproate, tiagabine, and topiramate.

Anticonvulsant drugs reduce the spontaneous "firing" of central motor neurons that causes seizures. This finding led researchers to note that these agents also decreased spontaneous firing of sensory neurons associated with pain. They are useful in the treatment of various painful conditions and some psychiatric conditions. They are discussed in more detail in Chapter 12.

BENZODIAZEPINES

Examples: clonazepam, diazepam, and lorazepam.

These tranquilizers may be useful for treating anxiety. They are discussed more completely in Chapter 14.

GLUCOCORTICOIDS

Examples: dexamethasone and prednisone.

Glucocorticoids have many concurrent uses in pain management. They may relieve nerve or spinal cord compression by reducing edema in tumor and nerve tissue. They may produce euphoria and increase appetite in severely ill patients. Long-term use produces weight gain, cushingoid appearance, osteoporosis, myopathy, and psychosis. When therapy is discontinued, glucocorticoids should be gradually withdrawn rather than abruptly stopped. These agents are discussed in more detail in Chapter 18.

LOCAL ANESTHETICS

Examples: capsaicin and lidocaine.

Topical lidocaine patches and nerve blocks have been used extensively in management of acute pain. Epidural and IV infusions of local anesthetics may be useful acutely but not for ongoing therapy. They are discussed in Chapter 12. Capsaicin is found in hot peppers. When applied topically in an ointment formulation, it relieves neuropathic pain and arthritic pain. These nonprescription formulations may be useful as adjunctive therapy.

AGENTS USED FOR METASTATIC BONE PAIN

Examples: bisphosphonates and radiotherapy.

Pamidronate disodium (Aredia) inhibits reduction of bone mass and has been shown to reduce skeletal complications such as pathologic fractures in metastatic bone lesions. It is administered as an IV infusion. Radiation of widespread bony metastases may be performed for pain relief, or targeted therapy may be performed with localized radiation using a radioactive isotope such as strontium, which may be taken up by the bony metastasis.

SKELETAL MUSCLE RELAXANTS

Examples: carisoprodol, cyclobenzaprine, and orphenadrine.

These agents may be useful in preventing pain from muscle spasms. They are sedating and may have anticholinergic side effects as well.

SPINAL CORD STIMULATOR IMPLANT AND INTRATHECAL PUMP IMPLANT

For many patients, a spinal cord stimulator is the best option for the control of pain. This implant uses small electrical pulses that are able to interfere with the nerve impulses that are ascending with pain sensations. It is usually used when pain is chronic and long-lasting and other methods have failed.

The intrathecal pump is a specialized device that delivers a concentrated amount of medication into the spinal cord through a catheter. It delivers medication around-the-clock and eliminates or diminishes breakthrough pain. In addition to cancer pain, this device is useful in the treatment of spastic disorders such as multiple sclerosis or spinal cord injuries associated with muscle spasms.

TRICYCLIC ANTIDEPRESSANTS

Examples: amitriptyline, desipramine, doxepin, imipramine, and nortriptyline.

These agents are used for treatment of neuropathic pain and for their antidepressant activity. Use of these agents alone is generally ineffective; they should be combined with other analgesics. Anticholinergic effects, such as dry mouth, urinary retention, constipation, sedation, and orthostatic hypotension, must be considered as potential side effects. Administration of these agents at bedtime may promote a better night's sleep and may minimize daytime side effects. They are discussed in more detail in Chapter 14.

PATIENT MEDICATION USE AGREEMENT

A written agreement made between the prescriber and the patient has become a useful tool in pain management. It has been found that a written agreement reinforces the serious nature of the patient's condition and points out the consequences if the patient does not comply with the agreed-on goals and conditions for long-term pain management. These agreements are generally written by the prescribing physician according to the needs of his or her practice and may include the statements shown in Figure 13-1.

Informed consent is an essential part of the documentation. These agreements are particularly recommended for patients with a history of substance abuse and patients receiving higher doses of opioids.

Random drug testing may not be necessary for every patient, but it may be extremely helpful for patients at risk for drug diversion activities or whose behavior seems unusual. Drug testing confirms that the patient is taking the medications prescribed and is not taking other controlled or illegal substances. Before discussing unusual drug test results with the patient, it may be helpful to speak to the laboratory technician to confirm the proper interpretation of the results. Drug testing techniques must follow acceptable standards to avoid mismanagement of samples.

****

Medication Agreement

1. I, _______________ understand that I have pain that has not been adequately controlled, and I understand that the purpose of pain management will be to relieve the pain. I understand that it may not be possible for the complete elimination of the painful condition.

2. I understand that the pain medication will only be prescribed by _________________ on the agreed upon schedule. I will not seek pain medication from any other practitioner, and will not take other medications without the knowledge and permission of _______________ .

3. Medication refills will be provided as written prescriptions only. No refills will be given prior to the next scheduled appointment date. No-show appointments may be cause for terminating the agreement. Forged or altered prescriptions, or diversion of the medications to any other person, will be cause for terminating the agreement.

4. Lost or stolen medications will not be replaced under any circumstances. It is my responsibility to secure my medication.

5. If recommended to see another specialist or take some other form of therapy, I understand it is my obligation to cooperate with these endeavors.

6. I agree to undergo random drug testing whenever it is requested.

7. I agree to fill my prescriptions only at the following pharmacy: ______________________ , address ___________________ . If I change pharmacies for any reason I will call the health care provider's office and inform him or her. I understand I cannot use more than one pharmacy at any one time. A copy of this agreement will be given to the pharmacist.

8. I understand that this agreement may be terminated if I am no longer receiving a reasonable therapeutic benefit from the medication, or if it is determined that I am no longer a good candidate to receive the medication.

9. I understand that by signing this agreement I must abide by the rules stated above and that failure to abide by these agreements will result in the possible termination of services from my health care provider.

(Patient)______________________________

Date_________________________________

(Health Care Provider)_________________

****

FIGURE 13-1 Sample medication use agreement.

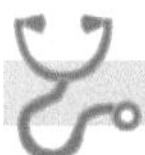

Clinical Implications

1. All members of the health care team are important when assessing a patient's pain and his or her response to medication.
2. Negative personal opinions concerning patients taking medications for chronic pain must be avoided.
3. Concurrent conditions such as depression or anxiety may need to be treated separately.
4. Apparent drug-seeking behavior may occur as a result of inadequate pain control rather than addictive behavior.
5. The use of analgesic medications should be progressive in nature, beginning with milder analgesics and moving to stronger agents as the severity of pain increases.
6. The patient should be encouraged to talk about his or her pain, including whether or not it is satisfactorily relieved, and should be taught to evaluate pain on a scale of 0 to 10.
7. A realistic goal for therapy is essential for a patient with chronic pain.
8. Patients should become familiar with the names of their medications, their actions, and their potential for side effects.
9. The patient may require a frank discussion of the differences between addictive use of opioids, generated by a search for euphoria, and the use of these agents for pain relief.
10. Physical dependence on an opioid may occur if it is used for more than 2 weeks; this is an expected effect and is not a matter of concern when treating chronic pain.
11. When an agent is discontinued, a gradual decrease in dosage minimizes withdrawal symptoms.
12. Methods of guarding against abuse of the opioids may include a medication use agreement and periodic drug testing.

CRITICAL THINKING QUESTIONS

1. A patient appears chronically ill and requests pain medication. He is pale and diaphoretic and was observed to be favoring his left leg when walking in. What questions would be important in the initial evaluation of his painful condition?
2. A patient is nervous and distracted and cannot answer most of the questions about his medical history. What additional considerations may be made with regard to his treatment?
3. A patient comes in with a grocery bag of medications. You notice there are many herbal remedies, cold products, antihistamines, and medications from several physicians. How would you approach this medical history?
4. A patient strongly resists a standard drug test as part of his medication agreement. He feels this means he is not trustworthy. How would you counsel him?

REVIEW QUESTIONS

1. A patient who watches the clock for each dose of pain medication may be:
   - **a.** a definite drug addict.
   - **b.** overtreated with pain medication.
   - **c.** undertreated with pain medication.
   - **d.** ignored.

2. With regard to an objective assessment of a patient's pain, the health care professional often:
   - **a.** overestimates the pain.
   - **b.** underestimates the pain.
   - **c.** needs the scale of 0 to 10 to assess the pain.
   - **d.** is totally accurate in her or his assessment.

3. An agent that may be given for mild pain is:
   - **a.** morphine.
   - **b.** codeine.
   - **c.** ibuprofen.
   - **d.** fentanyl.

4. A narcotic that can be given by the transdermal route is:
   - **a.** pentazocine.
   - **b.** ketorolac.
   - **c.** codeine.
   - **d.** fentanyl.

5. A dose of oral oxycodone that is equivalent to 10 mg of morphine intramuscularly is:
   - **a.** 10 mg.
   - **b.** 20 mg.
   - **c.** 30 mg.
   - **d.** 60 mg.

6. A coanalgesic is an agent that:
   - **a.** can be used instead of narcotics for relief of severe pain.
   - **b.** is responsible for codependency.
   - **c.** can be used to make the patient cooperate with pain relief.
   - **d.** can be used to potentiate pain relief.

7. A mechanism that helps avoid inappropriate use of or dependence on narcotics is:
   - **a.** the use of a medication agreement between the patient and physician.
   - **b.** periodic drug testing.
   - **c.** the use of only one pharmacy for prescriptions.
   - **d.** all of the above.

8. The person best qualified to assess the patient's pain is the:
   - **a.** patient.
   - **b.** health care professional.
   - **c.** family.
   - **d.** physician.

9. An agent that may be used for short-term breakthrough pain when a patient is already receiving a long-acting narcotic is:
   - **a.** Tylenol.
   - **b.** hydrocodone.
   - **c.** OxyContin.
   - **d.** rofecoxib.

10. An agent that is often necessary when a patient is receiving daily opioids is:
    - **a.** a laxative.
    - **b.** an antidiarrheal agent.
    - **c.** an antihistamine.
    - **d.** an anticholinergic agent.

Answers to the review questions can be found at the back of the book.

evolve Additional questions and activities can be found at *http://evolve.elsevier.com/asperheim/pharmacology*.

Tranquilizers and Antidepressants

CHAPTER 14

Objectives

After completing this chapter, you should be able to do the following:

1. Become familiar with the conditions for which tranquilizers and antidepressants are used.
2. Become familiar with the various types of drugs used to treat psychiatric disorders.
3. Distinguish between a monoamine oxidase inhibitor and a tricyclic antidepressant, and give two examples of each type.
4. Discuss adverse effects of the phenothiazine type of antipsychotic drugs.
5. Discuss important uses for the phenothiazine type of antipsychotic agents.
6. List indications for the temporary use of tranquilizers.
7. List the symptoms of a major depressive disorder.
8. Summarize important responsibilities of the health care professional for the administration of monoamine oxidase inhibitors.
9. Summarize important responsibilities of the health care professional for the administration of antidepressants.

Key Terms

Antidepressant (ăn-tī-dē-PRĔS-ănt), p. 133
Anxiolytic (ĂNGK-sē-ō-LĬT-ĭk) **agents,** p. 136
Depression, p. 133
Monoamine oxidase inhibitors (MAOIs), p. 134
Sedatives, p. 129
Selective serotonin reuptake inhibitors (SSRIs) (SĔR-ē-TŌ-nĭn rē-ŬP-tāk), p. 133
Selective serotonin and norepinephrine reuptake inhibitors (SNRIs), p. 134
Tranquilizers (TRĂNG-kwĕ-LĪZ-ĕrs), p. 130

Many agents have become available for the temporary and long-term treatment of psychosomatic and mental illnesses. The most satisfactory management would be aimed at the prevention of these disorders, but achieving this goal would be difficult for many and varied reasons. Until we provide a happy, peaceful environment for ourselves and our offspring, devoid of practices that lead to emotional trauma and instability, many emotional and mental disorders will persist. The religious, socioeconomic, educational, and political factors involved in rectifying the basic problems are so numerous and complicated that progress in the prevention campaign will undoubtedly be very slow. A much more practical solution would be to learn to adjust to our problems and difficulties rather than constantly seeking to be rid of them.

As research continues in the field of mental illness, more information is obtained about the direct effect of hormone levels on the brain and the mood of the individual. This research has led to the development of many new drugs that are known to function by altering brain chemistry.

Psychotherapy and psychoanalysis, with or without concomitant drug therapy, have been used to help patients uncover the underlying issues associated with their thoughts and behaviors. Electroconvulsive shock therapy may still be used for selected patients who do not respond to pharmacologic agents.

Among the first drugs used for these illnesses were simple **sedatives,** which served to calm or quiet nervous excitement and sometimes induced sleep. The treatment was merely a symptomatic approach, however, for it did nothing to remove the conditions causing the illness in the first place, and it did not help the patient to adjust to the circumstances.

TRANQUILIZERS

Tranquilizers were developed to calm or tranquilize individuals without making them too sedated to perform activities of daily living. There are several categories of tranquilizers based on their mechanism of action.

BENZODIAZEPINES

Benzodiazepines are mid-level anxiolytics and sedatives. They have a relatively low abuse potential and are not highly toxic in overdose.

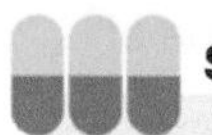

Special Considerations
Benzodiazepines

Benzodiazepines are metabolized through the cytochrome P-450 (CYP) 3A isoenzyme. Clearance of these drugs is inhibited by grapefruit, some calcium channel blockers, macrolide antibiotics, selective serotonin reuptake inhibitors (SSRIs), and human immunodeficiency virus (HIV) protease inhibitors. Concurrent use of these agents may produce a relative overdose of benzodiazepines.

alprazolam (Xanax). Alprazolam should be used only for the short-term relief of panic attacks and other anxiety disorders. More than the other agents in this class, alprazolam is very habit-forming, and continued use should be periodically evaluated. The efficacy of use longer than 4 months has not been evaluated. It is preferable to transfer to other, less limiting benzodiazepines when possible. Alprazolam should be withdrawn gradually to prevent withdrawal symptoms.
Dosage: Adults only: (Oral) 0.25 to 3 mg three times daily.

chlordiazepoxide hydrochloride, USP-NF, BP (Librium). Chlordiazepoxide is indicated when fear, anxiety, and other emotional upsets complicate the medical picture. In low oral doses, it is effective in mild to moderate anxiety and tension, although with the advent of shorter acting benzodiazepines, its use has declined. It is regulated by the Controlled Substances Act. Drowsiness, confusion, and ataxia (impaired coordination) have been reported in some patients after administration of this drug, but such effects can be avoided in almost all instances by proper dosage control.
Dosage: Adults: (Oral) 5 to 25 mg three to four times daily.
Children older than 6 years: (Oral) 5 to 10 mg two to four times daily.

clorazepate dipotassium (Tranxene). Clorazepate is used in the treatment of mild anxiety and tension states. It is not recommended for severely depressed or psychotic patients. Side effects include dizziness, nervousness, headache, ataxia, dry mouth, skin rashes, and decreases in blood pressure. The possibility of dependence must be considered when this agent is prescribed for a long period.
Dosage: Adults: (Oral) 7.5 mg four times daily.
Children: Dosage has not been established.

diazepam, USP-NF, BP (Valium). Diazepam is useful in the treatment of anxiety reactions stemming from stressful circumstances or whenever illness is complicated by emotional factors. It may be given to patients in psychoneurotic states manifested by anxiety, tension, fear, and fatigue and to patients in acute agitation resulting from alcohol withdrawal. It seems to be useful in the alleviation of muscle spasms associated with cerebral palsy and athetosis. It is of little use in psychotic patients. Diazepam has a tendency to be habit-forming. Side effects include drowsiness, nausea, dizziness, blurred vision, headache, incontinence, slurred speech, and skin rash. It is contraindicated for infants, patients with a history of convulsive disorders, and patients with glaucoma.
Dosage: Adults: (Oral, IM, IV) 2 to 10 mg two to three times daily.
Children: (Oral, IM, IV) 0.12 to 0.8 mg/kg/day in three to four divided doses.

flurazepam hydrochloride (Dalmane). Flurazepam hydrochloride is used as a hypnotic and is administered at bedtime.
Dosage: Adults only: (Oral) 15 to 30 mg at bedtime.

lorazepam (Ativan). Lorazepam is used to manage anxiety disorders.
Dosage: Adults only: (Oral) 1 to 10 mg divided two to three times daily or 2 to 6 mg at bedtime only; (IM) 0.05 mg/kg by deep IM injection before surgery.

midazolam hydrochloride (Versed). Midazolam is generally given parenterally and is used for procedural sedation. It may be given orally, intramuscularly, or by IV infusion.
Dosage: Adults: (Oral, IM) 2 to 3 mg before surgery; (IV) As infusion, 1.5 mg over 2 minutes, then titrated further to a total dosage of 5 mg.
Children: (IV) As infusion in dose of 50 to 100 mcg/kg to a total dose of 600 mcg/kg.

oxazepam. Oxazepam is often used for alcohol withdrawal and anxiety disorders.
Dosage: Adults only: (Oral) 10 to 15 mg three to four times daily.

temazepam (Restoril). Temazepam is used for short-term treatment of insomnia.
Dosage: Adults only: (Oral) 7.5 to 30 mg at bedtime.

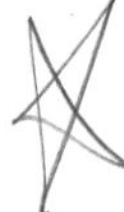

triazolam (Halcion). Triazolam is used as a hypnotic for short-term treatment of insomnia.
Dosage: Adults only: (Oral) 0.125 to 0.5 mg at bedtime.

ANTIPSYCHOTICS

PHENOTHIAZINES

Phenothiazines generally are used for symptomatic management of more severe psychiatric disorders.

chlorpromazine hydrochloride, USP-NF, BP (Thorazine). The quieting, relaxing effect of this drug was quickly appreciated, and it has been used extensively. It shows great tranquilizing effects in severe emotional upsets, in conditions characterized by hyperactivity and agitation, and in certain types of schizophrenia. The important feature of chlorpromazine and similar agents is that they make the patient more amenable to psychotherapy. Treatment may be all but impossible because of the inability even to communicate with the patient, much less reason with him or her, but on administration of the drug the patient is able to discuss problems and fears in a calm and sensible manner.

Chlorpromazine is useful in alleviating nausea and vomiting caused by certain conditions such as carcinoma, acute infections, radiation sickness, ingestion of certain drugs (e.g., nitrogen mustard), and postoperative effects. Possible side effects include tachycardia, hypothermia, dryness of the mouth, parkinsonism, jaundice, liver damage, blood dyscrasias, and rashes.
Dosage: Adults: (Oral, IM, IV) 200 to 600 mg/day in one to four divided doses.
Children: (Oral, IM) 0.5 to 1 mg/kg every 6 hours.

fluphenazine hydrochloride, USP-NF, BP (Prolixin). Fluphenazine hydrochloride, a structural derivative of the phenothiazine agents, may be administered orally or intramuscularly to relieve agitation associated with schizophrenia. This agent has a slight increase in extrapyramidal side effects compared with earlier phenothiazines. Sedation, nausea, polyuria (excreting large amounts of urine), headache, glaucoma, and urinary and fecal retention occur with use.
Dosage: Adults and children older than 12 years: (Oral) 0.5 to 10 mg daily in three to four divided doses; (IM) 2.5 to 10 mg in three to four divided doses. For prolonged therapy, the decanoate salt may be given every 2 to 4 weeks.

prochlorperazine maleate, USP-NF, BP (Compazine). Although effective as a tranquilizing agent, prochlorperazine maleate is rarely used for long-term therapy because of a high incidence of extrapyramidal symptoms such as gait disturbances, restlessness, and aberrations in muscle contraction. Occasionally, opisthotonos occurs even on the first dose of this drug, with arching of the back, inability to speak, and loss of muscle control. This reaction has been confused with a certain type of epileptic seizure but is seen to differ from it on close observation. This drug is used primarily for its antinauseant effects, particularly postoperatively. It may be given orally, intramuscularly, or rectally.
Dosage: Adults: (Oral, IM, IV) 5 to 10 mg three to four times daily; (Rectal) 25 mg two times daily.
Children 2 to 12 years: (Oral, Rectal) 2.5 mg every 8 to 12 hours; (IM) 0.13 mg/kg/dose.

trifluoperazine hydrochloride, USP-NF, BP (Stelazine). Trifluoperazine hydrochloride is also chemically quite similar to chlorpromazine, but it is more potent and can be given in lower doses. Lower doses are given to outpatients; higher doses are usually reserved for hospitalized patients.
Dosage: Adults: (Oral, IM) 1 to 10 mg twice daily.
Children older than 6 years: (Oral) 1 mg one to two times daily.

thioridazine hydrochloride, USP-NF, BP (Mellaril). The wide range of doses available with thioridazine makes it useful as an antipsychotic drug for patients who fail to respond to other agents. It should be avoided in patients who have cardiac problems and should not be used with other drugs that prolong the Q–T interval. Life-threatening arrhythmias have occurred.
Dosage: Adults: (Oral) 20 to 800 mg/day in divided doses.
Children: (Oral) 0.25 mg/kg four times daily.

NONPHENOTHIAZINES

aripiprazole (Abilify). Aripiprazole is used to treat schizophrenia. It should be used with caution in combination with other centrally acting drugs. It is not a controlled substance.
Dosage: Adults: (Oral) 15 to 30 mg once daily.

haloperidol, USP-NF, BP (Haldol). This phenothiazine derivative is primarily used to treat schizophrenia. Side effects resemble those of fluphenazine.
Dosage: Adults: (Oral) 0.5 to 5 mg two to three times daily; (IM) 2 to 5 mg. Additional doses may be administered every 30 to 60 minutes until control is obtained.
Children: Dosage has not been established.

haloperidol decanoate (Haldol). This injectable form of haloperidol is used for long-term parenteral treatment of schizophrenia and psychotic states. After IM injection, there is a slow and sustained release of the medication, with plasma concentration reaching a peak after 6 days from the time of the injection. The half-life is about 3 weeks.
Dosage: Adults: (IM) 50 to 100 mg every 4 weeks.

loxapine (Loxitane)
Dosage: Adults: (Oral) 20 to 100 mg daily in two to four divided doses.

molindone hydrochloride (Moban)
Dosage: Adults: (Oral) 50 to 100 mg daily in divided doses.

olanzapine (Zyprexa)
Dosage: Adults: (Oral) 5 to 20 mg daily; (IM) 2.5 to 10 mg every 2 to 4 hours as necessary to a maximum of 30 mg/day.

pimozide (Orap)
Dosage: Adults: (Oral) 7 to 10 mg/day at bedtime.
Children: (Oral) 2 to 4 mg/day at bedtime.

quetiapine fumarate (Seroquel)
Dosage: Adults: (Oral) 25 mg twice daily to a maximum of 800 mg daily.

risperidone (Risperdal)
Dosage: Adults: (Oral) 1 mg twice daily to a maximum of 8 mg daily.

thiothixene, USP-NF, BP (Navane)
Dosage: Adults: (Oral) 2 mg three times daily to a total of 15 mg/day; (IM) 4 mg two to four times daily.

OTHER SEDATING AGENTS

eszopiclone (Lunesta). Eszopiclone is a hypnotic agent that has a rapid onset of action. It should be taken just before going to bed or after the patient has gone to bed and is having difficulty going to sleep. Common adverse effects include an unpleasant taste in the mouth, headache, and dry mouth.
Dosage: Adults: (Oral) 1 to 3 mg at bedtime.

hydroxyzine hydrochloride, USP-NF, BP (Atarax, Vistaril). This drug is an antihistaminelike agent that is used to manage anxiety and tension and to treat pruritic dermatologic conditions. It is quite effective as an antipruritic agent.
Dosage: Adults: (Oral, IM) 25 to 100 mg three to four times daily.
Children: (Oral) 50 mg daily in divided doses; (IM) 0.5 mg/kg every 6 hours.

lithium carbonate, USP-NF, BP (Eskalith, Lithane, Lithonate). Lithium carbonate has been found to be highly effective in the control of bipolar disorder. Although the exact mechanism of action is unknown, it is believed to alter the metabolism of norepinephrine in the brain. The full effect of this drug is not seen until after 6 to 10 days of treatment; other pharmacologic agents with a more rapid onset of action are often prescribed with lithium in the early phase of treatment. Serum lithium levels should be measured frequently to avoid toxic levels of this drug. Fine hand tremor, polyuria, thirst, nausea, and diarrhea are seen at therapeutic levels of this agent. At toxic levels, serious neurologic and cardiovascular effects are seen. Table 14-1 lists drugs that interact with lithium.
Dosage: Adults and children older than 12 years: (Oral) Initially 600 mg three times daily, then reduced to 300 mg three times daily.
Children 6 to 12 years: (Oral) 15 to 60 mg/kg/day in three to four divided doses.
Children under 6 years: Not recommended.

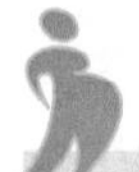

Considerations for Pregnant and Nursing Women

Lithium

Lithium can cause fetal toxicity when administered to pregnant women. Administration of lithium to pregnant and nursing women is appropriate only in life-threatening situations or with severe disease for which safer drugs are ineffective. When possible, lithium should be withdrawn for at least the first trimester. Monitor serum lithium concentrations carefully during pregnancy.

Table 14-1 Drug Interactions with Lithium

Drug	Effect on Lithium Level	Management
Thiazide diuretics	Increased	Monitor, adjust dosage
NSAIDs	Increased	Monitor, adjust dosage
ACE inhibitors	Increased	Monitor, adjust dosage
Calcium channel blockers	Increased or decreased	Monitor, adjust dosage

ACE, Angiotensin-converting enzyme; *NSAIDs,* nonsteroidal anti-inflammatory drugs.

meprobamate, USP-NF, BP. Meprobamate has a depressant effect on the transmission of nerve impulses inside the spinal cord and possibly in certain areas of the brain. It has a relaxant action on the skeletal muscles because of this depressant action. It is effective as a tranquilizer in moderately tense and anxious patients. Side effects are rare and minor; they include skin eruptions, fever, chills, weakness of skeletal muscles, and occasionally a decrease in blood pressure. There is a mild addiction with prolonged use of this drug, but withdrawal effects are minimal if the drug is tapered off rather than discontinued suddenly.

Dosage: Adults: (Oral) 400 mg three to four times daily.

Children older than 6 years: (Oral) 100 to 200 mg two to three times daily.

ramelteon (Rozerem). Ramelteon is indicated in the treatment of insomnia characterized by difficulty or delay in sleep onset. In contrast to most other drugs in this class, it is not a controlled drug. It has been approved for long-term use and has not been shown to have any habit-forming potential.

Dosage: Adults only: (Oral) 8 mg at bedtime.

ANTIDEPRESSANTS

Depression is a mental state characterized by feelings of sadness, often accompanied by psychomotor retardation. Clinical depression, or major depressive disorder, must be separated from despondency or sadness that is the direct result of life events. The latter is generally founded in difficult situations; it is temporary, and it is naturally reversed in time.

Endogenous depression, or depression without obvious external causes, is greatly underdiagnosed. Fearing the social stigma of mental illness, people would much rather blame their malaise on physical symptoms such as back pain, allergies, abdominal distress, headaches, fatigue, ulcers, and other disorders. The treatment of the secondary disorder is rarely completely successful if an underlying depression is not first discovered and treated. The tendency to see a patient's disease as a puzzle to be solved, and not to see the concerns of the patient, is common in all aspects of health care. Diseases are not independent and separate from the patient as a person. Depression in particular can alter the success of many treatments.

One in six people in the United States has a major episode of depression at some point in his or her lifetime. Except for coronary artery disease, no chronic physical illness results in more disability than depression. Diagnostic criteria for a major depressive episode are as follows:

1. Depressed mood
2. Anhedonia (loss of interest or pleasure)
3. Recurrent thoughts of death or suicide
4. Indecisiveness or decreased concentration
5. Fatigue or loss of energy
6. Feelings of worthlessness or guilt
7. Overall slowness or agitation
8. Insomnia or hypersomnia
9. Significant weight loss or gain

A patient must have five of these nine symptoms to be diagnosed as having a major depressive episode. Major depressive disorder may be diagnosed after the presence of one or more major depressive episodes that cannot be better accounted for by bipolar disorder or by schizophrenia or a related disorder.

An **antidepressant** is any agent used to counteract depression. Running can be used as a simple antidepressant. The production of natural endorphins after vigorous exercise has been shown to give an antidepressant or even euphoric effect. This effect is known as the "runner's high." Some institutions are now experimenting with vigorous physical exercise as an adjunct to the treatment of mental illness.

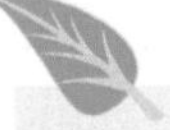

Herb Alert

St. John's Wort

St. John's wort has been used to treat mild to moderate depression. It is now a component of various herbal remedies for the treatment of anxiety and depression. St. John's wort reduces the effects of theophylline, coumarin, digoxin, indinavir, cyclosporine, and oral contraceptives. It seems to enhance the effects of SSRIs and tricyclic antidepressants. It should be avoided in patients taking monoamine oxidase inhibitors (MAOIs). See Chapter 28 for more information on St. John's wort.

Because antidepressant drugs work indirectly by increasing or decreasing the levels of certain naturally occurring brain hormones, 2 to 3 weeks may be needed to see an effect. These agents should be used with caution when other therapeutic agents are administered because there are many drug interactions and untoward side effects in such combinations.

SELECTIVE SEROTONIN REUPTAKE INHIBITORS

The main effect of all **selective serotonin reuptake inhibitors (SSRIs)** is the specific and potent inhibition of serotonin reuptake on the presynaptic neuron, which increases serotonin availability at the synapse. This effect causes increased concentration of serotonin in the central nervous system, and this is believed to be responsible for the antidepressant effect. The antidepressant effect is due to an increased supply of an intrinsic, or naturally occurring, brain hormone.

SSRIs are generally tolerated well. They are simple in their dosage requirements—starting slowly and gradually increasing the dose to the desired effect—and they are generally trouble-free. There is generally no advantage to starting immediately at a high dose because the adverse effects may become evident before enough time has elapsed to see whether the agent is effective against the depression. If no response occurs to an agent by about 8 weeks, it is best to switch to another drug in the same class. Long-term treatment seems to produce the most stable remission rates.

Long recognized side effects include gastrointestinal disturbances, particularly at the beginning of treatment; headache; sexual dysfunction; and anorexia. More recently, some symptoms have been recognized when the drug is abruptly stopped after the patient takes it for several months. These symptoms include vertigo, gastrointestinal symptoms, anxiety, crying spells, flulike symptoms, and insomnia. These are generally mild and usually resolve in 2 weeks. The dose should be tapered over at least 5 to 7 days when an SSRI is withdrawn to avoid or minimize these symptoms.

In addition to depression, other indications for SSRIs include obsessive-compulsive disorder, panic disorder, post-traumatic stress disorder, and premenstrual syndrome. Drugs in this class are summarized in Table 14-2. Table 14-3 lists drugs that interact with SSRIs.

Considerations for Older Adults

Paroxetine (Paxil)

There is evidence that older patients taking paroxetine may develop hyponatremia and a transient syndrome of inappropriate secretion of antidiuretic hormone (SIADH). Monitor serum sodium concentrations in older adults taking paroxetine, particularly in the first few months of therapy.

Table 14-2 Selective Serotonin Reuptake Inhibitors (SSRIs)

Generic Name	Trade Name	Dosage
citalopram	Celexa	10-60 mg/day
escitalopram	Lexapro	10-20 mg/day
fluoxetine	Prozac, Sarafem	20-80 mg/day
fluvoxamine	Luvox	25-300 mg/day
paroxetine	Paxil	10-60 mg/day
sertraline	Zoloft	50-200 mg/day

Table 14-3 Drug Interactions with Selective Serotonin Reuptake Inhibitors (SSRIs)

Drug	Interaction	Management
alprazolam (Xanax)	Increased alprazolam level	Monitor, reduce dosage
carbamazepine (Tegretol)	Increased carbamazepine level	Monitor and adjust dosage
cimetidine (Tagamet)	Increased SSRI level	Monitor clinically and adjust
phenytoin (Dilantin)	Possible phenytoin toxicity	Monitor phenytoin level
warfarin (Coumadin)	Increased warfarin level	Monitor, adjust dosage
beta blockers	Increased beta blocker effects	Adjust dosage

SELECTIVE SEROTONIN AND NOREPINEPHRINE REUPTAKE INHIBITORS

Selective serotonin and norepinephrine reuptake inhibitors (SNRIs) inhibit norepinephrine uptake as well as serotonin. They are useful as antidepressants and may be effective in circumstances where SSRIs were ineffective.

desvenlafaxine succinate (Pristiq). Desvenlafaxine is used to treat major depressive disorders in adults.
Dosage: Adults only: (Oral) 50 mg daily. Maximum dose is 400 mg daily.

duloxetine hydrochloride (Cymbalta). Duloxetine hydrochloride is used to treat major depressive disorders in adults. It is sometimes used as an adjunct in the treatment of fibromyalgia and neuropathic pain.
Dosage: Adults only: (Oral) 30 to 120 mg once daily.

venlafaxine hydrochloride (Effexor). Although most often used to treat major depressive disorders, venlafaxine has also been used to treat general anxiety disorders, social phobia, and panic disorders.
Dosage: Adults only: (Oral) 75 to 375 mg daily in two to three divided doses.

MONOAMINE OXIDASE INHIBITORS

Monoamine oxidase inhibitors (MAOIs) inhibit monoamine oxidase, a naturally occurring hormone that is involved in the breakdown of several neurotransmitters in the brain, including epinephrine, dopamine, and serotonin. These agents are effective antidepressants but have many untoward reactions with food substances. MAOIs may not be taken with foods that are high in amines such as cheeses, chicken liver, avocados, pickled herring, figs, and alcoholic beverages. If these are combined with an MAOI, a severe increase in blood pressure occurs.

phenelzine sulfate, USP-NF, BP (Nardil). The best results obtained with phenelzine sulfate are seen when it is used for true depressive states: patients who are sad, worried, and sleepless and who have gloomy thoughts and feel useless. This agent takes 1 to 2 weeks to attain the full therapeutic effect. Optic damage, constipation, urinary retention, hypotension, liver damage, and skin rashes have been observed with the use of this agent.
Dosage: Adults only: (Oral) 15 mg three times daily.

tranylcypromine sulfate, USP-NF, BP (Parnate). This antidepressant, similar to phenelzine, is an MAOI, and its actions, effects, and side effects are similar. The food and wine restrictions mentioned earlier apply to the use of this drug also.
Dosage: Adults only: (Oral) 20 to 30 mg/day in divided doses.

TRICYCLIC ANTIDEPRESSANTS

The term *tricyclic* describes the chemical structure of these compounds. Tricyclic antidepressants are composed of two aromatic hydrocarbon rings connected by a seven-member ring.

amitriptyline hydrochloride, USP-NF, BP (Elavil). In addition to serving as a mood elevator, this agent has a tranquilizing component that helps alleviate the anxiety that often accompanies depression. Many physicians customarily treat anxious or agitated and depressed patients with a combination of an antidepressant and a tranquilizer. This practice is seldom necessary when amitriptyline is used. Side effects, when they occur, are usually mild. Dizziness, nausea, excitement, hypotension, tremors, headache, heartburn, dryness of the mouth, and blurring of vision have been reported.
Dosage: Adults and children older than 12 years: (Oral) 25 to 150 mg/day once daily or in divided doses.
Children younger than 12 years: Not recommended.

desipramine hydrochloride, USP-NF, BP (Norpramin). This antidepressant is useful in the treatment of mild to moderate depressive states. Side effects include blurred vision, urinary retention, weakness, lethargy, nightmares, and euphoria.
Dosage: Adults and children older than 12 years: (Oral) 75 to 300 mg/day in divided doses.

doxepin hydrochloride, USP-NF, BP (Adapin, Sinequan). Doxepin has been shown to be beneficial as an antidepressant and antianxiety agent and is recommended in the treatment of alcoholism, depression neuroses, anxiety associated with various organic diseases, and some forms of insomnia. The maximum effect may not occur for 2 weeks after therapy is begun. Side effects are drowsiness, tachycardia, hypotension, extrapyramidal symptoms, nausea, vomiting, and paresthesias. It is administered orally.
Dosage: Adults: (Oral) 25 to 100 mg three times daily, or the entire daily dose may be administered at bedtime.
Children: Dose has not been established.

imipramine hydrochloride, USP-NF, BP (Tofranil). Although similar in effect to phenelzine, this agent has the singular property of not stimulating the central nervous system unless the individual is actually depressed. It has very little or no effect on an individual without depression. Because of this property, it has been used frequently for routine treatment of older patients. On days when an older individual is depressed, this agent has a mood-brightening effect; when the individual is not depressed, it does not produce overstimulation. It has been used with variable success in the treatment of enuresis (uncontrolled passing of urine).

Transient atropinelike effects, especially dryness of the mouth, are common during the initial phase of therapy, but they disappear with continued administration. Tachycardia, constipation, dizziness, and parkinsonism occasionally occur. Improvement is often seen within 3 to 4 days, and the maximum effect is seen within 2 weeks.
Dosage: Adults: (Oral) 75 to 300 mg daily in divided doses; (IM) 100 mg/day in divided doses.
Children older than 6 years: (Oral) For enuresis, 25 to 50 mg once daily 1 hour before bedtime.

nortriptyline hydrochloride, USP-NF, BP (Aventyl, Pamelor). Nortriptyline hydrochloride is a metabolite of amitriptyline and is used to treat mild to moderate depressive states. Side effects resemble those of desipramine.
Dosage: Adults and children older than 12 years: (Oral) 75 to 150 mg/day in divided doses.

protriptyline hydrochloride, USP-NF, BP (Vivactil). The action and effects of protriptyline resemble those of desipramine.
Dosage: Adults and children older than 12 years: (Oral) 15 to 60 mg/day in divided doses.

trimipramine maleate (Surmontil). Trimipramine is indicated for the treatment of depression. Side effects include hypotension, tachycardia, and paresthesias of the extremities.
Dosage: Adults: (Oral) 75 mg daily initially in divided doses, increased as necessary to 200 mg daily.

OTHER ANTIDEPRESSANTS

bupropion hydrochloride (Wellbutrin, Zyban). Bupropion hydrochloride, chemically unrelated to the other antidepressants, is used as a long-term antidepressant. It has also been shown to be effective as an adjunct to smoking cessation. When it is discontinued, it does not need to be tapered.
Dosage: Adults: (Oral) 150 to 300 mg daily in two to three divided doses.

mirtazapine (Remeron). Mirtazapine is used to treat major depressive disorders. Its activity is similar in potency to tricyclic antidepressants, although it is not related chemically.
Dosage: Adults: (Oral) 15 mg, up to a maximum of 45 mg, once daily at bedtime.

nefazodone. Nefazodone is indicated for use in the treatment of depression. Reported side effects include priapism, hepatotoxicity, postural hypotension, and mania.
Dosage: Adults: (Oral) 100 to 600 mg daily in two divided doses.

NONPSYCHIATRIC USES OF ANTIDEPRESSANTS

It has become evident in recent years that the concomitant use of antidepressants may help many patients cope with pain. The mechanism of antidepressant drug action in chronic pain syndromes is unclear. The increased serotonin and norepinephrine levels that these drugs produce are associated with increased analgesia, and decreased serotonin is associated with hyperalgesia. Antidepressants can be only one component of a comprehensive therapeutic program, and it is essential that a patient with chronic pain have other goals as well (i.e., returning to work, hobbies, or other daily activities).

Currently, there are insufficient data to support the choice of one antidepressant over another for certain types of pain. Amitriptyline and doxepin have been studied most thoroughly.

Antidepressants have also been used prophylactically to prevent migraine headaches and premenstrual syndrome. In addition, they are used with other agents in the treatment of other painful conditions such as shingles (varicella zoster), cancer, fibrositis, postherpetic neuralgia, and diabetic neuropathy.

ANXIOLYTIC AGENTS

Anxiolytic agents relieve anxiety and are used primarily for disorders caused by anxiety. These agents are generally less sedating than tranquilizers and lend themselves to more long-term treatment with fewer side effects.

buspirone hydrochloride (BuSpar). The principal pharmacologic effect of this drug is relief of anxiety. It has no anticonvulsant or muscle-relaxing properties, does not significantly depress psychomotor function, and has little sedative effect. For these reasons, it is generally the drug of choice for older patients. It is used for the management of anxiety disorders and has been shown to be useful for long-term therapy without losing its effectiveness. Dizziness, headache, nausea, and tachycardia have been reported in some patients. It has a slow onset of action; 3 to 4 weeks is required before optimal clinical results are noted.
Dosage: Adults only: (Oral) 10 to 30 mg daily in divided doses.

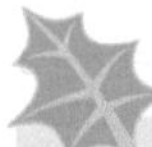

Considerations for Older Adults
Buspirone

Buspirone is the agent of choice as a tranquilizer for older patients because it is nonsedating and is not associated with memory impairment.

USE OF ANTICONVULSANTS IN ANXIETY DISORDERS

Despite progress in understanding of the pharmacotherapy of anxiety disorders, the response rate to drug therapy remains suboptimal in many cases. Anticonvulsants that are used to treat epilepsy are a class of agents with an emerging role in the treatment of anxiety disorders. The anatomic center for anxiety appears to be in the hippocampus and amygdala. The sensory input that is sent via the thalamus to the amygdala is known to be crucial for the evaluation of stress and fear and apparently is involved in some anxiety disorders. Anticonvulsants are in the treatment of anxiety disorders and post-traumatic stress disorder.

carbamazepine (Tegretol)
Dosage: Adults: (Oral) 800 to 1200 mg/day.

divalproex (Depakote)
Dosage: Adults: (Oral) 1000 mg/day (serum level 70 mcg/mL).

gabapentin (Neurontin)
Dosage: Adults: (Oral) 1190 mg/day.

topiramate (Topamax)
Dosage: Adults: (Oral) 400 mg/day.

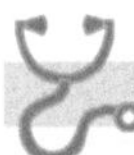

Clinical Implications

1. Psychotherapeutic agents are among the most overprescribed medications.
2. Natural, temporary situations promoting sadness, anxiety, or restlessness need not always be treated by a psychotherapeutic agent.
3. Endogenous depression—a generalized sadness and listlessness without apparent cause—may be alleviated by antidepressants.
4. A proper diet, vigorous physical exercise, and a pleasant environment should be incorporated in the treatment of emotional disorders.
5. Anxiety that interferes with normal functioning may be effectively treated with a tranquilizer.
6. The health care professional should be willing to discuss a patient's anxiety about his or her condition or reason for hospitalization. The patient's fears often can be calmly discussed and alleviated. The patient may fear that the physician is not telling the patient everything and that the condition is worse than he or she is being told.
7. Older patients generally require lower doses of psychotherapeutic agents and may experience excessive sedation when these drugs are administered.
8. Guardrails and assistance in ambulation should be added to a patient's care when tranquilizers are first administered.
9. Self-administered medication such as antihistamines and cough preparations may cause excessive sedation when combined with tranquilizers.
10. Alcohol or sedatives should not be combined with tranquilizers.
11. In most instances, 2 to 3 weeks is required before a therapeutic effect of an antidepressant is seen. The patient should be advised of this delay when these agents are administered.
12. The potential for abuse and addiction is high when tranquilizers are administered for an extended period.
13. A patient should not take more than the prescribed dose when these agents are administered. The patient should be counseled to this effect, particularly when ready for discharge from the hospital.
14. Monoamine oxidase inhibitors (MAOIs) may cause life-threatening reactions if combined with wine, cheese, or other substances containing amines.
15. Combining two or more psychotherapeutic agents may cause many untoward effects.
16. Current information on drug interactions may be obtained from the pharmacist. Information on untoward effects is computerized, constantly updated, and available to pharmacists online. Pharmacists should be consulted when the patient is taking many different medications.

CRITICAL THINKING QUESTIONS

1. A patient has been hospitalized in the state mental hospital for 6 months and is considerably improved after therapy and treatment with Thorazine. He has begun to walk with an increased shuffle lately, and at rest his fingers have a pill-rolling movement. Is this serious? Does the medication need to be discontinued? What could help him?
2. An older patient has been crying and upset since the sudden death of her husband. She states that her fatigue is increasing daily, and many days she does not even get out of bed and dress. She does not feel like cooking for herself and usually just has tea and toast during the day. What medication could be beneficial? Any other suggestions?
3. A patient recently lost his executive position as a result of company downsizing. His wife brought him in to the office today. In contrast to his previous appearance, he is now unshaven, his clothes are in some disarray, and he sits sullenly on the examining table, answering very few questions using only monosyllables. What medication could be beneficial?
4. A patient begins sobbing hysterically. She states that she and her husband are having marital troubles, her teenage son has been experimenting with drugs and is now at the Drug Abuse Center, and her in-laws are coming to stay for 2 weeks. She feels that if she could just get by the next few weeks, things may straighten themselves out. What medication might be beneficial in this situation?
5. A patient describes herself as having too many "highs" and "lows." Last night she did not sleep at all and instead reorganized all her closets and cleaned the house from top to bottom. At other times, she says she can hardly get out of bed for most of the day. What condition does she describe? What drug may help?

REVIEW QUESTIONS

1. What property does buspirone have that makes it useful in older patients?
   a. More sedating
   b. Less sedating
   c. Antiparkinsonian effect
   d. Antipsychotic

2. Which drug would not be expected to interact with lithium?
   a. hydrochlorothiazide
   b. ibuprofen
   c. penicillin
   d. enalapril

3. Serotonin levels may be increased by which drug?
   a. nortriptyline
   b. amitriptyline
   c. phenobarbital
   d. citalopram

4. An antidepressant that is used in smoking cessation therapy is:
   a. buspirone.
   b. bupropion.
   c. nortriptyline.
   d. sertraline.

5. An anticonvulsant that is used in the treatment of anxiety disorders is:
   a. gabapentin.
   b. buspirone.
   c. fluoxetine.
   d. doxepin.

6. When treating an older patient with a sedative, the dose may need to be:
   a. higher.
   b. lower.
   c. unchanged.
   d. combined with another drug.

7. Lithium is prescribed to treat:
   a. schizophrenia.
   b. chronic depressive disorders.
   c. hyperactivity in children.
   d. bipolar disorder.

8. Parkinsonism has been observed as a side effect of:
   a. diazepam.
   b. buspirone.
   c. bupropion.
   d. chlorpromazine.

9. Which tranquilizer is also effective as a muscle relaxant?
   a. chlorpromazine
   b. diazepam
   c. nefazodone
   d. trifluoperazine

10. A side effect of chlorazepate may be:
    a. hypertension.
    b. hypotension.
    c. hypersalivation.
    d. diarrhea.

Answers to the review questions can be found at the back of the book.

evolve Additional questions and activities can be found at *http://evolve.elsevier.com/asperheim/pharmacology*.

Prostaglandins and Prostaglandin Inhibitors

CHAPTER 15

Objectives

After completing this chapter, you should be able to do the following:

1. Recognize the drugs that are known as prostaglandins, and understand their effects in the body.
2. Recognize the effect that a prostaglandin inhibitor would have on a given body tissue.
3. Understand bodily functions that are carried out by prostaglandins.
4. Recognize inflammation as a function of prostaglandins.
5. Become familiar with the anti-inflammatory effects of prostaglandin inhibitors.
6. Become familiar with COX-2 inhibitors as anti-inflammatory agents and recognize their advantages.

Key Terms

COX-2 inhibitors, p. 142
Cyclooxygenase-2, p. 142
Nonsteroidal anti-inflammatory drugs (NSAIDs), p. 140
Prostaglandin (PRŌS-tă-GLĂN-dĭn) **inhibitor,** p. 140
Prostaglandins (PRŌS-tă-GLĂN-dĭns), p. 139

Prostaglandins are potent unsaturated fatty acids that act in exceedingly low concentrations on local target organs. They are physiologically active substances and are found in many tissues. The drugs in this class of pharmacologic agents were at first believed to exert their effects through the central nervous system because of the analgesic and anti-inflammatory effects exhibited by many of these agents. Early drugs, such as aspirin, were long believed to be central nervous system analgesics but are now known to exert their effects through the prostaglandin system.

The first report of the prostaglandins occurred in the 1930s when New York gynecologists Kurzrok and Lieb noted that human semen had an ability to produce strong contraction or relaxation of the uterus. It was soon found that this unknown substance, named prostaglandin because it was believed to be produced by the prostate gland, could affect other types of smooth muscle as well.

The term *prostaglandin* was found to be a misnomer because these substances are widely distributed in many tissues and body fluids. They are produced close to their sites of action and are rapidly metabolized when circulating through the body. For simplicity, these agents are named alphabetically—prostaglandin A, B, C—and abbreviated as PGA (prostaglandin A), PGB, PGC, and so on.

ACTIONS OF THE PROSTAGLANDINS

In this section, the known prostaglandins are discussed according to the body system that they affect.

REPRODUCTIVE TRACT

In men, prostaglandins are believed to assist in the emptying of the seminal vesicles, aiding in ejaculation. In women, prostaglandin release is believed to aid in uterine contraction during menstruation. Commercially produced prostaglandins are used to induce uterine contractions in elective abortions.

dinoprostone (Cervidil Vaginal Insert, Prepidil Cervical Gel, Prostin E_2 Suppositories). Dinoprostone is generally administered vaginally or, in the case of the cervical gel, directly into the external cervical os. It is given to terminate a pregnancy from the 12th to the 20th week of gestation. It may also be used to evacuate a uterus when a missed abortion or fetal death has occurred. Adverse effects include dizziness, vomiting, diarrhea, urine retention, headache, and cardiac arrhythmia.
Dosage: Adults: (Vaginal) 20 mg by suppository every 2 to 3 hours, or 10 mg as a vaginal insert for slow release; (Cervical) 0.5 mg/3 gm application.

mifepristone (Mifeprex). Mifepristone may be administered orally for the medical termination of a pregnancy that is up to 49 days from the last menstrual period. It is given in a single dose and should be administered in a clinic setting. Adverse effects include excessive vaginal bleeding, infections, abdominal pain, and nausea.
Dosage: Adults only: (Oral) 600 mg as a single dose.

CIRCULATORY SYSTEM

Cardiac output is generally increased by prostaglandins E, F, and A, but the therapeutic use of these agents has not been perfected as of yet. The primary purpose of prostaglandin E has been to keep the ductus arteriosus open (patent) in newborn infants. Infants with certain congenital heart deformities rely on a patent ductus arteriosus to supply oxygenated blood until they are old enough or stable enough to undergo corrective heart surgery. (Conversely, prostaglandin inhibitors such as indomethacin, discussed later in the chapter, are used to close a patent ductus arteriosus when natural processes fail to do so in an otherwise healthy infant; this has greatly reduced the necessity for surgery in many infants.)

alprostadil sterile solution (Prostaglandin E, Prostin VR Pediatric Injection). This agent is administered by intravenous (IV) infusion to keep the ductus arteriosus open. Infants with certain congenital heart deformities rely on a patent ductus arteriosus to supply oxygenated blood until they are old enough or stable enough to undergo corrective heart surgery. This agent should not be used in infants with respiratory distress syndrome. It has been noted to cause cortical proliferation of the long bones with long-term use.
Dosage: Infants: (IV) As a continuous infusion providing 0.1 mcg/kg/min.

GASTROINTESTINAL TRACT

misoprostol (Cytotec). Misoprostol, a synthetic analog of prostaglandin E (alprostadil), is a gastric antisecretory agent with protective effects on the gastric mucosa. It is used for the prevention of gastric ulcers induced by nonsteroidal anti-inflammatory drugs (NSAIDs). It should be administered for the duration of NSAID therapy. It is an abortifacient (causes abortion), and it is contraindicated in pregnancy.
Dosage: Adults: (Oral) 200 mcg four times daily taken with food.

URINARY TRACT

alprostadil (Caverject or Edex Injections, MUSE Suppositories). Alprostadil is a naturally occurring form of prostaglandin E. It is a vasodilator and a platelet aggregation inhibitor. It is used in a transurethral delivery system and is administered as needed to obtain an erection. The onset of action is within 5 to 10 minutes; the duration of action is 30 to 60 minutes. It may also be used as a direct intercavernosal injection for the treatment of erectile dysfunction. Urethral burning, bleeding, and testicular pain are reported as side effects.
Dosage: Adults only: (Transurethral) 125 mcg to 1 mg inserted into the urethra. Dosage is initially titrated in a medical setting. (Intracavernosal Injection) 1.25 to 60 mcg. Dosage is initially titrated in a medical setting.

ALLERGY AND IMMUNOLOGY

In high doses, prostaglandins prevent the release of histamine from sensitized cells. Very low doses of prostaglandins provoke the opposite response, however, and enhance histamine release. No therapeutic agents have yet been developed to exert a predictable response in the treatment of allergies.

PROSTAGLANDIN INHIBITORS

NONSTEROIDAL ANTI-INFLAMMATORY DRUGS

Many therapeutic agents exert their effects through inhibition of the prostaglandin systems. These agents are referred to as **prostaglandin inhibitors,** or antiprostaglandins. Although the exact action of prostaglandins in many areas of the body remains uncertain, it has been found that prostaglandins figure prominently in the process of inflammation and are found in inflammatory exudates. The mechanism of action of many anti-inflammatory agents is actually to prevent the synthesis of prostaglandins at the site of inflammation. These prostaglandin inhibitors are referred to as **nonsteroidal anti-inflammatory drugs (NSAIDs).** Many old and new agents are prostaglandin inhibitors.

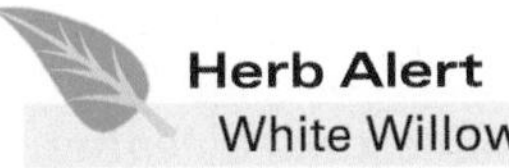

Herb Alert
White Willow

White willow is used in the treatment of rheumatism, inflammation, and fever. It reduces the effects of probenecid and enhances the antiplatelet action of NSAIDs and warfarin; it should not be taken with warfarin or NSAIDs. It also enhances the action of phenytoin and methotrexate. Use of white willow should be avoided in patients with preexisting bleeding tendencies. See Chapter 28 for more information on white willow.

aspirin, USP-NF; acetylsalicylic acid, BP. Although long used as an analgesic and anti-inflammatory agent, it is only more recently that the true mechanism of action of aspirin was found. It is now known that aspirin inhibits the synthesis of prostaglandins.

Aspirin is used to relieve mild to moderate pain; treat headaches; act as an anti-inflammatory medication in arthritic conditions; and reduce platelet aggregation, preventing blood clot formation. For this last use, low doses of aspirin are taken daily.

A relationship has been established in children between taking aspirin and the development of Reye's syndrome, an often fatal condition characterized by encephalopathy and liver damage. It is now recommended that aspirin not be given to children for minor febrile conditions. Aspirin is still used in inflammatory conditions, however, such as juvenile rheumatoid arthritis.

Dosage: Adults: (Oral, Rectal) 325 to 650 mg every 4 hours.

Children: (Oral) 65 mg/kg/day for inflammatory conditions only.

diclofenac (Voltaren)

Dosage: Adults only: (Oral) 150 to 200 mg in two divided doses.

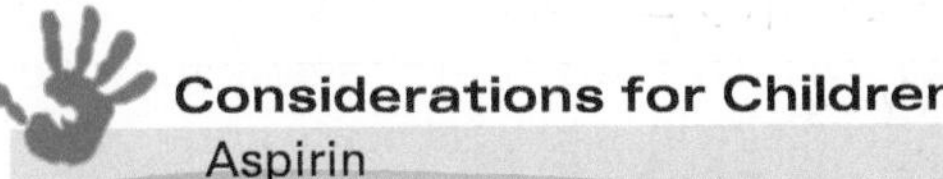

Considerations for Children
Aspirin

Avoid administering aspirin to children younger than 18 years old. Aspirin given to infants and young children is associated with the development of Reye's syndrome. Other NSAIDs, such as ibuprofen (Motrin), do not have this association.

diflunisal, USP-NF, BP (Dolobid)

Dosage: Adults only: (Oral) 1000 mg initially, followed by 500 mg every 12 hours.

etodolac (Lodine)

Dosage: Adults only: (Oral) 200 to 400 mg every 6 to 8 hours, or, as the long-acting (XL) form, 400 to 1000 mg once daily.

fenoprofen calcium, USP-NF, BP (Nalfon)

Dosage: Adults only: (Oral) 600 mg four times daily.

flurbiprofen (Ansaid)

Dosage: Adults only: (Oral) 200 to 300 mg daily in two to four divided doses.

ibuprofen, USP-NF, BP (Advil, Motrin). In addition to its use as an anti-inflammatory drug, ibuprofen is frequently used in the treatment of menstrual cramps and ovulation pain.

Dosage: Adults: (Oral) 200 to 800 mg four times daily.

Children: (Oral) 10 mg/kg per dose four times daily.

indomethacin, USP-NF, BP (Indocin). Used orally in the treatment of arthritis, indomethacin is also injected intravenously in newborns to induce closing of the ductus arteriosus. This agent should not be used in older patients because the incidence of gastrointestinal bleeding is high.

Dosage: Adults: (Oral) 25 mg three times daily.

Newborns: (IV) 0.2 mg/kg, may be given up to three times.

ketoprofen (Oruvail)

Dosage: Adults only: (Oral) 150 to 300 mg daily in three to four divided doses.

ketorolac tromethamine. This agent can be administered intramuscularly or intravenously for the relief of acute pain. In pain management studies, the overall analgesic effect of 30 mg of ketorolac was equivalent to 6 to 12 mg of morphine or 100 mg of meperidine. When administered by the intramuscular (IM) route, it is very effective for postoperative pain, and the patient does not experience the sedation that accompanies narcotic analgesia. Orally, ketorolac effectively treats mild to moderate pain and has been used for headaches, dental pain, and other disorders with chronic recurrent pain.

Dosage: Adults only: (Oral) 10 to 20 mg every 4 hours, maximum daily dose 40 mg; (IM) 30 to 60 mg as a loading dose, then 15 to 30 mg every 4 to 6 hours, maximum daily dose 150 mg.

meclofenamate

Dosage: Adults only: (Oral) 200 to 400 mg/day in three to four divided doses.

mefenamic acid (Ponstel)

Dosage: Adults only: (Oral) 500 mg initially, followed by 250 mg every 6 hours.

meloxicam (Mobic)

Dosage: Adults only: (Oral) 7.5 to 15 mg once daily.

nabumetone
Dosage: Adults only: (Oral) 500 mg to 1 gm once daily.

naproxen, USP-NF, BP (Naprosyn)
Dosage: Adults: (Oral) 200 mg two to three times daily to a maximum of 1250 mg daily.

Children: (Oral) 5 to 10 mg/kg/day in two divided doses.

naproxen sodium (Aleve, Anaprox)
Dosage: Adults only: (Oral) 220 mg two to three times daily to a maximum of 1250 mg/day.

oxaprozin (Daypro)
Dosage: Adults only: (Oral) 600 to 1200 mg once daily.

piroxicam, USP-NF, BP (Feldene). The main advantage of piroxicam is that it has a prolonged half-life in the body and can be taken in a once-daily dose for the treatment of inflammatory conditions.
Dosage: Adults: (Oral) 20 mg once daily.

sulindac, USP-NF, BP (Clinoril)
Dosage: Adults only: (Oral) 400 mg daily in two divided doses.

tolmetin sodium, USP-NF, BP (Tolectin). This agent is used for arthritis and more localized inflammatory conditions such as bursitis and tennis elbow.
Dosage: Adults: (Oral) 400 mg three times daily, increased as necessary to 2 gm/day.

Children: (Oral) 10 to 30 mg/kg/day in three divided doses.

CYCLOOXYGENASE-2 INHIBITORS

Cyclooxygenase-1 (COX-1) and **cyclooxygenase-2** (COX-2) are enzymes that are involved in the inflammatory process. The original NSAIDs inhibit both COX-1 and COX-2. **COX-2 inhibitors** preferentially inhibit the COX-2 enzyme over COX-1. Knowledge of the particular function and differentiation of these enzymes is beyond the scope of this text. However, these agents are described as a class by this function, so it is necessary to recognize the term.

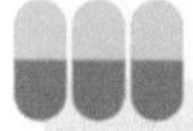

Special Considerations
NSAIDs

The simultaneous use of two NSAIDs, which includes the combination of a COX-2 inhibitor and low-dose daily aspirin, is a significant risk factor for gastrointestinal bleeding.

The main advantage of this group of NSAIDs is that they have considerably less antiplatelet effect, and there are fewer bleeding tendencies as a side effect. The prolonged use of the original NSAIDs that is generally necessary for arthritic conditions causes a high rate of severe gastrointestinal tract complaints, including abdominal pain and gastrointestinal bleeding. COX-2 inhibitors are effective as anti-inflammatories, particularly for arthritis and other inflammatory conditions, but have a greatly reduced adverse effect on the gastrointestinal tract. These agents are used orally for adults only.

celecoxib (Celebrex)
Dosage: Adults only: (Oral) 100 to 200 mg twice daily.

AGENTS USED IN THE TREATMENT OF GOUT

Gout is a condition in which crystals of monosodium urate are deposited in tissues—generally the joints of the feet and toes. It is caused by an increase in serum uric acid generally greater than 9 mg/100 mL. Uric acid is formed as a metabolite when a rich diet high in purines is eaten, and it may be artificially elevated if there is increased breakdown of red blood cells or if the exit pathway for the uric acid is altered secondary to taking a medication such as a thiazide diuretics. The goal of treatment is to obtain a serum concentration of uric acid of less than 6 mg/100 mL.

AGENTS TO TREAT ACUTE GOUT

colchicine, USP-NF (Colcrys). Colchicine is a uricosuric agent prescribed orally to treat acute gout flares by increasing the excretion of uric acid via the kidneys. The most common adverse effects include abdominal pain, vomiting, and diarrhea. It is contraindicated in patients who have hepatic impairment.
Dosage: Adults only: (Oral) Dosage varies according to the condition; 1.2 mg may be given initially followed by 0.6 mg 1 hour later. Dose may be repeated in 3 days.

probenecid, USP-NF. This uricosuric agent may be used alone or with colchicines to treat acute gout. Nausea and abdominal distress that may be caused by this agent are minimized if it is taken with food.
Dosage: Adults only: (Oral) 250 mg twice daily for 1 week, followed by 500 mg twice daily.

AGENTS USED TO PREVENT GOUT

allopurinol (Zyloprim). This agent is used to maintain a lower serum uric acid level in the blood and prevent attacks of acute gout. Allopurinol may be started after the acute attack of gout is treated with colchicine or probenecid. Adverse effects include skin rash, elevation of liver enzymes, and leukopenia.
Dosage: Adults only: (Oral) 100 to 600 mg daily.

febuxostat (Uloric). This agent is a xanthine oxidase inhibitor and is used for the long-term management of hyperuricemia in patients who have recurrent attacks of gout. Adverse effects include acute flares of gout after the medication is begun owing to increased mobilization of uric acid from tissues. Skin rashes, nausea, and liver enzyme elevations have been reported.

Dosage: Adults only: (Oral) 40 to 80 mg daily.

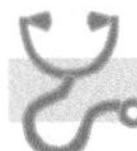

Clinical Implications

1. Aspirin and other antiprostaglandin agents have gastric irritation as their main side effect. Patients should be observed for signs of gastric distress when these agents are administered.
2. Routine use of aspirin and similar drugs should be discontinued before surgical procedures because bleeding complications occur with prolonged use. Surgical patients should be questioned about self-administration of aspirin-containing drugs.
3. Patients who are allergic to aspirin should be cautioned about aspirin-containing drugs such as Fiorinal, Robaxisal, and many other such combinations and antihistamine-analgesic combinations.
4. Patients should be cautioned about signs of bleeding disorders, such as bleeding gums, black stools, and petechiae, which are side effects of antiprostaglandin agents.
5. Fluid retention and visual problems occur as side effects of prostaglandin inhibitors. Patients should be assessed for these problems.
6. NSAIDs are best taken about an hour before meals to allow sufficient time for drug dissolution; the coating effect that food provides helps to prevent gastric irritation.
7. In children, acetaminophen is generally preferred to aspirin because of the association between aspirin intake and the development of Reye's syndrome.
8. Some prostaglandin inhibitors have a cross-sensitivity with aspirin, and these should be avoided in aspirin-sensitive patients.
9. In addition to anti-inflammatory medications, the application of warm compresses and physical therapy measures may increase joint mobility in the treatment of arthritic conditions.
10. Elevations in blood pressure, which may be observed as a side effect of NSAIDs, may signify fluid retention.
11. Parents should be advised to keep aspirin and other drugs safely out of the reach of children.
12. Prostaglandins given to affect one body system may have a series of untoward effects on other systems.
13. The COX-2 type of NSAIDs may be used if there is a history of abdominal distress with nonselective NSAIDs.

CRITICAL THINKING QUESTIONS

1. A patient complains of severe menstrual cramps. What agents may be prescribed to relieve her symptoms? She states she has used many over-the-counter preparations without relief.
2. A patient has been using acetaminophen (Tylenol) tablets without relief for her arthritis. Her physician advised her to get ibuprofen (Motrin) at the drugstore, but she states that this irritates her stomach and she wants to take Tylenol instead. How could you explain the difference in these drugs to her?
3. A patient has a long history of peptic ulcers. He now has rheumatoid arthritis and must take an NSAID. Which agent may be best and why?

REVIEW QUESTIONS

1. Prostaglandins are:
   - **a.** located only in the prostate gland.
   - **b.** active in many bodily tissues.
   - **c.** useful as an oral contraceptive.
   - **d.** useful in opening the ductus arteriosus in an infant.
2. An agent that has a protective effect on the gastric mucosa is:
   - **a.** ibuprofen.
   - **b.** mefenamic acid.
   - **c.** naproxen.
   - **d.** misoprostol.
3. Which drug is contraindicated in pregnancy?
   - **a.** misoprostol
   - **b.** erythromycin
   - **c.** penicillin
   - **d.** acetaminophen
4. The advantage of COX-2 inhibitors when used for arthritis is:
   - **a.** increased secretion of acid in the stomach.
   - **b.** more efficient reduction of joint swelling.
   - **c.** reduced gastric irritation.
   - **d.** less sedation.
5. Aspirin is contraindicated for use in young children because it is implicated in causing:
   - **a.** birth defects.
   - **b.** clotting disorders.
   - **c.** Reye's syndrome.
   - **d.** diarrhea.
6. An injectable agent that has analgesic properties similar to morphine is:
   - **a.** ibuprofen.
   - **b.** ketorolac.
   - **c.** piroxicam.
   - **d.** tolmetin.
7. An example of a COX-2 inhibitor is:
   - **a.** meclofenamate.
   - **b.** diclofenac.
   - **c.** celecoxib.
   - **d.** indomethacin.
8. Which agent may be used to induce an abortion?
   - **a.** dinoprostone
   - **b.** epoprostenol
   - **c.** estrogen
   - **d.** alprostadil
9. Which agent is used to treat congenital heart deformities?
   - **a.** dinoprostone
   - **b.** allopurinol
   - **c.** alprostadil
   - **d.** epoprostenol
10. The main disadvantage of COX-2 inhibitors compared with ibuprofen is generally increased:
    - **a.** gastric irritation.
    - **b.** platelet aggregation.
    - **c.** cost.
    - **d.** side effects.

Answers to the review questions can be found at the back of the book.

evolve Additional questions and activities can be found at *http://evolve.elsevier.com/asperheim/pharmacology*.

Drugs That Affect the Autonomic Nervous System

CHAPTER 16

Objectives

After completing this chapter, you should be able to do the following:

1. Explain the major effects of drugs on the autonomic nervous system.
2. Define the effects of sympathetic stimulation.
3. Give an example of an adrenergic drug.
4. Give an example of an adrenergic blocking agent.
5. Define and describe cholinergic effects.
6. Give an example of a cholinergic agent.
7. Give an example of a cholinergic blocking agent.
8. Become familiar with the different classes of antihypertensive agents.

Key Terms

Acetylcholine (ăs-ē-tĭl-KŌ-lēn), p. 146
Adrenergic (ĂD-rĭ-NŬR-jĭk), p. 146
Autonomic (ăw-tō-NŎM-ĭk) **nervous system,** p. 145
Cholinergic (KŌ-lĭn-ŬR-jĭk), p. 146
Epinephrine, p. 146
Ganglion (GĂNG-glē-ŏn), p. 145
Neuron (NUR-on), p. 145
Norepinephrine, p. 146
Parasympathetic (păr-ă-sĭm-pă-THĔT-ĭk) **nervous system,** p. 145
Sympathetic (sĭm-pă-THĔT-ĭk) **nervous system,** p. 145
Synapse (SIN-aps), p. 145

SYMPATHETIC AND PARASYMPATHETIC SYSTEMS

The **autonomic nervous system** is composed of nerves leading from the central nervous system (CNS) that innervate and control smooth muscle, cardiac muscle, and glands (Fig. 16-1). It controls many organ systems automatically; its actions are not generally under voluntary control. The autonomic nervous system is divided into two parts: the **sympathetic nervous system** and the **parasympathetic nervous system.** Generally, if one system stimulates a function, the other inhibits it. The systems oppose one another in governing the functions of smooth muscle and glands in many parts of the body. Some of the major effects of the two systems are compared in Table 16-1.

From Table 16-1, it can be seen that the sympathetic nervous system is the body's defense mechanism for emergency situations. The release of sympathetic hormones is increased at these times, enabling the body to run, fight, or meet the situation at hand (the "fight or flight" response). Sympathetic hormones may be given to relieve an asthmatic attack because of their relaxing effect on the smooth muscle of the bronchi. The parasympathetic system is more concerned with maintaining the normal "status quo" of body operations.

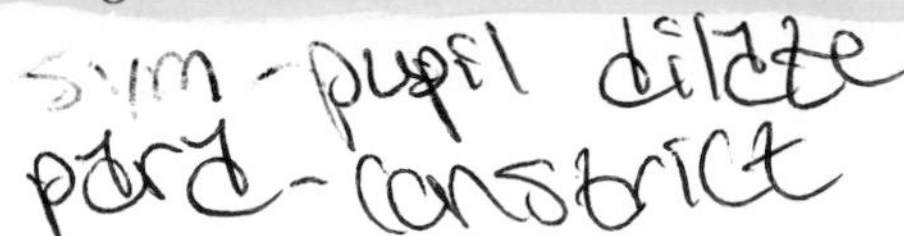

A **neuron,** or nerve cell, is the functional unit of the nervous system. Messages from the brain to various tissues and organs are transmitted as impulses along neurons. The junction (membrane-to-membrane contact) of any two neurons is called a **synapse;** a group of synapses is called a **ganglion** (Fig. 16-2).

In both the sympathetic and the parasympathetic nervous systems, two neurons function together to enable the CNS to control the muscles or glands. The first is a preganglionic (before the ganglion) neuron that leaves the CNS and travels toward the muscle or organ that is under control of the autonomic nervous system. At a certain point outside the CNS, this neuron joins (forms a synapse) with the second postganglionic

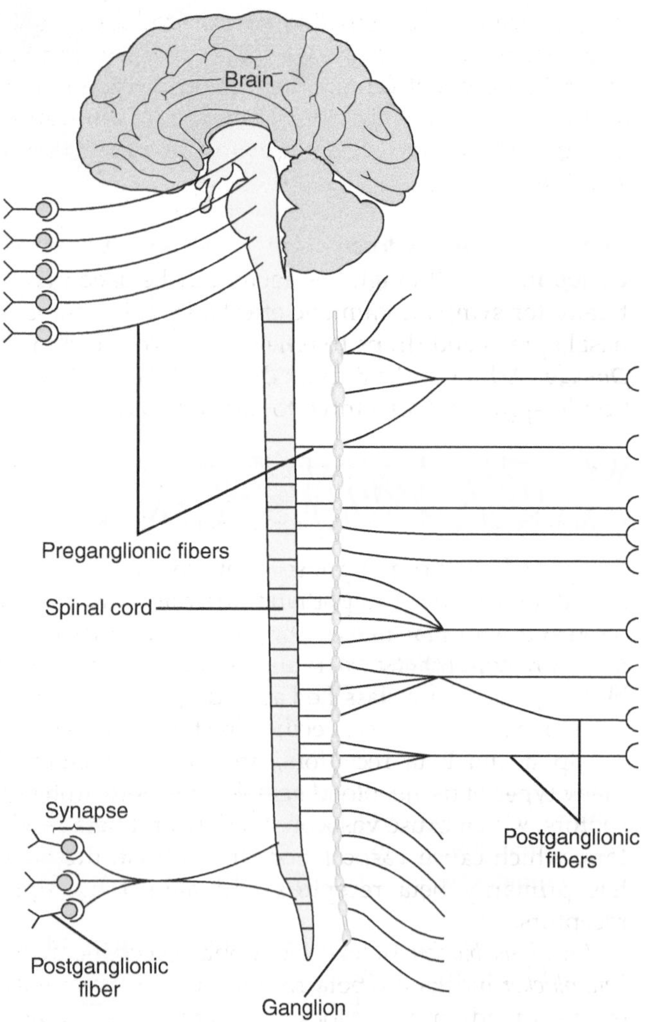

FIGURE 16-1 The autonomic nervous system.

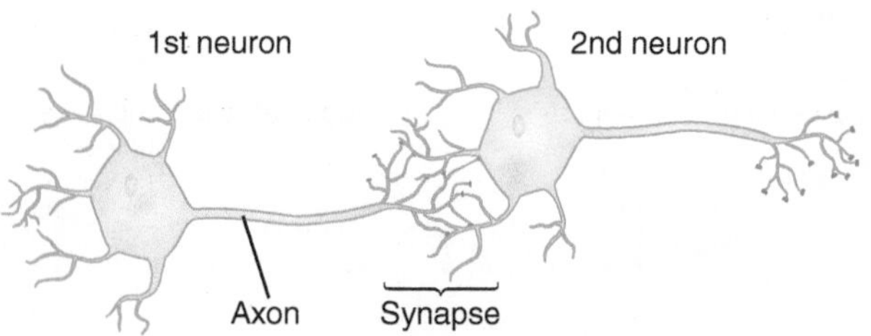

FIGURE 16-2 Junction of two neurons (nerve cells).

(after the ganglion) neuron that travels on to the muscle or organ in question. Because more than one neuron may travel to a given muscle or organ, several synapses occur at the junctions, forming a ganglion.

There is evidence that the transfer of nerve impulses at the synapse is carried out by chemicals liberated at the junctions. A neurotransmitter agent called **acetylcholine** is liberated at the ganglia of both systems and at the postganglionic parasympathetic nerve endings; cells that release acetylcholine are termed **cholinergic. Epinephrine** and **norepinephrine,** also neurotransmitter agents, are liberated at the postganglionic sympathetic nerve endings; the cells that release epinephrine and norepinephrine are referred to as **adrenergic.** It is thought that these chemicals exist in the tissues and are activated or released by an impulse carried along the nerve.

The activity of these chemicals after they are liberated is short-lived. Acetylcholine is rapidly inactivated by the enzyme acetylcholinesterase, and epinephrine is inactivated by the enzyme monoamine oxidase.

Drugs can act in four ways on the autonomic nervous system. They may stimulate or inhibit the sympathetic system, or they may stimulate or inhibit the parasympathetic system. Because the two systems oppose each other in action, a drug that acts by inhibiting the action of one system (e.g., the parasympathetic system) would have the same net effect as stimulation of the other system (i.e., the sympathetic system in this case).

Table 16-1 Major Effects of Sympathetic and Parasympathetic Systems

Sympathetic Effects	Parasympathetic Effects
Increase in cardiac rate and output*	Decrease in cardiac rate and output
Constriction of blood vessels in skin and viscera*	Dilation of blood vessels in skin and viscera
Elevation of blood pressure*	Lowering of blood pressure
Elevation of blood glucose*	No effect on blood glucose
Relaxation of smooth muscle in bronchi	Constriction of smooth muscle in bronchi
Decrease in peristalsis	Increase in peristalsis
Tightening of sphincters	Relaxation of sphincters
Promotion of urinary retention	Decrease in urinary retention
Dilation of pupils	Constriction of pupils

*These are emergency reactions of the body.

SYMPATHOMIMETIC (ADRENERGIC) AGENTS

Sympathomimetic agents produce or "mimic" the effects of stimulation of the sympathetic nervous system.

epinephrine hydrochloride, USP-NF, BP (Adrenalin, Epi-Pen). Epinephrine, as well as norepinephrine, is naturally produced by the adrenal medulla and at most sympathetic nerve endings. In stress situations, the adrenal medulla secretes an increased amount of epinephrine. The stress reaction, or the "fight or flight" response, consists of the sympathetic effects mentioned previously.

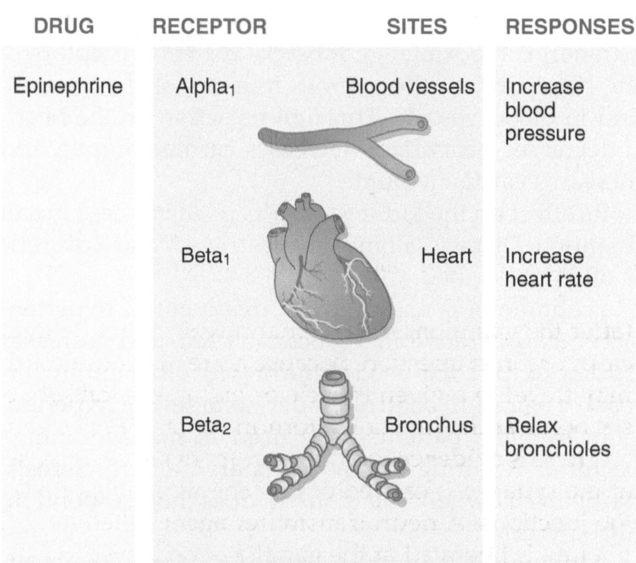

FIGURE 16-3 Epinephrine affects three different receptors: alpha$_1$, beta$_1$, and beta$_2$. (From Kee JL, et al: *Pharmacology: a nursing process approach*, ed 6, St. Louis, 2009, Saunders.)

Therapeutically, epinephrine is used to constrict blood vessels in the eye and nasal mucosa and to treat acute bronchial asthma and severe allergic reactions. It is perhaps the best heart stimulant in cases of heart block or acute heart failure (Fig. 16-3).

Epinephrine is a very potent drug, and care should be taken to be very accurate in the dosage given. It is used in advanced cardiac life support procedures. When large dosages are given, cardiac dilation, pulmonary edema, and cerebrovascular accident may occur. Death may also result from ventricular fibrillation as a result of overstimulation of the myocardium.

Dosage: Adults: (Subcut) 0.3 mg every 20 minutes or as necessary.

Children: (Subcut) 0.01 mg/kg every 20 minutes or as necessary.

metaraminol bitartrate, USP-NF, BP (Aramine). Metaraminol is often preferred over norepinephrine in the treatment of hypotension because it is not nearly as damaging to skin if it is accidentally extravasated into the surrounding tissues. If intravenous (IV) administration is not feasible, it may be given via the intramuscular (IM) route.

Dosage: Adults: (IM, IV) 0.5 to 5 mg as necessary to control blood pressure.

norepinephrine bitartrate, levarterenol bitartrate injection, USP-NF, BP (Levophed). Chemically related to epinephrine, this agent acts as an overall vasoconstrictor when given intravenously. It is used to treat hypotension and shock and may be given slowly in IV solutions for as long as it is needed for this purpose.

Caution must be taken to prevent the solution from infiltrating the skin of the surrounding areas because the powerful vasoconstriction that is produced would cause sloughing of the tissues. The best antidote for infiltration is phentolamine (Regitine), a sympatholytic agent that is injected directly into the area of infiltration.

Dosage: Adults: (IV) 1 to 2 mcg/min diluted in 1000-mL solution.

phenylephrine hydrochloride, USP-NF, BP (Neo-Synephrine). Although this agent may be used parenterally for sympathomimetic effects, its chief use is in nasal sprays and drops to relieve nasal congestion.

Dosage: Adults and children: (Nasal) 0.5% to 1% solution in spray or drops three to four times daily.

SYMPATHOLYTIC (ADRENERGIC BLOCKING) AGENTS

Sympatholytic drugs oppose or nullify the effect of stimulation of the sympathetic nervous system. The net result is similar to that obtained on stimulation of the parasympathetic nervous system. Adrenergic blocking agents are classified according to the receptor for which they are most specific. The two types, known as alpha and beta receptors, are found together in many types of tissue. Blood vessels have both alpha receptors, which cause vasoconstriction, and beta receptors, which cause vasodilation. In contrast, the heart has primarily beta receptors and almost no alpha receptors.

An *alpha blocker* blocks the alpha receptors, and a *beta blocker* blocks the beta receptors. The therapeutic effects of adrenergic blocking agents vary greatly. Many of these agents are discussed in other chapters as well because they have effects on the eye, the gastrointestinal tract, and the circulatory and other systems.

atenolol (Tenormin). Atenolol is a beta blocker that is used alone or with other agents to treat hypertension. It reduces cardiac output and systolic and diastolic blood pressures.

Dosage: Adults only: (Oral) 50 mg daily in one dose; may be increased to 100 mg daily.

clonidine hydrochloride, USP-NF, BP (Catapres). This agent produces inhibition of adrenergic receptors, after initially stimulating them. It reduces blood pressure in both the supine and the standing positions; orthostatic hypotension on rising is mild and infrequent. It is used in the treatment of hypertension either alone or with other agents such as diuretics. Side effects include dry mouth, sedation, dizziness, headache, nightmares, and depression.

Dosage: Adults: (Oral) 0.1 mg twice daily, increased as necessary to a maximum of 1.2 mg daily in divided doses.

Children: Dosage has not been established.

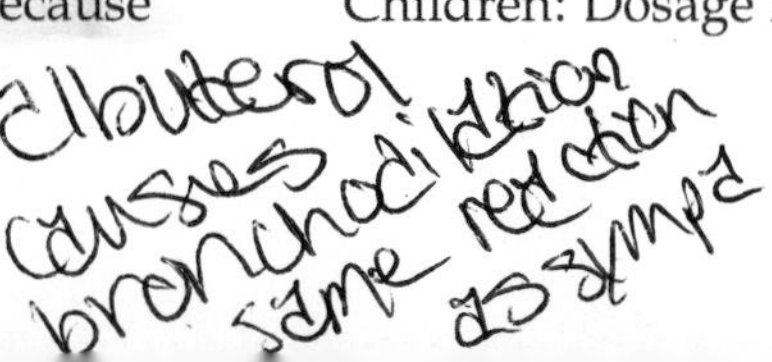

methyldopa, USP-NF, BP (Aldomet). Methyldopa is an antihypertensive drug that acts by interfering with the formation of the pressor amines norepinephrine and serotonin. It is used for patients with sustained, moderately severe hypertension. It is not used in pheochromocytoma and is usually not used in the milder forms of hypertension that may be treated with sedatives and diuretics. It is administered orally. Side effects include hemolytic anemia, drug fever, drowsiness, weakness, aggravation of angina pectoris, dryness of the mouth, and nasal stuffiness. Methyldopa should be used with caution in patients with a history of liver disease.
Dosage: Adults: (Oral) 500 mg to 2 gm daily in two to four divided doses.

methyldopa plus hydrochlorothiazide (Aldoril). This antihypertensive compound is available in two dosage sizes: Aldoril 15, which contains 250 mg methyldopa and 15 mg hydrochlorothiazide in each tablet, and Aldoril 25, which contains 250 mg methyldopa and 25 mg hydrochlorothiazide in each tablet. The combination of the antihypertensive and a thiazide diuretic provides potentiation of the hypotensive effect.
Dosage: Adults: (Oral) 2 to 4 of the combination tablets daily, based on individual requirements.

metoprolol tartrate, USP-NF, BP (Lopressor). This blocking agent has a preferential effect on the beta receptors in the myocardium of the heart. It is given to reduce systolic blood pressure and has the effect of reducing the heart rate and cardiac output as well.
Dosage: Adults only: (Oral) 100 mg daily in two divided doses; may be increased to 400 mg daily.

nadolol, USP-NF, BP (Corgard). Nadolol is used to treat hypertension and angina pectoris. It is a beta-blocking agent.
Dosage: Adults only: (Oral) 40 mg daily; may be increased to 240 mg daily.

prazosin hydrochloride, USP-NF, BP (Minipress). This oral agent is often used along with a diuretic in the treatment of hypertension. It may also be combined with other antihypertensive agents. The most notable side effect of this drug is a sudden loss of consciousness, or "drop attack." This side effect may be minimized by administering low initial doses with subsequent gradual increases. Vomiting, diarrhea, nervousness, skin rashes, and insomnia have been reported.
Dosage: Adults only: (Oral) 1 mg three times daily, gradually increased to a total of 15 mg/day in divided doses.

propranolol hydrochloride, USP-NF, BP (Inderal). This adrenergic blocking agent blocks the beta receptors in the heart, within the smooth muscles of the bronchi, and in blood vessels. Through its action on the heart, it decreases heart rate, decreases cardiac output, and increases cardiac volume.

Its effect on the kidneys results in an increase in salt retention. Dietary salt must be restricted, and a diuretic is often prescribed.

Propranolol is useful in the treatment of hypertension because it inhibits vasoconstriction and decreases cardiac output. It is used alone or with other antihypertensive agents to control moderate to severe hypertension. In some patients, it is used to manage angina pectoris resulting from coronary atherosclerosis, particularly when the patient does not respond to nitroglycerin.

Although it is not the drug of choice in the treatment of cardiac arrhythmias, propranolol has been used in the management of patients with arrhythmias. In some cases in which digitalis toxicity is present, this drug has been used to counteract the effects of digitalis excess.

The most common side effect is bradycardia, which may be accompanied by hypotension or shock. Severe bradycardia may be treated with atropine. Propranolol should be used with caution in patients with coronary artery disease because congestive heart failure may be precipitated. Fluid retention, ataxia, dizziness, hearing loss, visual disturbances, abdominal distress, rashes, and transient blood dyscrasias have been noted. When terminating therapy, discontinue propranolol slowly to avoid rebound effects.
Dosage: Adults: (Oral) For hypertension: initially, 80 mg/day in divided doses, then slowly increased to a maximum of 640 mg/day. For angina pectoris: 10 to 20 mg three to four times daily, increased as necessary. For arrhythmias: 10 to 30 mg three to four times daily; (IV) 0.5 to 3 mg at a rate not exceeding 1 mg/min.

Children: (Oral) 0.2 to 4 mg/kg/day in divided doses; (IV) 10 to 20 mcg/kg infused over 10 minutes.

ERGOT ALKALOIDS

Although ergot alkaloids do not lend themselves readily to classification as typical sympatholytic agents, they nevertheless are included in this category. With the exception of ergotamine, ergot alkaloids are used almost exclusively in obstetrics and are discussed in Chapter 18. Because of the similarity in the names of the ergot alkaloids *ergotamine* (used to treat migraines) and *ergonovine* (used to stimulate contraction of the uterus), serious errors can occur if the drugs are confused.

ergotamine tartrate, USP-NF, BP (Gynergen). Ergotamine is used to treat migraine headaches because of its ability to constrict the cerebral blood vessels. The periodic excruciating pain of migraine headaches, often associated with factors such as stress and food allergies, is accompanied by dilation of the cerebral arterioles and later by edematous swelling of the walls. The pain is relieved by the vasoconstrictive effect of ergotamine.

Dangerous side effects can accompany prolonged or too frequent use of this drug. Over time, the constriction of the blood vessels in the toes, fingers, hands, and feet can cause gangrene, resulting in death of the tissues and loss of the affected body parts. Constriction of the vessels in the retina of the eye may cause blindness.

Dosage: Adults: (Oral) 2 mg at the onset of headache. Dosage may be repeated one or two times if necessary for relief. No more than 3 doses per day or 10 doses per week should be given.

PARASYMPATHOMIMETIC (CHOLINERGIC) AGENTS

Parasympathomimetic agents "mimic" the effect of stimulation of the parasympathetic nervous system. Because acetylcholine is so rapidly inactivated by the enzyme acetylcholinesterase, it is not used therapeutically. Although synthetic analogs of acetylcholine produce the parasympathomimetic effects of the natural hormone, they are more resistant to the inactivating influence of the enzyme. Some drugs directly mimic the effects of acetylcholine, whereas others act by inhibiting acetylcholinesterase and prolonging the action of natural acetylcholine.

bethanechol chloride, USP-NF, BP (Urecholine). Bethanechol is similar in action to acetylcholine but is less active and less toxic. It is chiefly used in the treatment of postoperative abdominal distention, urinary retention, and retention of gastric contents (Fig. 16-4).

Dosage: Adults only: (Oral) 10 to 30 mg three to four times daily; (Subcut) 2.5 to 5 mg at 15- to 30-minute intervals to a maximum of four doses.

edrophonium chloride, USP-NF, BP. The main use of this acetylcholinesterase inhibitor is as an antidote for curare and similar drugs. It increases the tone of skeletal muscles, and it overcomes the excessive relaxation produced by curariform agents. It has been used in the treatment of myasthenia gravis.

Dosage: Adults: (IM, IV) 10 mg.

Children: (IM, IV) 1 to 5 mg; the dosage is individualized.

neostigmine methylsulfate, USP-NF, BP; neostigmine bromide, USP-NF (Prostigmin). Similar to physostigmine, neostigmine inhibits acetylcholinesterase. It is not as potent as physostigmine, but it is often preferred when a drug to restore peristalsis or treat atony of the bladder is indicated. It may be used in the treatment of postoperative abdominal distention, urinary retention, and myasthenia gravis.

Dosage: Adults: (Oral, IM, IV) 0.25 to 15 mg three times a day depending on indications.

pilocarpine nitrate, USP-NF, BP; pilocarpine hydrochloride, USP–NF. By stimulating the effector cells associated with the parasympathetic nerves, pilocarpine notably increases secretions, especially sweat, saliva, and nasal secretions. It is used mainly in the eye to produce miosis and to relieve pressure within the eye caused by glaucoma.

Dosage: Adults and children: (Ophthalmic) 1 to 2 drops of a 1% to 2% solution every 3 to 4 hours.

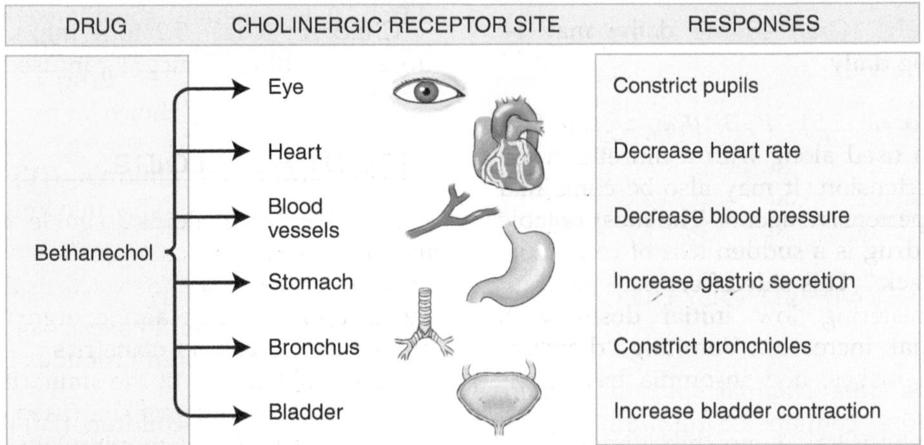

FIGURE 16-4 **Cholinergic receptors are located in the bladder, heart, blood vessels, stomach, bronchi, and eyes.** (From Kee JL, et al: *Pharmacology: a nursing process approach,* ed 6, St. Louis, 2009, Saunders.)

PARASYMPATHOLYTIC (CHOLINERGIC BLOCKING) AGENTS

Parasympatholytic agents oppose or nullify the effect of stimulation of the parasympathetic nervous system; they have the same net effect as stimulation of the sympathetic nervous system.

BELLADONNA

Three alkaloids are obtained from the natural plant belladonna: atropine, hyoscyamine, and scopolamine. These drugs make tissues insensitive to acetylcholine, paralyzing the effects of the parasympathetic nerves. Atropine is the alkaloid most often used, although there is not a great deal of difference among the actions of the three drugs.

atropine sulfate, USP-NF, BP (AtroPen). Perhaps the most important action of atropine is on the smooth muscles and the secretory glands. These drugs make tissues insensitive to acetylcholine, paralyzing the effects of the parasympathetic nerves. The gastrointestinal tract is relaxed, and there is decreased peristalsis and muscle tone; atropine is used as an antispasmodic in many of the various "colics." The smooth muscle of the bronchi is also relaxed, and this is accompanied by a decreased amount of secretion from the nose, pharynx, and bronchi.
Dosage: Adults: (Subcut) Atropine—0.5 mg every 4 to 6 hours, Scopolamine—0.6 mg every 4 to 6 hours, Hyoscyamine—0.5 mg every 4 to 6 hours.

ATROPINE POISONING

Usually the first indications of atropine poisoning are headache, dryness of the throat and skin, dilated pupils, and dimness of vision. The skin is flushed, and a rash may appear. The temperature increases because of decreased perspiration, and the pulse is rapid.

ANTIDOTE

Gastric lavage, along with parasympathomimetic drugs such as pilocarpine or tannic acid (tea), are used to treat atropine poisoning. The patient should be catheterized to prevent reabsorption of the drug from the urine. The symptoms are then treated (e.g., cold sponging for fever, administration of respiratory stimulants).

OTHER PARASYMPATHOLYTIC AGENTS

clidinium bromide plus chlordiazepoxide (Librax). Each capsule of Librax contains 2.5 mg clidinium bromide and 5 mg chlordiazepoxide. This combination of the anticholinergic agent with chlordiazepoxide, a mild tranquilizer, is beneficial in the treatment of spastic colitis and as an adjunct in the treatment of peptic ulcer. It is contraindicated in patients with glaucoma or bladder neck obstruction. Drowsiness, blurred vision, nausea, constipation, and blood dyscrasias have been reported as side effects. This drug should not be combined with alcohol or other sedative agents.
Dosage: Adults only: (Oral) 1 capsule four times daily.

dicyclomine hydrochloride (Bentyl). Dicyclomine is used to treat functional disturbances of gastrointestinal motility such as irritable bowel syndrome. It can be used alone or with phenobarbital to treat symptoms of infant colic.
Dosage: Adults: (Oral) 20 to 40 mg four times daily; (IM) 20 mg four times daily.
Children: (Oral) Syrup containing 10 mg/5 mL, 1.5 to 5.0 mL before feedings three to four times daily.

NEUROMUSCULAR BLOCKING AGENTS

pancuronium bromide (Pavulon). This synthetic, nondepolarizing neuromuscular blocking agent is used to provide short-term skeletal muscle relaxation to facilitate procedures such as endotracheal intubation, endoscopic examinations, ventilator therapy, or surgery.
Dosage: Adults and children: (IV) 0.04 to 0.1 mg/kg given as needed. Repeat dose every 25 to 60 minutes.

succinylcholine chloride (Anectine). This agent is used for the same indications as pancuronium. In addition, it is generally considered to be the drug of choice for orthopedic manipulations and for electroconvulsive therapy. The drug is very short-acting, making it the drug of choice for procedures lasting less than 3 minutes.
Dosage: Adults and children: (IV) 0.3 to 1.5 mg/kg in diluted solution. The maximum adult dose is 150 mg.

vecuronium bromide. Pharmacologically, this agent is similar to pancuronium bromide. The indications for use are the same.
Dosage: Adults and children: (IV) 0.08 to 0.1 mg/kg. Duration of effect is usually 25 to 30 minutes.

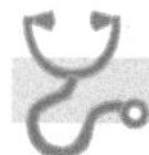

Clinical Implications

1. The drugs that affect the autonomic nervous system are not very specific; adverse effects may be observed frequently, according to which segment of the system is affected.
2. Assess the pulse and blood pressure for changes or irregularity when autonomic drugs are administered.
3. Weakness, nausea, vomiting, diarrhea, and abdominal cramps are frequent side effects of these agents. Patients should be carefully observed for these adverse effects, which should be duly reported.
4. Blurred vision is a frequent side effect of these agents because there are both adrenergic and cholinergic receptors in the eye.
5. Nursing procedures may be used to alleviate certain side effects (e.g., dry mouth can be treated by the use of gum, hard candy, or lemon-glycerin mouth swabs).
6. Constipation, as a side effect of anticholinergic drugs, should be carefully monitored, and laxatives should be requested as necessary.
7. Eye discomfort or pain should be immediately reported if a patient is taking anticholinergic drugs because there may be underlying and unsuspected glaucoma.
8. If flushing and elevated temperature are observed, alert the physician because these may be possible untoward effects of these agents.
9. When beta blockers are administered, bradycardia and congestive heart failure may occur as serious toxic effects.
10. Beta blockers may increase blood glucose levels in diabetic patients receiving these medications.
11. When peripheral vasodilators are given for the treatment of peripheral vascular diseases, signs of improvement in the patient's condition may be decreased blanching of the extremities, decreased paresthesia, and improved nail bed color.
12. Postural hypotension is a common side effect of some antihypertensive medications. Patients should not be allowed out of bed without assistance, particularly in the early days of treatment.
13. Patients should be observed carefully for any signs of urinary retention when taking anticholinergic drugs.
14. Patients should be observed carefully for side effects of autonomic drugs.

CRITICAL THINKING QUESTIONS

1. A patient has been feeling tired lately and having morning headaches. He has not been to a physician for 10 years. He works hard, drinks alcohol excessively at times, and is 30 lb overweight, but otherwise has no significant medical history. His blood pressure is noted to be 160/110 mm Hg. As he leaves the office, he comments that he hopes his blood pressure gets cured fast because he does not want to be on medication when he goes to Europe this fall. How should he be counseled regarding his medication?
2. A patient has just been diagnosed as having a duodenal ulcer. Her physician prescribed a bland diet, an antacid (Maalox), and cimetidine (Tagamet). She expresses to you her annoyance with her bland diet (she is a gourmet cook) and secretly worries that she will become a drug addict. How would you help her understand her treatment?
3. A patient has been taking propranolol hydrochloride for hypertension. She states that lately she has been feeling weak and listless. When taking her vital signs, you notice her pulse is 58 beats/min. Is this related to her medication? Should the physician be notified?

REVIEW QUESTIONS

1. A significant characteristic of the autonomic nervous system is that:
   a. it is tightly controlled by the CNS.
   b. it is ordinarily not under voluntary control.
   c. it controls voluntary muscles.
   d. it is overactive in depressive disorders.

2. All of the following are sympathetic effects except:
   a. lowering of blood pressure.
   b. decrease in peristalsis.
   c. tightening of sphincters.
   d. elevation of blood glucose.

3. All of the following are parasympathetic effects except:
   a. increase in peristalsis.
   b. constriction of pupils.
   c. hypertension.
   d. vasodilation.

4. Adrenergic agents have an effect that:
   a. counteracts the sympathetic nervous system.
   b. mimics the sympathetic nervous system.
   c. mimics the voluntary nervous system.
   d. mimics the parasympathetic nervous system.

5. The "fight or flight" response is a function of the:
   a. parasympathetic nervous system.
   b. musculoskeletal system.
   c. sympathetic nervous system.
   d. anticholinergic system.

6. Which agent is an adrenergic blocking agent?
   a. metaraminol
   b. phenylephrine
   c. norepinephrine
   d. propranolol

7. Hypertension may be treated with:
   a. metaraminol.
   b. norepinephrine.
   c. clonidine.
   d. diazepam.

8. A beta blocker commonly used in the treatment of hypertension is:
   a. atenolol.
   b. ergot.
   c. bethanechol.
   d. edrophonium.

9. What untoward effect may occur after a large dose of epinephrine?
   a. Pulmonary edema
   b. Slowing of the heart
   c. Hypotension
   d. Bronchial constriction

10. Beta blockers are often used in the treatment of:
    a. hypotension.
    b. irritable bowel disease.
    c. hypertension.
    d. duodenal ulcers.

Answers to the review questions can be found at the back of the book.

evolve Additional questions and activities can be found at *http://evolve.elsevier.com/asperheim/pharmacology.*

Drugs That Affect the Digestive System

CHAPTER 17

Objectives

After completing this chapter, you should be able to do the following:

1. Have a general understanding of the function of the gastrointestinal (GI) system and the drugs that affect it in various ways.
2. Identify the drug groups that affect the digestive system.
3. Become familiar with specific disorders of the GI tract, such as peptic ulcer disease and irritable bowel syndrome, and recognize the drugs used for these conditions.
4. Become familiar with the way antisecretory agents and antacids reduce the acidity of the stomach.
5. List the various types of cathartics, and give an example of each one.
6. List the antiemetics, and become familiar with their uses.
7. Explain how fecal softeners achieve their effects.
8. Discuss responsibilities of the health care provider related to the use of antacids and laxatives.

Key Terms

Antacids (ănt-ĂS-ĭds), p. 156
Antiemetics (ăn-tī-ē-MĔ-tĭks), p. 158
Cathartics (kă-THĂR-tĭks), p. 159
Constipation (cŏn-stĭ-PĀ-shŭn), p. 159
Diarrhea (dī-ăh-RĒ-ă), p. 161
Digestants (dī-JĔS-tĕnts), p. 157
Digestion (dī-JĔST-yŭn), p. 153
Emetics (ĕ-MĔ-tĭk), p. 158
Laxatives (LĂK-să-tĭvs), p. 159
Ulcers, p. 154

The digestive system is composed of organs or structures that enable food to be ingested (introduced into the system), digested (broken down into the basic components of the food), and absorbed (passed into the bloodstream). **Digestion** is a mechanical, chemical, and enzymatic process whereby food is converted to material suitable for use in the body. The bloodstream transports nutrients to various sites for use in manufacturing tissue or producing energy.

Simply stated, the digestive system consists of a tube within the head and trunk of the body with two external openings (Fig. 17-1). Food is considered to have entered the body only after it is digested, has left the tube, and its components have passed through a membrane into the bloodstream.

The tube is not one size throughout. There are enlargements and constrictions in some areas and characteristic qualities at different places. From the cells of its glands come enzymes and various chemical reagents that transform crude masses of food into simpler compounds suited for use by the body. The intestinal part of the gastrointestinal (GI) tract is in almost continuous movement and carries on its functions without the knowledge of the individual except in terms of the appreciation of the strength and well-being gained from food or the periodic removal of residue from the GI tract.

When food is taken into the mouth, it is cut and ground by the teeth and thoroughly mixed with saliva. The saliva performs three functions: (1) It acts as a solvent (making taste possible), (2) it initiates digestion, and (3) it lubricates the food so that it can be swallowed. Saliva contains the enzyme ptyalin, which reduces more complex carbohydrates to simpler forms. In some cases, saliva also contains maltase, which breaks maltose down into glucose.

The gastric juice encountered in the stomach normally contains mucin; hydrochloric acid; and the

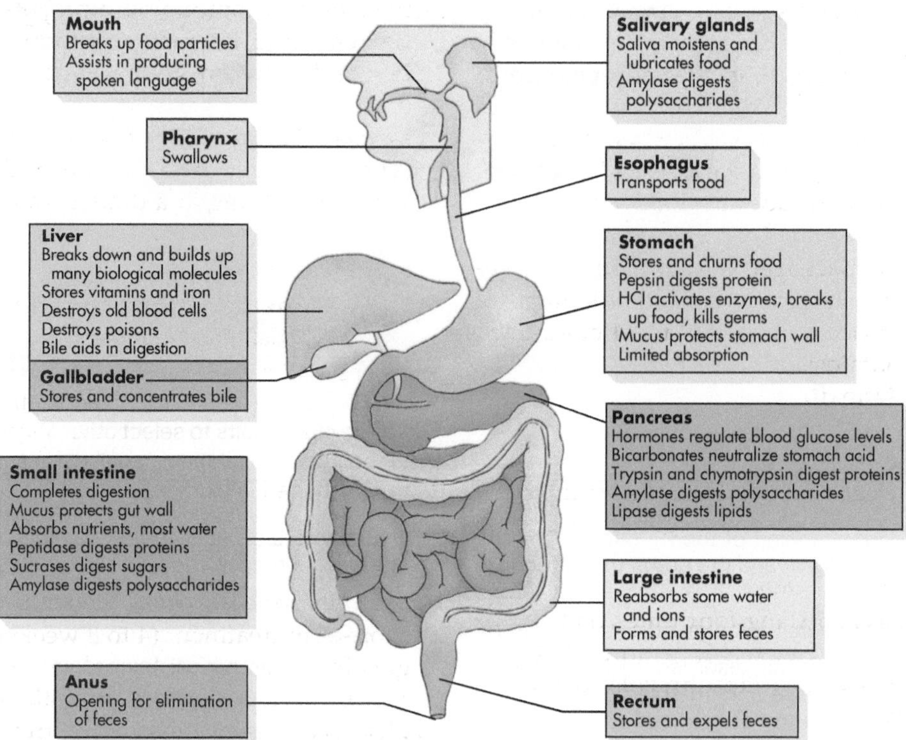

FIGURE 17-1 The digestive system. (From Patton KT, Thibodeau GA: *Mosby's handbook of anatomy and physiology*, St. Louis, 2000, Mosby.)

enzymes pepsin, rennin, and lipase. Mucin is a thick, sticky fluid that tends to cling to the surface of the mucosa, serving to protect it from injury by coarse particles of food and, to a certain extent, from the action of the enzymes and hydrochloric acid. The enzymes pepsin and lipase act on protein and fat to break these molecules into smaller, usable fractions. Rennin coagulates milk, producing a clumped mass, wool-like in appearance, called *curd*, and a clear fluid called *whey*. (Rennin obtained from calves' stomachs is used in making cheese because of its ability to coagulate milk.) Hydrochloric acid is necessary to provide an acid environment for the action of pepsin and to kill or inhibit many of the microorganisms that find their way into the stomach via food or other ingested materials.

Sometimes the acid becomes so strong that it can actually wear down an area of the stomach lining by its dissolving action. Ordinarily, the stomach is peculiarly resistant to this digestive action because of a protective coat of mucus, but under certain conditions, such as excessive or prolonged secretion of hydrochloric acid during periods of worry or stress, a small area of the surface membrane breaks down. The underlying connective tissue of the wall of the stomach is not nearly as resistant to acid as the lining membrane. The gastric juice may eat away at the tissue and cause a lesion through skin or mucous membrane, usually accompanied by inflammation. These lesions are known as **ulcers,** and lesions that occur in the gastric system are often called *peptic ulcers*.

It is necessary to neutralize the hydrochloric acid over weeks to allow the ulcer to heal. The goal is to re-establish the natural resistance of the intact lining membrane to the action of the hydrochloric acid.

HELICOBACTER PYLORI AND PEPTIC ULCER DISEASE

Peptic ulcer disease is believed to be caused by a high level of gastric secretion, in some cases aggravated by stress or drug therapy with gastric irritants such as nonsteroidal anti-inflammatory drugs (NSAIDs). An infectious agent, *Helicobacter pylori*, has been found in 75% of duodenal ulcers. Most of the remaining 25% of ulcers are caused by NSAIDs. Research has shown that many people are infected with *H. pylori*, but most do not develop an ulcer.

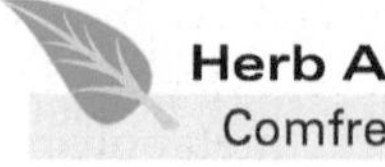

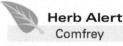

Herb Alert
Comfrey

Comfrey is used for the treatment of gastritis and peptic ulcers and for inflammatory conditions. However, this herb is hepatotoxic, or damaging to liver cells. Long-term oral use is not advisable, and it should not be used by patients with preexisting liver disease. See Chapter 28 for more information on comfrey.

In chronic peptic ulcer disease, treatment to kill the microorganism prevents ulcer relapse in about 95% of cases. In addition, there is increasing evidence of a relationship between *Helicobacter* infection and adenocarcinoma of the stomach. In some cases, eradication of the microorganism has cured malignancies. Treatment for *Helicobacter* infection includes the following options.

Prevpac. This is a prepackaged dosage form that provides patients with the following combination of drugs, to be taken twice daily for 10 to 14 days. Each twice-daily dose contains:

1 gm amoxicillin (Amoxil)
500 mg clarithromycin
30 mg lansoprazole

An alternative treatment for *Helicobacter* infection would be a 14-day or 21-day regimen with the following:

tetracycline, 500 mg four times daily
metronidazole (Flagyl), 500 mg four times daily
bismuth (Pepto-Bismol), 2 tablets four times daily
proton pump inhibitor (e.g., lansoprazole, pantoprazole), twice daily

ANTISECRETORY AGENTS

Although most anticholinergic agents currently used as adjuncts in the treatment of peptic ulcer inhibit gastric secretion indirectly, direct inhibition of gastric secretion, particularly secretion of hydrochloric acid, is now possible.

cimetidine, USP-NF, BP (Tagamet). Cimetidine inhibits the effect of histamine on the parietal cells that produce hydrochloric acid; it greatly reduces acid output in the stomach. It is used to treat peptic ulcers and Zollinger-Ellison syndrome (a combination of peptic ulcer and pancreatic tumors). Treatment is usually continued for 4 to 6 weeks. This agent is usually administered orally; however, intravenous (IV) therapy may be used in certain instances. Antacids may be used as well to reduce pain. Cimetidine is not the drug of choice for elderly patients because they show an increased susceptibility to the mental disturbances that may occur with this agent.

Many side effects of cimetidine are caused by its inhibition of some microsomal enzyme systems in the liver. As a result, it interferes with the metabolism of certain drugs by the liver, which causes the drugs to have an enhanced or prolonged effect on the body and can inadvertently cause toxic effects as well. This effect is more pronounced in older adults. Drugs whose effects may be enhanced or prolonged by their concurrent use with cimetidine include coumarin, phenytoin, propranolol, alprazolam, and diazepam. Current drug interaction information should always be checked when giving cimetidine with any other drug.

Dosage: Adults and children older than 12 years: (Oral) 300 mg four times daily with meals and at bedtime; (IV) 300 mg in a diluted solution every 6 hours.

Considerations for Older Adults

Cimetidine (Tagamet)

Older adults are more susceptible to the central nervous system effects of cimetidine (Tagamet) than younger adults. Advise older adults to select other antisecretory agents. Mental confusion, agitation, psychosis, and hallucinations have been reported in older adults and seriously ill patients taking cimetidine.

esomeprazole (Nexium). Esomeprazole is used for the short-term treatment (4 to 8 weeks) of erosive esophagitis from gastroesophageal reflux disease (GERD). It may be used in conjunction with amoxicillin and clarithromycin as an alternative treatment for *H. pylori* ulcer disease.

Dosage: Adults only: (Oral) 20 to 40 mg once daily.

famotidine (Pepcid). This agent is used to treat active duodenal or gastric ulcers and GERD and as maintenance therapy for duodenal ulcers and hypersecretory conditions. It is generally well tolerated. Headache, dizziness, constipation, and diarrhea have been reported.

Dosage: Adults only: (Oral) 20 mg twice daily.

lansoprazole (Prevacid). This agent is used for short-term treatment of active duodenal ulcers and gastric ulcer disease. It may be used for short-term (up to 8 weeks) treatment of GERD.

Dosage: Adults: (Oral) 15 to 30 mg once daily.
Children 1 to 11 years: (Oral) 15 mg once daily.

misoprostol (Cytotec). Misoprostol, which is also discussed in Chapter 15 with the prostaglandins, has both antisecretory and mucosal protective properties. It is particularly effective in counteracting the erosive effects of NSAIDs on the GI tract. NSAIDs are antiprostaglandin agents, and they diminish bicarbonate and mucus secretion in the intestine, contributing to mucosal damage. Misoprostol counteracts these effects. The most frequent side effects are diarrhea and abdominal pain. Misoprostol is a prostaglandin abortifacient (an agent that causes abortion), and it is contraindicated in pregnant women.

Dosage: Adults: (Oral) 200 mcg four times daily with food.

nizatidine (Axid). Nizatidine is an antisecretory agent used to inhibit acid secretion of the parietal cells. It is indicated for treatment of active duodenal ulcers for up to 8 weeks and may be used for maintenance therapy at a reduced dose. Sweating, urticaria, and somnolence are infrequent side effects.
Dosage: Adults: (Oral) 300 mg daily in one or two divided doses; 150 mg orally may be taken at bedtime or as a maintenance dose.

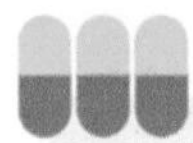

Special Considerations
Antisecretory Agents

Prolonged use of antisecretory agents may promote or worsen osteoporosis.

omeprazole (Prilosec). Omeprazole is indicated for the short-term treatment of active duodenal ulcers. It may be used in combination with other agents for the treatment of *Helicobacter* infections.
Dosage: Adults: (Oral) 20 mg once daily.

pantoprazole (Protonix). This antisecretory agent is used to treat erosive gastritis, erosive esophagitis, and GERD.
Dosage: Adults: (Oral) 40 mg daily.

ranitidine, USP-NF, BP (Zantac). The primary use of ranitidine is to inhibit gastric acid secretion. It is used to assist in the healing of peptic ulcers and associated conditions. Ulcers are generally healed in 2 weeks. Ranitidine minimally inhibits the liver metabolism of drugs, so it does not share the drug interactions of cimetidine. It is better tolerated than cimetidine by older patients.
Dosage: Adults and children older than 12 years: (Oral) 150 mg twice daily for 2 to 4 weeks.

ANTACIDS

Antacids destroy the gastric acid, either wholly or in part, by neutralizing or absorbing it and rendering it inactive.

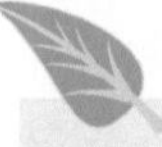

Herb Alert
Ginger

Ginger has been used for centuries for heartburn, as an antiemetic, as an anti-inflammatory, and as a laxative. It has also been used to treat motion sickness and morning sickness in pregnancy. Ginger enhances the antiplatelet action of NSAIDs and warfarin, and it enhances the effects of digitalis. Its use should be avoided in patients with gallstones or bleeding disorders. See Chapter 28 for more information on ginger.

aluminum hydroxide gel, USP-NF, BP (Amphojel, Creamalin). This gel is formed when aluminum oxide is added to water. It is insoluble and contains colloidal particles that do not precipitate out of the gel; it does not have some of the undesirable effects of sodium bicarbonate. Because it is insoluble and not absorbed, it does not interfere with the acid-base balance of the blood, and its neutralization reaction is slower; the acid rebound caused by the faster acting baking soda is eliminated. Carbon dioxide is not produced, and abdominal distention does not occur.

The colloidal particles possess absorptive properties. Hydrochloric acid adheres to the surface of these particles and is inactivated in this way, in addition to the chemical neutralization that occurs. Aluminum hydroxide gel is a mild astringent and demulcent. These qualities are helpful for local action in protecting and soothing the ulcer. The main disadvantage of this drug is the constipation produced, and it may produce a bowel obstruction in persons prone to constipation.
Dosage: Adults: (Oral) 600 to 1200 mg between meals and at bedtime.

magnesium oxide, USP-NF, BP. This agent is used quite frequently in powder form for its protective and antacid properties. In small doses, it is an antacid; in large doses, it is a laxative.
Dosage: Adults: (Oral) As an antacid—250 mg three to four times daily; as a laxative—500 mg to 1 gm daily.

sodium bicarbonate, USP-NF, BP (baking soda). Sodium bicarbonate is the home remedy used most often for gastric hyperacidity and heartburn. Heartburn is a burning sensation caused when some of the acid from the stomach is regurgitated into the esophagus.

Sodium bicarbonate has been greatly overused by the general public for numerous ailments. There are many disadvantages to the use of sodium bicarbonate as an antacid. Because of its solubility, it rapidly neutralizes all the acid present in the stomach and just as rapidly passes out of the stomach into the intestines. This action frequently results in "acid rebound," or a very high level of secretion of stomach acid after the rapid neutralization, which produces alkalinization of the stomach; this may cause considerable distress shortly after the administration of the antacid. Unknowingly, thinking the distress is a recurrence of the indigestion, the individual may consume more sodium bicarbonate, causing the whole cycle to repeat itself. The alkaline reaction produced in the stomach also inhibits the action of pepsin because hydrochloric acid is needed to activate this enzyme.

Another undesirable effect is caused by the absorption of sodium bicarbonate from the intestine, which produces a disturbance in the acid-base balance in the blood known as alkalosis. Alkalosis results in stress on the kidneys as they attempt to maintain the blood in stable acid-base balance. Renal failure may occur if the disturbance is prolonged. A further disadvantage is the production of gas in the stomach as a result of the neutralization reaction:

$$HCl + NaHCO_3 \rightarrow NaCl + H_2O + CO_2$$

The carbon dioxide produced causes distention of the stomach, a symptom that is quite uncomfortable and may be dangerous, particularly if the patient has an ulcer near the perforation point. Oral use of sodium bicarbonate is not recommended. It is used intravenously to correct acidosis in cardiac emergencies and other conditions.

Dosage: Adults: (IV) 1 mEq/kg, then titrated as necessary. Doses of 0.5 mEq/kg may be repeated as necessary.
Children: (IV) 0.5 to 1 mEq/kg, then titrated as necessary.

sucralfate (Carafate). This complex of sucrose and aluminum hydroxide aids the healing of ulcers with its topical, soothing effect. It adheres to the ulcer itself, acting as a mechanical protectant against the action of acid and digestive enzymes.

Dosage: Adults only: (Oral) 1 gm four times daily.

DIGESTANTS

Digestants are drugs that promote the process of digestion in the GI tract and constitute a type of replacement therapy in deficiency states.

Herb Alert
Cayenne (Capsicum)

Cayenne is taken orally as a digestive aid. It stimulates the production of gastric juices and helps relieve gas. In addition, various antimicrobial effects have been shown after administration of cayenne pepper. Capsaicin, the active ingredient of the pepper, can be applied topically to relieve the pain of diabetic neuropathy and for topical treatment of muscle and joint disorders. Cayenne reduces the effect of antihypertensive medications. See Chapter 28 for more information on cayenne.

hydrochloric acid, USP-NF, BP (diluted as 10% solution). A deficiency of hydrochloric acid in the stomach can result from (1) deficient secretion of the acid; (2) excess secretion of mucus, which neutralizes the acid; (3) regurgitation of alkaline substances from the intestine; (4) pernicious anemia; or (5) carcinoma of the stomach. If there is decreased secretion of hydrochloric acid from the stomach gland, the condition is known as *hypochlorhydria*. If there is no secretion, it is known as *achlorhydria*. Achlorhydria is common in carcinoma and is observed in pernicious anemia, infections, renal disease, and diabetes. Occasionally, achlorhydria occurs in individuals apparently otherwise normal in every respect. Dilute hydrochloric acid may be given to combat these conditions. It is taken in water through a glass straw to protect the enamel of the teeth.

Dosage: Adults: (Oral) 4 mL of the dilute acid.

lactase enzyme (Lactaid). Lactase is the enzyme that digests lactose, or milk sugar. It may be given to individuals with lactose intolerance to enable them to consume milk and milk products. It is supplied in caplets, chewable tablets, and in the form of drops to be added directly to milk.

Dosage: Adults and children: (Oral) Drops: 5 to 15 drops per quart of milk; Caplets: 1 to 3 caplets (3000 units each) with the milk product.

pancreatin, USP-NF, BP (Donnazyme, Kutrase). This commercial preparation from the pancreas tissue of hogs and oxen contains all the pancreatic digestive enzymes. It is used to replace pancreatic enzymes in conditions such as cystic fibrosis and various malabsorption syndromes.

Dosage: Adults and children: (Oral) 1000 mg three times daily with meals and 1000 mg between meals.

pancrelipase, USP-NF, BP (Creon, Ku-Zyme, Pancrease, Ultrase, Viokase). This standardized pancreas enzyme replacement is made from hog pancreas. It has more digestive enzymes on a weight basis than the cruder product pancreatin. It is used in the treatment of cystic fibrosis and other disorders of pancreatic dysfunction.

Dosage: Adults: (Oral) 900 mg with each meal and 300 mg with each snack.

APPETITE STIMULANT

megestrol acetate (Megace). This agent is a synthetic derivative of the female hormone progesterone. It enhances the appetite and is used in the treatment of cachexia from serious illnesses and anorexia. Its use as an antineoplastic agent is discussed in Chapter 21. Some adrenal suppression has been observed after use of this agent, as has exacerbation of diabetes. Other side effects include vomiting, diarrhea, rash, and headache.

Dosage: Adults: (Oral) 800 mg once daily.

ABSORPTION INHIBITOR

orlistat (Xenical). Orlistat is a lipase inhibitor for obesity management. It acts by blocking absorption of dietary fats. When present in the lumen of the stomach, it forms a covalent bond with gastric and pancreatic lipases. The inactivated enzymes are unable to digest fat. It should be used with a reduced-calorie diet and exercise plan. Side effects include weight loss, vitamin deficiencies, abdominal discomfort, and diarrhea.

Dosage: Adults: (Oral) 120 mg three times daily with each meal.

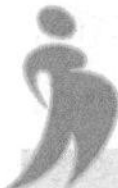

Considerations for Pregnant and Nursing Women
Orlistat (Xenical)

Orlistat (Xenical) is not recommended for pregnant or nursing women. The drug may reduce gastric absorption of fat-soluble vitamins and beta-carotene. It is unknown whether orlistat is distributed in breast milk, but it is not recommended for nursing mothers.

EMETICS

Emetics produce vomiting. They are used primarily as a first aid measure, when prompt emptying of the stomach is essential. Large amounts of tepid water distends the stomach and produce this effect, and 2 teaspoonfuls of salt or mustard in the tepid water hastens emesis. Mild soapsuds solution is also used.

The use of emetics should be avoided in cases of poisoning with a corrosive or caustic substance (a strong acid or alkali that can cause burns and tissue damage) because damage to the mouth, pharynx, and esophagus is increased by the second passage of the material over these structures. The use of emetics at the present time is limited because they have been widely replaced by gastric lavage using a stomach tube.

ipecac syrup, USP-NF, BP. Ipecac syrup is administered orally to produce vomiting when indicated in the management of acute poisonings. After oral administration, almost all patients vomit within 30 minutes. To increase the effectiveness of the drug, it is important to give additional fluids, ideally 200 to 300 mL of a clear liquid, after the dose of ipecac. Milk inhibits the effect of ipecac.

Emesis should not be produced when caustic substances, such as lye, have been ingested or after ingestion of petroleum distillates, such as gasoline, fuel oil, or paint thinners. If the second dose does not produce emesis within 30 minutes, gastric lavage should be performed. No more than two doses should be given.

Currently, the use of this agent is discouraged unless recommended by a health care professional. Ipecac syrup is available without a prescription.

Dosage: Adults and children older than 12 years: (Oral) 30 mL; may repeat in 20 minutes.

Children 1 to 11 years: (Oral) 15 mL; may repeat in 20 minutes.

Children 6 months to 1 year: (Oral) 5 mL; may repeat in 20 minutes.

All doses should be followed by copious clear liquids to increase the effectiveness.

ANTIEMETICS

Antiemetics relieve nausea and vomiting. Numerous preparations have been used, but ordinarily the cause of the nausea must be considered before the most effective treatment can be chosen. Vomiting may be attributed to irritation of the gastric mucosa, stimulation of the vomiting center in the brain, or possibly a combination of both. Antiemetics readily available for home use are carbonated drinks and hot tea.

Herb Alert
Chamomile

Chamomile is a popular remedy for nervous stomach and is known for its calming effect on the smooth muscle of the intestinal tract. Used externally, it relieves skin irritations and hemorrhoids. Used as a mouthwash, it may relieve the pain of toothache. Chamomile enhances the effects of sedatives and warfarin and the antiplatelet effects of NSAIDs. See Chapter 28 for more information on chamomile.

Certain types of vomiting are relieved by administering central depressants such as bromides or barbiturates. Other agents used include the following.

dimenhydrinate, USP-NF, BP (Dramamine). Dimenhydrinate inhibits vomiting and causes sedation. It is frequently used to relieve motion sickness and to control the nausea, vomiting, and vertigo associated with other conditions and medical treatments, such as electroconvulsive therapy, radiation sickness, and hypertension.

Dosage: Adults: (Oral) 50 to 100 mg every 4 to 6 hours to a maximum of 400 mg/day.

Children 6 to 12 years: (Oral, IM) 25 to 50 mg every 6 to 8 hours.

Children 2 to 5 years: (Oral, IM) 12.5 to 25 mg every 6 to 8 hours.

granisetron hydrochloride (Kytril). This centrally acting antiemetic is used to prevent nausea and vomiting associated with chemotherapy. It may be administered orally or intravenously.

Dosage: Adults and children older than 2 years: (IV) 10 mcg/kg as a 5-minute infusion.

Adults only: (Oral) 1 mg twice daily.

meclizine hydrochloride, USP-NF, BP (Antivert, Bonine). This drug prevents nausea and vomiting of motion sickness, and it is used to treat the vertigo associated with labyrinthitis.

Dosage: Adults: (Oral) 25 mg three times daily.

Children: Not recommended.

ondansetron hydrochloride (Zofran). The antiemetic activity of ondansetron is believed to be mediated by the central nervous system. It is administered intravenously and is effective in controlling nausea and vomiting caused by cancer chemotherapy and postoperative nausea and vomiting. It should not be used for routine prophylaxis.

Dosage: Adults: (IV) 32 mg infused over 15 minutes.

Children older than 3 years: (IV) 0.15 mg/kg infused over 15 minutes.

prochlorperazine maleate, USP-NF, BP (Compazine). In addition to its tranquilizing effect, prochlorperazine is very effective in controlling vomiting. It is used postoperatively for this purpose. It may also be given orally in tablet or liquid form.

Dosage: Adults: (Oral, Rectal, IM, IV) 5 to 10 mg three to four times daily.

Children: (Oral) 2.5 to 5 mg two times daily.

trimethobenzamide hydrochloride, USP-NF, BP (Tigan). This agent is closely related to the antihistamines. It acts centrally on the vomiting center to decrease nausea and vomiting. It is effective when administered orally, rectally, or parenterally.

Dosage: Adults: (Oral) 300 mg one to four times daily; (IM, Rectal) 200 mg three to four times daily.

Children: (Oral) 100 mg three times daily; (Rectal) 100 mg every 8 hours.

CATHARTICS

Cathartics relieve **constipation**, the condition in which bowel movements are infrequent or incomplete. Constipation occurs when fecal material remains too long in the large intestine and too much water is absorbed from it. The fecal material becomes hardened, and the lower bowel becomes distended. Constipation usually results from one or more of the following causes: (1) an improper diet that leaves too little residue in the intestinal tract, (2) insufficient fluid intake, (3) nervous tension and worry, (4) lack of exercise (an important factor in hospitalized patients), or (5) failure to respond to the normal defecation impulses. In most cases, correction of one or more of these simple health problems takes care of the constipation problem. In other cases, cathartics should be given as an adjunct.

There is no set time limit between bowel movements. Many parents become extremely upset when a child does not develop a regular habit of moving the bowels once every 24 hours. Continually lecturing the child about regularity can create an emotional problem in the child as well as constipation. As long as the stool is of normal consistency and as long as there is no discomfort resulting from distention after elimination, there is no constipation. Many healthy individuals may have normal eliminations no more often than every 3 or 4 days. The administration of laxatives or cathartics of any kind must be absolutely avoided in the presence of abdominal pain, nausea, vomiting, or similar symptoms that may indicate the presence of appendicitis.

BULK-INCREASING LAXATIVES

Laxatives are cathartics that evacuate the bowel by a mild action. Bulk-increasing laxatives act by swelling when in the presence of water and mechanically stimulate the intestine to contract because of the increased volume. They usually take 24 to 48 hours for action. Bulk-increasing laxatives generally substitute for fiber that should be part of a good diet. Information on natural fiber is presented in Chapter 6.

agar. This is a hydrophilic colloid obtained from seaweed. It swells in water to form a mucilaginous (moist and sticky) mass that is soothing to the gastric mucosa. It increases the bulk and keeps the intestinal contents moist and soft. It is contained in the commercial preparation Agoral.

Dosage: Adults: (Oral) 4 gm once daily.

methylcellulose, USP-NF, BP (Citrucel). This compound is made synthetically from cellulose. It swells in water to form a gel. It is available in tablet or liquid form and is found in the commercial preparations Cellothyl, Cologel, and Hydrolose.

Dosage: Adults: (Oral) 1 to 2 gm one to three times daily.

psyllium seed. The powdered mucilaginous portion of these seeds swells in water to form a gel. Psyllium seed has a soothing effect on the mucosa and produces a soft, moist stool. It can be found in the commercial preparation Metamucil.

Dosage: Adults: (Oral) 2 to 6 capsules or 1 tbsp in 8 oz of water, taken once.

LUBRICANT LAXATIVES

Lubricant laxatives act by mixing with and softening the fecal mass but do not increase the bulk. They take 12 to 18 hours for action.

mineral oil, USP-NF, BP. A mixture of hydrocarbons obtained from petroleum, mineral oil is indigestible and not absorbed. It is purely a mechanical lubricant. However, one disadvantage to its continued use is that it prevents absorption of fat-soluble vitamins and carries them through the intestinal tract. If mineral oil is aspirated when swallowing, lipid pneumonia may result; this may be a problem particularly in older patients.

Dosage: Adults: (Oral) 15 to 45 mL once daily.

SALINE CATHARTICS

Saline cathartics are highly water-soluble substances that are poorly absorbed from the GI tract. Because of their high osmotic pressure, they hold water in the GI tract and cause more water to be absorbed into the tract from other tissues. This water greatly increases the bulk in the intestine and promotes contraction of the smooth muscle.

In addition to their use as laxatives, these agents may be used to treat edematous conditions and food poisoning in which the most rapid evacuation possible is desired. They act in 1 to 4 hours, but considerable gripping (severe spasms of pain in the abdomen) may be produced.

Osmosis is the passage of water through a semipermeable membrane from a less concentrated to a higher concentrated area; this tends to dilute the more highly concentrated solution and to equalize the concentrations of the solutions on either side of the semipermeable membrane.

Osmotic pressure may be best explained by an example. An aqueous solution of sugar or salt is placed in a small, closed semipermeable (permeable to water; impermeable to the dissolved molecules) sac made of cellophane, parchment, or sausage skin and immersed in a container of water. Water from the container is drawn into the sac by osmosis, but the sugar or salt solution does not pass out. The pressure within the sac increases because of the increased volume of water; the walls of the sac become distended and may rupture. The force created in this way is referred to as the osmotic pressure.

electrolytes for oral solution (NuLYTELY, GoLYTELY). Polyethylene glycol combined with sodium chloride, sodium bicarbonate, and potassium chloride is reconstituted in a 4-L jug for bowel cleansing before colonoscopy or barium enema examinations. It induces diarrhea, which rapidly cleanses the bowel, usually within 4 hours. Side effects include nausea, abdominal distention, and pain, although these effects are generally mild.
Dosage: Adults: (Oral) 4 L at a rate of 8 oz every 10 to 15 minutes.

Children: (Oral) 25 mL/kg/hr until rectal effluent is clear.

magnesia magma, USP-NF, BP (milk of magnesia). The mildest of the saline cathartics, this is the agent preferred for children. In addition to its use as a laxative, it is an effective antacid in smaller doses.
Dosage: Adults and children: (Oral) As an antacid—5 to 15 mL up to four times a day; as a laxative—15 mL at bedtime.

magnesium citrate solution, USP-NF, BP (citrate of magnesia). This is a fast-acting saline cathartic in liquid form. Because the solution contains a considerable amount of sugar, it should not be given to a diabetic unless this sugar is taken into consideration.
Dosage: Adults: (Oral) 6 to 12 oz.

sodium phosphate monobasic monohydrate (Visicol). This combination of salts is used in a tablet form as a bowel evacuant before colonoscopy or barium enema examination. It should be used with caution in patients with impaired renal function. Side effects include abdominal distention and pain.
Dosage: Adults only: (Oral) Two doses of 30 gm approximately 12 hours apart.

IRRITANT CATHARTICS

These agents act by irritating the mucosa of the intestinal tract; they produce contraction of the muscle and elimination.

bisacodyl (Dulcolax). This commercial irritant laxative is used in either tablet or suppository form.
Dosage: Adults: (Oral, Rectal) 10 mg once daily.

castor oil, USP-NF, BP. Castor oil is broken down in the intestine (hydrolyzed), similar to any other digestible fat, to glycerin and a fatty acid. This fatty acid is responsible for the irritation and the laxative effect of the oil. It is given in larger doses than are strictly needed for the laxative effect (laxation) because as soon as enough oil is hydrolyzed, laxation is produced, and the remainder of the unhydrolyzed oil gives a soothing effect to the mucosa as the mass moves through the tract.
Dosage: Adults: (Oral) 15 mL.

senna, USP-NF, BP (Senokot). Senna consists of the dried leaf of *Cassia acutifolia*. It contains glucosides, which are stimulant cathartics. It is only slightly absorbed from the small intestine and produces a bowel movement generally in 6 to 12 hours.
Dosage: Adults and children older than 12 years: (Oral) 15 mg once daily; (Rectal) 30 mg one to two times daily.

Children 6 to 12 years: (Oral) 8.6 mg once daily.

FECAL SOFTENERS

Fecal softeners are surface-active agents (surfactants) or detergents. Their action is accomplished by mixing with the fecal material, causing it to be "wetted" by the water in the GI tract, emulsifying and softening it for easier elimination. These agents gain the desired effect without irritating the gastric mucosa and without increasing the bulk content of the intestine. For these reasons, they are the agents of choice for cardiac patients.

Fecal softeners take 1 to 3 days for action; they cannot be used when a faster elimination is desired. Occasionally, the surface-active agent is combined with one or more of the other laxatives for a faster effect.

FECAL SOFTENERS USED AS SINGLE AGENTS

docusate calcium (Dioctyl, Surfak)
Dosage: Adults: (Oral) 240 mg/day.

docusate sodium (Colace, Correctol, Modane)
Dosage: Adults: (Oral) 50 to 300 mg/day.

FECAL SOFTENERS IN COMBINATION

docusate sodium, 100 mg, plus casanthranol, 30 mg (Doxidan, Peri-Colace)
Dosage: Adults: 1 to 2 capsules daily.

OTHER LAXATIVES

lubiprostone (Amitiza). Lubiprostone is a fatty acid that activates the intestinal chloride channels and increases intestinal fluid secretion. It is used to treat idiopathic constipation in adults. Side effects include nausea, diarrhea, headache, and abdominal pain.
Dosage: Adults: (Oral) 24 mcg twice daily.

ANTIDIARRHEALS

Antidiarrheals are used to treat **diarrhea,** a disorder associated with too-rapid passage of intestinal content, gripping action, and abnormally frequent, watery stools. Some causes of diarrhea are (1) contaminated or partially decomposed food, (2) intestinal infection, (3) nervous disorders, (4) circulatory disturbances, and (5) inflammatory conditions of the adjacent viscera. In view of these numerous causes, the treatment of diarrhea varies greatly. In some cases, a cathartic that brings about emptying of the entire bowel may relieve the diarrhea because it removes the irritating material. If diarrhea is caused by an infection, treatment must be directed toward killing the invading organism.

AGENTS USED FOR SIMPLE DIARRHEA

DEMULCENTS

Demulcents have a soothing effect on the irritated membrane of the GI tract. Boiled starch and boiled milk are convenient home remedies of this type. Others are acacia, glycyrrhiza, and glycerin.

ADSORBENTS

Adsorbents act by adsorbing the irritating material on the surface of the GI tract and removing it. Examples of this type are activated charcoal, kaolin, and kaolin-pectin mixture (Kaopectate). The last mixture combines the adsorbing properties of kaolin with the demulcent effect of pectin. Sometimes an agent that decreases peristalsis is added to these preparations, such as paregoric or belladonna alkaloids. Antibiotics may be combined with the adsorbents also.

AGENTS USED FOR SEVERE DIARRHEA

alosetron hydrochloride (Lotronex). Alosetron is indicated *only* for women with severe, diarrhea-prominent irritable bowel syndrome. It should not be used in patients with constipation. Side effects include abdominal discomfort, nausea, abdominal distention, hemorrhoids, and tachycardia.
Dosage: Adults: (Oral) 0.5 to 1 mg twice daily.

diphenoxylate hydrochloride plus atropine sulfate (Lomotil). Diphenoxylate acts on the smooth muscle of the GI tract in a manner similar to morphine, inhibiting GI motility. Although this drug in standard dosages has essentially no analgesic effect, the administration of opioid antagonists may precipitate a withdrawal syndrome in patients who take it regularly.

Atropine is added to diphenoxylate as a deterrent to overdose. In higher doses, the atropine produces an unpleasant tachycardia along with the other symptoms of atropine overdose (see the discussion of atropine in Chapter 16).

Each tablet or 5 mL of the liquid contains diphenoxylate hydrochloride 2.5 mg with atropine sulfate 0.025 mg. The following dosages are of diphenoxylate only.
Dosage: Adults: (Oral) 5 mg four times daily.
Children 2 to 12 years: 0.3 to 0.4 mg/kg/day.

loperamide hydrochloride (Imodium). Loperamide slows GI motility by exerting a direct effect on the nerve endings of the intestinal wall. It prolongs the transit time of the intestinal contents and reduces fecal volume, diminishing loss of fluid and electrolytes.
Dosage: Adults: (Oral) 4 mg initially, then 2 mg after each unformed stool.
Children: (Oral) 0.08 to 0.24 mg/kg/day in two to three divided doses.

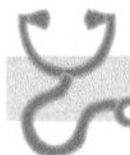

Clinical Implications

1. Antacids interfere with the absorption of many drugs, particularly antibiotics. The ideal time for administration of antacids is 2 hours after a meal, when the acid rebound that follows the completion of digestion of food occurs. They should be given alone or at the time when other drugs are administered.
2. Many drugs that affect the gastrointestinal (GI) tract are liquids. They should be shaken well before administration.
3. Observe the patient for symptomatic relief when GI drugs are being administered; this is generally noted as reduced gastric pain and abdominal distention.
4. Dietary habits should be discussed with patients. A bland diet that eliminates fried or spicy foods and any beverages that contain alcohol or caffeine should be encouraged.
5. Liquid antacids may cause either constipation or diarrhea, depending on their composition. The patient should be observed for these effects.
6. The usual side effects of antiemetic drugs are dry mouth, blurred vision, and urinary retention. Patients should be observed for these effects.
7. Injectable antiemetics should be administered into a large muscle mass because they are often irritating to tissues.
8. The primary side effect of antiemetic agents is central nervous system depression. Patients should be cautioned about this effect. Concurrent administration with other depressants, such as alcohol and sedative or hypnotic agents, should be avoided if possible.
9. The health care professional can instruct patients in changing their diet to include substances such as bran and fiber to eliminate the need for routine laxative therapy.
10. Laxatives are often necessary in hospitalized patients because inactivity and bed rest alter normal bowel function.
11. Laxatives are generally given to hospitalized patients at bedtime to promote effects the following morning.
12. Antidiarrheal preparations may be habit-forming. Patients should be instructed not to overuse these agents.
13. Laxatives may be overused by patients to have a "normal" bowel movement every morning. The health care professional should discuss the range of "normal" with regard to bowel habits.
14. Hyperemesis may be associated with eating disorders.
15. Peptic ulcer disease often has an infectious cause and can be treated specifically.

CRITICAL THINKING QUESTIONS

1. A 12-year-old girl is brought to the physician by her mother, who reports that despite every laxative and food program she could think of, the child is "constantly constipated," having a bowel movement only every 3 or 4 days. There never seems to be any problem or pain associated with the stools, but the mother is concerned that her daughter become "regulated." What is your advice?
2. A patient had a heart attack 2 months ago and is now doing well except for constipation. He calls the office to speak to you because he does not want to bother the doctor. He is just about to take a big dose of Epsom salts to "flush out his system," but his wife made him call to check with you first. What is your advice?
3. A patient calls the physician's office, nearly frantic because her 2-year-old has eaten half a bottle of baby aspirin. The physician is not back from lunch yet. What would you advise?

REVIEW QUESTIONS

1. A frequent cause of peptic ulcer disease is:
   a. infection with *Escherichia coli.*
   b. infection with *Pseudomonas* organisms.
   c. hypertension.
   d. infection with *Helicobacter pylori.*

2. A drug that is often implicated in peptic ulcer disease is:
   a. penicillin.
   b. misoprostol.
   c. ibuprofen.
   d. clarithromycin.

3. A drug that inhibits the secretion of gastric hydrochloric acid is:
   a. ibuprofen.
   b. cimetidine.
   c. pancreatin.
   d. magnesium oxide.

4. A digestant is intended to:
   a. digest food directly.
   b. counteract stomach acid.
   c. replace deficient enzymes of the GI tract.
   d. heal peptic ulcers.

5. An agent used to promote weight loss is:
   a. dimenhydrinate.
   b. orlistat.
   c. pancrelipase.
   d. omeprazole.

6. An agent that prevents vomiting associated with chemotherapy is:
   a. dimenhydrinate.
   b. meclizine.
   c. trimethobenzamide.
   d. granisetron.

7. A cathartic may be necessary if:
   a. there has been no bowel movement for 24 hours.
   b. the stool is of normal consistency.
   c. there is discomfort associated with elimination.
   d. the stools are too loose.

8. An example of a fecal softener is:
   a. magnesium sulfate.
   b. docusate.
   c. ondansetron.
   d. loperamide.

9. An agent that slows intestinal motility is:
   a. docusate.
   b. loperamide.
   c. castor oil.
   d. mineral oil.

10. All of the following are causes of diarrhea *except:*
    a. emesis.
    b. food poisoning.
    c. nervous disorders.
    d. bowel inflammation.

Answers to the review questions can be found at the back of the book.

evolve Additional questions and activities can be found at *http://evolve.elsevier.com/asperheim/pharmacology.*

The Endocrine Glands and Hormones

CHAPTER 18

Objectives

After completing this chapter, you should be able to do the following:

1. Name the glands that are included in the endocrine system.
2. State the function of each endocrine gland.
3. Identify conditions caused by abnormal functioning of each endocrine gland.
4. Identify contraceptives, how they function, and some contraindications for their use.
5. Identify agents used to promote ovulation.
6. Identify oxytocic agents, and discuss precautions to be observed when these are administered.
7. Become familiar with the different types of diabetes and the agents used to treat them.
8. Understand replacement therapy for gonadal dysfunction.

Key Terms

Bioidentical hormone replacement therapy, p. 174
Cortisone (KŎR-tĭ-sōn), p. 167
Endocrine (ĔN-dō-krĕn) **gland,** p. 164
Estrogen (ĔS-trō-jĕn), p. 173
Follicle-stimulating hormone (FSH), p. 172
Hormones (HŎR-mōns), p. 164
Hydrocortisone (hī-drō-KŎR-tĭ-sōn), p. 167
Insulin (ĬN-sū-lĭn), p. 168
Luteinizing (LŪ-tē-ĭn-Ī-zĭng) **hormone (LH),** p. 172
Oxytocic (ŏk-sē-TŌ-sĭk) **agents,** p. 176
Progesterone (prō-JĔS-tē-rōn), p. 172
Testosterone (tĕs-TŎS-tē-rōn), p. 177

The **endocrine glands** do not possess ducts or any openings to the exterior but rather secrete internally. Their secretions, called **hormones,** are chemical substances that pass into the bloodstream and are carried to the various tissues of the body, on which they exert their action—altering the function or activity of that target organ.

The organs of the endocrine system, although separated physically, are unified and well integrated (Fig. 18-1). The main organs belonging to this group of structures that furnish internal secretions to the body are the pituitary, thyroid, parathyroids, adrenals, gonads, and pancreatic islets of Langerhans. The endocrine glands, mammary glands, and growth of the body's skeletal system are under the control of the anterior lobe of the pituitary gland, sometimes called the "master gland."

PITUITARY GLAND

The anterior lobe of the pituitary, a small gland located at the base of the brain, secretes regulating hormones that control the action of other endocrine glands of the body. These regulating hormones are called the *tropic hormones* and are named according to the gland they affect (e.g., the thyrotropic hormone affects the thyroid gland, the adrenocorticotropic hormone affects the cortex of the adrenal glands). These regulating hormones cause the endocrine glands to secrete their respective hormones into the bloodstream.

THYROID GLAND

The thyroid gland is composed of two lobes located on either side of the larynx. The thyrotropic hormone (also known as thyroid-stimulating hormone [TSH]) from

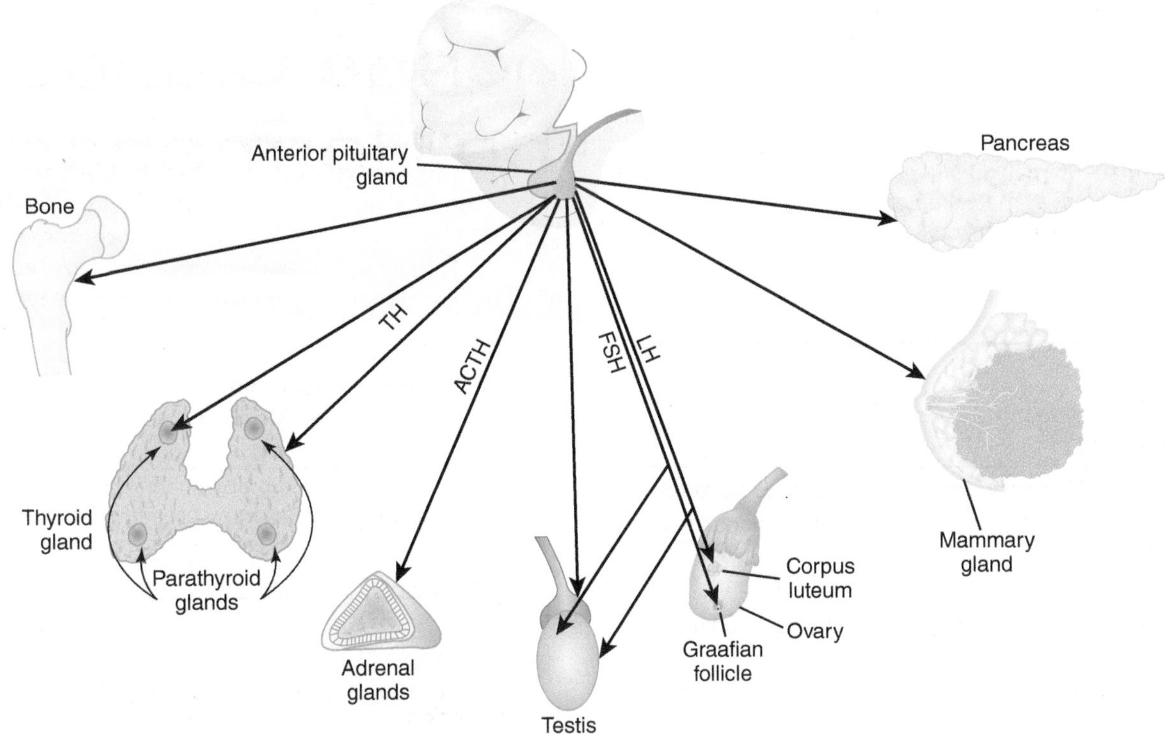

FIGURE 18-1 The endocrine system. *ACTH*, adrenocorticotropic hormone; *FSH*, follicle-stimulating hormone; *LH*, luteinizing hormone; *TH*, thyroid hormone.

the anterior pituitary stimulates the thyroid gland to secrete the thyroid hormones. These hormones, thyroxine (T_4) and triiodothyronine (T_3), affect the metabolism, growth, and development of the body.

Hypothyroidism refers to reduced activity of the thyroid gland. If the thyroid gland of a growing child does not function adequately, the child fails to develop normally. The child has pronounced mental retardation and slow sexual development, and the skin is thickened, dry, and wrinkled. The tongue is thick and protrudes from the mouth, the abdomen protrudes, the legs are short, the hands and feet are poorly developed, and the body musculature is weak. Such a child is known as a cretin; the disorder is called *cretinism*.

Cretinism develops whenever the thyroid gland fails to function properly during the formative years of a child's development. For the most part, it occurs in regions having a deficiency of iodine in the drinking water and food. Cretinism may be corrected if thyroid hormone therapy is given in early infancy. If therapy is not begun until later, permanent mental retardation results.

Severe and prolonged hypothyroidism in an adult can lead to myxedema, which is characterized by a gradual slowing of mental and physical functions. The hands and feet are puffy, the skin is thick and leathery, and the patient is hypersensitive to cold. Good results are usually obtained by treatment with thyroid hormone because full mental and physical development has already been achieved.

Hyperthyroidism, or overactivity of the thyroid, is characterized by an enlargement of the thyroid gland, protruding eyes, elevation of the basal metabolic rate, disturbance of carbohydrate metabolism, nervousness, and hyperactivity. The condition is most commonly caused by the autoimmune disorder Graves' disease. Hyperthyroidism may be treated with an antithyroid drug such as propylthiouracil (100 mg), methimazole (10 mg), or radioactive iodine, or part of the gland may be removed surgically.

Hashimoto's disease, also known as chronic lymphocytic thyroiditis or chronic autoimmune thyroiditis, is caused by an autoimmune process. The serum of these patients contains antibodies to one or more of the thyroid antigens, and it is presumed that the destruction of the thyroid is caused by the antigen-antibody process. Thyroid treatment should be started based on the thyroid studies as soon as the disease is diagnosed. The prognosis is excellent.

Goiter is the term applied to an enlarged thyroid gland. This increase in size may be caused by hyperthyroidism (overactivity of the gland), or it may be caused by hypothyroidism, the growth resulting from a body "reflex" to compensate for the inefficiency of the gland. It is impossible to predict which thyroid abnormality is causing the enlarged appearance of the gland.

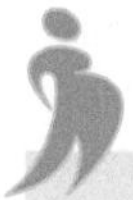

Considerations for Pregnant and Nursing Women

Thyroid Agents

Thyroid agents do not readily cross the placenta and can be administered during pregnancy. However, thyroxine levels are lower than normal during pregnancy, and monitoring generally includes a measurement of serum thyrotropin (TSH), to ensure accurate dosing. Although only minimal amounts of thyroid agents are secreted in breast milk, breast-feeding is generally discouraged for women taking thyroid products.

THYROID PREPARATIONS

Thyroid drugs are either natural or synthetic preparations containing hormones that are naturally produced in the thyroid gland. The synthetic products permit a greater accuracy and predictability when treating thyroid dysfunction.

thyroid, USP-NF, BP. Thyroid is cleaned and dried thyroid gland, obtained primarily from hogs. It may be used in varied dosages as necessary to attain thyroid function in the normal range.

The T_4 level is often used to evaluate thyroid function and therapy. The normal range is 5 to 12 mcg/dL, with the most effective range 7 to 10 mcg/dL. Full thyroid replacement of normal function is 180 mg/day. Partial hypothyroidism requires smaller doses.
Dosage: Adults and children: (Oral) 30 to 60 mg daily, up to 180 mg daily. Dosage is individualized.

SYNTHETIC THYROID PREPARATIONS

There is natural variability in the amount of thyroid in the pulverized crude gland. A more accurate form of thyroid replacement can be achieved with synthetic preparations. They have various potencies; a comparative dosage scale is shown in Table 18-1.

Direct substitution between the thyroid preparations is impossible. Patients may metabolize or excrete one thyroid agent differently than they metabolize another. There have even been some untoward reactions when substituting a generic drug for a formerly used brand-name drug.

Table 18-1 Thyroid Equivalent Dosage

Thyroid Agent	Equivalent Dose
thyroid	60 mg
levothyroxine (Levoxine, Levothroid, Synthroid, T_4)	100 mcg
liothyronine (Cytomel, T_3)	25 mcg

ANTITHYROID AGENTS

Hyperthyroidism is a condition resulting from an overproduction of thyroid hormone. It is also a condition that must be treated medically or surgically. The symptoms of hyperthyroidism include protruding eyes, weight loss, increased appetite, tachycardia and palpitations, nervousness, diarrhea, abdominal cramps, increased pulse and blood pressure, headache, intolerance to heat, fever, and menstrual irregularities.

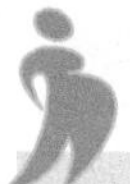

Considerations for Pregnant and Nursing Women

Antithyroid Agents

Antithyroid agents such as propylthiouracil and methimazole (Tapazole) should not be taken by pregnant women because these drugs can induce goiter and hypothyroidism in the developing fetus.

methimazole, USP-NF, BP (Tapazole). Methimazole inhibits the synthesis of thyroid hormones by preventing the incorporation of iodine into the hormone. It is used for palliative treatment of hyperthyroidism and preoperatively before surgical or radiation procedures.
Dosage: Adults: (Oral) 15 to 60 mg daily.

Children: (Oral) 0.4 mg/kg initially, then decreased.

propylthiouracil, USP-NF, BP. Propylthiouracil also interferes with the incorporation of iodine into the thyroid hormone molecule. It is used both for suppression of the thyroid gland before surgical procedures and for medical suppression.
Dosage: Adults: (Oral) 300 to 1200 mg daily in divided doses.

Children 6 to 10 years: (Oral) 50 to 150 mg/m^2 daily in three divided doses.

PARATHYROID GLANDS

There are four parathyroid glands, which are usually located at the poles of the thyroid gland. They are responsible for bone metabolism and for the regulation of calcium between the blood and bone. *Hyperparathyroidism*—increased activity in the parathyroid glands (usually associated with a tumor in one or more of the glands)—causes too much calcium to move away from the bones, giving a moth-eaten appearance to the bones on x-rays. The increase of the calcium level in the blood gives rise to renal and other calculi. Generalized aches and pains are also a part of the syndrome. Hyperparathyroidism is diagnosed by the parathyroid hormone level in the blood.

teriparatide (Forteo). Teriparatide is a biosynthetic (recombinant DNA origin) peptide fragment of human parathyroid hormone. It is used to treat osteoporosis in men and women. It should be used with caution in patients who have had renal calculi. Orthostatic hypotension has also been reported.
Dosage: Adults only: (Subcut) 20 mcg daily for up to 2 years.

Other agents to treat osteoporosis are discussed in Chapter 24.

ADRENAL GLANDS

The adrenal glands are located directly above the kidneys and are composed of two parts: an outer portion, the cortex, and an inner part, the medulla. The medullary portion secretes epinephrine and norepinephrine. The cortex secretes numerous hormones that are essential to life. Death can result when this cortex is removed or severely impaired.

Some hormones secreted by the adrenal cortex are cortisone, hydrocortisone, aldosterone, and deoxycorticosterone. These hormones are secreted when the gland is activated by the adrenocorticotropic hormone from the anterior pituitary. The most important functions of these hormones in the body are (1) regulation of water and salt metabolism, (2) regulation of carbohydrate metabolism, and (3) production of anti-inflammatory effects.

Addison's disease is a destructive disease of the adrenal cortex in humans. If untreated, it is gradually progressive, and death occurs within 2 or 3 years. This condition is characterized by weight loss, weakness, and disturbed carbohydrate and mineral metabolism; in addition, there is increased pigmentation of the skin in certain areas. The skin may be mottled, with areas of depigmentation adjacent to areas of overpigmentation. Addison's disease may be treated by administering deoxycorticosterone along with a diet high in sodium and low in potassium.

Cortisone and **hydrocortisone** are potent anti-inflammatory drugs. When irritation or inflammation is present anywhere in the body, there is an increase in the production of these hormones by the adrenal cortex. If the inflammation is very severe, the adrenals may be unable to secrete an adequate supply to overcome the effects. Additional hormones may be administered to the patient from another source, increasing their levels in the circulation and affording symptomatic relief. Cortisone and hydrocortisone are useful in the suppression of the symptoms of rheumatoid arthritis, bursitis, and various types of skin diseases. The anti-inflammatory properties of these agents have made them useful in the treatment of multiple sclerosis. They can shorten the duration of a relapse and accelerate recovery. The effect on the long-term course of the disease is questionable. Neither cortisone nor hydrocortisone, or any of their derivatives, cures the disease or causes any real improvement. They merely suppress the symptoms; on withdrawal of the drug, symptoms recur.

With continued use of these adrenocorticoid agents, many side effects occur. These side effects are primarily salt and water retention, "moon facies," muscular weakness, hirsutism, acne, and occasionally mental disturbances. Because their action is to suppress the inflammatory response of the body, this suppression occurs also when it is not desired; hence ulcers may be perforated before the patient is aware of them, and tuberculosis may advance at an alarming rate. These drugs should be used with caution in patients with peptic ulcers, and they are contraindicated in patients with tuberculosis or other severe infectious diseases. Newer synthetic compounds are similar in action to cortisone and hydrocortisone, but they have lessened the number and severity of the side effects produced to a great extent.

betamethasone, USP-NF, BP (Celestone).
Dosage: Adults: (Oral) 0.6 to 7.2 mg/day in two to four divided doses; (IM) 0.5 to 9 mg/day in two to four divided doses.

budesonide (Entocort). Budesonide is used for the management of mild to moderate Crohn's disease. In the delayed-release form, it is intended to be released in the terminal ileum and ascending colon, which are the sites of inflammation. It has topical anti-inflammatory and immunosuppressant effects. Adverse effects include nausea, vomiting, and abdominal pain.
Dosage: Adults only: (Oral) 6 mg daily for up to 3 months.

cortisone acetate, USP-NF, BP (Cortogen, Cortone).
Dosage: Adults: (Oral) 25 to 300 mg/day.

dexamethasone, USP-NF, BP (Decadron).
Dosage: Adults: (Oral) 0.75 to 9 mg/day in two to four divided doses; (IM, IV) 0.5 to 24 mg/day; (Intra-articular) 0.4 to 0.6 mg/day.

fludrocortisone acetate (Florinef).
Dosage: Adults: (Oral) 0.1 to 0.2 mg/day.

fluocinolone A, USP-NF, BP (Synalar).
Dosage: Adults: (Topical) 0.01% two to four times daily.

flurandrenolide ointment, USP-NF, BP (Cordran).
Dosage: Adults: (Topical) 0.05% two to three times daily.

hydrocortisone, USP-NF, BP (Cortef, Hydrocortone, Solu-Cortef).

Dosage: Adults: (Oral) 25 to 300 mg/day; (IM, IV, Intrathecal) 100 to 500 mg per dose over 8 hours or as ordered.

methylprednisolone, USP-NF, BP (Medrol, Solu-Medrol).

Dosage: Adults: (Oral) 4 to 60 mg/day; (IM, IV) 10 mg to 1.5 gm daily.

prednisolone, USP-NF, BP (Cotolone, Prelone).

Dosage: Adults: (Oral) 5 to 60 mg/day.

prednisone, USP-NF, BP (Deltasone, Sterapred).

Dosage: Adults: (Oral) 5 to 60 mg/day.

triamcinolone acetonide, USP-NF, BP (Aristocort, Kenalog).

Dosage: Adults: (Oral) 4 to 48 mg/day; (Intralesional, Intra-articular) 2 to 20 mg per dose as ordered.

PANCREAS

Clusters of cells known as the islets of Langerhans are found on the pancreas and are the sources of the hormone known as **insulin**. In a healthy individual, insulin serves three purposes: (1) It aids in the use of glucose as energy, (2) it stores excess glucose as glycogen in the liver, and (3) it is responsible for the conversion of glucose to fat. When the pancreas does not secrete sufficient insulin to carry out these reactions or body cells are resistant to the effects of insulin, the glucose level in the blood becomes quite high after ingestion of carbohydrates. This condition is known as diabetes mellitus.

If diabetes is not treated, sugar spills over into the urine, and acidosis and ketosis occur as a result of the metabolism of fat for energy, resulting in the creation of ketones as by-products. If untreated, a patient in ketosis eventually becomes comatose and dies.

INSULIN THERAPY

The dose of insulin required to treat this condition varies from individual to individual. It is determined by four factors: (1) the weight of the patient, (2) the metabolic rate, (3) physical activity, and (4) any residual function of the pancreas. It is very important to be accurate in the dosage of insulin because an overdose can lead to insulin shock, and too small a dose can result in diabetic coma (Table 18-2). For mild cases,

Table 18-2 Symptoms of Hyperglycemic and Hypoglycemic Reactions

Diabetic Coma	Regular Insulin Reaction	Protamine Zinc or NPH Insulin Reaction
ONSET		
Slow (days) in adults	Sudden, rapid (minutes)	Insidious, slow (hours)
Fairly rapid in children	Reaction occurs in daytime	Reaction occurs in evening
SYMPTOMS		
Weakness, mental dullness	Trembling, mental confusion, weakness, drowsiness, nervousness	Weakness, drowsiness, nervousness, trembling, irritability
FREQUENTLY	FREQUENTLY	OCCASIONALLY
Nausea, vomiting	No nausea	Nausea, vomiting
No appetite	Hunger	Frequently
Thirst	No abdominal pain	Headache
Hot, dry skin	Cold, clammy skin	Hunger
Abdominal pain	Double vision	No abdominal pain
Dim vision	Normal or shallow breathing	Cold, clammy skin
Deep, labored breathing	Loss of consciousness	Double vision
Air hunger		Normal or shallow breathing
Loss of consciousness		Loss of consciousness
Fruity odor on breath		
TREATMENT		
Check blood glucose—will be high.	Check blood glucose—will be low.	Check blood glucose—will be low.
Call physician, who will prescribe regular insulin.	Keep awake: Give sugar or orange juice.	Give sugar or orange juice for fast effect and milk, crackers, or bread for prolonged effect.
	Call physician.	Call physician.

diet therapy alone may be sufficient, along with regulated exercise to maintain the blood glucose level. In more severe cases, oral hypoglycemics or insulin must be given.

Insulin that is used for therapy is structurally the same as human insulin, but it is not extracted from humans. It is prepared biosynthetically using recombinant DNA technology and special laboratory strains of microorganisms, usually *Escherichia coli*. Insulin from pork is still available, but it is rarely used. Table 18-3 presents a comparison of the different types of insulin.

New technology continues to change the way diabetes is treated. The transplantation of new islet cells from human organ donors has achieved limited but encouraging success thus far. It seems to offer promise for the future.

Insulin requirements vary, based on individual needs. Many diabetic patients are treated successfully on 40 to 60 units of insulin per day. In certain cases, insulin resistance occurs, however, and very high doses are required, in some cases up to 100 units/day. This resistance may be due to cirrhosis of the liver, hemochromatosis, allergy, or infection. In many cases, the cause of the insulin resistance is unknown. The U-500 dosage form is used for patients with high insulin requirements. Most patients use the U-100 strength, which is 100 units/mL.

When added to the diabetic regimen, angiotensin-converting enzyme inhibitors (ACE inhibitors) have been shown to reduce the cardiovascular complications of diabetes. In completed studies, the risk of myocardial infarction, strokes, and renal pathology seems to be reduced significantly. ACE inhibitors are discussed in more detail in Chapter 11.

Table 18-3 Comparison of the Types of Insulin

Insulin Type	Onset (hr)	Peak (hr)	Duration (hr)
RAPID-ACTING			
regular insulin (Humulin R)	½-1	2-3	4-8
insulin lispro	½-1	2-3	4-8
INTERMEDIATE-ACTING			
isophane insulin (Humulin N)	1½	4-12	Up to 24
lente insulin zinc (Humulin L)	2½	7-15	Up to 24
LONG-ACTING			
ultralente insulin (Humulin U)	4-8	12-18	Up to 28
insulin glargine (Lantus)	4	Steady	24

INDIVIDUAL INSULIN PRODUCTS

human insulin, USP-NF, BP. This biosynthetic insulin can be prepared in various forms to lower blood glucose rapidly or over a prolonged time. Dosages vary widely based on individual needs.

The family of human insulins is structurally identical to the insulin produced by the human body. It is synthesized by a special non–disease-producing strain of *E. coli* that has been genetically altered by the addition of the gene for human insulin production.

human insulin injection, regular (Humulin R, Novolin R). This product consists of zinc-insulin crystals that are dissolved in a clear fluid. Nothing has been added to change the speed or duration of its activity. It takes effect rapidly and generally lasts 4 to 6 hours. It is given by subcutaneous injection. It may not be given as an IM injection, but it may be given as an IV injection.

Regular insulin is the only insulin form that may be given intravenously. The effect of regular insulin, regardless of the mode of administration, lasts only a few hours.

The Novolin R PenFill and Humulin R cartridges contain 100 units of regular insulin and are easily carried for self-administration of regular insulin.

human insulin injection, isophane (Humulin N, Novolin N). Also known as isophane insulin, or NPH, this is an intermediate-acting insulin containing a suspension of zinc-insulin crystals and protamine sulfate. The onset of action is within 1½ hours, peak activity is expected from 4 to 12 hours, and the duration of action is up to 24 hours. It is given subcutaneously only; it may not be given intramuscularly or intravenously. The Novolin N PenFill and Humulin N Pen contain 100 units of isophane insulin for self-administration.

lente human insulin zinc injection (Humulin L, Novolin L). This intermediate-acting product is a mixture of crystalline and amorphous insulin in a ratio of 7:3. Onset of action is within 2½ hours, peak activity is from 7 to 15 hours, and duration of action is up to 24 hours. It is given subcutaneously only, not intramuscularly or intravenously.

ultralente human insulin injection (Humulin U). This long-acting insulin is a crystalline suspension of human insulin with zinc that provides a slower onset of action and a longer duration of activity. Onset of activity may be expected in 4 to 8 hours, peak activity is from 12 to 18 hours, and duration of action is up to 28 hours. It is given subcutaneously only, not intramuscularly or intravenously.

INSULIN ANALOGS

insulin aspart (Novolog). This analog of human insulin is a rapid-acting insulin that is prepared using recombinant DNA technology. It may be administered alone or in combination with insulin aspart protamine (Novolog Mix 70/30). Dosage must be individualized. It may be administered by continuous infusion and is available in multidose vials and in a FlexPen.

insulin detemir (Levemir). Manufactured from a recombinant DNA biosynthetic origin, this insulin is long-acting and may be administered once or twice daily. When administered once daily, it should be given at the time of the evening meal.

insulin glargine (Lantus). This biosynthetic (recombinant DNA origin) agent is a long-acting human insulin analog. It is administered once daily at the same time of day using a regular insulin syringe or the OptiPen.

insulin glulisine (Apidra). Also of recombinant DNA origin, this is a rapid-acting insulin. It may be administered by subcutaneous injection or by a continuous insulin infusion device.

insulin lispro (Humalog). This analog of human insulin has undergone a slight change from the human insulin molecule. It has a slightly more rapid onset of action when given subcutaneously or intravenously, but for all practical purposes it is interchangeable with regular insulin. There is also a Humalog KwikPen for self-injection that contains 100 units of insulin.

COMBINATION INSULIN PRODUCTS

Humulin 50/50. This product is a combination of 50% regular and 50% isophane insulin.

Humulin 70/30 and Novolin 70/30. These products have combinations of 70% isophane and 30% regular insulin.

INSULIN PUMP THERAPY

Insulin pump therapy, or continuous subcutaneous insulin infusion, is designed to simulate normal pancreatic beta-cell function and deliver both basal and bolus insulin doses in patients with type 1 diabetes. The use of insulin pumps for diabetics was first reported in the late 1970s and demonstrated the possibility of achieving strict glucose control in a select group of individuals. Since then pumps have become dramatically smaller, safer, and easier to use. Current models have electronic memory, multiple basal rates, several bolus options, and a remote control. They are worn on the belt and are now about the size of a pager compared with the large backpack required with the earliest models.

Several factors are key to successful treatment with insulin pumps. The most important is the frequency of blood glucose monitoring. Monitoring blood glucose three or more times a day allows for better control. Other important factors in the success of the pump include logbook recording of insulin doses and blood glucose results, counting carbohydrates, and use of the long-acting insulin lispro with regular insulin. These pumps are now being used with great success for pediatric patients as well.

Some pumps are waterproof and immersible to a depth of 8 feet, allowing patients to swim while wearing one. They can be disconnected during exercise, if desired.

The most serious adverse effect of intensive insulin therapy is severe hypoglycemia. Patients who have had type 1 diabetes for more than 5 years often lose their counterregulatory mechanism for identifying and reversing hypoglycemia. They commonly develop a condition known as hypoglycemic unawareness and no longer recognize the symptoms of low blood glucose levels such as fatigue, sweating, dizziness, palpitations, and impaired cognition. One strategy for preventing hypoglycemia is to set a higher target blood glucose level, using a lower basal insulin delivery rate and eliminating the wide glycemic swings.

Available insulin pumps are the Medtronic MiniMed, Disetronic, Animas, and Deltec.

INCRETIN MIMETIC

exenatide (Byetta). This synthetic glucagonlike agent is used as an adjunct to therapy. It is generally used with metformin or other oral hypoglycemic agents and is administered subcutaneously twice daily. Its actions include slowing the gastric emptying, which slows the meal-derived increase in glucose, and lowering the serum glucagon secretion during periods of hyperglycemia.
Dosage: Adults only: (Subcut) 5 mcg twice daily 60 minutes before morning and evening meals.

ORAL HYPOGLYCEMIC AGENTS

More recent developments in diabetes research have produced oral hypoglycemic agents. These are not insulin derivatives but agents that lower the glucose level in the blood through various actions.

acarbose (Precose). Acarbose inhibits enzymes, known as the alpha-glucosidase enzymes, that break down complex carbohydrates into glucose and other monosaccharides. In a diabetic patient, inhibition of these enzymes results in delayed carbohydrate breakdown, delayed glucose absorption, and a resultant reduction in postprandial hyperglycemia. Acarbose may be used singly or in combination with other agents for the management of type 2 diabetes.
Dosage: Adults: (Oral) 25 mg with the first bite of each meal three times daily.

chlorpropamide, USP-NF, BP (Diabinese). Although a potent oral hypoglycemic agent, this is not a routine insulin substitute. It acts on the pancreatic cells to cause them to release residual insulin. Not all patients with diabetes are suitable candidates for chlorpropamide therapy. It is essential that patients be carefully selected by the physician because the drug would be of little value if the pancreatic cells contained little or no residual insulin to release. This drug should not be used alone in the juvenile type of diabetes (type 1) or when the disease is complicated by acidosis, coma, infection, surgical procedures, or severe trauma. In these cases, insulin is indispensable. A physician prescribing chlorpropamide should insist that the patient report at least once weekly for the first month of therapy because the initial test period should be carefully controlled. The main indication for the use of this agent is uncomplicated diabetes of the stable, mild, or moderately severe maturity-onset or adult type (type 2). However, it may be used in other types of the disease to decrease insulin requirements.
Dosage: Adults: (Oral) 100 to 250 mg/day.

glipizide (Glucotrol). Similar to other sulfonylurea agents, glipizide lowers blood glucose levels in diabetic and nondiabetic patients. It is used as an adjunct to dietary control in the management of non–insulin-dependent (type 2) diabetes.
Dosage: Adults only: (Oral) 2.5 to 40 mg daily in divided doses.

glyburide (Diabeta, Glynase, Micronase). In addition to lowering blood sugar, this agent produces a mild diuresis. It is used along with dietary management to control non–insulin-dependent diabetes.
Dosage: Adults only: (Oral) 1.25 to 20 mg daily in divided doses.

metformin hydrochloride (Glucophage). Metformin is ineffective in the absence of some endogenous insulin. It is believed to improve sensitivity to insulin at the receptor sites. It may be used alone or with another agent.
Dosage: Adults: (Oral) 500 mg twice daily or 850 mg once daily, up to 2550 mg/day in three divided doses with meals.

tolazamide. Tolazamide is used to help in the management of mild to moderate type 2 diabetes. A transition period is not required when transferring to this agent from other oral hypoglycemic agents.
Dosage: Adults only: (Oral) 250 to 500 mg daily.

tolbutamide, USP-NF, BP (Orinase). Tolbutamide is recommended as an adjunct to diet and exercise in the treatment of type 2 diabetes. Its effect is similar to chlorpropamide.
Dosage: Adults: (Oral) 500 mg to 3 gm/day.

OTHER ORAL HYPOGLYCEMICS

All dosages for the following agents are oral dosages and for adults only.

glimepiride (Amaryl).
Dosage: 1 to 4 mg once daily.

miglitol (Glyset).
Dosage: 25 to 300 mg three times daily, taken before meals.

nateglinide (Starlix).
Dosage: 60 to 120 mg three times daily, taken before meals.

pioglitazone (Actos).
Dosage: 15 to 30 mg/day.

repaglinide (Prandin).
Dosage: 0.5 to 16 mg three times daily, taken before meals.

rosiglitazone maleate (Avandia).
Dosage: 4 to 8 mg/day.

COMBINATION ORAL HYPOGLYCEMICS

glipizide plus metformin (Metaglip). This combination is available in three strengths of glipizide/metformin: 2.5 mg/250 mg, 2.5 mg/500 mg, and 5 mg/500 mg.
Dosage: Adults only: Usual maximum dosage is 20 mg glipizide/2000 mg metformin daily.

glyburide plus metformin (Glucovance). This combination comes in three strengths of glyburide/metformin: 1.25 mg/250 mg, 2.5 mg/500 mg, and 5 mg/500 mg.
Dosage: Adults only: Dosage is individualized; not to exceed a daily dose of 20 mg glyburide/2000 mg metformin taken before meals.

rosiglitazone plus metformin (Avandamet). This combination is available in five strengths of rosiglitazone/metformin: 1 mg/500 mg, 2 mg/500 mg, 4 mg/500 mg, 2 mg/1000 mg, 4 mg/1000 mg.
Dosage: Adults only: Usual maximum dosage is 8 mg rosiglitazone/2000 mg metformin.

GONADS

The gonads (sex glands) of the female are the ovaries, and the gonads of the male are the testes. These gonads, under the stimulation of the gonadotropic hormones from the anterior pituitary gland, release the sex hormones. The same gonadotropic hormones are produced in both males and females, but they naturally act on different organs, and the sex hormones released by the respective glands are different. The gonadotropic hormones from the anterior pituitary are **follicle-stimulating hormone (FSH)** and **luteinizing hormone (LH)**.

FEMALE HORMONES

Figure 18-2 shows a cross section of the female reproductive organs. At maturity, FSH stimulates the maturation of the graafian follicles in the ovaries. These follicles are developed from the germinal epithelial cells that cover the surface of the ovary. Small groups of cells separate from the columns and become arranged with a large cell in the center and others in a single layer around it. These primary graafian follicles are found in great numbers in fetal ovaries and in the ovaries of children. The large central cell is called a primitive ovum. Under the influence of FSH, the cells around the ovum produce the female hormone estradiol, which is responsible for (1) the changes in the accessory organs of reproduction during the first part of the menstrual cycle and (2) the development of the secondary sex characteristics.

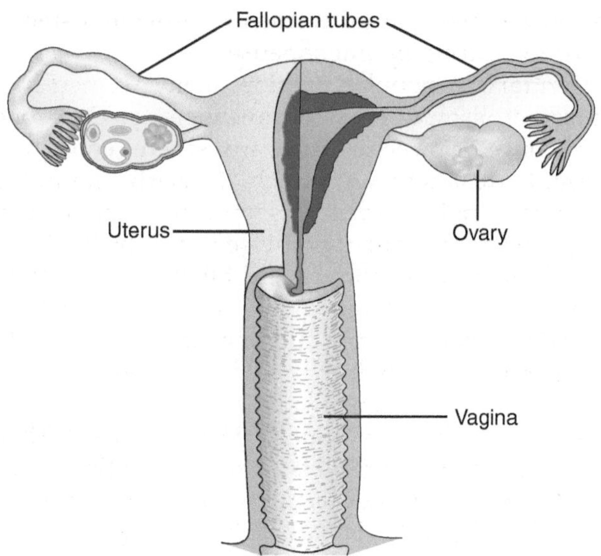

FIGURE 18-2 Female reproductive organs.

The removal of the ovaries in a young girl prevents her from becoming sexually mature. The accessory organs fail to develop, menstruation does not occur, secondary sex characteristics do not appear, and the sex instinct is never manifested. Injection of the female sex hormone estradiol corrects all the effects of ovariectomy.

As the follicle matures or ripens, it becomes distended by the accumulation of fluid and moves outward to the surface of the ovary. It projects from the surface of the ovary as a small cystlike swelling that eventually bursts and discharges the ovum. In women, this process is known as ovulation and occurs about every 28 days (Fig. 18-3).

The cavity of the ruptured follicle becomes filled with a clot of blood that is soon replaced by a mass of cells filled with a yellow, fatlike material called lutein. The structure is now called the corpus luteum, and under the developmental stimulation of LH, the corpus luteum produces **progesterone,** a hormone that prepares the uterus for the reception of the ovum.

Progesterone is responsible for (1) the uterine changes characteristic of the first half of the menstrual cycle (e.g., thickening of the uterine wall, increased supply of blood vessels); (2) the development of the placenta (the organ that enables the embryo to receive nourishment from the mother during pregnancy; after the birth of a child, the placenta is expelled from the uterus as the "afterbirth"); (3) the maturation of the mammary glands during pregnancy; (4) the multiplication of the uterine muscle fibers; and (5) the inhibition of uterine contraction. In short, progesterone induces favorable conditions for the growth and development of the fetus.

If fertilization occurs, the corpus luteum continues to increase in size until the later months of pregnancy, and its hormone continues to exert an influence on the growth and functional integrity of the placenta and uterus. As the conclusion of pregnancy approaches, the corpus luteum disintegrates, the uterus contracts because the inhibiting influence of progesterone is no longer present, and parturition (birth) occurs.

Progesterone may be given parenterally in cases of threatened abortion. If the corpus luteum disintegrates early or if progesterone is not produced naturally, full-term pregnancy can be brought about by administration of the deficient hormone.

If fertilization does not occur, the corpus luteum disintegrates, and the unfertilized ovum and the thickened uterine lining pass off in the menstrual flow. Figure 18-4 is a diagram of the menstrual cycle, showing the fluctuations in hormone concentrations in the blood, the growth of the follicle and corpus luteum,

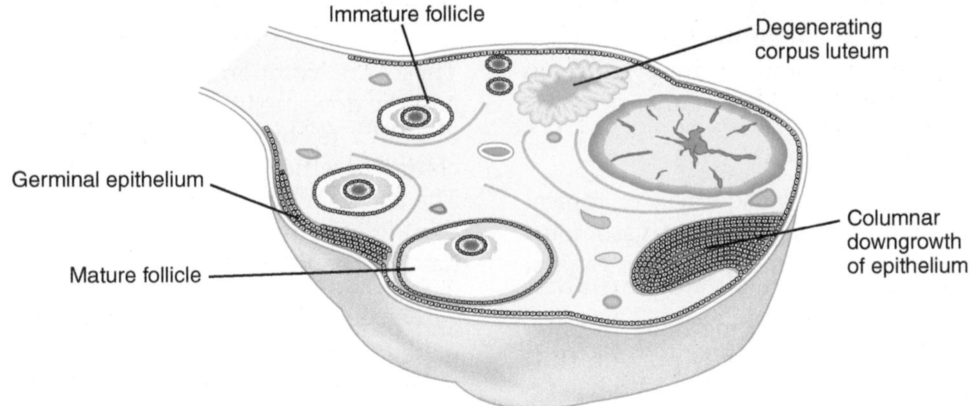

FIGURE 18-3 Ovulation.

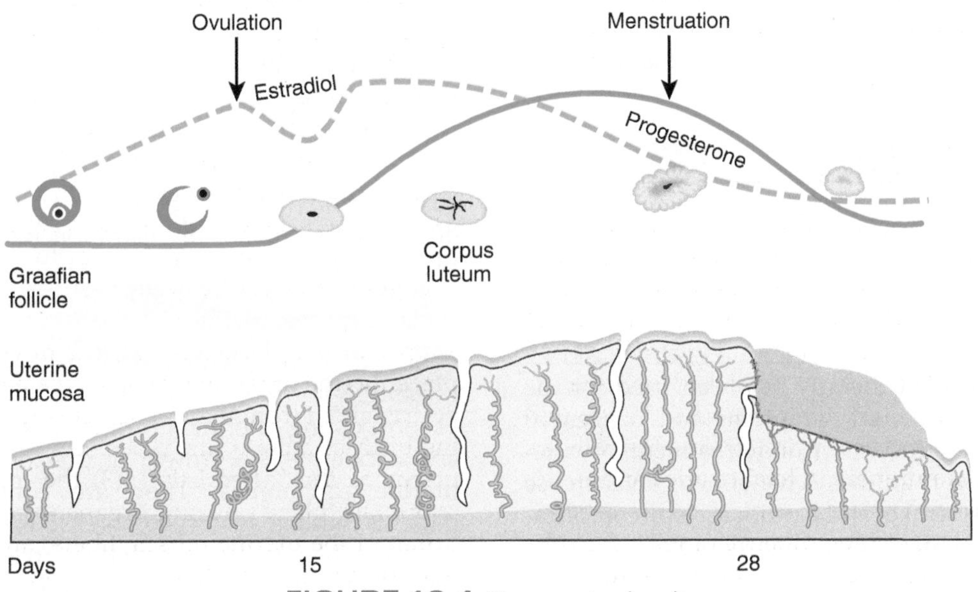

FIGURE 18-4 The menstrual cycle.

and the changes in the uterine lining during the menstrual cycle.

Estradiol is the naturally occurring female hormone in humans and other mammals. The term **estrogen** is a generic term referring to natural and synthetic agents that exert the biologic effect of estradiol.

If fertilization occurs, the placenta produces hormones that are similar to the gonadotropins produced by the anterior pituitary gland. These hormones are called the anterior pituitary–like hormones or the chorionic gonadotropins, named after the chorion, which is the part of the placenta that develops around the fetus. The presence of these hormones in the urine is the basis for pregnancy tests.

It is necessary to provide female sex hormone therapy in cases in which a known deficiency of this hormone is present because therapy brings about a normal physiologic state. Estrogen is used to treat conditions such as sexual infantilism and senile vaginitis and in perimenopausal women to provide a smooth transition during perimenopause.

Contrary to popular opinion, many women have almost no symptoms at perimenopause. Only one-third have symptoms that are severe enough to warrant treatment. Although formerly hormones were used only during this transition phase, now longer term hormone therapy seems to be beneficial in preventing osteoporosis and other tissue changes in postmenopausal women and so is often routinely prescribed both during perimenopause and after the menopause. An increased risk of breast cancer (8 per 10,000 women increase) was observed in one study after continued hormone use. There continues to be controversy regarding this subject. Cardiovascular issues seem to increase, but much variability depends on family history and maintenance of good cholesterol, blood pressure, and body weight.

It has also been found that estrogens in high concentration in the blood tend to inhibit the female organs. Commercial estrogenic preparations may be given postpartum to inhibit lactation if the mother does not choose to breastfeed the infant.

estradiol, USP-NF, BP. Oral, transdermal, or topical estradiol is used for the management of vasomotor symptoms associated with menopause and for vaginal atrophy.
Dosage: Adults only: (Oral) 1 to 2 mg daily, supplemented with progestin if the uterus is present; (IM) 1 to 5 mg (cypionate salt) once every 3 to 4 weeks; (Vaginally) 25 mcg daily for 2 weeks.

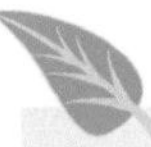

Herb Alert
Black Cohosh

Black cohosh is an herbal remedy used to treat the hot flashes of menopause, premenstrual tension, and dysmenorrhea (painful menstruation). Black cohosh must not be used during pregnancy because it is associated with an increased risk of spontaneous abortion (miscarriage). Black cohosh enhances the effects of antihypertensives and diuretics and the antiplatelet action of warfarin and nonsteroidal anti-inflammatory drugs. See Chapter 28 for more information on black cohosh.

HORMONE REPLACEMENT THERAPY

Estrogen replacement therapy has been used for the treatment of menopausal symptoms and urogenital dryness and the prevention and treatment of osteoporosis. However, studies have shown an increase in breast cancer, stroke, and cardiovascular complications with the use of replacement therapy.

estrogens, conjugated, USP-NF, BP (Premarin).
Dosage: Adults: (Oral) 0.625 to 2.5 mg daily; (IV) 25 mg daily; (Vaginal) As a cream once daily.

esterified estrogens tablets, USP-NF (Estratab).
Dosage: Adults: (Oral) 0.3 to 1.25 mg daily.

ESTROGEN AGONIST-ANTAGONISTS

raloxifene hydrochloride (Evista). Raloxifene is an estrogen agonist-antagonist. It is used as an alternative to cyclic estrogen/progestogen treatment in postmenopausal women. It is believed that this agent has a lower incidence of breast cancer as a side effect than the cyclic estrogen replacement.
Dosage: Adults: (Oral) 60 mg/day.

BIOIDENTICAL HORMONE REPLACEMENT THERAPY

The term **bioidentical hormone replacement therapy,** or natural hormone therapy, is an ill-defined term. It generally refers to the use of hormones that are identical to endogenous hormones in the body. These are compounded by pharmacists to order, and the dose prescribed is determined through blood or saliva testing. Many authorities believe that the claims of efficacy are exaggerated and unfounded. The accuracy of the saliva and blood levels in determining effective levels of estrogen and progesterone has not been determined.

Specific hormones used include estrone, estradiol, and progesterone. They would be expected to have the same issues and side effects as the commercially available hormone preparations. The term is also used to mean "plant derived,"—hence "natural"—but these plant substances are not bioidentical with human hormones.

ORAL CONTRACEPTIVES

Oral contraceptives are agents that prevent pregnancy by virtue of their estrogen content. Estrogens act to prevent ovulation by suppressing the release of FSH from the anterior pituitary. Estrogens are administered in combination with progesterone to prevent the side effects of estrogen administration (i.e., breakthrough bleeding and prolonged menses).

Side effects of oral contraceptives include breast changes, loss of scalp hair, dermatoses, headache, nervousness, thromboembolic disorders, and emotional instability. Oral contraceptives accelerate the growth of preexisting uterine fibroids and cervical polyps and accelerate the growth of preexisting breast and uterine carcinomas. They are contraindicated in patients with a history of breast or genital cancer; thrombophlebitis; myocardial infarction or coronary artery disease; or preexisting liver, kidney, or heart dysfunction. They should be used with extreme caution in patients with epilepsy. An important side effect when oral contraceptives are used is that they become *less* effective in preventing ovulation when the patient is also taking antibiotics.

levonorgestrel plus ethinyl estradiol (Seasonale). This is an extended-cycle oral contraceptive consisting of 84 active tablets and 7 inert tablets per cycle. It is based on a 91-day regimen that reduces the number of menstrual periods from 12 to 13 per year to 4 per year. Because there are fewer menstrual cycles with this product, pregnancy should be ruled out before it is started. The side effects are the same as the general oral contraceptives. Active ingredients are 0.15 mg levonorgestrel and 30 mcg ethinyl estradiol per tablet.

levonorgestrel plus ethinyl estradiol (Triphasil). This oral contraceptive consists of three different drug combinations to be taken at appropriate times during the

Table 18-4 Oral Contraceptives

Brand Name	Component Drugs	Dose			
Enovid	norethynodrel mestranol	5 mg 0.075 mg			
Enovid-E	norethynodrel mestranol	2.5 mg 0.1 mg			
Ortho Novum (three strengths)	norethindrone mestranol ethynodiol diacetate	2 mg 2 mg 0.1 mg		1/50 1 mg 0.05 mg	1/80 1 mg 0.08 mg
Ovulen	mestranol ethinyl estradiol	1 mg 0.1 mg			
Demulen	ethynodiol diacetate ethinyl estradiol	50 mcg 1 mg			
Norlestrin (two strengths)	norethindrone acetate ethinyl estradiol	50 mcg 1 mg	*or*	50 mcg 2.5 mg	
Ovral	norgestrel ethinyl estradiol	50 mcg 500 mcg			
Lo/Ovral	norgestrel	0.03 mg 0.3 mg			

month. It more nearly replicates the natural hormone variations.

Phase 1 (6 tablets): Each tablet contains 0.05 mg levonorgestrel and 30 mcg ethinyl estradiol.

Phase 2 (5 tablets): Each tablet contains 0.075 mg levonorgestrel and 40 mcg ethinyl estradiol.

Phase 3 (10 tablets): Each tablet contains 0.125 mg levonorgestrel and 30 mcg ethinyl estradiol.

For other oral contraceptives, see Table 18-4.

INJECTABLE AND TRANSDERMAL CONTRACEPTIVES

ethinyl estradiol and etonogestrel ring (NuvaRing). This soft flexible ring may be inserted into the vagina by the patient. Its exact positioning is not important. When used for the first time, it should be inserted 5 days after the menstrual period starts. If accidentally expelled, it can be rinsed with cool water and reinserted. If it has been out of the vagina more than 3 hours, a back-up method of contraception should be used. Withdrawal bleeding usually occurs 2 to 3 days after removal of the ring.

Dosage: Adults: (Intravaginal) Ring should be inserted for 3 weeks each cycle followed by a 1-week free period. The same day of the week should be used for insertions and removals.

etonogestrel subdermal implant (Implanon). One implant is placed subdermally for 3 years of contraception.

Dosage: Adults only: (Subdermal) 68 mg.

levonorgestrel intrauterine device (Mirena). Within 7 days of menses onset, this intrauterine device (IUD) may be inserted in the uterus. It provides 5 years of contraception.

Dosage: Adults only: (IUD) 52 mg.

medroxyprogesterone acetate, USP-NF, BP (Depo-Provera). Medroxyprogesterone is administered intramuscularly every 3 months for contraception. The level of this progesteronelike hormone is sufficient to prevent ovulation.

Menses may cease entirely or become irregular with the administration of this agent. Statistically, it is 99% effective in preventing pregnancies and is useful for women who do not wish to take oral contraceptives. There is a warning for this agent, however. It is now recommended that it be used no longer than 2 years unless other contraceptive methods are unavailable. It causes loss of bone mineral density, which may not be entirely reversible when the agent is discontinued.

Dosage: Adults: (IM) 150 mg every 3 months.

norelgestromin plus ethinyl estradiol (Ortho Evra). This contraceptive transdermal patch is placed on weekly for 3 weeks and then left off for 1 week. Each patch contains 6 mg norelgestromin and 0.75 mg ethinyl estradiol. It releases 150 mcg of norelgestromin and 20 mcg of ethinyl estradiol into the bloodstream per 24 hours.

Although not having to remember to take an oral contraceptive daily is an advantage, the transdermal patch also has its disadvantages. Reportedly, about 2% to 6% of the patches detached completely. They are less satisfactory in warm, humid climates.

EMERGENCY CONTRACEPTION

Immediate use of an emergency contraceptive agent reduces a woman's risk of pregnancy to 1% to 2%. Various methods are used. Because these agents, with the exception of levorgestrel (Plan B), are available by prescription only and not yet available over-the-counter, they must be prescribed in advance of need. Levorgestrel (Plan B) is available without a prescription to women 18 years old and older.

High Doses of a Combination Oral Contraceptive

The first dose should be taken within 72 hours of unprotected intercourse.

ethinyl estradiol plus levonorgestrel (Preven). Each tablet contains 100 mcg of ethinyl estradiol and 0.5 mg of levonorgestrel.
Dosage: Adults: (Oral) 2 tablets within 72 hours of unprotected intercourse and 2 tablets 12 hours later.

levonorgestrel plus ethinyl estradiol (Ovral). Two of the standard Ovral contraceptive tablets equal the dose of Preven.
Dosage: Adults: (Oral) 2 tablets within 72 hours of unprotected intercourse and 2 tablets 12 hours later.

Progestin-Only Regimen

levonorgestrel (Plan B). Single tablets contain 0.75 mg levonorgestrel.
Dosage: Adults: (Oral) 2 tablets once or 1 tablet within 72 hours of unprotected intercourse and 1 tablet 12 hours later.

AGENTS TO PROMOTE OVULATION

Agents to promote ovulation are used in an attempt to promote pregnancy in a woman previously unable to conceive. Only one agent is approved for use in the United States at this time.

clomiphene citrate, USP-NF, BP (Clomid). Clomiphene is a synthetic, nonsteroidal compound that may be administered orally to promote ovulation in women who have been anovulatory. It is believed to act by promoting the release of pituitary gonadotropins, which promote ovulation. Multiple conceptions (including triplets, quadruplets, quintuplets, and sextuplets) increase 10-fold when this drug is used. Infant mortality is very high in the multiple conceptions, often because of premature delivery. This drug is contraindicated in patients with a history of liver disease and patients with abnormal uterine bleeding. Side effects include blurred vision, hot flashes, abdominal discomfort, nausea, vomiting, breast engorgement, headache, dizziness, and skin reactions.
Dosage: Adults: (Oral) 50 mg daily for 5 days. Dosage is then individualized.

OXYTOCIC AGENTS

Although many drugs may be used during the course of pregnancy and delivery and immediately postpartum, the drugs specifically related to uterine function are the **oxytocic agents,** which are uterine stimulants. Oxytocic drugs are so named because they resemble the action of oxytocin, a hormone secreted from the posterior pituitary gland.

dinoprostone (Prostin E_2). This naturally occurring prostaglandin is prepared synthetically for commercial use. It is used intravaginally to induce abortion during the second trimester of pregnancy. Abortion generally occurs within 12 to 14 hours after intravaginal administration.
Dosage: Adults: (Intravaginal) 20 mg every 3 to 5 hours until abortion occurs.

dinoprostone cervical gel (Prepidil). This gel is administered endocervically. Its purpose is to stimulate the myometrium of the gravid uterus to contract. It also has a softening or effacement effect on the cervix, enhancing dilation. It is used in pregnant women at or near term with a medical or obstetric need for labor induction.
Dosage: Adults: 0.5 mg endocervically via catheter. Dosage may be repeated once in 6 hours.

ergonovine maleate, USP-NF, BP (Ergotrate). The dangerous similarity in names between this ergot alkaloid and ergotamine, a drug used to treat migraine headaches, is discussed in Chapter 16.

Similar to oxytocin, this drug has a constricting effect on uterine muscles, although it seems to have a greater selective action on the uterus, causing less peripheral vasoconstriction, and it acts more quickly than oxytocin. It is used for the treatment of postpartum and postabortion hemorrhage. Long-term use of this drug may produce ergotism, a prolonged constriction of the blood vessels in other parts of the body that may lead to gangrene and loss of the affected parts of the body.
Dosage: Adults: (Oral, IM, IV) 0.2 mg every 2 to 4 hours for a total of five doses.

methylergonovine maleate, USP-NF, BP (Methergine). This synthetic drug may be administered orally or parenterally to cause constriction of the uterus. Its action is similar to ergonovine, but it is more potent and has a more prolonged duration of action. In addition, it has less tendency to elevate blood pressure; it is preferred for patients with threatened eclampsia.
Dosage: Adults: (Oral, IM, IV) 0.2 mg every 2 to 4 hours for a total of five doses.

mifepristone (Mifeprex, RU-486). This oral abortifacient was used for some time in Europe before being approved in the United States. It may be taken orally anytime before the 8th week of pregnancy. When the tablets are absorbed, they block receptors of progesterone, a hormone needed to maintain pregnancy.
Dosage: Adults: (Oral) 3 tablets (200 mg each) taken on day 1 and 2 tablets of misoprostol (200 mcg each) taken on day 3. A post-treatment examination is necessary on day 14.

oxytocin injection, USP-NF, BP (Pitocin, Syntocinon). Oxytocin stimulates the uterine muscles and produces rhythmic contractions. Sensitivity to this drug increases as a pregnancy progresses. It is contraindicated in the first stage of labor because severe laceration and trauma are likely if used when the cervix is undilated and rigid.

Overdose of oxytocin may produce uterine tetany. The drug must be given with great caution to patients with cardiovascular disease or a previous cesarean section or when there is a malpresentation of the fetus or threatened uterine rupture for any reason.

This drug is administered in small doses as an IV drip to induce labor, but this procedure must be carried out under close medical supervision. An infusion pump is necessary for precise control of this medication when given intravenously.
Dosage: Adults: (IM) 3 to 10 units; (IV) 0.5 to 2 milliunits/min.

sodium chloride 20% injection. Injected directly into the amniotic fluid, this concentrated sodium chloride solution is useful in the induction of second-trimester abortions. When the injection is performed correctly, little sodium chloride is absorbed by the mother. However, it is recommended that at least 2 L of water be given to the mother before the abortion is induced. Side effects include a sensation of heat, thirst, and mental confusion, and there have been reported maternal deaths as a result of hypernatremia.
Dosage: Adults: (IV) 200 to 250 mL by transabdominal intra-amniotic catheter.

urea 40% to 50% injection (carbamide). Hypertonic urea, especially in conjunction with IV oxytocin, induces fetal death and abortion. When the procedure is performed correctly, there is little risk. However, the patient should take fluids during the procedure to facilitate urea excretion. Monitoring for signs of fluid and electrolyte imbalance should be performed throughout the procedure.
Dosage: Adults: (IV) 200 to 250 mL by transabdominal intra-amniotic catheter.

MALE HORMONES

In the human male, as already stated, the same two gonadotropic hormones are produced by the anterior pituitary as are found in females. In males, however, FSH causes production of spermatozoa, and LH causes development of the interstitial cells that produce **testosterone,** the male hormone.

Testosterone is responsible for normal development of the male reproductive tract and maintains the secondary sex characteristics. It plays a role in the development of the penis, the seminal vesicles, and the prostate gland and in the descent of the testes from the abdominal cavity. The accessory sexual characteristics affected by testosterone are the depth of the voice, the distribution of facial and body hair, and the development of the masculine skeletal muscles. Muscular strength and endurance are also increased by administration of the male hormone.

Testosterone confers a sense of "well-being" and restores mental equilibrium and energy. It can also increase the resistance of the central nervous system to fatigue. It may be used therapeutically in the following instances: (1) when a deficiency of the hormone is known, (2) in females to treat certain ovarian dysfunctions such as menorrhagia and dysmenorrhea, and (3) in females to treat breast engorgement and suppress lactation. (Some commercial preparations contain a combination of estrogen and androgen for this purpose.)

testosterone gel (AndroGel). This clear gel provides a continuous transdermal delivery of testosterone after a single application to clean, dry skin. It is used for testosterone replacement therapy in men.
Dosage: Adults: 5 gm gel delivering 5 mg testosterone applied to clean, dry skin once daily.

testosterone transdermal system (Androderm). This patch is applied once every 24 hours and delivers testosterone for the 24-hour period. It is used as replacement therapy in men.
Dosage: Adults: (Transdermal patch) 2.5 or 5 mg, applied daily.

Agents that treat erectile dysfunction are discussed in Chapter 19.

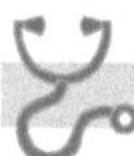

Clinical Implications

1. When preparing a vial of insulin before giving an injection, rotate the bottle between the palms. Vigorous shaking produces bubbles, which interfere with accurate dosage.
2. Carefully measure the exact dose of insulin to be administered, using a calibrated insulin syringe or a tuberculin syringe.
3. The sites of injection are to be rotated. Chart the site of injection for effective rotation.
4. Finger-stick blood samples for blood glucose levels should be used to determine the patient's status and response to insulin.
5. It is necessary for a diabetic to follow his or her diet closely. The health care professional should be familiar with dietary requirements and be available to answer any questions that the patient may have regarding the diet.
6. Vigorous exercise alters the requirements for insulin and dietary requirements in a diabetic.
7. A patient who is vomiting or who has missed a meal should have the insulin dosage reduced to prevent insulin shock.
8. Infection, surgery, and physical and emotional stresses alter the requirements for insulin.
9. Diabetic patients should become familiar with MedicAlert tags and wear one at all times.
10. Thyroid tablets deteriorate with excessive exposure to light and moisture. Patients should be instructed in their proper storage.
11. Excessive thyroid medication produces symptoms of hyperthyroidism, including hypertension, tachycardia, chest pain, and heat intolerance.
12. The symptoms of Cushing's syndrome are similar to the side effects experienced when adrenocorticoid drugs are administered to a patient.
13. Patients should be instructed about taking oral contraceptives daily as prescribed. Pregnancy can result if pills are missed during the month. If a period does not occur at the end of the cycle, the patient should be instructed not to resume the oral contraceptive and to consult her physician.
14. Symptoms of breakthrough bleeding midcycle are seen with some oral contraceptives; this can often be corrected by increasing the strength of the contraceptive.

CRITICAL THINKING QUESTIONS

1. A patient is brought to the office by her daughter for a checkup. She is afraid of doctors and has not seen one since her last child was born 25 years ago. She is noted to speak slowly, she has dry hair that is thinning in the central scalp, and her skin has a puffy appearance. What may be her problem?
2. A patient has received dexamethasone for his rheumatoid arthritis for the last 6 months. He is noted to have a rounder face than previously and has gained 8 lb, although he states he has not changed his eating habits. His arthritis is improved, but he is afraid the physician will stop the medication because of his "side effects." What would you tell him?
3. A pediatric patient was diagnosed as having diabetes mellitus 1 year ago. Since yesterday, he has been vomiting and is unable to eat. This morning his mother gave him his regular insulin dose. Now, 3 hours later, the mother calls to say he is sweaty, trembling, and nervous. What is the most likely diagnosis? What should the mother do before she brings her son to the office? After the boy has recovered, the mother wants to know if his medication can be changed to the diabetic "pills" that she has heard about so that he would not have all this trouble with insulin anymore. What is your answer?
4. A patient has been married 1 month and comes to the office with her husband, who states that she cries all the time, although they are "deliriously happy." She has been on oral contraceptives for 4 months now and takes no other medication. She also states she does not know why she acts this way and wants a mood elevator. What other steps might be taken?
5. A patient has had recurrent problems with varicose veins for 8 years. Her surgeon is now speaking about vein stripping in the near future. She wants to know if she can be placed on oral contraceptives because a pregnancy would be inconvenient now that surgery is a possibility. How do you respond to this question?

REVIEW QUESTIONS

1. The master gland of the body is the:
   - **a.** anterior pituitary.
   - **b.** posterior pituitary.
   - **c.** adrenal cortex.
   - **d.** adrenal medulla.

2. All of the following are symptoms of hypothyroidism *except:*
   - **a.** enlarged thyroid gland.
   - **b.** hypersensitivity to heat.
   - **c.** slowing of mental functions.
   - **d.** slowing of physical functions.

3. Insulin is secreted in the body by the:
   - **a.** islets of Langerhans.
   - **b.** adrenal medulla.
   - **c.** sympathetic nervous system.
   - **d.** anterior pituitary.

4. If not treated with insulin, a diabetic would be unable to:
   - **a.** metabolize sugar.
   - **b.** metabolize fat.
   - **c.** metabolize cholesterol.
   - **d.** digest fiber.

5. A side effect of oral contraceptives is:
   - **a.** ovulation.
   - **b.** thromboembolic disorders.
   - **c.** increased fertility.
   - **d.** hirsutism.

6. Which of the following is an estrogen agonist-antagonist?
   - **a.** estradiol
   - **b.** conjugated estrogens
   - **c.** raloxifene
   - **d.** Ortho Evra

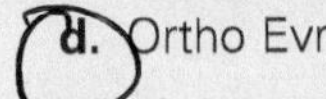

7. An agent that promotes ovulation is:
   - **a.** conjugated estrogens.
   - **b.** testosterone.
   - **c.** clomiphene.
   - **d.** medroxyprogesterone.

8. An agent that stimulates the uterine muscles and promotes rhythmic contractions of the uterus is:
   - **a.** esterified estrogens.
   - **b.** acarbose.
   - **c.** OxyContin.
   - **d.** oxytocin.

9. A hormone that is given via transdermal patch is:
   - **a.** testosterone.
   - **b.** raloxifene.
   - **c.** pancrelipase.
   - **d.** oxytocin.

10. Which of the following may be used to treat diabetes?
    - **a.** liothyronine
    - **b.** medroxyprogesterone
    - **c.** clomiphene
    - **d.** glimepiride

Answers to the review questions can be found at the back of the book.

evolve Additional questions and activities can be found at *http://evolve.elsevier.com/asperheim/pharmacology.*

CHAPTER 19

Diuretics and Other Drugs That Affect the Urinary System

Objectives

After completing this chapter, you should be able to do the following:

1. Understand the function of the kidney.
2. Understand the role of the kidney in selectively regulating output and its importance in drug excretion.
3. Explain the importance of antidiuretic hormone in regulating urine output.
4. Become familiar with the different classes of diuretics and how they are used.
5. Identify drugs used to treat urinary tract infections.
6. Identify drugs used to treat enuresis.
7. Become familiar with the action of drugs that treat benign prostatic hypertrophy and erectile dysfunction.
8. Discuss nursing responsibilities in the administration of diuretics.

Key Terms

Antihypertensive (ăn-tī-hī-pĕr-TĔN-sĭv) **drugs,** p. 182
Diuresis (dī-ŭ-RĒ-sĭs), p. 180
Enuresis (ĕn-ū-RĒ-sĭs), p. 184
Incontinence (ĭn-KŎN-tĭĭ-nĕns), p. 185
Steroid (STĬR-ōyd) **antagonists,** p. 182
Thiazide diuretics, p. 181

The kidney is the principal organ involved in maintaining the water balance of the body. If the output of water from the body exceeds the water intake, the body is said to be in a negative water balance. This imbalance leads to dehydration of the body. At the other extreme, a positive water balance occurs when the intake of water exceeds the output. Ordinarily, the body maintains a balance between the water ingested and the water excreted.

In addition to excretion via the kidney, water may be lost through perspiration. Perspiration may occur by diffusion through the skin, termed *insensible perspiration* because it is not noticed. Alternatively, perspiration may involve the sweat glands, producing sensible perspiration that is recognized as sweat. Sweat consists of a weak solution of sodium chloride and a few other substances. It is possible to lose 3000 mL of water through the skin in 24 hours when both sensible and insensible perspiration routes are active.

The kidney has the ability to regulate its output according to the amount of fluid ingested and the amount lost by other routes from the body. In very warm weather when perspiration is greater, the output from the kidneys is considerably less than it is in cool weather.

The kidney consists of more than 1 million functional units, or nephrons (Fig. 19-1). The nephron is composed of a tuft of capillaries, called a glomerulus, that is encapsulated in a cuplike structure known as Bowman's capsule. Water, salts, and waste products can filter through the thin walls of the capillaries into Bowman's capsule and through the series of collecting tubules to the pelvis of the kidney. The renal pelvis opens into the ureter, the ureter leads to the bladder, and excretion from the bladder is accomplished via the urethra.

A great deal more fluid is filtered into Bowman's capsule than is excreted in the urine. Much of the fluid is reabsorbed where the collecting tubule from Bowman's capsule circles back through another capillary bed on its way to the renal pelvis. It is estimated that for every 125 mL of fluid filtered through the glomerulus, only 1 mL is eventually secreted.

Reabsorption of the filtered fluid is largely due to the influence of the antidiuretic hormone from the posterior pituitary gland. Diabetes insipidus is a disease in which this hormone is missing or present in inadequate amounts. This disease is characterized by **diuresis** (the formation and excretion of increased amounts of urine); in this case, copious amounts of

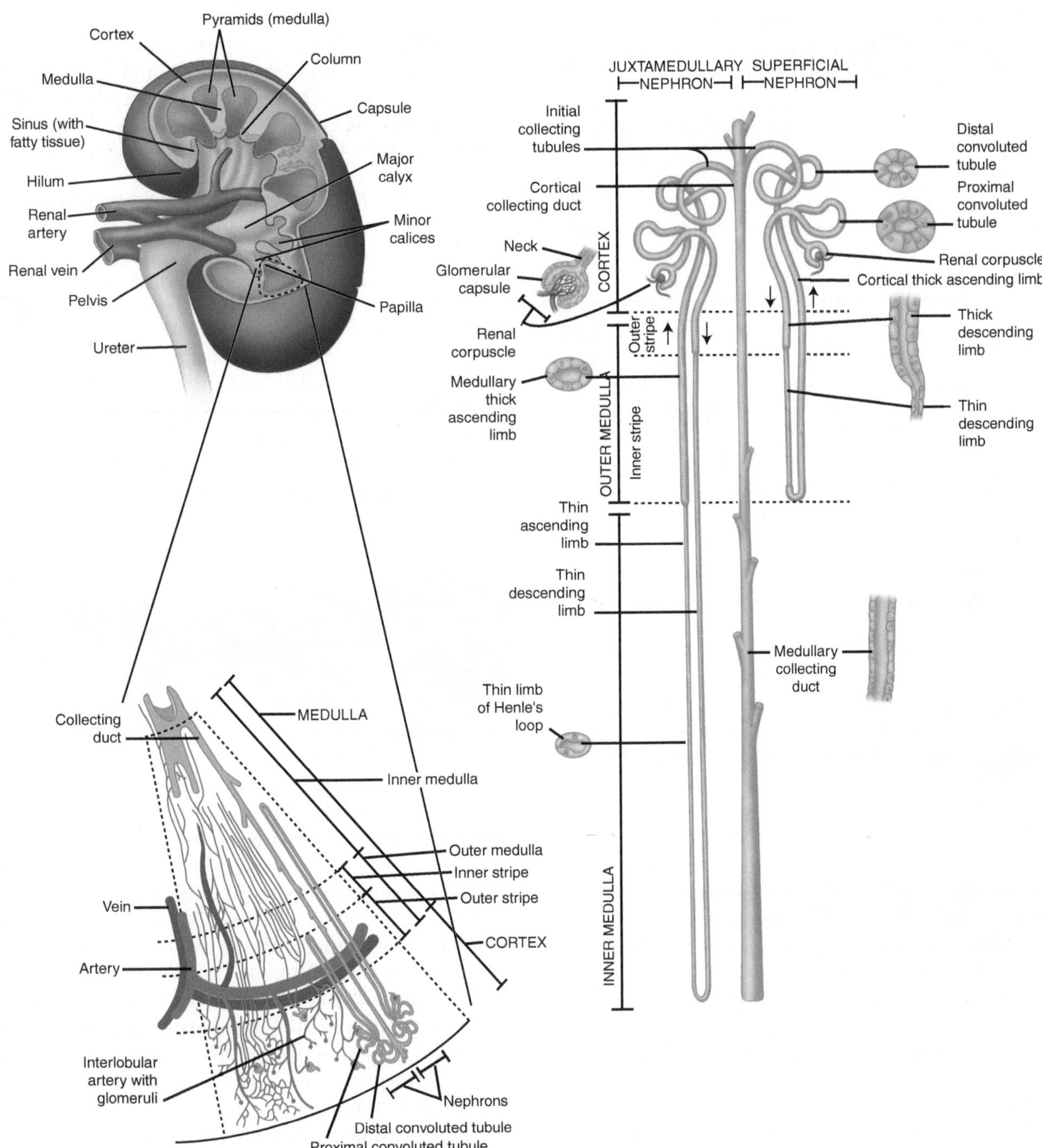

FIGURE 19-1 The structure of the kidney. (From *Dorland's illustrated medical dictionary*, ed 31, Philadelphia, 2007, Saunders.)

urine are produced—sometimes 10 to 12 L a day. Diabetes insipidus is treated by the administration of posterior pituitary hormone.

DIURETICS

A diuretic is a drug that increases the flow of urine. If sodium and fluids are retained in excessive amounts, edema, particularly of the extremities, results. Fluid accumulation in the lungs results in pulmonary edema. There are several classes of diuretics; all work in different areas of the urinary tract.

THIAZIDE (BENZOTHIADIAZINE) DIURETICS

Thiazide diuretics, although they act in part by inhibiting the enzyme carbonic anhydrase, also exert action directly on the collecting tubules of the kidney and promote the excretion of sodium, potassium, chloride, and bicarbonate along with the necessary excretion of water. Potassium depletion is often a problem when thiazide diuretics are used over a prolonged period; a potassium supplement or foods high in potassium, such as oranges and bananas, are often added to the diet.

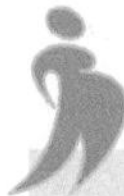

Considerations for Pregnant and Nursing Women

Thiazide Diuretics

Thiazide diuretics are generally contraindicated in pregnant women. These agents cross the placental barrier and appear in cord blood. Thrombocytopenia and jaundice are among the effects in the newborn that have been attributed to the use of thiazide diuretics during pregnancy.

In addition to their activity as diuretics, thiazides are effective as **antihypertensive drugs** (i.e., they lower high blood pressure). This action is separate from their effect on diuresis, and it is not completely understood. When thiazides are used by themselves, their action in lowering blood pressure is mild; when combined with other drugs, however, they are a useful adjunct in the treatment of hypertensive patients because they greatly increase the activity of these drugs.

Side effects of these drugs include alterations in the body chemistry such as hypokalemia, hypochloremic alkalosis, hypotension, tachycardia, aplastic anemia, jaundice, hyperuricemia, glycosuria, muscle cramps, and weakness. They should be used with caution in patients known to have gout or liver or kidney disorders. Potassium supplements are recommended when these agents are prescribed.

chlorothiazide, USP-NF, BP (Diuril). Chlorothiazide was the first diuretic to be synthesized in the thiazide group. It is used as a diuretic in patients with heart failure, in pregnant patients, and in patients with premenstrual fluid retention. It is also used as an adjunct in the treatment of hypertension.
Dosage: Adults: (Oral) 500 mg one to two times daily.
Children: (Oral) 10 mg/kg two times daily.

hydrochlorothiazide, USP-NF, BP (HydroDIURIL). A small alteration in the chemical structure of chlorothiazide greatly increases the potency of this compound. Much smaller doses provide diuretic effects comparable to chlorothiazide.
Dosage: Adults: (Oral) 25 to 100 mg one to two times daily.
Children: (Oral) 1 mg/kg twice daily.

THIAZIDELIKE DIURETICS

Thiazidelike diuretics are structurally similar to thiazide diuretics and work in a similar way. Potassium depletion may occur after prolonged use.

chlorthalidone (Thalitone). Chlorthalidone may be used alone or in combination with another agent in the control of hypertension or edema.
Dosage: Adults: (Oral) 12.5 to 100 mg daily.
Children: (Oral) 0.3 mg/kg daily. Alternatively, 2 mg/kg three times weekly may be given.

indapamide (Lozol). Indapamide is used to manage edema and salt retention in patients with congestive heart failure and in the treatment of hypertension.
Dosage: Adults only: (Oral) 1.25 to 5 mg daily.

metolazone (Zaroxolyn). Metolazone is used to manage edema in patients with congestive heart failure and renal diseases (i.e., nephritic syndrome). It is more effective than some other agents in managing edema from impaired renal function.
Dosage: Adults only: (Oral) 5 to 10 mg once daily. Up to 20 mg daily has been used.

STEROID ANTAGONISTS

Steroid antagonists are diuretics that act by inhibiting aldosterone, an adrenal hormone that promotes the retention of sodium and the excretion of potassium. The excretion of sodium and chloride caused by steroid antagonists is accompanied by an appropriate amount of water.

eplerenone (Inspra). Eplerenone is used to treat edema after myocardial infarction and left ventricular failure. It may be used alone or in combination with other drugs in the treatment of hypertension.
Dosage: Adults only: (Oral) 25 to 50 mg once daily.

spironolactone plus hydrochlorothiazide (Aldactazide). Aldactazide is a combination of 25 mg of hydrochlorothiazide and 25 mg of spironolactone per tablet. The combined form of the two drugs is more effective as a diuretic than either of the two used alone because the reabsorption of fluids and electrolytes in the kidney is blocked by two methods.
Dosage: Adults: (Oral) One tablet four times daily (25 mg of each drug).
Children: (Oral) 1.5 to 3 mg/kg of each drug daily in two to four divided doses.

spironolactone, USP-NF, BP (Aldactone). Spironolactone is used to treat edema associated with congestive heart failure, hepatic cirrhosis with ascites and nephritis, and edema of unknown origin. Side effects observed with the use of this drug include mild headache, confusion, dermatitis, drowsiness, ataxia, and mild abdominal pain.
Dosage: Adults: (Oral) 50 to 400 mg daily.
Children: (Oral) 1.5 to 3 mg/kg daily in two to four divided doses.

MISCELLANEOUS DIURETICS

amiloride hydrochloride (Midamor). Structurally unrelated to the other drugs that are used as diuretics, this agent differs also in its action in that it is potassium-sparing. It does not cause potassium depletion when used as a diuretic. Side effects include nausea, flatulence, and mild rash, but it is generally well tolerated.
Dosage: Adults: (Oral) 5 to 20 mg/day.
Children: (Oral) 0.625 mg/kg/day.

ethacrynic acid, USP-NF, BP (Edecrin). Similar to furosemide, this agent works throughout the nephron tubules to prevent the reabsorption of sodium and water. The potency of ethacrynic acid and furosemide is approximately equal.
Dosage: Adults: (Oral) 50 to 400 mg daily; (IV) 0.5 to 1 mg/kg. Single IV doses should not exceed 100 mg.
Children: (Oral) Initially 25 mg, then stepwise increments until results are achieved; (IV) 1 mg/kg. IV dosing is not generally recommended.

furosemide, USP-NF, BP (Lasix). Furosemide is a diuretic that has been shown to act throughout the collecting tubules of the nephron, particularly on the ascending limb of the loop of Henle, to prevent the reabsorption of—and hence cause the excretion of—sodium and chloride. Although usually administered orally, it may be administered via the intramuscular or IV route.

Furosemide may be used in congestive heart failure associated with liver or kidney disease. It is of particular value when other, less potent diuretics have failed to decrease edema. Side effects are electrolyte depletion, dizziness, weakness, jaundice, leg cramps, vomiting, and confusion.
Dosage: Adults: (Oral) 20 to 80 mg once daily; (IM, IV) 20 mg to 1 gm daily.
Children: Dosage has not been established.

mannitol (Osmitrol). Mannitol is an osmotic diuretic and is used to promote diuresis for the prevention or treatment of acute renal failure. Renal failure may occur after massive blood loss, trauma, shock, burns, or mismatched blood. It is used in neurosurgery to reduce intracranial pressure and in certain instances to reduce the intraocular pressure of acute glaucoma. Diuresis may occur in 1 to 3 hours after administration. Adverse effects include nausea, acidosis, tachycardia, and thrombophlebitis.
Dosage: Adults: (IV) Dosages range greatly; may begin with 0.2 gm/kg or 12.5 gm as a 15% to 20% solution infused over 3 to 5 minutes to test response. 50 to 100 gm may be given.

metolazone (Zaroxolyn). This drug is structurally similar to the thiazide diuretics and generally has the same side effects. Hyperuricemia and gout, fluid depletion, nausea, and headaches have been described.
Dosage: Adults only: (Oral) 5 to 20 mg daily.

torsemide (Demadex). Torsemide is used to manage edema associated with congestive heart failure or hepatic or renal disease. It may be used alone or in combination with other agents in the treatment of hypertension.
Dosage: Adults only: (Oral) 5 to 100 mg daily; (IV) 5 to 10 mg daily.

triamterene, USP-NF, BP (Dyrenium). Triamterene is often combined with hydrochlorothiazide because the diuretic and hypotensive effects are increased by the combination. Nausea, vomiting, headache, and weakness occur occasionally with the use of this drug.
Dosage: Adults: (Oral) 100 mg one to two times daily.
Children: (Oral) 4 mg/kg/day in two divided doses.

triamterene plus hydrochlorothiazide (Dyazide). Dyazide is a commercial preparation containing a combination of 37.5 mg of triamterene and 25 mg of hydrochlorothiazide per capsule.
Dosage: Adults: (Oral) 1 capsule daily.

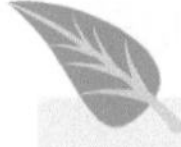

Herb Alert
Juniper

Juniper is used as a diuretic when administered orally. Juniper also has an antihypertensive effect and enhances the effects of lithium. However, prolonged oral administration may result in nephrotoxicity, and it should be avoided in patients with preexisting liver disease. See Chapter 28 for more information on juniper.

URINARY ANTISEPTICS

Bacterial infections of the urinary tract are the causative agents of various symptomatic conditions that may be described as cystitis, pyelitis, or pyelonephritis. These terms merely refer to the location of the infection or the source of the symptoms related to the infection.

Many patients who have had a single urinary tract infection have recurrences after asymptomatic periods. For this reason, they are often placed on long-term drug therapy. Most sulfonamides and antibiotics such as tetracyclines, chloramphenicol, erythromycin, streptomycin, kanamycin, and cephalothin may be used to treat these conditions. Because these drugs have been discussed previously in other chapters, this section is reserved for drugs used more exclusively as urinary antiseptics.

co-trimoxazole (trimethoprim-sulfamethoxazole; TMP/SMX) (Bactrim, Septra). The commercial preparations of Bactrim and Septra contain identical formulations, with tablets consisting of a combination of 80 mg of trimethoprim and 400 mg of sulfamethoxazole. Each manufacturer also produces a double-strength tablet labeled *DS* (i.e., Bactrim DS, Septra DS).

The combination of a sulfonamide with the synthetic antibacterial compound trimethoprim has been shown to be very effective against chronic urinary tract infections, primarily pyelonephritis, pyelitis, and cystitis. Its use should be reserved for chronic infections, however, because untoward effects do occur from this drug. The use of these agents in upper respiratory infections is discussed in Chapter 10, and their use for other indications is discussed in Chapter 7.

The patient should be warned to report sore throat, fever, pallor, purpura, or jaundice to the physician immediately because these may be early signs of blood dyscrasias that may occur with this drug. Adequate fluid intake should be maintained during therapy to prevent the formation of renal calculi. The drug should be used with caution in patients with impaired renal or liver function. It is contraindicated in pregnant women.

Dosage: Adults: (Oral) 1 to 2 tablets every 12 hours for 10 to 14 days (or 1 tablet of the double-strength form every 12 hours).

Children: (Oral) 8 mg/kg trimethoprim and 40 mg/kg sulfamethoxazole daily in two divided doses.

methenamine mandelate, USP-NF, BP (Mandelamine). This combination of methenamine and mandelic acid is a well-tolerated urinary antiseptic and is particularly useful for chronic, resistant, or recurrent infections. It is effective against almost all strains of microorganisms that are causative agents in urinary tract infections and may be effective even against strains resistant to antibiotics or sulfonamides. It may be given alone or in combination with other drugs. Sensitization in the form of allergic reactions rarely occurs with this drug, but it is contraindicated in patients with severe hepatitis or renal insufficiency.

Dosage: Adults: (Oral) 1 gm four times daily.

Children older than 6 years: (Oral) 50 to 75 mg/kg (mandelate salt) in three to four divided doses daily.

Children younger than 6 years: (Oral) 18 mg/kg four times daily.

nitrofurantoin, USP-NF, BP (Furadantin, Macrobid, Macrodantin). This synthetic drug has a spectrum of activity that encompasses most urinary tract infective agents. After oral administration, approximately 45% of the dose is excreted in the urine, imparting to it a brown color. The drug should continue to be administered for at least 3 days after sterility of the urine has been achieved, to minimize the possibility of recurrent infections. Nausea, vomiting, or sensitivity reactions may occur with administration of this drug. Gastrointestinal symptoms may be minimized if the dose is given with food or milk.

Dosage: Adults and children older than 12 years: (Oral) 50 to 100 mg four times daily.

Children 1 month to 12 years: (Oral) 5 to 7 mg/kg/day in four divided doses to a maximum of 400 mg/day.

phenazopyridine hydrochloride, USP-NF, BP (Pyridium). This drug acts promptly to produce an analgesic effect on the urinary tract mucosa. It usually acts within 30 minutes to relieve the symptoms of pain, burning, urgency, and frequency associated with urinary tract infections. This drug is compatible with any antibacterial or with other corrective therapy for infections of this nature. The patient should be informed that phenazopyridine causes the urine to turn a reddish color.

Dosage: Adults: (Oral) 200 mg three times daily.

Children: Dosage has not been established.

DRUGS USED TO TREAT ENURESIS

Enuresis is the involuntary discharge of urine and most commonly occurs at night; this is known as nocturnal enuresis, or "nighttime bedwetting." Enuresis is a common problem in children. Without treatment, the percentage of bedwetters gradually decreases by the age of 21 years, but a small percentage are still wetting at that age.

It is well established that withholding fluids in the evening, many nightly awakenings by the parent, and other behavioral techniques may give temporary improvement, but 100% relapse occurs as soon as these interventions cease. Various alarms and early warnings of wetting have been devised, also without real improvement. The problem seems to be a small or spastic bladder that is stimulated to empty automatically when a certain volume of urine is present, much as an infant's bladder empties. Various drugs are useful for this problem.

desmopressin acetate (DDAVP Nasal Spray). This is an antidiuretic agent that affects renal water conservation. It is an analog of vasopressin (antidiuretic hormone) that is used as a nasal spray. Side effects include headache, increase in blood pressure, nosebleed, and sore throat.

Dosage: Children 6 years and older: 10 to 40 mcg by nasal spray pump at bedtime.

imipramine hydrochloride (Tofranil). This agent, which acts as an antidepressant as well, may improve the symptoms of enuresis in some children. The mechanism of action in the improvement of enuresis is thought to be separate from its antidepressant effect.
Dosage: Children older than 12 years: (Oral) 75 mg at bedtime.

Children 6 to 12 years: (Oral) 25 mg at bedtime.

oxybutynin chloride (Ditropan). This agent has a direct antispasmodic effect on the smooth muscle and relaxes bladder smooth muscle in patients with involuntary bladder symptoms. It may be used for day and night wetting. Side effects include drowsiness, decreased tearing, dry mouth, constipation, and palpitations.
Dosage: Adults and children older than 12 years: (Oral) 5 mg three times daily.

Children 5 to 12 years: (Oral) 5 mg twice daily.

DRUGS USED TO TREAT INCONTINENCE

The inability to control the discharge of excretions, either urine or feces, is referred to as **incontinence.** Urinary incontinence affects 10% to 35% of community-dwelling adults and 50% to 70% of patients in nursing homes. It is twice as common in women as in men. Certain age-related physiologic and anatomic factors increase the risk of incontinence, including the following:

- Nocturia, or excessive urination during the night
- Decline in bladder capacity
- Decrease in urethral closure pressure
- Increase in postvoiding residual volume
- Loss of elasticity or stiffening of the bladder tissue such as produced after radiotherapy
- Benign prostatic hypertrophy (BPH) in men
- Decreased pelvic muscle tone after childbirth in women

Although supportive treatment may help, incontinence is generally treated medically with anticholinergic drugs.

oxybutynin chloride (Ditropan XL). This agent exerts a direct antispasmodic effect on smooth muscle, relaxing the bladder smooth muscle. Side effects include dry mouth, dry eyes, somnolence, and constipation.
Dosage: Adults: (Oral) 5 to 15 mg once daily.

tolterodine tartrate (Detrol, Detrol LA). By relaxing the smooth muscle of the bladder, this agent increases bladder capacity and decreases urge urinary incontinence. Side effects are the same as for oxybutynin.
Dosage: Adults: (Oral) 2 mg twice daily. For the long-acting form (Detrol LA), dosage is 2 to 4 mg once daily.

DRUGS USED TO TREAT BENIGN PROSTATIC HYPERTROPHY

BPH, or benign prostatic hyperplasia (an increase in the number of cells), is an abnormal enlargement of the prostate gland that occurs in most men 55 years old or older. It produces symptoms such as weakened urinary stream, difficulty in initiation of urination, urinary frequency, and urgency. Surgery, in the form of a transurethral resection of the prostate or newer minimally invasive techniques, is the treatment of choice, but if surgery is not an option, some cases of BPH respond to drug therapy. The potential coexistence of carcinoma of the prostate makes a careful differential diagnosis necessary.

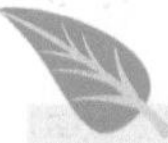

Herb Alert

Saw Palmetto

Saw palmetto has been used to suppress the symptoms of BPH, including urinary hesitancy, nocturia, and urinary frequency. However, its use may mask coexisting prostate cancer, which should always be ruled out when symptoms of prostate obstruction are present. Saw palmetto reduces the effects of estrogens, androgens, adrenergic drugs, and oral contraceptives. Although it is used primarily by men, its use should be avoided by women during pregnancy and lactation. See Chapter 28 for more information on saw palmetto.

alfuzosin hydrochloride (Uroxatral). Alfuzosin is used to reduce urinary obstruction and relieve symptoms associated with BPH. It is contraindicated in patients with severe hepatic impairment. Postural hypotension has been reported with use.
Dosage: Adults only: (Oral) 10 mg daily after a meal.

dutasteride (Avodart). Dutasteride is used to reduce prostate size and relieve associated symptoms of BPH. It may be used alone but is often combined with tamsulosin for long-term treatment.
Dosage: Adults only: (Oral) 0.5 mg daily.

finasteride (Proscar). Finasteride is used to reduce prostate size and the associated symptoms of urinary obstruction. It is generally well tolerated. Side effects include impotence, decreased volume of ejaculate, abdominal pain, diarrhea, and flatulence.
Dosage: Adults only: (Oral) 5 mg once daily.

silodosin (Rapaflo). Silodosin relieves the urinary frequency, urgency, and nocturia associated with BPH. It improves the urinary flow rates.
Dosage: Adults only: (Oral) 8 mg daily.

tamsulosin hydrochloride (Flomax). This agent is used to relieve mild to moderate obstructive manifestations of BPH. Side effects include rash, urticaria, and angioedema of the tongue, lips, and face.
Dosage: Adults only: (Oral) 0.4 mg daily.

DRUGS USED TO TREAT ERECTILE DYSFUNCTION

Erectile dysfunction is a subjective diagnosis. It is defined as the persistent or repeated inability to maintain an erection sufficient for satisfactory sexual performance. Before prescribing a drug for this problem, it is important to rule out other causes of erectile dysfunction such as hypertension and the use of antihypertensive drugs, thyroid disease, cardiovascular disease, diabetes mellitus, and psychological disorders.

sildenafil citrate (Viagra). Sildenafil is an oral agent that is effective in the temporary treatment of erectile dysfunction. It acts as a vasodilator and increases the tumescence, or swelling, and duration of the penile erection. Before this agent is used, it is important to obtain a careful medical history. If the patient has cardiac decompensation, this agent may have serious or even fatal effects. It potentiates the vasodilating effects of nitrites, producing potentially life-threatening hypotension. It is contraindicated in patients taking organic nitrates or nitrites such as nitroglycerin.
Dosage: Adults only: (Oral) 50 mg 1 hour before sexual activity.

tadalafil (Cialis). The advantage of this agent is that it has a duration of action of up to 36 hours. The precautions and contraindications are similar to vardenafil (discussed next). Priapism may occur. Current drug interaction information should be obtained if the patient is taking other medications because tadalafil has many interactions with other drugs.
Dosage: Adults only: (Oral) 10 mg once daily before sexual activity. Dosage range is 2.5 to 20 mg.

vardenafil HCl (Levitra). This agent also prolongs the duration of penile erections. It should be avoided in patients with unstable angina; hypotension; and a recent history of stroke, arrhythmia, or myocardial infarction. Many drugs are incompatible with vardenafil, and current information should be obtained if the patient is taking other medications. A partial list of incompatible drugs includes alpha blockers, nitrates, quinidine, procainamide, amiodarone, nifedipine, and many antiviral agents.
Dosage: Adults only: (Oral) 10 mg 1 hour before sexual activity; may increase to 20 mg. Dosage can be taken up to once daily.

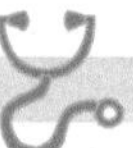

Clinical Implications

1. Diuretics are generally administered in the morning so that diuresis does not interfere with sleep.
2. The patient should be observed for the intended effects of diuretic medication, which include increased urine volume, lessening of edema about the face and extremities, and weight loss.
3. Patients receiving a diuretic should be instructed in the importance of a low-sodium diet. Sodium promotes fluid retention and counteracts the desired effect of the diuretic.
4. Potassium loss is an untoward effect of many diuretics. Patients may receive potassium supplements or be instructed to consume foods that are high in potassium such as raisins, oranges, and bananas.
5. Fluid and electrolyte changes that occur with diuretics may cause postural hypotension. The patient should be instructed to be observant if he or she experiences dizziness on rising or in ambulation.
6. Diuretics are often given to aid in the management of hypertension and to diminish the fluid and sodium content of the body.
7. Diuretics are of great value in the treatment of congestive heart failure when the weakened heart cannot mobilize excessive bodily fluids.
8. When a patient is receiving urinary antiseptics, it is often advisable to maintain an acidic urine to aid the drug in its intended effect. Large doses of vitamin C, cranberries, and prunes promote an acidic urine. Carbonated beverages and citrus fruits produce an alkaline urine as a result of the metabolic by-products of sodium citrate and sodium bicarbonate.
9. Certain agents given for urinary tract infections, such as Urised and Pyridium, cause discolorations of the urine. Patients should be counseled to expect this effect.
10. Maintaining an adequate fluid volume intake should be encouraged in patients who are being treated for a urinary tract infection.
11. The most common side effect of urinary tract antiseptics is a skin rash. Patients should be observed for this effect. Other untoward reactions include headache, nervousness, and drug fever. An elevation of temperature may be a drug reaction, not a worsening of the infection.
12. Patients should be observed for signs of improvement of urinary tract infection (i.e., less dysuria, frequency, and hesitancy on urination). The urine volume often increases as the infection is eradicated.
13. Withholding fluids before bedtime is not effective in treating enuresis.
14. All men older than 55 years should be questioned about symptoms of prostate hypertrophy (i.e., difficulty in starting the urine flow and frequent nocturia).
15. Older patients should be questioned about symptoms of incontinence and advised that effective treatments are available.

CRITICAL THINKING QUESTIONS

1. A patient has been taking hydrochlorothiazide (HydroDIURIL) for hypertension for 1 year, and she now complains of fatigue and weakness and many somatic symptoms including nonspecific malaise. Her blood pressure is 130/80 mm Hg. The physician orders serum electrolyte determinations. The results are sodium, 145 mEq/L; potassium, 2.8 mEq/L; chloride, 110 mEq/L; and carbon dioxide, 28 mEq/L. What may be her problem? How can it be helped?
2. A patient has had nausea and vomiting since he has been taking nitrofurantoin (Furadantin) for a urinary tract infection. He is now concerned that he is coming down with an intestinal virus and asks you to see if the physician will give him some trimethobenzamide hydrochloride (Tigan), which he says usually works for him. Would you have any other recommendations?
3. A patient wants the physician to give him a prescription for sildenafil citrate (Viagra). What questions should be asked about his medical history?
4. A boy is brought to the office by his mother. She expresses a great deal of annoyance with the child because no matter "what she does," he continues to wet the bed. The mother has tried withholding fluids after 5 p.m., waking him up three times a night, and setting alarm clocks for him to wake up. Nothing seems to work. What discussion would be appropriate with this mother?
5. A patient presents with pitting edema of the lower extremities that has slowly worsened over the last 3 days. He is worried because he cannot take "water pills"; his potassium goes down too low. Which of the diuretics may be useful?

REVIEW QUESTIONS

1. The functional unit of the kidney is the:
   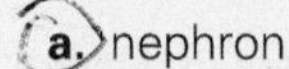
   a. nephron.
   b. renal artery.
   c. ureter.
   d. posterior pituitary hormone.

2. An example of a thiazide diuretic is:
   a. spironolactone.
   b. amiloride.
   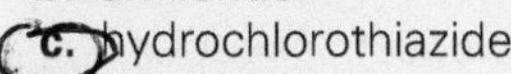
   c. hydrochlorothiazide.
   d. Aldactazide.

3. Spironolactone functions as a diuretic by:
   a. causing potassium depletion.
   b. increasing the output of Bowman's capsule.
   c. inhibiting aldosterone.
   d. inhibiting corticosteroids.

4. The most common side effect of thiazide diuretics is:
   a. hypertension.
   b. cirrhosis of the liver.
   c. hypokalemia.
   d. sodium retention.

5. An example of a urinary antiseptic is:
   a. metolazone.
   b. furosemide.
   c. spironolactone.
   d. nitrofurantoin.

6. A drug that turns the urine a reddish color is:
   a. phenazopyridine.
   b. co-trimoxazole.
   c. sulfamethoxazole.
   d. pyribenzamine.

7. A drug used to treat urinary incontinence is:
   a. sulfamethoxazole.
   b. oxybutynin.
   c. diazepam.
   d. sildenafil.

8. A drug used to treat erectile dysfunction is:
   a. desmopressin.
   b. oxybutynin.
   c. imipramine.
   d. sildenafil.

9. Desmopressin acetate is useful in the treatment of:
   a. urinary tract infections.
   b. prostatic hypertrophy.
   c. enuresis.
   d. erectile dysfunction.

10. Reabsorption of filtered urine is under the influence of:
    a. diuretic hormone from the anterior pituitary.
    b. antidiuretic hormone from the posterior pituitary.
    c. glomerular stimulating hormone.
    d. thiazide diuretics.

Answers to the review questions can be found at the back of the book.

evolve Additional questions and activities can be found at *http://evolve.elsevier.com/asperheim/pharmacology*.

CHAPTER 20

Immunizing Agents and Immunosuppressives

Objectives

After completing this chapter, you should be able to do the following:

1. Become familiar with immunization schedules for children.
2. Understand the difference between agents that provide active immunity and agents that provide passive immunity.
3. Be aware of side effects of immunizing agents.
4. Understand the action of immunosuppressive agents, and know why they are used.
5. Be aware of side effects of immunosuppressive agents.
6. Discuss responsibilities of the health care provider for patients receiving immunosuppressive agents.

Key Terms

Active immunity, p. 188
Immunity, p. 188
Immunizing agent, p. 188
Immunosuppressives, p. 192
Passive immunity, p. 188
Vaccine, p. 188

Immunity, the status of being protected against an infectious disease, may be brought about by actual contact with the disease or by the administration of a substance called a vaccine. A **vaccine,** or **immunizing agent,** is a preparation that uses an altered or killed microorganism to produce active immunity to a disease. Immunity may be gained by using a vaccine without the accompanying adverse effects of the disease itself.

Active immunity is achieved when the antigen, or altered microorganism, is injected into the body, and natural antibodies are produced against it. **Passive immunity** is obtained when previously formed antibodies are injected into the body. This provides a faster immunity; however, it is short lived, lasting only a few weeks or months.

Because of the proven success of vaccines against infectious diseases, childhood immunization is now required by law, generally before admission to school (see Figs. 20-1 and 20-2 at the end of the chapter). Usually only minor complications occur from childhood vaccines. Rare serious effects do occur, but considering the illness and death previously associated with these diseases in infants and children, there is no doubt that the vaccines provide a safe and effective way to ensure the health of the population.

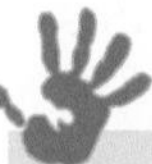

Considerations for Children

Immunizations

Encourage parents to have their children immunized in a timely manner. Immunity to some diseases may not develop if booster doses of the immunizing agents are not given at the recommended intervals. Explain the importance of the immunization schedule during well-baby and well-child checkups.

Despite the effectiveness of immunization in adults, diphtheria/tetanus, pertussis, influenza, hepatitis A and B, and pneumococcal vaccines continue to be underused. Health care workers should encourage the use of adult vaccines (see Figs. 20-3 and 20-4 at the end of the chapter).

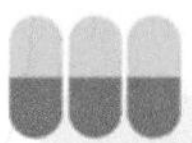

Special Considerations
Immunizations

Immunizations are not just for children anymore. Everyone should receive tetanus toxoid every 10 years. Older adults should also receive pneumococcal vaccine. Health care workers, older adults, and anyone with an underlying respiratory illness should receive an annual influenza vaccine (flu shot). The hepatitis B vaccine series is required for most health care workers. Hepatitis A vaccine is recommended for people in endemic areas.

AGENTS THAT PROVIDE ACTIVE IMMUNITY

diphtheria and tetanus toxoids, adsorbed (DT, Td). This agent is used for boosting immunity to diphtheria and tetanus when pertussis immunization is unnecessary. It is used in late childhood and adulthood.
Dosage: Adults and children older than 7 years: (IM) 0.5 mL.

diphtheria and tetanus toxoids and acellular pertussis vaccine (DTaP) (Daptacel, Infanrix, Tripedia). This vaccine differs from earlier DPT vaccine in that the pertussis vaccine is prepared from inactivated acellular pertussis. It produces fewer adverse reactions than the whole-cell pertussis vaccine, while retaining the immunogenic properties. Side effects include local reactions of erythema and swelling at the injection site, mild fever, and malaise after injection. Immunocompromised individuals have a diminished immunologic response.
Dosage: Children 6 weeks to 6 years: (IM) 0.5 mL.

diphtheria and tetanus toxoids, acellular pertussis, and inactivated poliovirus vaccine (Kinrix). This combination is used for the fifth DTaP and fourth IPV in children 4 to 6 years old whose previous DTaP doses have been with Infanrix or Pediarix.
Dosage: Children 4 to 6 years: (IM) 0.5 mL.

diphtheria and tetanus toxoids, acellular pertussis, inactivated poliovirus, and* Haemophilus *b vaccine (Pentacel). This agent has five antigens and may be used in the vaccine schedule to reduce the number of injections.
Dosage: Children: (IM) 0.5 mL.

diphtheria and tetanus toxoids, acellular pertussis, inactivated poliovirus, and hepatitis B vaccine (Pediarix). This was the first 5-in-l vaccine available, and it has the ability to reduce greatly the number of vaccine injections necessary for infants and young children. Side effects include injection-site reactions such as pain, swelling, redness, and fever. This agent is associated with higher rates of febrile reactions than are seen with the separately administered vaccines. It is contraindicated in infants with known sensitivity to any component of the vaccine, including yeast, neomycin, and polymyxin B. It should not be administered to any infant before 6 weeks of age or to any child older than 7 years. It is a suspension and should be shaken vigorously before administration. It should not be used if all the material in the vial is not in the form of a suspension.
Dosage: Children up to 7 years: (IM) Three 0.5-mL injections at 2, 4, and 6 months of age.

Haemophilus *b conjugate vaccine (Hib).* This vaccine is a noninfectious, bacteria-derived vaccine used to prevent *Haemophilus influenzae* infections in infants and young children. Several different types of conjugated vaccines (vaccines made by linking the inactivated bacteria to a carrier molecule) are available. They may differ in the protein carrier, the polysaccharide carrier, and the method of conjugation. Whatever type is chosen, it should be continued for the duration of the immunization schedule. The PedvaxHIB, ActHIB, and HibTITER vaccines all may be used in infants and children up to 5 years of age. The ProHIBiT vaccine may be used in children 15 months to 5 years old.
Dosage: Children up to 5 years: (IM) 0.5 mL.

Haemophilus *b and hepatitis B vaccine (Comvax).* This combination vaccine may be used in children younger than 5 years of age. It should not be administered to any infant younger than 6 weeks of age. If one dose of the hepatitis B vaccine was administered to the child as a newborn, this combination may still be used for the subsequent doses on the same schedule as follows.
Dosage: Children 6 weeks to 5 years: (IM) 0.5 mL at 2 months, 4 months, and 12 to 15 months of age.

hepatitis A virus vaccine, inactivated (Havrix, VAQTA). This vaccine is a noninfectious inactivated virus vaccine recommended for all children 12 to 23 months of age. The two vaccines have different unit strengths, and the dose is given for each. A series of two doses is given.
Dosage: Havrix: Adults: (IM) 1440 units; repeat in 6 to 12 months.
Children 1 to 18 years: (IM) 720 units; repeat in 6 to 12 months.
VAQTA: Adults: (IM) 50 units; repeat in 6 to 18 months.
Children 1 to 18 years: (IM) 25 units; repeat in 6 to 18 months.

hepatitis B vaccine (Engerix-B, Recombivax HB). Hepatitis B vaccine (recombinant) is a noninfectious subunit viral vaccine containing hepatitis B surface antigen. It is prepared from a strain of *Saccharomyces cerevisiae* using recombinant DNA technology. The strain of *Saccharomyces* used has been genetically altered to contain the hepatitis B virus gene coding. Immunization is given to infants beginning at birth and should be given to all high-risk groups, particularly individuals in the health professions.

At least 90% of children and adults develop antibodies with this vaccine, but the duration of the immunity has not been established. Further booster doses may be necessary in the future. Recombivax HB and Engerix-B have different unit strengths, so their dosages are given separately. Three doses are necessary, the first two given 1 month apart and the third given 6 months after the first dose, according to the schedule in Figure 20-1.

Dosage:
Recombivax: Infants to 19 years: (IM) 5 mcg.
Adults older than 20 years: (IM) 10 mcg.
Before undergoing dialysis: (IM) 40 mcg.
Engerix-B: Infants to 19 years: (IM) 10 mcg.
Adults older than 20 years: (IM) 20 mcg.
Before undergoing dialysis: (IM) 40 mcg.

human papillomavirus vaccine (Gardasil). This vaccine, intended for females between ages 11 and 26 years, protects against four types of human papillomavirus (HPV), which is now recognized as the primary risk factor in developing cervical cancer. There are more than 100 subtypes of the virus. The four types included in the vaccine are recognized as the subtypes most closely associated with cervical and vulvar cancer.

Dosage: Children and young adults 9 to 26 years: (IM) 0.5 mL. Three injections, with the second injection 2 months after the first, and the third injection 6 months after the first.

influenza virus vaccine, USP-NF, BP (Fluvirin, Fluzone). This vaccine contains virus material from several different strains of influenza A and B. It is prepared anew every year based on the influenza viruses seen at various places in the world, which presumably will be responsible for the following year's epidemic. It is given annually and is no longer restricted to elderly individuals and patients with respiratory diseases. It is recommended annually even for children.

Dosage: Adults and children 8 years and older: (IM) 0.5 mL in the autumn, annually.

Infants and children younger than 8 years: (IM) 0.25 mL one month apart.

influenza virus vaccine live, intranasal (FluMist). The intranasal form of influenza vaccine is recommended for persons 5 to 49 years of age (Fig. 20-5 at the end of the chapter). The effectiveness of the vaccine compares favorably with the injectable form. Immunized individuals should avoid contact with immunocompromised persons in the same household. Its safety in patients with asthma and reactive airway disease has not been established.

Dosage: Adults and children 9 to 49 years: (Intranasal) 0.2 mL once annually.

Children 2 to 8 years previously vaccinated with influenza vaccine: (Intranasal) 0.2 mL once annually.

Children 2 to 8 years not previously vaccinated with influenza vaccine: (Intranasal) two doses of 0.2 mL 1 month apart.

measles, mumps, and rubella virus vaccine, live, USP-NF, BP (MMR) (M-M-R II). Although all these virus vaccines are available as single vaccines, it has been shown that immunity is conferred just as effectively with the triple live virus vaccine. Immunity is suboptimal if the vaccine is administered before 12 months of age. If it is administered early because of a community epidemic, the dose must be repeated between 12 and 15 months of age. Side effects are minimal with this vaccine; however, occasionally the patient may experience a low-grade fever and light pink rash 10 to 14 days after administration.

Dosage: Children: (Subcut) 0.5 mL initial dose at 12 to 15 months, then second dose at 4 to 6 years.

meningococcal vaccine (Menactra, Menomune). Two types of meningococcal vaccine are available: a conjugated vaccine (MCV4) that is administered intramuscularly and an unconjugated vaccine (MPSV4) that is given subcutaneously. Both vaccines contain four antigens from the meningitis bacteria. Routine immunization is not recommended at this time for children younger than 11 years old, but certain children 2 to 10 years old in an endemic area or in an area where the disease is widespread may be vaccinated. Primary vaccination is recommended after age 12. Military recruits and college students who plan to live in dormitories should be vaccinated. The necessity for booster doses has not been established.

Dosage: Adults and children 12 to 55 years: Menactra (MCV4) (IM) 4 mcg of each antigen/0.5 mL; Menomune (MPSV4) (Subcut) 50 mcg of each antigen/0.5 mL.

pneumococcal vaccine, polyvalent (Pneumovax 23). Polyvalent pneumococcal vaccine is a sterile solution containing antigenic polysaccharides extracted from *Streptococcus pneumoniae*. It is used to stimulate immunity to 23 types of pneumonia that are represented in the vaccine. The polysaccharides in the vaccine promote production of antibody-specific immunity for each type. Antibody levels remain protective for at least 5 years after immunization. It is recommended for adults, particularly adults older than 50 years.

Dosage: Adults and children older than 2 years: (IM) 0.5 mL.

pneumococcal 7-valent conjugate vaccine (Prevnar). This agent is used for active immunization of infants and toddlers against invasive disease caused by *S. pneumoniae*. It is recommended for administration at 2 months, 4 months, 6 months, and 12 to 15 months of age. This agent is *not* to be used for adults. It is *not* to be substituted for the pneumococcal polysaccharide vaccine in older adults. Not all individuals establish immunity after administration of this vaccine.
Dosage: Children only: (IM) 0.5 mL.

poliovirus vaccine, inactivated (IPV, Salk vaccine) (IPOL). Inactivated poliovirus vaccine is a noninfectious suspension containing three strains of poliovirus. It may be administered intramuscularly or subcut. The major disadvantage of the formerly used live oral polio vaccine was the risk of associated paralytic poliomyelitis in vaccine recipients and their contacts. It has been replaced by the injectable inactivated form. The duration of immunity when using the inactivated virus has not yet been determined.
Dosage: Adults and children: (IM, Subcut) 0.5 mL.

rotavirus vaccine, live oral (RotaTeq). This live oral vaccine stimulates immunity to rotavirus gastroenteritis. The current vaccine contains five live rotaviruses representing the serotypes most likely to infect humans. It is supplied in 2-mL single dose units, and three doses are required.
Dosage: Children: (Oral) 2 mL initial dose at 6 to 12 weeks of age, followed by two more doses at 4- to 10-week intervals. It should not be given after 32 weeks of age.

tetanus toxoid, USP-NF; tetanus vaccine, BP. Tetanus toxoid is a preparation of the formaldehyde-treated by-products of the tetanus bacillus *Clostridium tetani*. Although it is given routinely in childhood in combination with other vaccines in the DPT and DT series, the tetanus toxoid alone is often chosen for periodic boosters after childhood. An effective serum level is sustained for 10 years after the booster dose; however, boosters can be given as often as every 5 years if there is concern that the patient may develop tetanus from an extremely dirty wound.
Dosage: Adults: (IM) 0.5 mL.

tetanus toxoid, reduced diphtheria toxoid, and acellular pertussis vaccine (Tdap) (Adacel). This product may be used for immunization of adults when a reduced diphtheria component is desired. The antigens for tetanus and pertussis are the same as in other vaccines.
Dosage: Adults: (IM) 0.5 mL.

varicella virus vaccine, live (Varivax). This vaccine stimulates immunity to varicella virus, or chickenpox. Long-term studies are necessary to determine the duration of protection after the use of this vaccine. Development of antibodies after vaccination does not occur in all cases, and breakthrough epidemics may still occur.
Dosage: Children older than 12 months: (IM) 0.5 mL.

zoster vaccine live (Zostavax). Zoster vaccine is indicated for the prevention of varicella zoster in individuals 60 years old and older. It should not be administered to individuals allergic to gelatin or neomycin or to patients with immunodeficiency states.
Dosage: Adults older than 60 years: (Subcut) 19,400 units/0.65 mL.

AGENTS THAT PROVIDE PASSIVE IMMUNITY

Various preparations of antibodies are available to provide short-lived but immediately effective protection against disease.

botulism immune globulin, USP-NF, BP. This agent is used for infant botulism.
Dosage: Infants: (IV) 50 mg/kg as a single infusion.

crotalidae polyvalent immune Fab (CroFab). This polyvalent snake antivenin is used to treat North American pit viper envenomation. The antivenin should be used within 6 hours of the snakebite. The Rocky Mountain Poison and Drug Center should be consulted for specific treatment recommendations.
Dosage: By diluted IV infusion, using the recommended number of reconstituted vials.

cytomegalovirus immune globulin (CytoGam). This product is used to provide passive immunity to cytomegalovirus. It may be used prophylactically in kidney transplant recipients to prevent cytomegalovirus.
Dosage: By diluted IV infusion, 150 mg/kg.

hepatitis B immune globulin
Dosage: Adults: (IM) 0.06 mL/kg within 7 days of exposure.

immune human serum globulin, USP-NF, BP
Dosage: Adults: (IM) Prophylactic: 1.3 to 2 mL/kg every 6 to 8 weeks; Therapeutic: for dysgammaglobulinemia therapy, 20 to 50 mL monthly.

Rho(D) immune human globulin, USP-NF (RhoGAM). This antibody preparation is used to desensitize Rh-negative mothers after delivery of an Rh-positive infant. The sensitization of the mother occurs when infant blood cells enter the mother's bloodstream, resulting in antibody formation. The antibodies cause erythroblastosis fetalis in subsequent Rh-positive infants that she may carry.

When administered within 72 hours of delivery, the immune globulin diminishes antibody formation in the mother. Slight temperature elevations and mild local reactions at the site of injection may occur after administration.

Dosage: Adults: (IM) 300 mcg.

tetanus immune human globulin, USP-NF, BP

Dosage: Adults: (IM) Prophylactic: 250 units; Therapeutic: 3000 to 6000 units.

The immune system has its origins in the fetal thymus gland. A process occurs during intrauterine life whereby the infant recognizes certain substances and tissues as its own and develops two types of lymphoid cells, T cells and B cells, which are activated to recognize and destroy foreign substances and tissues.

For the successful development of organ transplants, the body's attempts to reject foreign tissue had to be prevented. A great deal of improvement has occurred in the matching of tissue samples to provide the person receiving a transplant with an organ that matches his or her own tissues as closely as possible. This process, similar to but much more complex than typing blood, has improved the outcome of organ transplants. However, **immunosuppressives**—agents that interfere with the development of antibody response to a foreign substance—are also needed to prevent organ rejection.

General complications of immunosuppressive agents include increased susceptibility to infections and potentially fatal adverse effects when otherwise minor illnesses such as chickenpox are contracted. Central nervous system toxicity may be observed; symptoms include dizziness, headache, confusion, slurred speech, and paresthesias. Jaundice from liver damage and symptoms of bone marrow suppression, such as sore throat, oral mucosal lesions, and excessive bruising, may also occur. Immunosuppressed patients may contract poliomyelitis from the live virus shed by infants after oral administration of live poliovirus vaccine. Family members of immunocompromised patients are generally administered the inactivated or Salk vaccine for this reason.

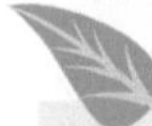

Herb Alert

Echinacea

Echinacea is taken to prevent or reduce the severity of colds. *Echinacea* reduces the effects of immunosuppressants, cyclosporine, and azathioprine. It should be avoided in patients with autoimmune disorders and multiple sclerosis. See Chapter 28 for more information on *Echinacea*.

CORTICOSTEROIDS

The synthetic corticosteroids prednisone, prednisolone, and dexamethasone are used most often for immunosuppression. Side effects specific to this group include salt and water retention, with the characteristic moon facies and fat distribution noted as the administration is prolonged.

dexamethasone

Dosage: Adults: (Oral) 0.75 to 9 mg daily in divided doses.

Children: (Oral) 0.3 mg/kg daily in divided doses.

prednisone and prednisolone

Dosage: Adults: (Oral) 10 to 100 mg daily in divided doses.

OTHER IMMUNOSUPPRESSIVE AGENTS

azathioprine, USP-NF, BP (Imuran). Because of its similarity to the naturally occurring purines, this agent acts as an antagonist to RNA and DNA synthesis, interfering with cell metabolism. This agent is primarily used in the treatment of renal transplant patients to prevent rejection. It is occasionally used in the treatment of other autoimmune disorders, such as systemic lupus erythematosus, hemolytic anemias, and idiopathic thrombocytopenia. Liver damage, increased susceptibility to infection, and bone marrow suppression are the most common side effects of azathioprine.

Dosage: Adults and children: (Oral) 3 to 5 mg/kg daily initially, then 1 to 2 mg/kg daily as a maintenance dosage.

cyclophosphamide, USP-NF, BP (Cytoxan). By interfering with DNA and RNA activities, this agent disrupts cellular function and destroys multiplying lymph cells. It is used to treat autoimmune disorders, such as systemic lupus erythematosus, rheumatoid arthritis, and nephrotic syndrome, and to prevent organ transplant rejection. Cyclophosphamide is also discussed in Chapter 21 in its role as an antineoplastic agent.

Dosage: Adults and children: (Oral, IV) 1 to 5 mg/kg daily.

cyclosporine (Sandimmune). This agent acts primarily against T lymphocytes and inhibits the factors that stimulate T-lymphocyte growth. For this reason, it is used to prevent rejection of organ and bone marrow transplants. Other uses include the treatment of rheumatoid arthritis, psoriasis, and other conditions that have an immunologic basis. Administration of this drug with grapefruit juice apparently causes decreased serum clearance of cyclosporine, increasing the serum levels of the drug. Bioavailability has been increased by 20% to 200% in various studies of this effect.
Dosage: Adults and children: (Oral) 10 to 25 mg/kg daily in one to two divided doses. The dosage varies widely based on its use.

tacrolimus (Prograf). This agent can be used orally or intravenously for its immunosuppressive effect. It is used to prevent rejection of kidney transplants, generally in combination with other agents. Side effects include nephrotoxicity, neurotoxicity, insomnia, paresthesias, and psychological disorders.
Dosage: Adults only: (Oral, IV) 0.03 to 0.05 mg/kg/day.

Multiple sclerosis is a chronic, progressive neurologic disorder. Lesions develop in the brain and spinal cord that accumulate during the course of the disease. It is believed that the individual's immune system attacks the nerve cells in the central nervous system and impairs their ability to function properly. Several immunomodulating agents are used in the treatment of multiple sclerosis.

glatiramer acetate (Copaxone). This agent is a synthetic mixture of polypeptides that has an immunomodulating activity in multiple sclerosis. It reduces the frequency of relapses in the relapsing-remitting form of the disease. Injection-site reactions may occur, as may transient chest pain.
Dosage: Adults: (Subcut) 20 mg daily.

interferon beta-1a (Avonex, Rebif). Interferons are proteins that possess complex antiviral, antineoplastic, and immunomodulating activities. This biosynthetic (recombinant DNA origin) form of human interferon has beneficial effects in the treatment of multiple sclerosis. It reduces the frequency of clinical relapses. Complete blood count and liver function should be checked every 3 months. Elevated liver enzymes and abnormal blood counts may occur.
Dosage: Adults: (Subcut) 22 or 44 mcg three times a week.

interferon beta-1b (Betaseron). This agent is used to treat multiple sclerosis and is believed to act principally by inhibiting the production of interferon gamma, thought to be involved in the increase in severity of the disease. The frequency and severity of relapses is lower in the treated patients than in the controls. Complete blood count and liver function should be checked every 3 months. Elevated liver enzymes and abnormal blood counts may occur.
Dosage: Adults: (Subcut) 250 mcg every other day, with rotation of injection sites.

mitoxantrone (Novantrone). Mitoxantrone has been shown to reduce neurologic disability and the frequency of clinical relapses in patients with relapsing multiple sclerosis. Cardiac evaluation should be performed before treatment. Medication for nausea should be given before infusions. Bone marrow suppression, menstrual abnormalities, and gastrointestinal disturbances have been reported.
Dosage: Adults: (IV) 12 mg/m^2 IV infusion every 3 months.

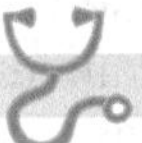

Clinical Implications

1. The health care professional should be familiar with the childhood and adult diseases now prevented by the routine immunizations. All health care professionals should be familiar with both childhood and adult immunization schedules.
2. The health care professional has an important and effective role in promoting adherence to routine infant immunization.
3. When administering immunizations, the health care professional should shake the vial carefully before withdrawing the required dose.
4. All biologic agents have an expiration date; this should be checked before administration of a vaccine.
5. Immunizations are often withheld when a patient is receiving corticosteroids or antineoplastic agents. In some cases, immunization is deferred when close family members are immunologically compromised.
6. Before administration of a biologic vaccine from an animal source, a patient should be closely questioned for allergic reactions.
7. Patients should be counseled about expected side effects of vaccines (i.e., pain, erythema, and swelling at the site of injection and a fever that may last 24 to 48 hours).
8. When patients are receiving immunosuppressive medications, they should be observed for side effects such as fever, sore throat, bone marrow suppression, and bleeding disorders.
9. Oral hygiene should be maintained when a patient is receiving immunosuppressive agents. Lemon-glycerin swabs may be used in lieu of vigorous toothbrushing to prevent gingival bleeding.
10. The health care professional should observe a patient who is receiving immunosuppressive agents for signs of

renal toxicity, which include dark urine, decreased urine output, and peripheral edema.

11. Liver damage as a side effect of immunosuppressive agents is manifested by jaundice, dark urine, clay-colored stools, and abdominal pain or swelling.

12. Patients should be observed for signs of skin rashes or petechiae when receiving immunosuppressive agents.

13. Foods such as grapefruit juice enhance the activity of certain drugs such as cyclosporine.

Vaccine ▼ Age ►	Birth	1 month	2 months	4 months	6 months	12 months	15 months	18 months	19–23 months	2–3 years	4–6 years
Hepatitis B*	HepB	HepB			HepB						
Rotavirus*			RV	RV	RV*						
Diphtheria, Tetanus, Pertussis*			DTaP	DTaP	DTaP	*	DTaP				DTaP
Haemophilus influenzae type b*			Hib	Hib	Hib*	Hib					
Pneumococcal*			PCV	PCV	PCV	PCV				PPSV	
Inactivated Poliovirus*			IPV	IPV	IPV						IPV
Influenza*					Influenza (Yearly)						
Measles, Mumps, Rubella*						MMR			*		MMR
Varicella*						Varicella			*		Varicella
Hepatitis A*						HepA (2 doses)				HepA Series	
Meningococcal*										MCV4	

Range of recommended ages for all children

Range of recommended ages for certain high-risk groups

This schedule includes recommendations in effect as of December 21, 2010. Any dose not administered at the recommended age should be administered at a subsequent visit, when indicated and feasible. The use of a combination vaccine generally is preferred over separate injections of its equivalent component vaccines. Considerations should include provider assessment, patient preference, and the potential for adverse events. Providers should consult the relevant Advisory Committee on Immunization Practices statement for detailed recommendations: **http://www.cdc.gov/vaccines/pubs/acip-list.htm.** Clinically significant adverse events that follow immunization should be reported to the Vaccine Adverse Event Reporting System (VAERS) at **http://www.vaers.hhs.gov** or by telephone, **800-822-7967.** Use of trade names and commercial sources is for identification only and does not imply endorsement by the U.S. Department of Health and Human Services.

* For complete information go to http://www.cdc.gov/vaccines/recs/schedules.

FIGURE 20-1 Recommended 2011 U.S. immunization schedule for children 0 to 6 years old. (From U.S. Department of Health and Human Services, Centers for Disease Control and Prevention. Accessed February 11, 2011.)

Vaccine ▼ Age ►	7–10 years	11–12 years	13–18 years
Tetanus, Diphtheria, Pertussis*		Tdap	Tdap
Human Papillomavirus*	*	HPV (3 doses)(females)	HPV Series
Meningococcal*	MCV4	MCV4	MCV4
Influenza*	Influenza (Yearly)		
Pneumococcal*	Pneumococcal		
Hepatitis A*	HepA Series		
Hepatitis B*	Hep B Series		
Inactivated Poliovirus*	IPV Series		
Measles, Mumps, Rubella*	MMR Series		
Varicella*	Varicella Series		

Range of recommended ages for all children

Range of recommended ages for catch-up immunization

Range of recommended ages for certain high-risk groups

This schedule includes recommendations in effect as of December 21, 2010. Any dose not administered at the recommended age should be administered at a subsequent visit, when indicated and feasible. The use of a combination vaccine generally is preferred over separate injections of its equivalent component vaccines. Considerations should include provider assessment, patient preference, and the potential for adverse events. Providers should consult the relevant Advisory Committee on Immunization Practices statement for detailed recommendations: **http://www.cdc.gov/vaccines/pubs/acip-list.htm.** Clinically significant adverse events that follow immunization should be reported to the Vaccine Adverse Event Reporting System (VAERS) at **http://www.vaers.hhs.gov** or by telephone, **800-822-7967.**

* For complete information go to http://www.cdc.gov/vaccines/recs/schedules.

FIGURE 20-2 Recommended 2011 U.S. immunization schedule for children and adolescents 7 to 18 years old. (From U.S. Department of Health and Human Services, Centers for Disease Control and Prevention. Accessed February 11, 2011.)

VACCINE▼ AGE GROUP▶	19–26 years	27–49 years	50–59 years	60–64 years	≥65 years
Influenza*			1 dose annually		
Tetanus, diphtheria, pertussis (Td/Tdap)*	Substitute 1-time dose of Tdap for Td booster; then boost with Td every 10 years				Td booster every 10 years
Varicella*			2 doses		
Human papillomavirus (HPV)*	3 doses (females)				
Zoster*				1 dose	
Measles, mumps, rubella (MMR)*	1 or 2 doses		1 dose		
Pneumococcal (polysaccharide)*		1 or 2 doses			1 dose
Meningococcal*			1 or more doses		
Hepatitis A*			2 doses		
Hepatitis B*			3 doses		

For all persons in this category who meet the age requirements and who lack evidence of immunity (e.g., lack documentation of vaccination or have no evidence of previous infection)

Recommended if some other risk factor is present (e.g., based on medical, occupational, lifestyle, or other indications)

No recommendation

* For complete information, go to http://www.cdc.gov/vaccines/recs/schedules.

FIGURE 20-3 Recommended 2011 U.S. immunization schedule for adults by vaccine and age group. (From U.S. Department of Health and Human Services, Centers for Disease Control and Prevention. Accessed February 11, 2011.)

INDICATION ▶ / VACCINE▼	Pregnancy	Immunocompromising conditions (excluding human immunodeficiency virus [HIV])*	HIV infection* CD4+T lymphocyte count <200 cells/μL	HIV infection* CD4+T lymphocyte count ≥200 cells/μL	Diabetes, heart disease, chronic lung disease, chronic alcoholism	Asplenia* (including elective splenectomy) and persistent complement component deficiencies	Chronic liver disease	Kidney failure, end-stage renal disease, receipt of hemodialysis	Health-care personnel
Influenza*					1 dose TIV annually				1 dose TIV or LAIV annually
Tetanus, diphtheria, pertussis (Td/Tdap)*	Td				Substitute 1-time dose of Tdap for Td booster; then boost with Td every 10 years				
Varicella*	Contraindicated					2 doses			
Human papillomavirus (HPV)*						3 doses through age 26 years			
Zoster*	Contraindicated						1 dose		
Measles, mumps, rubella*	Contraindicated					1 or 2 doses			
Pneumococcal (polysaccharide)*					1 or 2 doses				
Meningococcal*		1 or more doses							
Hepatitis A*				2 doses					
Hepatitis B*						3 doses			

For all persons in this category who meet the age requirements and who lack evidence of immunity (e.g., lack documentation of vaccination or have no evidence of previous infection)

Recommended if some other risk factor is present (e.g., on the basis of medical, occupational, lifestyle, or other indications)

No recommendation

* For complete information, go to http://www.cdc.gov/vaccines/recs/schedules.

FIGURE 20-4 Recommended 2011 U.S. vaccines that might be indicated for adults based on medical and other indications. (From U.S. Department of Health and Human Services, Centers for Disease Control and Prevention. Accessed February 11, 2011.)

INDICATIONS AND USAGE

FluMist is a vaccine indicated for the active immunization of individuals 2-49 years of age against influenza disease caused by influenza virus subtypes A and type B contained in the vaccine.

DOSAGE AND ADMINISTRATION

For intranasal administration by a health care provider.

Dosing Information

FluMist should be administered according to the following schedule:

Age Group	Vaccination Status	Dosage Schedule
Children age 2 years through 8 years	Not previously vaccinated with influenza vaccine	2 doses (0.2 mL* each, at least 1 month apart)
Children age 2 years through 8 years	Previously vaccinated with influenza vaccine	1 dose (0.2 mL*)
Children, adolescents and adults age 9 through 49 years	Not applicable	1 dose (0.2 mL*)

*Administer as 0.1 mL per nostril.

For children age 2 years through 8 years who have not previously received influenza vaccine, the recommended dosage schedule for nasal administration is one 0.2 mL dose (0.1 mL per nostril), followed by a second 0.2 mL dose (0.1 mL per nostril) given at least 1 month later.

For all other individuals, including children age 2-8 years who have previously received influenza vaccine, the recommended schedule is one 0.2 mL dose (0.1 mL per nostril).

FluMist should be administered prior to exposure to influenza. Annual revaccination with influenza vaccine is recommended.

Administration Instructions

Each sprayer contains a single dose of FluMist; approximately one-half of the contents should be administered into each nostril. See figures below for step-by-step administration instructions. Once FluMist has been administered, the sprayer should be disposed of according to the standard procedures for medical waste (e.g., sharps container or biohazard container).

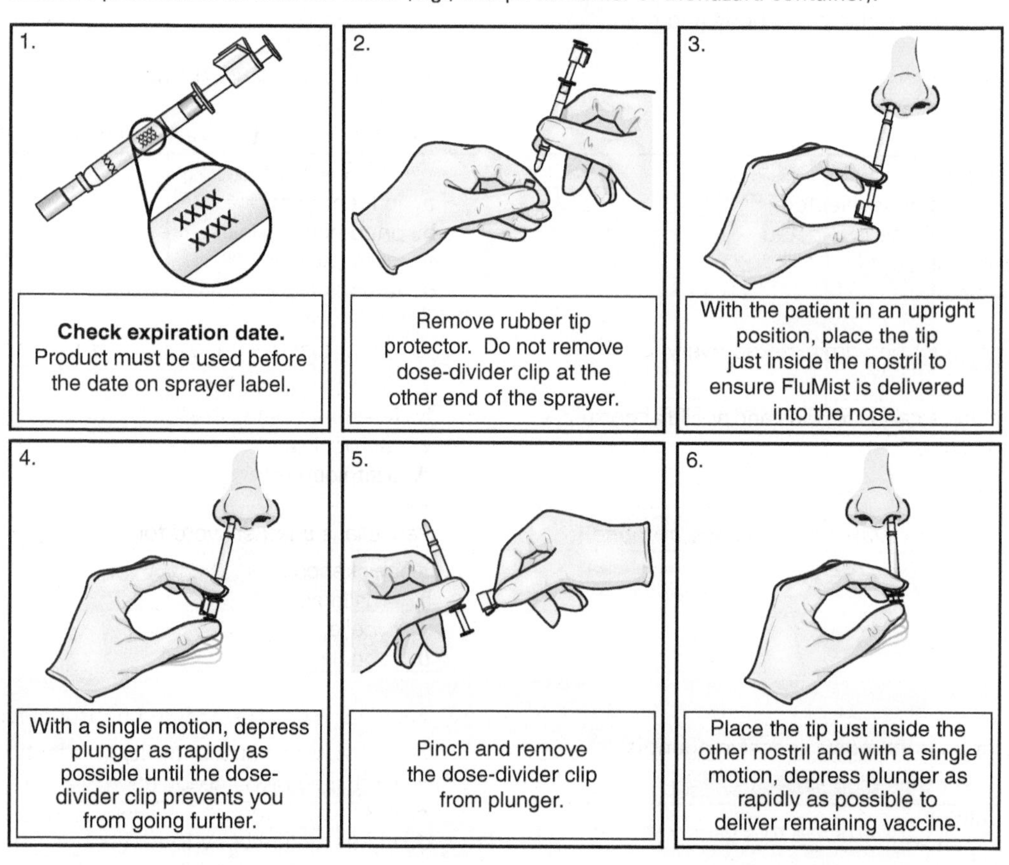

1.
XXXX
XXXX
Check expiration date.
Product must be used before the date on sprayer label.
2.
Remove rubber tip protector. Do not remove dose-divider clip at the other end of the sprayer.
3.
With the patient in an upright position, place the tip just inside the nostril to ensure FluMist is delivered into the nose.
4.
With a single motion, depress plunger as rapidly as possible until the dose-divider clip prevents you from going further.
5.
Pinch and remove the dose-divider clip from plunger.
6.
Place the tip just inside the other nostril and with a single motion, depress plunger as rapidly as possible to deliver remaining vaccine.

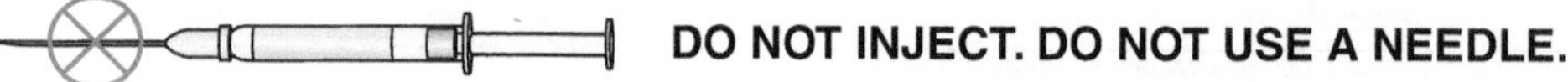

DO NOT INJECT. DO NOT USE A NEEDLE.

Note: Active inhalation (i.e., sniffing) is not required by the patient during FluMist administration

FIGURE 20-5 FluMist dosage and administration. (From FluMist package insert, MedImmune LLC, Gaithersburg, Maryland, 2010.)

CRITICAL THINKING QUESTIONS

1. Your neighbor, who has a 1-month-old daughter, is confused by what she hears regarding the dangerous effects of the "baby shots." She wants your honest opinion as to whether these are really necessary. How would you respond?
2. A patient is alarmed and dismayed at the fat face she now has after her kidney transplant. She is being treated with Imuran and prednisolone. How would you discuss this problem with her?
3. A patient has never had a tetanus injection or any other childhood immunizations. He has just sustained deep lacerations after a fall off his tractor. How do you think tetanus immunity would best be attained?
4. A patient is planning to travel extensively in the Middle East and do missionary work in small villages in India. He wants to know where to check for required immunizations. Where would he go in your community? Which of the vaccines discussed in this chapter would be beneficial, even if not required?

REVIEW QUESTIONS

1. Active immunity is produced when:
   a. the previously formed antibodies are injected into the body.
   b. the antigen is injected into the body and natural antibodies are formed.
   c. the person is exposed to a disease.
   d. an antiserum is injected.

2. Passive immunity is produced when:
   a. a live virus vaccine is injected.
   b. a killed virus vaccine is injected.
   c. an antitoxin is injected.
   d. a toxin is injected.

3. Which vaccine must be administered every year?
   a. Tetanus toxoid
   b. Diphtheria and tetanus toxoids and acellular pertussis
   c. Influenza vaccine
   d. Pneumonia vaccine

4. Which gland is responsible for an infant's immune system?
   a. Thyroid
   b. Thymus
   c. Parathyroid
   d. Adrenal glands

5. An example of an immunosuppressive agent is:
   a. hepatitis B immune globulin.
   b. tetanus antitoxin.
   c. diphtheria antitoxin.
   d. prednisone.

6. An agent that may be used to prevent rejection of kidney transplants is:
   a. RhoGAM.
   b. Energix-B.
   c. tacrolimus.
   d. lymphocytic live vaccine.

7. Adults should get periodic injections of all of the following *except:*
   a. influenza vaccine.
   b. pneumococcal vaccine.
   c. polio vaccine.
   d. tetanus toxoid.

8. An agent that may be used to treat multiple sclerosis is:
   a. cyclophosphamide.
   b. interferon beta.
   c. tacrolimus.
   d. azathioprine.

9. Varicella is another word for:
   a. chickenpox.
   b. smallpox.
   c. rubella.
   d. rubeola.

10. A serious side effect of immunosuppressive agents is:
    a. an increased susceptibility to infections.
    b. increased blood coagulation.
    c. rejection of foreign tissues.
    d. increased antibody formation.

Answers to the review questions can be found at the back of the book.

evolve Additional questions and activities can be found at *http://evolve.elsevier.com/asperheim/pharmacology.*

CHAPTER 21

Antineoplastic Drugs

Objectives

After completing this chapter, you should be able to do the following:

1. Identify antineoplastic drugs, and understand their different modes of action.
2. Explain the use of antineoplastic drugs in immunosuppressive therapy.
3. Understand the use of hormones in the treatment of certain tumors.
4. Understand and anticipate the toxic effects of antineoplastic agents.
5. Discuss nursing measures that provide supportive therapy for cancer patients.

Key Terms

Alkylating (ĂL-kĭ-LĀ-tĭng) **agents,** p. 199
Androgens (ĂN-drĕ-jĭns), p. 202
Antimetabolite (ăn-tĭ-mĕ-TĂB-ĕ-līt), p. 200
Antineoplastic drugs, p. 198
Carcinoma (KĂR-sĭ-NŌ-mĕ), p. 198
Corticosteroid (KŎR-tĭ-kō-STĬR-ŏyd), p. 202
Estrogens (ĔS-trō-jĭns), p. 202
Neoplasm (NĒ-ō-PLĂZ-ĕm), p. 198
Recombinant (rē-KŎM-bĭ-nĕnt), p. 206

Neoplastic diseases, or cancers, are caused by abnormal and uncontrolled growths known as **neoplasms.** Neoplasms that invade surrounding and distant healthy tissues or organs, interfering with function and capable of causing the death of the entire organism, are referred to as malignancies. A **carcinoma** is a malignancy arising from the epithelial cells. Of malignancies, 80% can be defined as carcinomas, but in common practice, the terms *malignancy* and *carcinoma* are often used interchangeably.

Surgery and radiation are still the primary treatment modalities for malignant diseases, but **antineoplastic drugs**—drugs used to treat cancer—have a very important role in the treatment of certain tumors. Systemic drug treatment is important when cancer is widespread or when the organ or tissue cannot be removed. Antineoplastic drugs are also used after surgical removal of a cancer to treat microscopic disease that may be left behind.

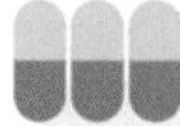

Special Considerations
Immunity

A patient receiving an antineoplastic agent has reduced immunity to infections. The patient should avoid contact with infected persons and anyone who has recently received a live virus vaccine.

Because the malignant cell is dividing more rapidly than normal cells, it is more sensitive than normal cells to antineoplastic agents, which interfere with cell growth or metabolism. The main disadvantage of cancer drugs is that they are often toxic to normal cells as well. The more rapidly dividing healthy tissues (e.g., gastrointestinal [GI] epithelium, oral mucosa, bone marrow, lymphoid tissue, and gonads) are the first to be affected by antineoplastic drugs, and too much tissue destruction in these areas can require withdrawal of the antineoplastic drug before the disease is brought under control.

Antineoplastic drugs may be classified as follows:

1. *Alkylating agents* attach "alkyl groups," or organic side chains, to the proteins or DNA within the cancer cell, interfering with its function.
2. *Antimetabolites* interfere with some phase of normal cellular metabolism. Antimetabolites are substances that compete with, replace, or antagonize a metabolic or bodily function.
3. *Hormones* may antagonize certain tumors of the reproductive tract and accessory sex organs by altering normal hormonal balance.
4. *Antitumor antibiotics* act usually by interfering with DNA or RNA synthesis.
5. *Enzyme inhibitors* interfere with tumor enzymes.
6. *Immunomodulating agents* enhance the body's own defense mechanisms to attack the cancer cells.
7. *Molecular medicine and targeted therapy* treat cancer at the cellular level with agents that are specifically developed to arrest cancer at the cellular level.
8. *Platinum-containing agents* disrupt the function of DNA and proteins because the platinum component of the drugs binds to the DNA and proteins.
9. *Vaccines* stimulate the individual's own immune system to destroy the cancer cells.
10. *Miscellaneous drugs* are a heterogeneous group of drugs having various mechanisms of action.

ALKYLATING AGENTS

Alkylating agents alter the chemical composition of proteins, probably the nucleoproteins, of the cell. The cell cannot function normally in the presence of these abnormal molecules. Alkylating agents were one of the first forms of antineoplastic therapy and have remained in use because of their undisputed effectiveness in the palliation of certain types of cancer. They are all highly toxic compounds, however, and produce many unpleasant and dangerous side effects with continued use.

busulfan, USP-NF, BP (Myleran). Busulfan is administered orally and is used primarily for malignancies of the blood-forming organs.

Dosage: Adults: (Oral) 4 to 8 mg daily.

Children: (Oral) 0.06 mg/kg daily.

carmustine (BiCNU). This alkylating agent is a derivative of nitrosourea. It is used primarily in the treatment of malignant brain tumors. The most serious and frequent side effect is a cumulative and delayed bone marrow toxicity that usually occurs 4 to 6 weeks after therapy. Nausea, vomiting, renal toxicity, hepatotoxicity, and skin rashes occur.

Dosage: Adults: (IV) 200 mg/m^2 body surface every 6 weeks.

chlorambucil, USP-NF, BP (Leukeran). Chlorambucil has its greatest effect on the blood-forming tissues; it is used primarily in the treatment of leukemias and malignancies of the lymphatic system. It is most commonly used in the treatment of chronic lymphocytic leukemia. Chlorambucil has an advantage over mechlorethamine in that it can be administered orally. Side effects include nausea, vomiting, diarrhea, bone marrow suppression, and dermatitis.

Dosage: Adults and children: (Oral) 0.1 to 0.2 mg/kg daily for 3 to 6 weeks. Maintenance dose is 2 to 4 mg daily.

cyclophosphamide, USP-NF, BP (Cytoxan). Cyclophosphamide may be administered orally, intramuscularly, intravenously, or as an intracavitary infusion. It is most often used in treatment of breast cancer, non-Hodgkin's lymphoma, chronic lymphocytic leukemia, ovarian carcinoma, sarcoma, and Wilms' tumors. It may also be used as an immunosuppressant in diseases such as lupus erythematosus. Side effects include nausea, vomiting, diarrhea, bone marrow suppression, and dermatitis. After administration, there is an increased risk of hemorrhagic cystitis and secondary malignancies such as bladder cancer.

Dosage: Adults: (Oral) 1 to 5 mg/kg daily; (IV) 60 to 120 mg/m^2 daily.

Children: (Oral) 2 to 8 mg/kg daily; (IV) 40 to 50 mg/kg daily.

ifosfamide (Ifex). Ifosfamide is structurally related to cyclophosphamide. It is particularly useful in the treatment of germ cell testicular neoplasms, sarcomas, and lymphomas. Side effects are similar to side effects of cyclophosphamide.

Dosage: Adults only: (IV) 1.2 gm/m^2 daily for 3 to 5 consecutive days every 21 to 28 days.

lomustine (CCNU). This agent is well absorbed from the GI tract and is generally administered orally, although it may be used as a topical application in certain cases. It is used in the treatment of brain tumors, lymphomas, and tumors of the GI tract and kidney. It has been used topically to treat mycosis fungoides and psoriasis. Delayed bone marrow toxicity, nausea, vomiting, alopecia, liver and kidney toxicity, and skin reactions occur with therapy.

Dosage: Adults and children: (Oral) 130 mg/m^2 body surface as a single dose. It is given at intervals of at least 6 weeks.

melphalan, USP-NF, BP (Alkeran). Melphalan is used alone and in combination with other antineoplastic agents to treat multiple myeloma and amyloidosis. Side effects include bone marrow toxicity, nausea, vomiting, alopecia, and liver and kidney toxicity.

Dosage: Adults: (Oral, IV) 0.15 mg/kg daily for 7 days. Dosage varies widely.

Children: Dosage has not been established.

procarbazine (Matulane). This agent is used in the treatment of brain tumors and lymphomas. It is a weak monoamine oxidase inhibitor and should not be used with tricyclic antidepressants, sympathomimetic drugs, alcohol, or foods high in tyramine. Concurrent use with central nervous system (CNS) depressants or antihistamines may lead to respiratory depression. Other side effects are similar to the side effects of the other drugs in this class and include nausea, vomiting, alopecia, and bone marrow toxicity.
Dosage: Adults only: (Oral) 60 to 100 mg/m^2 daily for 14 days.

temozolomide (Temodar). Temozolomide is used to treat brain tumors, such as glioblastoma multiforme, and melanoma. Thrombocytopenia and neutropenia are dose-limiting toxicities. Nausea, vomiting, and headache are also seen.
Dosage: Adults only: (Oral) 150 mg/m^2 daily for 5 consecutive days.

thiotepa, USP-NF, BP. Thiotepa is administered topically or as an intracavitary infusion as well as intravenously or intramuscularly. It is primarily used to treat cancer of the reproductive tract, lymphomas, leukemias, and bladder cancer. It is often instilled in the pleural space to decrease pulmonary effusions that occur with local neoplastic diseases. It is occasionally instilled in the bladder to aid in the treatment of small bladder tumors by topical action. Side effects are similar to the side effects of the other drugs within this group.
Dosage: Adults and children: (IM, IV) 30 to 60 mg/m^2 every 7 days; (Topical) 15 mg diluted with a small amount of water.

ANTIMETABOLITES

Antimetabolites are antineoplastic drugs that act by interfering with a specific phase of cell metabolism. Because neoplastic cells grow more rapidly than normal cells, theoretically they should be affected by these drugs at dosage levels that cause only minimal interruption in the metabolism of normal cells. This theory does not always prove to be true, however, and severe bone marrow suppression in particular occurs very often, requiring withdrawal of the drug. Loss of the GI epithelium and ulcers of the oral mucosa are also frequent side effects of antimetabolites.

azacitidine (Vidaza). This agent inhibits DNA methylation. It is approved for the treatment of myelodysplastic syndrome. Side effects include cytopenia, GI side effects, and elevated liver enzymes.
Dosage: Adults only: (IV) 75 mg/m^2 daily for 7 days every 4 weeks.

capecitabine (Xeloda). Capecitabine is an oral version of fluorouracil (5-FU) used to treat metastatic breast cancer and GI malignancies. This agent acts as a radiation sensitizer, and lower doses may be administered if given concurrently with radiation. Side effects include nausea, vomiting, diarrhea, abdominal pain, stomatitis, edema, paresthesias, and hyperbilirubinemia. Often the hands and feet become dry and painful. This side effect may be minimized if patients are encouraged to moisturize the hands and feet several times daily before symptoms occur. Capecitabine is contraindicated in patients allergic to 5-FU.
Dosage: Adults only: (Oral) 2500 mg/m^2 daily in two divided doses for 2 weeks on, 1 week off. With radiation, the dosage may be reduced to 1650/m^2 on days of radiation.

cladribine (Leustatin, 2-Cda). Cladribine is indicated for the treatment of hairy cell leukemia. Side effects include nephrotoxicity, bone marrow suppression, nausea, vomiting, headache, and edema.
Dosage: Adults only: (IV) 0.09 mg/kg/day for 7 days.

clofarabine (Clolar). This agent interferes with DNA replication and is given for relapsed or refractory acute lymphocytic leukemia. Side effects include myelosuppression (suppression of the bone marrow), edema, hypotension, nausea, vomiting, renal toxicity, and hepatotoxicity.
Dosage: Adults and children: (IV) 52 mg/m^2 daily for 5 days every 2 to 6 weeks.

cytarabine, USP-NF, BP (Ara-C, Cytosar-U). The antimetabolic effect of cytarabine seems to occur by interference with DNA formation. It is used primarily to treat acute myelocytic leukemia in adults, although it has been used to treat other adult and childhood leukemias. It may be used intrathecally for meningeal leukemia. Primary side effects are suppression of bone marrow and GI symptoms. Fever, rash, cellulitis, pain at the injection site, sore throat, conjunctivitis, and alopecia also occur frequently. Cerebellar side effects may be observed, and arachnoiditis is a common side effect when cytarabine is used intrathecally.
Dosage: Adults and children: (IV) 100 to 200 mg/m^2 daily for 7 days; (Intrathecal) 5 to 75 mg/m^2 or 30 to 100 mg once every 2 to 7 days. Dosage varies greatly.

dacarbazine (DTIC-Dome). This agent has many uses, including treatment of melanoma and Hodgkin's disease. Side effects include adverse hematologic, hepatic, and GI symptoms.
Dosage: Adults only: (IV) Wide dosage range from 2 mg/kg/day for 10 days to 375 mg/m^2/day, repeated every 15 days.

decitabine (Dacogen). Decitabine interferes with DNA replication and inhibits methylation of DNA. It is used in the treatment of myelodysplastic syndrome. Side effects include myelosuppression, nausea, vomiting, and elevated bilirubin.
Dosage: Adults only: (IV) 15 mg/m^2 daily every 8 hours for 3 days every 6 weeks.

floxuridine, USP-NF, BP (FUDR). By interfering with the synthesis of DNA, floxuridine has been found to be beneficial in certain malignancies. It is recommended only for intrahepatic arterial infusion and is used primarily for treatment of metastatic GI carcinoma confined to the liver. Side effects are generally related to the area where the drug was infused but can include oral stomatitis, esophagopharyngitis, duodenal ulcer, liver toxicity, and GI bleeding. Localized erythema, ataxia, blurred vision, and vertigo have also been noted.
Dosage: Adults: (Intra-arterial) 100 to 600 mcg/kg in diluted solution daily. Therapy is generally continued for 7 to 14 days.

fludarabine phosphate (Fludara). Many malignancies are treated with fludarabine, including chronic lymphocytic leukemia and non-Hodgkin's lymphoma. It has no activity in solid tumors. Side effects are dose-related and include neurotoxicity and myelosuppression.
Dosage: Adults only: (IV) 25 mg/m^2 daily for 5 days every 28 days.

fluorouracil, USP-NF (5-FU). 5-FU is a chemical analog of uracil, a component of RNA. When incorporated into the RNA molecule, it interferes with normal growth and metabolism of the cell. It is administered intravenously for the treatment of breast cancer, GI malignancies, head and neck cancer, and ovarian cancer. It may also be applied topically to treat actinic keratoses.
Dosage: Adults: (IV) 12 mg/kg once daily for 4 days, then 6 mg/kg every other day for four doses. Dosages vary widely. Maintenance dosage ranges from 10 to 15 mg/kg once a week; (Topical) 1% to 5% cream, applied twice daily to the lesion.

gemcitabine hydrochloride (Gemzar). Gemcitabine is used to treat adenocarcinoma of the pancreas and lung and bladder cancer. Side effects include hematologic toxicity. Gemcitabine should be given with caution to patients with renal and hepatic impairment.
Dosage: Adults only: (IV) 1 gm/m^2 once weekly.

mercaptopurine, USP-NF (Purinethol, 6-MP). Mercap topurine is an antimetabolite that inhibits the synthesis of purines (components of DNA). It is administered orally and is effective in the treatment of acute lymphoblastic leukemias, Hodgkin's disease, and other tumors of the lymphatic system. Toxicity includes immunosuppression with increased risk of infection and nausea and vomiting.
Dosage: Adults and children: (Oral) 2.5 mg/kg daily.

methotrexate, USP-NF, BP (Amethopterin). Metho trexate is a folic acid antagonist that exerts its action by interfering with the formation of the reduced or active form of folic acid in the body. It is particularly useful in the treatment of acute lymphocytic leukemias of childhood. The disease eventually becomes resistant to this compound, but often remissions lasting months or years may be obtained. In addition, methotrexate has been used effectively to treat uterine choriocarcinoma, breast cancer, sarcomas, adult leukemias, non-Hodgkin's lymphoma, bladder cancer, and carcinomatous meningitis. It is also effective in the treatment of psoriasis, psoriatic arthritis, and rheumatoid arthritis.

Methotrexate is commonly administered orally but is also available in a parenteral form that may be given intramuscularly, intravenously, intra-arterially, or intrathecally (within the spinal cord). Side effects include myelosuppression; mucositis; and renal, liver, lung, and neural toxicity. The dosage of this drug varies widely because of its many uses.
Dosage: Adults: (Oral, IM, IV) As an antineoplastic—(Oral) 2.5 to 30 mg daily; As an antipsoriatic—(Oral) 2.5 to 5 mg/day for 3 days every week; For rheumatoid arthritis—(Oral) 7.5 mg once weekly; High-dose therapy—(IV) 1 to 12 gm/m^2 over 3 to 24 hours every 1 to 3 weeks.

Children: (Oral, IM, IV) As an antineoplastic—(Oral) 0.12 mg/kg daily.

pemetrexed (Alimta). Pemetrexed is a folic acid antagonist that is used to treat small cell lung cancer and mesothelioma. The patient must be started on folic acid and vitamin B_{12} supplementation before starting the drug. Oral corticosteroids are generally administered before and after treatment to reduce the severity of the dermatologic reactions. Side effects include myelosuppression, GI distress, skin rash, and elevation of liver enzymes.
Dosage: Adults only: (IV) 500 mg/m^2 every 3 weeks.

6-thioguanine, 6-TG (Tabloid). This agent is used to treat acute myelogenous and lymphocytic leukemia, Hodgkin's lymphoma, multiple myeloma, and solid tumors. There is usually cross-resistance between mercaptopurine and thioguanine. Side effects include myelosuppression, pancytopenia, hyperuricemia, nausea, vomiting, intestinal necrosis, and perforations.
Dosage: Adults and children: (Oral) 2 mg/kg/day for 4 weeks.

HORMONES

Hormones have various uses in the treatment of malignant diseases. **Corticosteroids** (hormones produced by the adrenal cortex and their synthetic forms) have long been shown to be valuable in producing remissions of certain malignancies, notably acute lymphocytic leukemia of childhood. They are used either alone or in combination with other drugs. The mechanism of action is not fully understood.

Corticosteroids have been used with less effectiveness in the treatment of Hodgkin's disease, non-Hodgkin's lymphoma, chronic lymphocytic leukemia, prostate cancer, and multiple myeloma. Side effects are those of excessive administration of corticosteroids (i.e., salt and water retention, moon facies, edema, and striae). In many cases, dietary salt may have to be strictly curtailed during administration. Prednisone is perhaps used more than any other corticosteroid in treating malignancies, but other compounds, such as dexamethasone (Decadron), are similarly effective.

Sex hormones have been used to palliate carcinomas of the reproductive tract. **Estrogens,** steroids responsible for feminine characteristics, may be administered to men with carcinoma of the prostate. **Androgens,** substances causing masculinization, have been administered to premenopausal women with breast cancer. These agents are only palliative, not curative. Side effects are as expected: virilization (masculinization) when androgens are given to a woman and feminization when estrogens are given to a man.

ANTIANDROGENS

bicalutamide (Casodex). Generally, this agent is used in combination therapy for the treatment of metastatic cancer of the prostate. Side effects include hot flashes, loss of libido, impotence, gynecomastia, galactorrhea, GI symptoms, and occasionally elevation of the liver enzymes.
Dosage: Adults only: (Oral) 50 mg daily.

flutamide (Eulexin). Flutamide is an orally active antiandrogen used to treat metastatic cancer of the prostate. Side effects include hot flashes, loss of libido, impotence, galactorrhea, gynecomastia, impotence, drowsiness, anemia, and edema. A yellow-green urine may be noted.
Dosage: Adults only: (Oral) 250 mg three times daily.

nilutamide (Nilandron). Nilutamide is a nonsteroidal, orally active antiandrogen. It is used to treat metastatic prostate cancer. Side effects include hot flashes, loss of libido, impotence, gynecomastia, galactorrhea, hepatic impairment, respiratory insufficiency, and interstitial pneumonia.
Dosage: Adults only: (Oral) 150 to 300 mg daily.

ESTROGENS

estramustine phosphate sodium (Emcyt). Estramustine is a conjugate of 17-beta-estradiol and nornitrogen mustard. It is used to treat metastatic prostate cancer and exerts its effect by inhibiting cell division. Absorption is significantly decreased when it is given with dairy products or other calcium-rich foods. Side effects include nausea, vomiting, diarrhea, angioedema, thromboembolic disorders, and cardiovascular and hepatic effects.
Dosage: Adults only: (Oral) 14 mg/kg daily in three or four divided doses.

megestrol acetate (Megace). Chemically related to progesterone, megestrol is used to treat endometrial carcinoma, breast cancer, endometriosis, and prostatic hypertrophy. It is also used as an appetite stimulant for cachexia from various causes, including acquired immunodeficiency syndrome (AIDS) (see Chapter 17). Very few side effects occur with this agent. It should be used with caution in patients with a history of thrombophlebitis. It may be associated with a tumor flare (i.e., the tumor gets larger before reducing in size).
Dosage: Adults: (Oral) 160 mg daily in four divided doses. Dosage may be increased up to 800 mg daily for cachexia.

ANTIESTROGENS

fulvestrant (Faslodex). Fulvestrant is used to treat metastatic breast cancer in women who have had a recurrence after tamoxifen or aromatase inhibitor therapy. Side effects include hematologic disorders and GI effects of nausea, vomiting, diarrhea, and abdominal pain.
Dosage: Adults only: (IM) 250 mg monthly.

SELECTIVE ESTROGEN RECEPTOR MODULATORS

Within the antiestrogens is a group known as selective estrogen receptor modulators (SERMs). SERMs exert selective agonist or antagonist effects on various estrogen target tissues. These agents are chemically diverse but possess a tertiary structure that allows them to bind to the estrogen receptor.

Because of their estrogen receptor–activating properties, SERMs can be used to prevent or treat diseases caused by estrogen deficiency, such as osteoporosis. Because of their estrogen receptor–blocking properties, they can also be used to prevent or treat diseases such as breast cancer. Currently available SERMs have two major limitations: They are only weak estrogen agonists, and they aggravate hot flashes. Side effects generally include nausea, vomiting, headache, hot flashes, constipation, and abdominal pain. In addition, there is an increased risk of blood clots, stroke, and endometrial carcinoma after administration. The patient should be monitored for cataracts.

tamoxifen citrate (Nolvadex). This antiestrogenic compound is similar to clomiphene. It competes with estradiol for receptor sites in tumors of the breast, uterus, and vagina and in other tumors with estrogen receptors. Its primary use is in the treatment of advanced breast cancer in postmenopausal women, but it has been studied in premenopausal women as well.

An important adverse effect should be noted with this drug. Many women with breast cancer are depressed and simultaneously treated for depression. If concomitant selective serotonin reuptake inhibitors are given with tamoxifen, the anticancer effect of this drug is cut in half. Selective serotonin reuptake inhibitors include citalopram, escitalopram, fluoxetine, paroxetine, and sertraline. Selective serotonin-norepinephrine reuptake inhibitors may be given with tamoxifen without adverse effect; these include desvenlafaxine, duloxetine, and venlafaxine. These agents are discussed in Chapter 14.

Dosage: Adults: (Oral) 20 to 40 mg daily in two divided doses.

toremifene citrate (Fareston). Toremifene is indicated for the treatment of metastatic breast cancer in postmenopausal women. Side effects include hypercalcemia, leukopenia, and vaginal bleeding. It should not be used in patients with a history of thromboembolic disease.

Dosage: Adults only: (Oral) 60 mg daily.

AROMATASE INHIBITORS

Aromatase inhibitors are used to treat advanced breast cancer in postmenopausal women or may be given after surgical removal of the tumor. Many breast cancers contain aromatase, an enzyme found primarily in adipose tissue that converts a naturally occurring adrenal hormone to additional estrogen. The activity of this enzyme leads to estrogen production even in postmenopausal women. This estrogen production is a disadvantage when treating breast cancer. Aromatase inhibitors interfere with this process of estrogen production and can lead to diminished tumor growth. The side effects are notably similar to menopausal symptoms: hot flashes, weight gain, mood changes, and most notably osteoporosis and fractures.

anastrozole (Arimidex)

Dosage: Adults only: (Oral) 1 mg daily.

exemestane (Aromasin)

Dosage: Adults only: (Oral) 25 mg once daily.

letrozole (Femara)

Dosage: Adults only: (Oral) 2.5 mg daily.

INHIBITORS OF PITUITARY HORMONES

goserelin acetate (Zoladex). Goserelin acetate is a synthetic analog of gonadotropin-releasing hormone that is used for its endocrine effects. It reduces the amount of testosterone or estrogen in the bloodstream. It is used for the treatment of prostate and breast cancer and for endometriosis and dysfunctional uterine bleeding. Side effects include hot flashes, sexual dysfunction, headaches, blood pressure instability, rash, dizziness, elevated serum cholesterol, and occasionally a tumor flare (temporary increase in the size of the tumor).

Dosage: Adults only: (Subcut Implant) 3.6 mg in implant every 4 weeks for breast cancer; may be increased to 10.8 mg. Subcut implant is administered every 3 months for prostate cancer.

leuprolide acetate (Eligard, Lupron, Viadur). Another synthetic analog of gonadotropin-releasing hormone, leuprolide can be used for its antineoplastic and endocrine effects. Its uses and side effects are similar to those of goserelin acetate, but it additionally is used to treat precocious puberty.

Dosage: Adults: (IM, Subcut) 3.75 to 30 mg approximately every 4 weeks based on serum levels.

Children: (IM, Subcut) 3.75 to 15 mg approximately every 4 weeks.

triptorelin pamoate (Trelstar). Also an analog of gonadotropin-releasing hormone, triptorelin pamoate has actions and uses similar to the other drugs in this category. It is used in the palliative treatment of prostate cancer.
Dosage: Adults only: (IM) 3.75 to 11.25 mg monthly.

ANTITUMOR ANTIBIOTICS

bleomycin sulfate, USP-NF, BP (Blenoxane). The antibiotic action of bleomycin apparently occurs by causing a splitting of the DNA chain. It is used in the treatment of Hodgkin's disease and squamous cell carcinomas of the skin, penis, vulva, head, neck, and larynx. In contrast to most antineoplastic agents, this drug has a very low incidence of bone marrow toxicity. The most serious toxic effect is interstitial pneumonitis. Skin or mucocutaneous lesions, alopecia, fever, chills, and hypotension have been reported. Liver enzymes must be checked monthly while a patient is receiving this drug.
Dosage: Adults: (IM, IV, Subcut, Intra-arterial, Intrapleural Injection) 0.25 to 0.5 units/kg weekly.

dactinomycin, USP-NF, BP (Actinomycin D, Cosmegen). Dactinomycin is an antibiotic that exerts its effect as an antineoplastic agent by interfering with both DNA and RNA synthesis. It also inhibits DNA replication. It is used in the treatment of Wilms' tumor of the kidney and for control of the metastases of this tumor. It has been used in combination with other agents in the treatment of metastatic tumors of the testes, choriocarcinoma, and certain lymphomas. Toxic effects include bone marrow suppression, liver and kidney toxicity, nausea, vomiting, oral stomatitis, anorexia, alopecia, and various skin eruptions.
Dosage: Adults and children: (IV) 15 mcg/kg daily for 5 days.

daunorubicin hydrochloride (Daunomycin). Daunorubicin works by inhibiting DNA and RNA synthesis and by inhibiting the unwinding of the DNA, a function necessary for replication. It is used primarily to treat acute myelogenous leukemia. It has also been used to treat lymphocytic leukemias and disseminated neuroblastoma. Side effects include myelosuppression, GI toxicity, red-orange discoloration of the urine and contact lenses, and alopecia. It may cause acute and delayed cardiotoxicity including arrhythmias and congestive heart failure. Care must be taken to avoid extravasation because it is a potent vesicant.
Dosage: Adults and children: (IV Infusion) 30 to 60 mg/m^2 daily for 3 to 5 days.

daunorubicin liposome (Daunoxome). This agent is daunorubicin with liposomal encapsulation. It is used as a first-line agent for human immunodeficiency virus (HIV)–associated Kaposi's sarcoma. The mechanism of action and side effects are similar to the parent compound.
Dosage: Adults only: (IV) 40 mg/m^2 every 2 weeks.

doxorubicin hydrochloride, USP-NF, BP (Adriamycin). Doxorubicin is an antibiotic produced by a strain of *Streptomyces*. As with the other antibiotics in this group, it has antibacterial properties but is generally considered to be too toxic to be used in this way. The drug works by inhibiting DNA and RNA synthesis and by inhibiting the unwinding of DNA necessary for replication. It is used to treat solid tumors of the breast, ovaries, bladder, lung, liver, thyroid gland, and bone. It is also valuable in the treatment of neuroblastoma; Wilms' tumor; Hodgkin's disease; Ewing's sarcoma; squamous cell tumors of the head, neck, cervix, and vagina; and carcinomas of the testes, prostate, and uterus. The major side effects are in the bone marrow and GI tract. The patient should be monitored for cardiotoxicity, as manifested by changes on the electrocardiogram. Facial flushing, edema, alopecia, fever, chills, and skin rashes also occur. Careful monitoring is advised to avoid extravasation.
Dosage: Adults: (IV) 60 to 75 mg/m^2 body surface as a single dose at 21-day intervals.

doxorubicin liposome (Doxil). This liposomal encapsulated version of doxorubicin has a mechanism of action and side effects similar to doxorubicin. It is used to treat Kaposi's sarcoma, ovarian carcinoma, and multiple myeloma.
Dosage: Adults only: (IV) 20 to 50 mg/m^2 every 21 to 28 days.

epirubicin hydrochloride (Ellence). Related to doxorubicin, epirubicin hydrochloride is used to treat breast cancer. Side effects are similar to the side effects of its parent compound.
Dosage: Adults only: (IV) 100 to 120 mg/m^2 every 3 to 4 weeks.

idarubicin hydrochloride (Idamycin). This agent is an analog of daunorubicin and also inhibits nucleic acid synthesis. It is used in combination with other antileukemic drugs to treat acute myeloid leukemia in adults. Side effects include tissue necrosis at the site of injection, myelosuppression, myocardial toxicity, nausea, vomiting, and peripheral neuropathy. Red discoloration of the urine may occur.
Dosage: Adults only: (IV) 8 to 12 mg/m^2 daily for 3 days.

mitomycin C, USP-NF, BP (Mutamycin). This antibiotic is used in conjunction with 5-FU or radiation therapy or both to treat adenocarcinoma of the stomach, pancreas, colon, and rectum; squamous cell carcinomas of the lungs, cervix, head, and neck; and malignant melanoma. Bone marrow suppression can lead to fatal sepsis if not monitored. Mouth ulcers, nausea, vomiting, and renal toxicity are among the side effects seen after administration. Hemolytic uremic syndrome has been reported.
Dosage: Adults: (IV) 10 to 20 mg/m^2 every 6 to 8 weeks.

mitoxantrone hydrochloride (Novantrone). This synthetic antineoplastic agent is used to treat acute myelogenous leukemia and advanced prostate cancer. It also has activity in malignancies such as breast cancer and non-Hodgkin's lymphoma. Side effects include bone marrow suppression, cardiotoxicity, nausea, vomiting, fatigue, and hemorrhage. There may be blue discoloration of the urine, sclera, and fingernails after 1 to 2 days of administration.
Dosage: Adults only: (IV) 12 mg/m^2 daily.

pentostatin (Nipent). Pentostatin is indicated for the treatment of hairy cell leukemia. Side effects include renal, liver, pulmonary, and CNS toxicities.
Dosage: Adults only: (IV) 2 to 4 mg/m^2 every other week.

streptozocin (Zanosar). This antibiotic is produced by *Streptomyces achromogenes*. It is used to treat pancreatic islet cell carcinoma, carcinoid tumor, Hodgkin's disease, and colorectal cancer. The most serious side effect is nephrotoxicity, which occurs in up to 75% of patients. Nausea, vomiting, bone marrow suppression, tissue necrosis, confusion, and depression have also been reported.
Dosage: Adults only: (IV, Intra-arterial) 500 mg/m^2 daily for 5 days.

valrubicin (Valstar). Valrubicin is a semisynthetic analog of doxorubicin. It is used for instillation into the urinary bladder for carcinoma in situ of the bladder. Side effects include bladder spasm, hematuria, incontinence, pelvic pain, vomiting, diarrhea, and peripheral edema.
Dosage: Adults only: (Intravesical) 800 mg once weekly for 6 weeks.

ENZYME INHIBITORS

asparaginase, L-asparaginase (Elspar). This enzyme, derived from *Escherichia coli*, is mainly used in combination chemotherapy for childhood acute lymphocytic leukemia, but it is used in adults as well. Side effects include skin rashes and various hepatic, renal, and hematologic effects.
Dosage: Adults and children: (IM, IV) 6000 units/m^2 every other day for 3 to 4 weeks.

etoposide, VP-16 (VePesid). Etoposide is a natural product of the mandrake plant. It inhibits an enzyme that is important in the unwinding of the DNA during replication. It is active in a broad range of tumors, including lung, testicular, and germ cell tumors and non-Hodgkin's lymphoma. Side effects include myelosuppression, hypersensitivity reactions, and alopecia.
Dosage: Adults: (IV) 100 mg/m^2 on treatment days per protocol.

imatinib mesylate (Gleevec). This inhibitor of tyrosine kinase is used primarily to treat chronic myelogenous leukemia. Side effects include neutropenia, hepatotoxicity, and fluid retention.
Dosage: Adults only: (Oral) 400 to 600 mg daily.

irinotecan hydrochloride (Camptosar, CPT-11). Originally isolated from the bark and wood of the Chinese tree *Camptotheca accuminata*, this agent inhibits the unwinding of DNA and is used in the treatment of GI, cervical, and lung cancers. Side effects include neutropenia, diarrhea, fever, and cardiovascular toxicity.
Dosage: Adults only: (IV) 125 mg/m^2 weekly.

pegaspargase (Oncaspar). A conjugated asparaginase, pegaspargase is used in the treatment of childhood acute lymphocytic leukemia. Side effects include hypotension, cough, epistaxis, malaise, nausea, and vomiting.
Dosage: Children and young adults: (IM) 2500 units/m^2 at 14-day intervals.

topotecan (Hycamtin). Topotecan is similar to irinotecan in mechanism of action and side-effect profile. It is used most commonly in the treatment of ovarian cancer and small cell lung cancer. Diarrhea is less prominent when using this agent, but some patients develop a flulike syndrome on the first day of therapy.
Dosage: Adults only: (IV) 1.5 mg/m^2 for 5 consecutive days in the 21-day protocol.

IMMUNOMODULATING AGENTS IN CANCER

In the 1950s when it was discovered that there was an interference phenomenon between viruses (subsequently labeled "virus-inhibitory factor"), there was no recognition that the scientists had stumbled on one of the arsenals of the body's own defense mechanism. This interference substance, later called interferon, was found to be produced by leukocytes (white blood cells), and it showed antitumor effects in tissue cultures and animal experiments. A newer form of cancer treatment has come into use with the development of interferons via **recombinant** DNA techniques—techniques in which a cell or organism receives genes from different parental strains.

aldesleukin (Proleukin). This human recombinant interleukin is used to treat metastatic renal cell carcinoma and metastatic melanoma in adults. Side effects include flu symptoms, hypotension, ventricular tachycardia, cardiac tamponade, renal failure, toxic psychosis, and GI bleeding.
Dosage: Adults only: (IV) 600,000 international units/kg/dose every 8 hours for 14 days.

interferon alfa (Alferon N, Intron A, Rebetron, Roferon-A). Interferon alfa is actually a family of proteins that possess complex antiviral, antineoplastic, and immunomodulating activities. Interferons for human use are of human origin, produced by means of cultured cells or recombinant techniques.

When used in cancer therapy, interferons have a growth-inhibiting effect on normal and malignant cells. Interferon alfa-2a and alfa-2b have been used in the treatment of hairy cell leukemia; Kaposi's sarcoma in patients with AIDS; renal cell carcinoma; bladder, cervical, and ovarian cancer; melanoma; and multiple myeloma. Interferon alfa is used after surgical resection of melanoma. Side effects include a flulike syndrome, myalgia, arthralgia, anorexia, mental disturbances, elevated liver enzymes, and skin rashes.
Dosage: Adults only: (IM, Subcut) 2 million units/m^2 three times per week.

MOLECULAR AND TARGETED THERAPIES

Continuing studies aimed at bringing treatment to the cellular level have produced many advances in cancer therapy. Treatment using agents developed through the techniques of molecular medicine and targeted therapy is often more specific for a certain type of cancer than is the case with the other classes of antineoplastic agents. These agents are discussed in Chapter 22.

PLATINUM-CONTAINING AGENTS

Platinum-containing agents exert their effect by binding elemental platinum to DNA and proteins, disrupting their function.

carboplatin (Paraplatin). This agent is used parenterally for the treatment of ovarian, cervical, breast, head and neck, bladder, esophageal, gastric, and lung cancers; Wilms' tumors; and testicular neoplasms. Side effects include bone marrow suppression, nausea and vomiting, renal toxicity, ototoxicity, and neuropathy.
Dosage: Adults only: (IV) Individualized based on glomerular filtration rate—300 mg/m^2 once every 4 weeks.

cisplatin (Platinol-AQ). Cisplatin is used to treat testicular tumors, advanced ovarian and bladder cancers, lung and GI tumors, and a wide variety of other neoplasms. Side effects include bone marrow suppression, nausea, vomiting, ototoxicity, neuropathy, and a metallic taste in the mouth. Renal function must be monitored and is often a dose-limiting factor.
Dosage: Adults only: (IV) 50 to 120 mg/m^2 every 3 weeks.

oxaliplatin (Eloxatin). This third-generation platinum compound is commonly used to treat colon cancer. It also has activity in pancreatic, esophageal, and gastric cancers and is often administered in combination with 5-FU. Neurotoxicity is the dose-limiting side effect, and neurologic symptoms are worsened by exposure to cold. Myelosuppression, nausea, vomiting, and diarrhea may also be seen.
Dosage: Adults only: (IV) 85 to 100 mg/m^2 every 2 to 3 weeks.

VACCINES USED IN THE TREATMENT OR PREVENTION OF CANCER

human papillomavirus vaccine (Gardasil). Gardasil is discussed in Chapter 20. It is used to immunize young women against human papillomavirus, the causative agent of cervical cancer.
Dosage: Children and young adults 9 to 26 years: (IM) 0.5 mL in a series of three injections. The second and third injections are administered 2 months and 6 months after the first.

sipuleucel-T (Provenge). This vaccine is given for metastatic prostate cancer. The patient's own mononuclear cells are removed through plasmapheresis; activated by exposure to a protein, which consists of prostatic acid fused to a granulocyte-macrophage colony-stimulating factor (GM-CSF); and administered back to the patient.
Dosage: Adults: (IV) Up to 50 million total cells administered back to the patient at 2-week intervals for three doses.

MISCELLANEOUS CANCER TREATMENT AGENTS

The following agents have many different modes of action, and many do not fit into the previously mentioned classes. For information on other miscellaneous agents, see Table 21-1.

docetaxel (Taxotere). This synthetic derivative of paclitaxel is effective in many tumor types, including breast, lung, esophageal, gastric, head and neck, ovarian, bladder, and testicular cancers. Side effects include neurotoxicity, bone marrow suppression, fluid retention, hypersensitivity reactions, alopecia, and rash.
Dosage: Adults only: (IV) 60 to 100 mg/m^2 every 3 weeks.

hydroxyurea, USP-NF, BP (Hydrea). This derivative of urea is an antineoplastic drug believed to act by interfering in the formation of DNA. Hydroxyurea is used orally in the treatment of essential thrombocytosis, polycythemia vera, and leukemias. In lower doses, it has been used in patients with sickle cell disease to reduce the number of crises. Side effects are bone marrow suppression, nausea, vomiting, diarrhea, lower extremity ulcers, and teratogenicity.
Dosage: Adults: (Oral) 20 to 30 mg/kg daily.
Children: Dosage has not been established.

mitotane, USP-NF, BP (Lysodren). Mitotane is believed to suppress the adrenal cortex and alter the use of steroids. It is used to treat adrenocortical carcinoma.. GI disturbances, somnolence, dizziness, anorexia, nausea, vomiting, and diarrhea have occurred after administration.
Dosage: Adults only: (Oral) 2 to 10 gm daily in three or four divided doses.

paclitaxel (Taxol). Paclitaxel, isolated from the bark of the Pacific yew tree, works by inhibiting cell division. It is used in the treatment of ovarian, breast, lung, head and neck, esophageal, gastric, and bladder cancers. Side effects include bone marrow suppression, acute hypersensitivity reactions, alopecia, neuropathy, cardiotoxicity with bradycardia, and nail bed deformity.
Dosage: Adults only: (IV) 135 to 175 mg/m^2 every 3 weeks.

Table 21-1 Other Miscellaneous Drugs for the Treatment of Cancer

Drug	Use	Adult-Only Dose
altretamine (Hexalen)	Ovarian cancer	260 mg/m^2
arsenic trioxide (Trisenox)	Acute myeloid leukemia	0.15 mg/kg IV daily
azacitidine (Vidaza)	Myelodysplastic syndrome	75 mg/m^2 subcut daily
bendamustine HCl (Treanda)	Chronic lymphocytic leukemia	100 mg/m^2 IV 2 days a month
bexarotene (Targretin)	T-cell lymphoma	300 mg/m^2 orally daily
bortezomib (Velcade)	Multiple myeloma	1.3 mg/m^2 IV twice weekly
cabazitaxel (Jevtana)	Prostate cancer	25 mg/m^2 orally every 3 weeks
dasatinib (Sprycel)	Myelogenous leukemia	70 mg orally twice daily
docetaxel (Taxotere)	Breast and lung cancer	60 to 100 mg/m^2 IV every 3 weeks
everolimus (Afinitor)	Renal cell cancer	10 mg orally once daily
gefitinib (Iressa)	Lung cancer	250 mg orally daily
histrelin acetate (Vantas)	Prostate cancer	50 mg per implant every 12 months
ipilimumab	Metastatic melanoma	3 mg/kg orally every 3 weeks
ixabepilone (Ixempra)	Metastatic breast cancer	40 mg/m^2 IV every 3 weeks
lapatinib ditosylate (Tykerb)	Breast cancer	2.5 mg orally daily
lenalidomide (Revlimid)	Multiple myeloma	25 mg orally daily
nelarabine (Arranon)	Leukemia	1500 mg/m^2 IV on alternate days
nilotinib (Tasigna)	Chronic myelogenous leukemia	400 mg orally twice daily
panitumumab (Vectibix)	Colorectal cancer	6 mg/kg IV every 2 weeks
pemetrexed disodium (Alimta)	Mesothelioma	500 mg/m^2 IV every 3 weeks
sorafenib tosylate (Nexavar)	Renal cell carcinoma	400 mg orally twice daily
sunitinib malate (Sutent)	Renal and gastrointestinal tumors	50 mg orally daily
temsirolimus (Torisel)	Renal cell cancer	25 mg IV once weekly
thalidomide (Thalomid)	Leprosy and multiple myeloma	100-200 mg orally daily at bedtime
tretinoin (Vesanoid)	Leukemia	45 mg/m^2 orally daily in 2 divided doses

paclitaxel nanoparticle albumin (Abraxane, nab-paclitaxel). Nab-paclitaxel is an albumin-bound version of paclitaxel with the same mechanism of action and side effects. The albumin-bound form gives this drug more specificity for the tumor cells than normal cells. It is used in the treatment of breast cancer after previous treatment failure.
Dosage: Adults only: (IV) 100 to 150 mg/m^2 weekly 3 out of 4 weeks.

vinblastine sulfate, USP-NF, BP (Velban). A derivative of the periwinkle plant, this drug acts primarily by interfering with cell division. It is also administered intravenously and has been used with limited success in the treatment of Hodgkin's disease, lymphosarcoma, and choriocarcinoma. It is of no practical value in the treatment of leukemias. Side effects include bone marrow suppression, neurologic symptoms, alopecia, vomiting, diarrhea, and abdominal pain.
Dosage: Adults: (IV) 4 to 20 mg/m^2 weekly.
Children: (IV) 2.5 mg/m^2 every 1 to 2 weeks.

vincristine sulfate, USP-NF, BP (Oncovin). Also a derivative of the periwinkle plant, vincristine acts by interfering with normal cellular division. It must be administered intravenously and is used in the treatment of acute lymphocytic leukemia, lymphomas, myeloma, sarcomas, and Wilms' tumors. Side effects include bone marrow suppression, neurologic symptoms, vomiting, diarrhea, and abdominal pain.
Dosage: Adults: (IV) 0.5 to 1.4 mg/m^2 weekly.
Children: (IV) 1.5 to 2 mg/m^2 weekly.

vinorelbine (Navelbine). This semisynthetic derivative of vinblastine is active in many tumor types, including breast, lung, head and neck, and ovarian cancers and Hodgkin's lymphoma. Side effects include bone marrow suppression, nausea, vomiting, diarrhea, alopecia, and abdominal pain.
Dosage: Adults only: (IV) 30 mg/m^2 weekly.

SUPPORTIVE AGENTS

Supportive agents are used to make the patient more comfortable during chemotherapy. This may include treating anemia, controlling nausea associated with chemotherapy, and stimulating the appetite in some cases to ameliorate the weight loss associated with cancer and its treatment. IV iron may be used to treat anemia, and blood transfusions are given when appropriate.

HEMATINIC AGENTS

darbepoetin alfa (Aranesp). This is a long-acting form of epoetin alfa that may be given on an every-2-week protocol. Side effects and uses are the same as the parent compound. It is used to treat chemotherapy-induced anemia.
Dosage: Adults only: (Subcut) 200 mcg every 2 weeks.

epoetin alfa (Epogen, Procrit). Epoetin alfa is a biosynthetic form of the hormone erythropoietin. It is used to treat chemotherapy-induced anemia. In some circumstances, it is also used to treat anemia associated with chronic renal failure, hemodialysis, and other conditions such as HIV infection. There is some potential for abuse by athletes, who may use it to increase the oxygen-carrying ability of cells. Side effects include hypertension, seizures, nausea, cardiovascular incidents, vomiting, and increased incidence of blood clots. There is some evidence that this agent may increase mortality in certain cases; its use should be monitored.
Dosage: Adults and children: (IV, Subcut) 150 units/kg three times weekly.

filgrastim (G-CSF, Neupogen). Filgrastim stimulates the formation of white blood cell precursors in the bone marrow. It is given starting the day after chemotherapy and continued on a daily basis for 7 to 10 days to reduce the chances of neutropenia. It may be used to stimulate stem cell production in donors for bone marrow transplants. Side effects consist mainly of bone pain.
Dosage: Adults only: (Subcut) 5 mcg/kg/day.

pegfilgrastim (Neulasta). This is a long-lasting form of filgrastim. It is given the day after chemotherapy as a one-time dose.
Dosage: Adults only: (Subcut) 6 mg one time.

sargramostim (GM-CSF, Leukine). This agent has the same uses and side effects as filgrastim.
Dosage: Adults only: (Subcut) 250 mcg/m^2/day.

ANTIEMETICS USED WITH CHEMOTHERAPY

Some routine antiemetics, such as prochlorperazine maleate (Compazine), promethazine (Phenergan), and scopolamine transdermal, may be used when they are sufficient. Generally, more powerful antiemetics are required before and during chemotherapy treatments. These agents generally act centrally through the CNS by antagonizing serotonin receptors. All doses are for adults. Some agents may be adapted for pediatric use.

aprepitant (Emend)
Dosage: (Oral) 125 mg 1 hour before chemotherapy, then 80 mg daily for 2 days.

dolasetron (Anzemet)
Dosage: (IV) 1.8 mg/kg before chemotherapy.

dronabinol (Marinol)
Dosage: (Oral) 2.5 mg every 12 hours as needed, maximum 20 mg/day.

granisetron (Kytril)
Dosage: (Oral) 1 mg every 12 hours for two doses; (IV) Before chemotherapy, an IV infusion of 10 mcg/kg is given as a 5-minute infusion. Dose is given 30 minutes before chemotherapy.

granisetron transdermal (Sancuso)
Dosage: (Transdermal) Each 24-hour patch has 3.1 mg of granisetron. Start 24 hours before chemotherapy; leave in place at least 24 hours after chemotherapy is completed.

ondansetron (Zofran)
Dosage: (IV) 32 mg before chemotherapy, or (Oral) 4-8 mg every 6 to 8 hours as needed for nausea.

palonosetron (Aloxi)
Dosage: (Oral) 0.5 mg or (IV) 0.25 mg before chemotherapy.

APPETITE AND ENERGY STIMULANTS FOR CANCER PATIENTS

Appetite and energy stimulants often improve the quality of life for cancer patients. They are meant to counteract the malaise, weight loss, and anorexia that accompany serious illnesses.

dronabinol (Marinol). This synthetic cannabinoid is derived from marijuana. It is used to treat anorexia associated with cancer conditions. It also relieves nausea and vomiting.
Dosage: Adults only: (Oral) 2.5 mg every 12 hours, maximum 20 mg/day.

dexamethasone (Decadron). This synthetic corticosteroid is used to stimulate the appetite. Side effects of cushingoid syndrome apply.
Dosage: Adults only: (Oral) 0.75 mg given Monday, Wednesday, and Friday; may increase as necessary.

megestrol acetate (Megace). This synthetic progestin may be used to treat anorexia and weight loss in cancer patients and patients with AIDS.
Dosage: Adults only: (Oral) 800 mg daily in a suspension.

methylphenidate (Ritalin). This CNS stimulant is used to improve the patient's sense of well-being.
Dosage: Adults only: (Oral) Up to 10 mg twice daily.

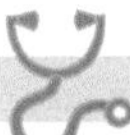

Clinical Implications

1. Patients receiving antineoplastic agents are often anxious and upset. Efforts should be made to provide emotional support to patients and their families.
2. The health care provider should instruct the patient about the importance of good nutrition and his or her nutritional requirements. A diet high in protein but low in saturated fat is optimal (e.g., fish, lean poultry, eggs, nonfat dairy products, nuts, seeds, and legumes). Healthy choices include whole grains, legumes, fruits, and vegetables. Dietary supplements may be beneficial but cannot replace a nutrient-rich diet.
3. Assess the patient's understanding of his or her illness and the possible side effects of medication.
4. Hair loss can be an emotional issue. Patients should be advised that hair grows back in time, even if total alopecia results from the treatments. A wig purchased in advance is a good idea.
5. Oral lesions and bleeding from the gums may result from treatment with antineoplastic agents. Good oral hygiene should be promoted, such as the use of lemon-glycerin swabs and the avoidance of irritating foods or acidic juices. Ice chips held in the mouth during chemotherapy administration can dilute these drugs in the oropharynx and decrease mucositis and the metallic aftertaste.
6. Common side effects of antineoplastic agents are fever, sore throat, blood dyscrasias, and infections. Patients should be monitored for these effects. Any fever should be reported to the physician immediately.
7. Patients receiving antineoplastic medications are susceptible to untoward effects from minor illnesses. Patients and families should be counseled about avoiding contact with possibly infected persons.
8. Sedation or antiemetic medication before the administration of intravenous agents may minimize the nausea and vomiting produced as side effects. Administration in the evening may allow remission of the nausea before the next morning. Patients should be encouraged to eat small, frequent meals.
9. The site of injection should be observed carefully for signs of extravasation because these agents may produce sloughing of tissues.
10. Observe patients for therapeutic effects, such as reduction in tumor size and weight gain.
11. A patient may be depressed as a result of having cancer. Observation for depression and recommendation for treatment, if indicated, help in the overall management of the patient.

CRITICAL THINKING QUESTIONS

1. A child is undergoing treatment for acute lymphocytic leukemia and is presently receiving methotrexate. She has noticed that her long hair is falling out rapidly and is very upset. What would you say to her?
2. A patient is receiving therapy with multiple antineoplastic agents for metastatic breast carcinoma. She has been resisting all attempts to brush her teeth because of extreme soreness in her mouth and throat. What nursing procedures may make her more comfortable?
3. A patient is in the office for a follow-up examination after treatment of a brain tumor with carmustine. He asks for a suggestion for a lotion to treat the rash that has appeared on his stomach and thighs. He had been putting Calamine lotion on the rash to no avail.
4. A patient is improving with antineoplastic agents but has become more and more quiet and listless. What may be the problem? What suggestions may be made?

REVIEW QUESTIONS

1. Neoplasms are caused by:
   a. carcinoma.
   b. uncontrolled cell division.
   c. cell growth of certain genes.
   d. rapidly dividing healthy tissues.

2. An antimetabolite, when used to treat cancer, works by:
   a. interfering with abnormal cell growth.
   b. alkylating the offending cells.
   c. interfering with some phase of normal cellular metabolism.
   d. interfering with abnormal metabolic processes.

3. An example of an antimetabolite is:
   a. carboplatin.
   b. thiotepa.
   c. methotrexate.
   d. nilutamide.

4. Androgens may be used to treat:
   a. breast cancer.
   b. leukemia.
   c. prostate cancer.
   d. testicular cancer.

5. An example of an antiandrogen is:
   a. testosterone.
   b. gemcitabine.
   c. nilutamide.
   d. nikethamide.

6. An example of an antitumor antibiotic is:
   a. goserelin.
   b. dactinomycin.
   c. angiotensin.
   d. amoxicillin.

7. Interferon alfa may be used to treat:
   a. melanoma.
   b. colon cancer.
   c. acute leukemia.
   d. myalgia.

8. An enzyme that is used in cancer chemotherapy is:
   a. pancrelipase.
   b. ptyalin.
   c. pegaspargase.
   d. asparaginase.

9. Hydroxyurea is believed to function in cancer therapy by:
   a. interfering with cell wall formation.
   b. suppressing cell metabolism.
   c. functioning as an immunosuppressive.
   d. interfering with the formation of DNA.

10. An agent used to treat anemia that often occurs after chemotherapy is:
    a. mitoxantrone.
    b. vitamin E.
    c. epinephrine.
    d. epoetin alfa.

Answers to the review questions can be found at the back of the book.

evolve Additional questions and activities can be found at *http://evolve.elsevier.com/asperheim/pharmacology*.

Molecular and Targeted Therapies

CHAPTER 22

Objectives

After completing this chapter, you should be able to do the following:

1. Understand the genetic basis of many diseases.
2. Obtain an overview of the methods used in gene and targeted therapies.
3. Become familiar with the terms used in gene and targeted therapies.
4. Understand the various mechanisms of action of genetically engineered drugs.
5. Understand the role of the health care provider in recognizing the serious side effects of these very potent agents.

Key Terms

Chimeric antibody, p. 213
Cytokine, p. 212
Double helix, p. 211
Deoxyribonucleic acid (DNA), p. 211
Gene therapy, p. 212
Genome (JĒ-nōm), p. 211
Monoclonal (MŎN-ĕ-KLŌ-nĕl) **antibody,** p. 212
Stem cells, p. 212
Targeted therapy, p. 212
Vector, p. 212

In 1953 Watson and Crick uncovered the structure of **deoxyribonucleic acid (DNA),** the substance of which genes are made, and changed biology forever. Only four bases—adenine, guanine, cytosine, and thymine—make up DNA in a twin-coil structure, or **double helix** (Fig. 22-1). Since this discovery, great advancements have been made in understanding of heredity (the genetic transfer of traits from parents to offspring), and the composition of the entire human **genome** (the complete set of chromosomes) has been determined. The challenge of transferring these novel discoveries to the bedside is just beginning.

GENETIC BASIS OF DISEASE

By understanding the genetic basis of disease, researchers can hope to develop predictive tests for the disease. If a diagnosis is made before the disease becomes apparent, treatment may be started early, and the disease may be prevented or at least treated more effectively.

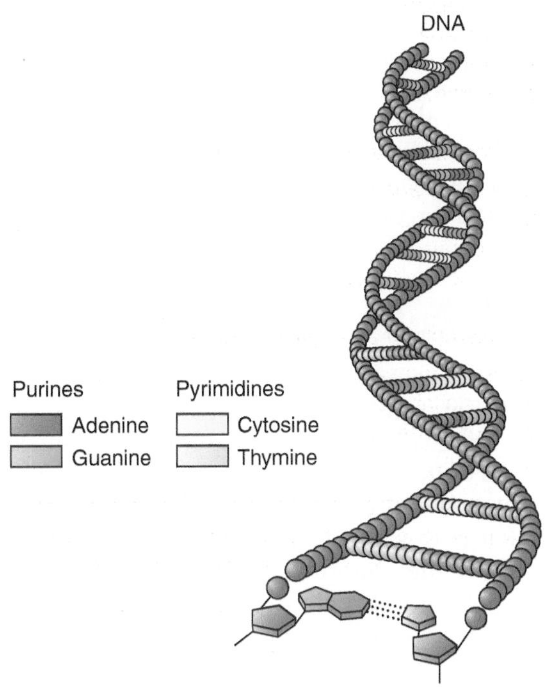

FIGURE 22-1 Double helix structure of DNA.

It is common knowledge that certain drugs affect individuals differently. Antihistamines may cause dangerous drowsiness in one individual and rarely affect another. Various side effects of drugs are more pronounced in certain individuals. The reason for these variations lies in the genome.

GENE THERAPY

The term **gene therapy** can be defined as the application of genetic principles to the treatment of human disease. Certain diseases occur because the body does not make a necessary substance, such as insulin or blood-clotting factors. If the faulty or missing gene that manufactures these substances within a cell could be replaced, the body could manufacture its own missing protein. Gene therapy in this instance would have as its goal the permanent replacement of the missing gene within the cells of the body. Viruses are known to invade the cells of the body and transfer their genetic material for further manufacture by the cell, so one approach to this gene transfer is the use of viral **vectors,** or carriers. The use of nonviral vectors is also under study.

STEM CELLS

Stem cells are primitive cells that have the potential to develop into any of the tissues of the body. They can be harvested from human embryos, from umbilical cords, from shed baby teeth, and in small numbers from peripheral blood. It is hoped that, when implanted, stem cells would manufacture a missing substance or create new tissue cells to replace damaged tissue. Research on the implantation of stem cells in the brains of patients with Parkinson's disease is now in its early stages. Stem cells are also used in bone marrow transplants to treat various disorders. Continuing research is expected to provide many developments in this field.

TARGETED THERAPY

Targeted therapy, or therapy directed specifically at an abnormal or missing site in the body, is a rapidly developing field of pharmacology. It has been shown to be a very effective method for cancer chemotherapy. Therapy is based on mechanisms that target critical molecular pathways of tumors. Examples include the targeting of the abnormal Philadelphia chromosome in patients with chronic myelogenous leukemia, the treatment of gene-specific breast cancer in women with the *BRCA1* and *BRCA2* genes, and the treatment of renal cell carcinoma.

Targeted therapy can also be used to treat certain disorders in which the body's immune system is misdirected toward its own tissues. These disorders include multiple sclerosis, rheumatoid arthritis, thyroiditis, and Crohn's disease. Immunosuppressives have become invaluable in treating these conditions. Other diseases with a confirmed genetic cause or link include cystic fibrosis, Huntington's disease, Alzheimer's disease, diabetes, hypertension, asthma, obesity, and certain heart disorders.

A monoclonal antibody is now available for the treatment of psoriasis that targets skin-infiltrating lymphocytes that express a certain **cytokine** (a protein secreted by certain cells that regulates immune response). Advances in the treatment of macular degeneration, in preventing the progression of calcific aortic stenosis, and in the treatment of autoimmune and inflammatory conditions have shown great progress with the use of targeted therapy.

Targeted therapy is useful outside pharmacology as well. When tumors are targeted with a radiolabeled substance, radiation therapy also becomes more effective. The radiation targets these radioactive substances and delivers lethal molecules directly into the tumor, sparing more of the surrounding normal tissues.

MONOCLONAL ANTIBODIES

Humans have the ability to make antibodies that recognize and bind to any antigen. Antibodies have been discussed previously in this text in their application as immunizing agents to protect against diseases (see Chapter 20). Human antibodies made in response to vaccines or in response to a disease or other antigen are often polyclonal—that is, they attach to many different receptors on the antigen.

A **monoclonal antibody** attaches to only one specific site or receptor; it may have more uses in the treatment of specific disorders. To manufacture a monoclonal antibody, mice are immunized with the desired antigen; in a complicated process, spleen cells from the mice then are used to produce the specific desired monoclonal antibodies from human myeloma cells. One problem with this technique has been that the mouse antibodies are seen as foreign, and often human patients mount an immune response against them, producing human antimouse antibody (HAMA). Not only does the production of HAMA cause the therapeutic antibodies to be quickly eliminated, but also the immune complexes that form can cause damage to the kidneys. Two approaches have been used in an attempt to reduce the problem of the HAMA response:

1. **Chimeric antibodies**—using genetic engineering, the antigen-binding part of the mouse antibody is fused to the part of a human antibody that controls its function. Infliximab and abciximab are examples.
2. Humanized antibodies—the mouse amino acids responsible for making the antigen-binding site are inserted into a human antibody molecule. Daclizumab, rituximab, Vitaxin, gemtuzumab, trastuzumab, and omalizumab are examples.

Monoclonal antibodies are used therapeutically in several ways, as follows:

1. As agents to suppress the immune system. The immune system may be prevented from rejecting an organ after transplant, or these agents may be given as disease-modifying drugs in conditions such as rheumatoid arthritis and Crohn's disease.
2. As agents to treat various types of cancer.
3. As agents with variable modes of action against disease processes. An example is the monoclonal antibody used in the treatment of psoriasis.

AGENTS USED TO SUPPRESS THE IMMUNE SYSTEM

In this discussion, there is necessarily some overlap with agents already presented. Some immunosuppressives, including azathioprine (Imuran), cyclophosphamide (Cytoxan), cyclosporine (Sandimmune), interferon beta (Betaseron), and tacrolimus (Prograf), are discussed in Chapter 20.

basiliximab (Simulect). This chimeric monoclonal antibody is used to prevent the rejection of transplanted kidneys. It is often used in conjunction with other agents such as cyclosporine and corticosteroids. Acute hypersensitivity reactions have occurred. Symptoms of hypersensitivity include hypotension, bronchospasm, tachycardia, and rash.
Dosage: Adults and children weighing more than 35 kg: (IV) 20 mg just before transplantation and a second dose 4 days later.

Children weighing less than 35 kg: (IV) 10 mg just before transplantation and a second dose 4 days later.

daclizumab (Zenapax). Daclizumab is used to prevent acute rejection of transplanted kidneys. It is often used as part of an immunosuppressive regimen that includes cyclosporine and corticosteroids. Generally mild adverse reactions occur in less than 5% of patients and include gastritis, renal insufficiency, nausea, diarrhea, and headache. This agent should be used with caution because it is unknown whether the drug will have a long-term effect on the ability of the body to react normally to an antigen first encountered after the patient has begun receiving daclizumab therapy.
Dosage: Adults and children: (IV) 1 mg/kg, diluted. The first dose is given no more than 24 hours before the transplant, then five doses are given at 14-day intervals.

mycophenolate mofetil hydrochloride (CellCept); mycophenolate sodium (Myfortic). The two salts of this agent may be used orally for the prevention of heart, liver, and kidney transplant rejection, generally in conjunction with cyclosporine and corticosteroids. The hydrochloride salt may also be given intravenously. Mycophenolate has also been used to treat Crohn's disease. Side effects include increased susceptibility to infection and the development of lymphoma. Gastrointestinal bleeding and neutropenia have been reported.
Dosage: Adults: (Oral, IV) 1 to 1.5 gm twice daily.

Children: (Oral) 600 mg/m^2 twice daily.

natalizumab (Tysabri). This recombinant monoclonal antibody is used in the management of multiple sclerosis. It is used to delay the accumulation of physical disability and to reduce the frequency of exacerbations. Natalizumab may be used with other agents such as interferon beta-1b (Betaseron). Natalizumab has also been used to treat Crohn's disease. Adverse effects include leukoencephalopathy, hypersensitivity reactions, and increased susceptibility to infections. Natalizumab can be prescribed in controlled distribution programs only.
Dosage: Adults only: (IV) 300 mg infusion every 4 weeks.

omalizumab (Xolair). This monoclonal antibody is used to control symptoms in patients with moderate to severe asthma who do not respond to corticosteroids. It binds to immunoglobulin E (IgE), preventing IgE from binding to mast cells. Adverse reactions include headache, sinusitis, anaphylaxis, and possibility of malignant neoplasms.
Dosage: Adults and children older than 12 years: (Subcut) 150 to 375 mg every 2 to 4 weeks.

sirolimus (Rapamune). This agent is a macrolide antibiotic, but it is used to prevent rejection of kidney transplants. Similar to the other agents in this class, it is generally advisable to use it in combination with cyclosporine and corticosteroids. Immunosuppression may potentially result in the development of hyperlipidemia, diarrhea, thrombocytopenia, or lymphoma.
Dosage: Adults only: (Oral) 6 mg loading dose, then 2 mg daily.

AGENTS USED TO TREAT RHEUMATOID ARTHRITIS AND CROHN'S DISEASE

abatacept (Orencia). Abatacept is used in the management of the signs and symptoms of rheumatoid arthritis. It is used to produce a clinical response and to slow the progression of structural damage from the disease. Live virus vaccines should not be administered during administration of this agent or within 3 months after its discontinuance. Hypotension, urticaria, and dyspnea have been reported.
Dosage: Adults only: (IV) 500 mg to 1 gm in diluted infusion at 2 weeks and 4 weeks, then at 4 week intervals.

adalimumab (Humira). Also used in the treatment of rheumatoid arthritis, this agent is similar to abatacept in its actions and adverse reactions.
Dosage: Adults only: (Subcut) 40 mg every other week.

anakinra (Kineret). Anakinra is used to manage the signs and symptoms of rheumatoid arthritis and to prevent the structural damage that can occur with the condition. It should not be combined with etanercept because the risk of serious infection and neutropenia is increased. Live virus vaccines should not be administered while taking this agent.
Dosage: Adults only: (Subcut) 100 mg once daily.

etanercept (Enbrel). Etanercept, which binds to tumor necrosis factor, has shown promise in the treatment of rheumatoid arthritis. It is used to reduce signs and symptoms and to inhibit the progression of structural damage in patients with severe rheumatoid arthritis, psoriatic arthritis, and juvenile rheumatoid arthritis. Etanercept can be used in combination with methotrexate in patients who do not respond adequately to methotrexate alone. Glucocorticoids, nonsteroidal anti-inflammatory drugs (NSAIDs), or analgesics may be continued during treatment. Adverse reactions include sepsis; allergic reactions; aplastic anemia; and neurologic disorders such as transverse myelitis, demyelinating diseases, and seizures.
Dosage: Adults: (Subcut) 25 mg given twice weekly 72 to 96 hours apart.

Children 4 to 17 years: (Subcut) 0.4 mg/kg (up to 25 mg) twice weekly 72 to 96 hours apart.

infliximab (Remicade). Infliximab binds specifically to human tumor necrosis factor. Elevated levels of this factor have been found in the joints of patients with rheumatoid arthritis and the stools of patients with Crohn's disease. In rheumatoid arthritis, treatment with infliximab reduced passage of the inflammatory cells into joints. In Crohn's disease, there is a reduction in passage of inflammatory cells in the intestine. After treatment, these patients had decreased levels of C-reactive protein and other inflammatory proteins. Adverse reactions include infusion-related reactions of dyspnea, flushing, headache, and rash. Anaphylactic reactions have occurred, including laryngeal edema, severe bronchospasm, and seizures.
Dosage: Adults: (IV) 3 to 5 mg/kg as an infusion, repeated in 2 weeks and 6 weeks.

leflunomide (Arava). This immunomodulating agent is used for the management of moderate to severe rheumatoid arthritis. It improves physical function and retards structural damage associated with the disease. Therapy often is in combination with NSAIDs and corticosteroids. Side effects include reversible elevations in liver enzymes, anemia, opportunistic infections, hypertension, and alopecia.
Dosage: Adults only: (Oral) 100 mg daily for 3 days, then 20 mg daily.

AGENTS USED TO TREAT CANCER

Viruses have been associated with cancers in animals for many years. Epstein-Barr virus has been accepted as a cause of lymphomas and certain cancers. Many people are infected with a given virus, but few develop the associated cancers. This pattern of individual immunity to infections and malignant diseases is well known but poorly understood. Gardasil, the vaccine for human papillomavirus (HPV), provides immunity to specific strains of the virus and prevents cervical cancer.

Genetic mutations, either inherited or spontaneous, can cause cancer. These mutations may enhance the function of genes that may promote cancer, or they may cause tumor suppressor genes to lose function. There is continuing evidence of abnormal silencing of genes in cancer cells. The aim is to bring the treatment of cancer to a cellular level by understanding these processes.

aldesleukin (Proleukin). A biosynthetic agent of recombinant DNA origin, this agent can be used to treat several types of cancer, including renal cell cancer and melanoma. It has complex antineoplastic and immunomodulating properties. Adverse effects include renal toxicity, hepatotoxicity, and cardiovascular effects.
Dosage: Adults only: (IV) 600,000 units/kg every 8 hours for 14 doses.

alemtuzumab (Campath). A DNA-derived monoclonal antibody, alemtuzumab is used to treat chronic lymphocytic leukemia. It binds to CD22, a molecule

found on white blood cells. Adverse effects include immunosuppressive complications, such as lymphopenia and infection.
Dosage: Adults only: (IV) 3 mg daily; may be increased to 30 mg/day 3 days a week.

bevacizumab (Avastin). This monoclonal antibody is used for metastatic colorectal cancer and for non–small cell lung cancer. Adverse effects include thromboembolism, wound healing problems, hemorrhage, and hypertension.
Dosage: Adults only: (IV) 5 mg/kg or 10 mg/kg every 2 weeks.

cetuximab (Erbitux). This chimeric monoclonal antibody binds to epidermal growth factor receptors. It is used in the treatment of colorectal cancer and head and neck cancer primarily. Adverse effects include dyspnea during the infusion and adverse cardiac and pulmonary events.
Dosage: Adults only: (IV) 400 mg/m^2 loading dose, then 250 mg/m^2 infusion once weekly.

denileukin diftitox (Ontak). Denileukin diftitox is a recombinant DNA–derived cytotoxic protein related to diphtheria toxin. It is used to treat T-cell lymphoma. Adverse effects include hypersensitivity reactions, hypotension secondary to vascular leak syndrome, and a predisposition to infections.
Dosage: Adults: (IV) 9 mcg/kg/day or 18 mcg/kg/day.

erlotinib hydrochloride (Tarceva). Erlotinib is an inhibitor of a human epidermal growth factor receptor. It is used to treat non–small cell lung cancer and pancreatic cancer. Adverse effects include nausea, vomiting, diarrhea, and muscle cramps.
Dosage: Adults only: (Oral) 100 to 150 mg once daily.

gemtuzumab ozogamicin (Mylotarg). This monoclonal antibody binds CD33, a cell surface molecule found on the cancerous cells in acute myelogenous leukemia. CD33 is not found on other cells. It should be used alone, not combined with other agents. Adverse effects include hypersensitivity reactions of chills, fever, nausea, hepatotoxicity, and respiratory distress syndrome. In most cases, hypersensitivity reactions occur during the transfusion or within 24 hours after the transfusion.
Dosage: Adults: (IV) 9 mg/m^2 administered as a 2-hour infusion. A second dose may be given in 14 days.

ibritumomab tiuxetan (Zevalin). Ibritumomab is a monoclonal antibody that is conjugated with tiuxetan and then chelated with the radioisotopes indium-111 and yttrium-90. Use is as a single course of treatment for relapsed non-Hodgkin's lymphoma. Adverse effects include infusion reactions, thrombocytopenia, hemorrhage, and infections. Secondary leukemia has been reported.
Dosage: Adults: (IV) Dosage expressed as the radioactive component 0.4 millicurie/kg.

imatinib mesylate (Gleevec). This antineoplastic agent is an inhibitor of the enzyme tyrosine kinase. It is used for the treatment of Philadelphia chromosome–positive myelogenous leukemia. It is often administered along with corticosteroids. Adverse effects include nausea, vomiting, diarrhea, and muscle cramps.
Dosage: Adults: (Oral) 400 to 800 mg daily.

rituximab (Rituxan). Rituximab binds to the CD20 molecule found on most beta cells and is used to treat beta cell non-Hodgkin's lymphomas. Adverse reactions include infusion reactions, which in some cases have resulted in death within 24 hours. Infusion reactions can include hypoxia, myocardial infarction, cardiogenic shock, and acute respiratory distress syndrome. Approximately 80% of infusion reactions occur with the first infusion.
Dosage: Adults: (IV) 375 mg/m^2 as an infusion once weekly for 4 to 8 weeks.

trastuzumab (Herceptin). Trastuzumab is the first monoclonal antibody that is effective against solid tumors. It binds to HER2, a receptor that is found on certain tumor cells (some breast cancers and some lymphomas). Adverse effects include the development of left ventricular dysfunction and congestive heart failure. Left ventricular function should be evaluated before treatment.
Dosage: Adults: (IV) 4 mg/kg as a 90-minute infusion, repeated weekly as 2 mg/kg per infusion.

MISCELLANEOUS AGENTS

abciximab (ReoPro). Abciximab binds to the glycoprotein receptor of human platelets and prevents clumping of the platelets. It is helpful in preventing recurrent obstruction of coronary arteries in patients after angioplasty. The risk of bleeding is increased with the use of this drug, particularly in the presence of anticoagulants.
Dosage: Adults: (IV) 0.25 mg/kg bolus followed by an infusion of 125 mcg/kg/min over 12 hours.

ranibizumab (Lucentis). Ranibizumab is a fragment of a monoclonal antibody; it binds to and inhibits all forms of vascular endothelial growth factor A. It is used to treat age-related macular degeneration. This agent is injected directly into the vitreous cavity of the eye; it prevents vision loss and improves visual acuity. Presently, ranibizumab needs to be injected monthly, and treatment is required indefinitely. It is contraindicated in the presence of ocular or periocular infections. Endophthalmitis, increased intraocular pressure, and thromboembolic events have occurred.

Dosage: Adults: (Intravitreal Injection) 0.5 mg monthly.

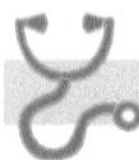

Clinical Implications

1. When the immune system is suppressed, a patient is susceptible to many common infections. The patient should be cautioned against exposure to infected individuals.
2. Immunocompromised patients should not be around individuals, particularly children, who are receiving vaccines. The shedding of antigens or viruses from the vaccines may infect immunocompromised patients.
3. The health care worker should provide general recommendations to encourage patients to maintain good lifestyle habits, including regular exercise, good nutrition, and a positive outlook on life.
4. Serious adverse effects occur during and after administration of many of these agents. The health care worker should become familiar with the adverse effects and prepare to report them as soon as possible.
5. Many other drugs and herbal products react adversely with these drugs. A careful history of prescription and over-the-counter drug use should be taken. Patients should be advised not to take any drug or herb without the practitioner's knowledge.
6. Expiration dates should be carefully checked on these agents, and recommendations for storage should be given (i.e., in a refrigerator, in a freezer, or at room temperature).
7. Patients should be observed frequently for skin rashes, signs of bleeding, or other untoward effects and should be questioned about their own observations of side effects.
8. The use of lemon-glycerin swabs is helpful in maintaining oral hygiene.
9. Many drug programs are sponsored by the pharmaceutical manufacturers for the administration of these agents to indigent or uninsured patients. Patients may need assistance in obtaining this information.
10. Older patients may be more susceptible to the adverse effects of these agents than younger patients.

CRITICAL THINKING QUESTIONS

1. A patient presents for his monthly infusion of infliximab (Remicade). In the general conversation, he reports that he has been to his dermatologist twice in the past month for his persistent skin rash, which he attributes to eating a lot of seafood lately. What advice may be given to him?
2. A patient has been taking ibuprofen for more than a year for rheumatoid arthritis. He is now going to begin treatment with etanercept (Enbrel). He wants to know if he has to stop the ibuprofen. How would you respond? He then admits he also takes herbal therapies. Should he stop taking those too?
3. A patient is receiving daclizumab (Zenapax). He had a mild headache and some nausea after the last treatment. He wants to know if this means he cannot take this drug anymore. How would you respond?

REVIEW QUESTIONS

1. The human gene is composed of:
   a. DNA strands.
   b. a genome.
   c. an oncogene.
   d. transfer RNA.

2. A monoclonal antibody is:
   a. the cause of genetic diseases.
   b. a curative agent for genetic diseases.
   c. a specific antibody that binds to one receptor only.
   d. more heterogeneous than a polyclonal antibody.

3. An agent that is used to treat rheumatoid arthritis is:
   a. aldesleukin.
   b. omalizumab.
   c. infliximab.
   d. Vitaxin.

4. A possible adverse effect of treatment with etanercept is:
   a. vomiting.
   b. renal toxicity.
   c. hypertension.
   d. sepsis.

5. Gene therapy means:
   a. using genetic knowledge to treat human diseases.
   b. giving genes by transplant.
   c. increasing the DNA in cells.
   d. suppressing all genomes.

6. Gene transfer into humans or animals can be made by:
   a. oral agents.
   b. viral vectors.
   c. insect vectors.
   d. combining cell nuclei.

7. An adverse reaction to daclizumab may be:
   a. hypertension.
   b. hypotension.
   c. gastritis.
   d. increased urine output.

8. Aldesleukin is used in the treatment of:
   a. melanoma.
   b. leukemia.
   c. lymphoma.
   d. brain neoplasms.

9. Simulect is an example of a(n):
   a. viral vector.
   b. angiogenesis inhibitor.
   c. immunosuppressive.
   d. antiplatelet agent.

10. Stem cells are:
    a. cells found in the stems of plants.
    b. cells found in the nucleus.
    c. specialized cells in the brain.
    d. cells that can develop in any tissue.

Answers to the review questions can be found at the back of the book.

evolve Additional questions and activities can be found at *http://evolve.elsevier.com/asperheim/pharmacology.*

CHAPTER 23

Drug Therapy in Women

Objectives

After completing this chapter, you should be able to:

1 Recognize that there are disorders of women that require specific pharmacologic intervention.
2 Recognize that there are many instances in which drugs behave differently in women.
3 Identify reasons why women may not seek prompt medical attention for symptoms.
4 Recognize that the incidence and morbidity of many disorders vary greatly in men and women.
5 Become more skilled in assessing the particular responses of women to medication.
6 Assist women in obtaining the necessary information about their health and medication.

Key Terms

Fibromyalgia, p. 220
Menstrual migraines, p. 223
Osteoporosis, p. 220
Perimenopausal, p. 219
Postpartum depression, p. 222
Premenstrual dysphoric disorder (PMDD), p. 222

Women constitute 50.9% of the population and account for 59.4% of medical visits in the United States, yet the health care needs of women have only more recently received adequate attention. The health care fields now recognize that women are not just "little men" in regard to their presentation of diseases and their absorption and metabolism of medications. Gender differences that occur in all aspects of the treatment of women are increasingly recognized.

In the past, women were excluded from most investigative trials, but they now must be included in all biomedical and pharmaceutical research supported by the National Institutes of Health. More information will be forthcoming in regard to specific pharmacologic responses of women as this research continues.

Women sometimes do not seek medical attention for their symptoms because of their many responsibilities or out of fear that their symptoms may be trivialized. Health care providers are expected to administer respectful treatment, use clear communication in understandable language, and provide referrals for issues that may need more attention. This chapter provides an overview of various conditions prevalent among women and of their treatment. In some cases, referral is made to other chapters in the text for further information.

CARDIOVASCULAR DISEASE IN WOMEN

Although cardiovascular disease is the leading cause of death in women, far outranking breast cancer (which is currently number 7 as a cause of death in women), women with cardiovascular disease are less likely than men to be diagnosed early or correctly. Women may not always present with common symptoms of heart disease, and their symptoms are often ascribed to other causes (i.e., fibromyalgia, depression, or nervous disorders). Women are much less likely than men to be referred for a cardiology consultation and are less likely to be transferred from community hospitals to tertiary medical centers for advanced care.

Women with cardiovascular disease or a myocardial infarction may not present with shortness of breath on exertion or sudden chest pain, symptoms commonly experienced by men, but instead often present with unusual fatigue; shortness of breath; or vague pain in the chest, upper back, shoulders, neck, or jaw. Women may also have symptoms of anxiety, sleep disturbances, and indigestion. Only 30% of women with heart disease present with chest pain. Once heart disease is correctly diagnosed, response of women to most medications is standard. Hypertension, obesity, lack of exercise, and diabetes may increase the risk for cardiovascular disease, and these conditions should be carefully monitored.

When women experience **perimenopausal** heart palpitations, they are usually benign and may be due to increased sympathetic activity at that time. Arrhythmias during the premenopausal years have a different etiology and are related to fluctuating hormone levels at various stages of the menstrual cycle. Arrhythmias are less frequent midcycle when estrogen levels are high and are more common just before the menstrual period when the hormone levels decline. The response to antiarrhythmic agents is satisfactory at general dosage levels.

DRUGS USED IN THE PREVENTION OF CARDIOVASCULAR DISEASE

Aspirin, in a dosage of one 81-mg tablet daily, has shown to be more helpful to women than men in preventing strokes.

Antilipemic agents should be given to maintain low-density lipoproteins (LDL) and high-density lipoproteins (HDL) at acceptable levels. LDL is now cited as the most significant risk factor in cardiovascular disease and should be maintained at less than 100 mg, and preferably less than 70 mg. HDL (the "good" cholesterol) may be increased by exercise and a healthy diet; the proper range is 40 to 60 mg. Triglycerides should be maintained at less than 150 mg. Women are underrepresented in the statin trials; however, this situation is being corrected with current research. Examples of antilipemic agents are lovastatin (Mevacor), simvastatin (Zocor), and atorvastatin (Lipitor); these are discussed in Chapter 11. A diet low in saturated fats and use of supplements such as flaxseed oil, omega 3, or fish oil supplements are advantageous as well.

Hypertension in women should be carefully monitored and treated. The blood pressure goal is equal to or less than 130/80 mm Hg. Sodium intake should be carefully monitored; this includes sodium in the diet, glucose-containing carbonated drinks and many processed foods. Antihypertensive agents include diuretics such as hydrochlorothiazide or chlorthalidone. Angiotensin-converting enzyme inhibitors (ACE inhibitors) include lisinopril (Prinivil), beta blockers such as atenolol (Tenormin), angiotensin receptor blockers such as olmesartan (Benicar), aldosterone inhibitors such as spironolactone (Aldactone), and renin inhibitors such as aliskiren (Valturna). These agents and others are discussed more thoroughly in Chapter 11.

Diabetes is also a risk factor, often occurring with obesity. The metabolic syndrome occurs before frank diabetes and may be screened for with a 2-hour postprandial glucose test. The 2-hour blood glucose value, which should be close to the fasting level in a nondiabetic, may be markedly elevated in a patient with the metabolic syndrome. This elevation shows a sluggish insulin response and may be an early sign of prediabetes. Diabetes is generally not diagnosed until the fasting blood glucose is greater than 126 mg, but there is often a span of many years of the metabolic syndrome or prediabetes when many steps may be taken to minimize unfavorable outcomes. Oral hypoglycemics and the various types of insulin are discussed in Chapter 18.

Estrogen has been shown to increase HDL and decrease LDL. However, estrogen has been shown to increase slightly the incidence of heart disease when given as hormone replacement therapy in postmenopausal women. Contrary to publicity, the increase in breast cancer is a very small one, only 8 per 10,000, and most researchers believe further studies should be done. There is also a contradictory report that estrogen tablets may reduce the amount of calcified plaque in the coronary arteries when given to women in their 50s. Although women should not take postmenopausal hormones to prevent heart disease, many studies are under way at the present time. Many experts in women's health believe that the withdrawal of estrogens from postmenopausal women was premature and not entirely justified. There is a trend by many experts to resume hormone replacement therapy. These agents are discussed in Chapter 18. There are strict federal labeling requirements for estrogen products, and descriptive inserts must be placed in each consumer package. Information is given on the benefits and risks of these products.

Prescription niacin may be used to reduce cholesterol if statins are poorly tolerated.

niacin (Niacor, Niaspan). This B vitamin may be used in high doses to regulate cholesterol. Side effects include flushing, pruritus, vomiting, and diarrhea. These symptoms can be minimized if the dose is started at the minimal effective level and is gradually increased. ***Dosage:*** Adults: (Oral) (Niacor) 1.5 to 3 gm daily in three divided doses; (Niaspan) 500 to 2000 mg at bedtime.

OSTEOARTHRITIS

Arthritis disproportionately affects women. Women with arthritis report greater prevalence of joint pain, activity and work limitations, and psychological distress than their male counterparts. Women have a greater risk of knee and hand osteoarthritis than men. Cartilage at the knee is thinner in women, so deterioration may occur at a more rapid rate. In this condition, cartilage breaks down, allowing bones to rub painfully against each other. Knee injuries that occur in sports are now known to have more serious and long-lasting effects in women and should be cared for aggressively when they occur.

Estrogen receptors have been detected within cartilage, indicating it is an estrogen-sensitive tissue. The role of estrogen in the prevention and treatment of osteoarthritis is unclear, but it is under investigation.

DRUGS USED FOR OSTEOARTHRITIS

Acetaminophen and nonsteroidal anti-inflammatory drugs (NSAIDs) have been shown to be effective in controlling the pain of osteoarthritis, although an anti-inflammatory effect is present only with aspirin and NSAIDs. The risk of gastrointestinal bleeding is significant with long-term use of NSAIDs.

Injection of the knee with intra-articular betamethasone or hyaluronic acid or both has been shown to be an effective treatment when other agents fail. Although intra-articular injection is less effective in women than men, the technique and use of these agents in women are being investigated.

betamethasone sodium phosphate and betamethasone acetate (Celestone). This synthetic glucocorticoid has anti-inflammatory and immunosuppressive properties. It may be administered intramuscularly but is generally administered as an intra-articular injection. Anti-inflammatory effects appear within 1 to 3 hours and may persist for 7 days. Side effects common to all corticosteroids are not too apparent with short-term intra-articular use. Many experts advise that no more than three corticosteroid injections should be given per year. Each 1 mL contains 3 mg of each salt of betamethasone.
Dosage: Adults and children: (IM, Intra-articular) 0.25 to 2 mL injection into the joint.

hylan G-F (Synvisc). This synthetic polymer of hyaluronic acid, a natural component of connective tissue, is injected into the joint to treat osteoarthritis. It is contraindicated if there is an infection or inflammation in the joint or if the patient has an allergy to feathers or egg products.
Dosage: Adults: (Intra-articular) 2 mL or variable dosage based on joint size, once weekly for 3 weeks.

OSTEOPOROSIS

Osteoporosis and its treatment are discussed in Chapter 24; however, a few specific points are made here. Contrary to the advertised incidence of hot flashes as a reason for hormone replacement therapy, the most serious and long-lasting effect of postmenopausal estrogen deprivation is osteoporosis. **Osteoporosis** is a progressive decrease in bone density and strength that can lead to painful fractures and bony collapse.

Although osteoporosis is generally uncommon in premenopausal women, it is being recognized with increasing frequency. Disorders most commonly associated with the disease in young women include premenopausal estrogen deficiency; amenorrhea for 6 months; anorexia nervosa; celiac disease; and exposure to drugs that cause bone loss, particularly glucocorticoids. A low trauma fracture may be the first sign that this condition is present and should be followed by a bone mineral density measurement and appropriate therapy.

The impact of osteoporosis on women is that 50% of women will experience an osteoporotic fracture, 25% will have a vertebral deformity, and 15% will have a hip fracture. All percentages increase with longevity. Postmenopausal bone loss is significant and continuous, amounting to an average ongoing 2% to 4% bone loss annually. The most rapid bone loss is during the first 5 years after menopause or the first 5 years after discontinuing hormone replacement therapy.

Secondary causes of osteoporosis include carbonated beverages, prolonged use of antisecretory agents for gastric distress, alcohol, smoking, poor nutrition, and excessive weight loss. After consumption of a carbonated beverage, phosphoric acid complexes with calcium in the intestine to block calcium absorption. There are calciuric (calcium loss in the urine) effects of high phosphorus and low calcium.

Therapy for the prevention of osteoporosis includes exercise and a healthy diet. The excessive dieting, near-cachexia, and malnutrition seen in many young women have lifelong deleterious effects on the bony matrix. Carrying sufficient weight—not obesity—gives women stronger bones and increased bony matrix. Estrogen replacement therapy is most useful for preventive therapy if the side effects can be monitored and tolerated.

Women should begin taking calcium salts in the amount of 1200 mg daily early in their adult lives to build stronger bones. Postmenopausally, the intake should be 1500 mg of calcium daily. Women should also take 400 units of vitamin D daily to enable absorption of the calcium.

Specific agents to treat osteoporosis are discussed in Chapter 24. These agents include alendronate (Fosamax), calcitonin (Miacalcin), raloxifene (Evista), risedronate (Actonel), ibandronate (Boniva), and zoledronic acid (Reclast).

FIBROMYALGIA SYNDROME

Although seen occasionally in men and children, fibromyalgia is primarily a disease of women, who constitute 80% to 90% of patients. **Fibromyalgia** comprises a complex set of painful signs and symptoms, and it is best understood as a central pain processing disorder. Diagnosis is difficult because there are no confirmatory laboratory tests, and the symptoms of pain and fatigue overlap with other conditions, such as cardiac disease, myofascial pain syndromes, irritable bowel syndrome, thyroid malfunction, and allergic disorders, which all must be ruled out first. In patients with fibromyalgia, fatigue and poor sleep are almost universal, and it is widely acknowledged that serotonin levels are abnormally low.

DRUGS USED FOR FIBROMYALGIA

Medications used in the treatment of fibromyalgia include the following:

- Analgesics such as acetaminophen, tramadol, and mild opioids
- NSAIDs such as aspirin and ibuprofen
- Antidepressants such as the tricyclics, including amitriptyline, doxepin, and nortriptyline, and selective serotonin reuptake inhibitors (SSRIs), including fluoxetine, paroxetine, and sertraline
- Benzodiazepines such as clonazepam (occasionally used to relax painful muscles)

milnacipran (Savella). After treatment with this agent, patients report a reduced pain level and an overall improvement in symptoms. Side effects include nausea, dizziness, dry mouth, palpitations, and diarrhea.
Dosage: Adults only: (Oral) 100 to 200 mg daily.

pregabalin (Lyrica). Pregabalin was first used as an antiseizure medication but has shown some effectiveness in the treatment of fibromyalgia as well. Dizziness, somnolence, and ataxia have been reported as side effects.
Dosage: Adults only: (Oral) 300 to 600 mg daily in divided doses.

CHRONIC FATIGUE SYNDROME

There has been a long and fruitless search for the causes of chronic fatigue syndrome, which is a disease almost exclusively of women. The symptoms defy a clear diagnosis and are confused with, and bundled with, depression, fibromyalgia, and mental illness. The disease is characterized by unexplained mental and physical exhaustion, memory lapses, muscle pain, insomnia, digestive distress, and other health problems. It has been a diagnosis of exclusion.

More recently, an obscure retrovirus has been discovered in two-thirds of patients diagnosed with this condition. It is a gammaretrovirus, XMRV; it is postulated that this arose from a mouse retrovirus that somehow jumped to humans. Other retroviruses, such as human immunodeficiency virus (HIV), are known to attack the immune system, and XMRV may affect immune cells in the blood as well. There may be some significant improvements in the treatment of this condition in the near future.

INSOMNIA

From the age of menarche through menopause, insomnia in women is often influenced by complex hormonal cycles. Sleep problems, whether caused by domestic or professional stressors, increase the risk for developing clinical depression.

Subjective sleep reports are often unreliable when gauging the sleep experience, but they remain an important clinical tool in the assessment of overall health. A study of women established the difference in symptoms reported for different countries and ethnic backgrounds. American women have the highest percentage of insomnia symptoms (32.2%), described as difficulty initiating sleep and difficulty maintaining sleep. Canadian women report 10.9%, and Mexican women report 16.4%. Women in the United Kingdom reported the lowest percentage (8.7%). All percentages in European countries were lower than the percentage reported in the United States. Factors that may be considered regarding insomnia include lifestyle with exercise habits, labor force participation, career types, vacation time, length of work day or work week, and psychological factors. Focusing attention on these factors may be beneficial.

Shift work can be especially problematic for women because this may be associated with irregular menstrual cycles and pregnancy difficulties. There is an often quoted association with an increased risk of breast cancer in women who routinely have their circadian rhythms disrupted by working the night shift.

Difficulties with sleep onset and sleep maintenance are common in menopausal women and are often reported symptoms of premenstrual dysphoric disorder. Daytime fatigue, mood lability, irritability, and memory lapses may result.

Remedies other than hypnotics that may be beneficial include magnesium and calcium supplements. One often reported reason that women crave and benefit from chocolate is believed to be its magnesium content because magnesium is a known sedative. Salty foods and carbonated drinks should be avoided because fluid retention exacerbates the condition. Other substances to avoid include caffeine, nicotine, and alcohol. Ginger, chamomile, and lemon balm teas at bedtime may be used to ease digestive problems. Pyridoxine (vitamin B_6), 100 mg daily, has also been shown to be beneficial. Warm milk and cookies at bedtime have a sedative effect. The cookies have an additive effect over the warm milk alone. It is believed that the amino acid tryptophan exerts a sedative effect. When pharmacologic help is needed to treat insomnia, various sedatives and hypnotics can be prescribed (see Chapters 12 and 14).

DEPRESSION

Women of all ages are more vulnerable to depressive disorders than men; this is especially true during the childbearing years. In addition to the general feeling of sadness, depression affects eating and sleeping habits, pain perception, cognition, memory, and self-esteem. Most women do not readily seek treatment, and a great deal of continued educational effort is needed in this area. Without treatment, symptoms of depression can last for years.

St. John's wort is readily available as an over-the-counter (OTC) remedy for mild to moderate depression. It is available alone and in combination with various herbal products. It is discussed in more detail in Chapter 28. Antidepressants are discussed in Chapter 14.

PREMENSTRUAL DYSPHORIC DISORDER

Some estimates are that 50% of women have symptoms of **premenstrual dysphoria disorder (PMDD)**, experienced as premenstrual tension such as anxiety, irritability, and emotional sensitivity, in the days leading up to their menstrual period. These symptoms may be severe enough to impair some aspects of the affected woman's life during the week before the onset of menstrual bleeding. The symptoms attenuate when the menstrual period begins or shortly thereafter. Clinically significant symptoms affect the woman's life in many areas, including interpersonal relationships, social behavior, work attendance, work productivity, and health-related quality of life. The economic burden is increased among women with PMDD.

Several studies have been done with women to determine if there is a difference in insulin sensitivity or carbohydrate intake across menstrual phases in women with PMDD. A craving for chocolate and other foods during the premenstrual phase is well recognized. These studies are inconclusive at the present time. A greater understanding of endocrine variables may assist in the management of this condition.

Research indicates a low level of serotonin as a cause of PMDD. SSRIs such as fluoxetine and sertraline have been shown to be effective in treating this disorder. These agents may be taken for short-term therapy during the premenstrual period or throughout the month as necessary.

DEPRESSION DURING PREGNANCY

A woman who is clinically depressed during pregnancy often requires medical intervention. If left untreated, depression may independently contribute to adverse obstetric, fetal, and neonatal outcomes. Medical illnesses such as thyroid disorders, anemia, carcinoma, inflammatory conditions, and obesity may contribute to the depressive symptoms and should be carefully assessed. Depression may contribute to exposure to illicit drugs, to poor self-care, or to alcohol and tobacco use. SSRIs have been used during pregnancy with few adverse outcomes on the fetus, although their use should be controlled and monitored.

POSTPARTUM DEPRESSION

Many women are particularly vulnerable to depression after giving birth. Significant depression is estimated to occur in 14.5% of women in the early postpartum period. The most significant factor in the duration of the depressive episode is delay in identification and treatment. All health care workers should be alert to the symptoms of depression in a new mother and encourage her to get treatment as necessary. Guilt, issues of self-worth as related to mothering, and other factors often cause a delay in treatment. The hormonal changes and the new responsibility can lead to a cascade of symptoms. Transient "baby blues" are common, often limited to a "good cry" or two, but the paralyzing effects of full **postpartum depression** must be treated with medication and counseling. SSRIs have been shown to be effective for this condition. Agents that act on both serotonin and norepinephrine (selective serotonin-norepinephrine reuptake inhibitors), such as venlafaxine and duloxetine, have also shown great benefit in treating postpartum depression. There are issues of safety for a nursing infant when the mother is receiving these agents. The introduction of formula and a bottle or two a day immediately after birth allows for flexibility in the feeding of the infant and the easy transfer to formula feeding if medications are necessary. The infant would then accept either breast or bottle if the mother is taking medications.

DRUG SAFETY DURING PREGNANCY AND LACTATION

Following the use of thalidomide for nausea during pregnancy and the resultant limb deformities and disastrous teratogenic effects, a category of safety was developed for drug safety during pregnancy and lactation. This category can be obtained for any drug in current use. A drug occasionally is approved for lactation but not pregnancy, or a different category is given.

There are five categories of safety, as follows:

A—Safe. Controlled human studies show no risk in the first, second, or third trimester of pregnancy or lactation.

B—Fetal harm possible but not likely. Generally, controlled human studies of the first trimester are unavailable, but no adverse fetal effects are seen in the second and third trimesters of pregnancy or during lactation.

C—Weigh possible fetal risk versus maternal benefit. Animal studies show adverse fetal effects, but no controlled human studies are available.

D—Positive evidence of human fetal risk. In some cases, maternal benefit may outweigh fetal risk. Use extreme caution when prescribing.

X—Absolutely contraindicated in pregnancy. Another category may be given for lactation in some instances, but the use is generally not advised.

MENSTRUAL AND PERIMENOPAUSAL MIGRAINES

Migraines are neurologic disorders with symptoms that can range from mild to severe and that may be disabling. They can have many causes, but this discussion is limited to migraines that are linked to the female sex hormones estrogen and progesterone as causative agents.

Migraines are more common in boys than girls until menarche, at which point they are about three times more common in girls. Obstacles to a clear diagnosis of **menstrual migraines** include a general lack of awareness of the cyclic nature and character of the headaches and confusion caused by the simultaneous administration of other agents such as NSAIDs for associated symptoms of cramps. An aura may or may not be present with these migraines. A careful history and increased awareness of the nature of the headaches are crucial to diagnosis and treatment and determine how aggressive the therapy needs to be. Menstrual migraines generally occur from 2 days before the period until day 3 of the menses in at least two of three menstrual cycles. The decrease in estrogen during the luteal phase is believed to be the most important trigger of menstrual migraines.

The onset of new and worsening headaches may occur in the perimenopausal period. During the transitional perimenopausal phase, which may begin in the mid-30s to late 30s and could last 10 years or more, there are episodic fluctuations in hormone levels, along with an overall decline in absolute levels. These fluctuations culminate in the symptoms of perimenopause, which may include fatigue, insomnia, irritability, irregular periods, night sweats, hot flashes, forgetfulness, a decrease in libido, and difficulty concentrating.

Patients with migraines may experience social ostracism, job loss, and disruptions in personal relationships. Missed work—an average of 4 to 6 work days per year—and impairment at work are the most determining factors in migraine.

Dietary triggers may increase the incidence of migraines. These include monosodium glutamate (a common ingredient in Chinese foods), alcohol, chocolate, aged cheese, and other food preservatives such as sulfites. Perfumes, bright lights, loud noises, lack of sleep, and physical or emotional distress may also act as triggers.

DRUGS USED FOR MENSTRUAL MIGRAINES

Treatment for the prevention of migraines may include the use of oral contraceptives, perimenstrual prophylaxis with NSAIDs or SSRIs, anticonvulsant therapy, beta blocker therapy, behavioral therapy, and biofeedback. OTC products that contain caffeine and black coffee are often effective when combined with the other available drugs.

The primary goals of acute therapies are to abort and reduce the severity and duration of attacks and to reduce the disability associated with an attack. Evidence suggests that there are higher response rates for acute treatment used earlier in an attack while the pain is still mild. The triptans, such as sumatriptan, zolmitriptan, and rizatriptan, have been found to be effective in the treatment of menstrual migraines. Cyclic prophylaxis using a triptan or an NSAID beginning 2 to 3 days before the menses can also be used.

Transdermal estradiol patches, such as Climara or Estraderm, which deliver estrogen for 24 hours, are recommended by some experts but have inconsistent efficacy. They are applied 1 to 2 days before the anticipated decrease in estrogen. Higher doses are more effective.

Hormone replacement therapy in perimenopause has had variable results in the treatment of migraines. It improves symptoms in some women and worsens the symptoms of others. Opioids or other analgesics are also used to treat menstrual migraines.

MIGRAINE PREVENTIVE THERAPY

Reasons for instituting migraine preventive therapy include the presence of recurrent migraines that interfere with functioning; more than three headaches per month; contraindications to acute therapy; adverse events from acute therapy; cost of acute and preventive therapy; and presence of unusual migraine conditions including hemiplegic migraine, basilar migraine, or migraine with prolonged aura. These medications are given on a daily basis, and the dose is often increased to tolerance; success is measured by the reduction in the frequency of migraines. Often trial and error must occur to choose an effective prophylactic agent.

BETA BLOCKERS

propranolol (Inderal). Side effects of propranolol include fatigue, nausea, and bradycardia. This agent is contraindicated in patients with asthma or preexisting cardiovascular disease.

Dosage: Adults: (Oral) May be given in a dose of 80 mg daily in divided doses, then progressed to 240 mg daily in a long-acting tablet. If no improvement occurs in 4 to 6 weeks, the dosage may be tapered and discontinued.

timolol. Side effects are similar to propranolol.

Dosage: Adults: (Oral) 10 mg twice daily to a maximum of 100 mg/day. If no response occurs in 6 to 8 weeks, taper dosage over 1 to 2 weeks to discontinue.

ANTICONVULSANTS

carbamazepine (Tegretol). Reported side effects include dermatologic reactions, blood disorders, and cardiac arrhythmias.

Dosage: Adults: (Oral) 100 mg twice daily, increasing by 200 mg per day to a maximum of 1200 mg daily.

divalproex (Depakote). Divalproex has been associated with dyspepsia, abdominal pain, and weight gain. There are three black box warnings for teratogenicity. It should not be given to pregnant women or used for hepatotoxicity and pancreatitis. Monitoring is essential.

Dosage: Adults: (Oral) 250 to 500 mg twice daily for migraine prophylaxis.

MENSTRUAL ABNORMALITIES

DYSMENORRHEA

Primary dysmenorrhea is a cramping pain in the lower abdomen that occurs at menstruation and in the absence of identifiable pelvic disease. Many women have dysmenorrhea at some time during their reproductive years, but 10% may be incapacitated with severe pain for 1 to 3 days each month. It is a frequent cause of absenteeism from school or work and can affect productivity.

Increased production of prostaglandins by the endometrium during menstruation is thought to be the likely cause of dysmenorrhea. It causes uterine hypercontractility and a high resting tone of contraction. Treatment with NSAIDs, especially ibuprofen and naproxen, is generally effective. The gastrointestinal side effects are reduced if the drug is taken ½ hour before a starchy meal. Heat applied to the abdomen using a hot water bottle or heating pad is beneficial as well.

MENORRHAGIA

Each woman's menstrual period is unique. Bleeding can be light or heavy and still be considered "normal." Menorrhagia is often a matter of perception. Actual blood loss is often less than perceived because the tissue is mixed with mucous as well. When women lost only 20 to 40 mL in a cycle, one-third believed they had menorrhagia. Similarly, when the actual loss was greater than 80 mL per cycle, one-third of women believed they had menorrhagia with two-thirds believing the cycle was normal. Heavy menstrual bleeding is most often caused by hormonal imbalances of estrogen and progesterone, which control menstruation. Hormones are more likely to be off-balance in adolescents and in perimenopausal women.

Measurement of hemoglobin is important in establishing menorrhagia and its need for treatment. A hemoglobin of less than 12 gm should be investigated. Underlying causes of a more serious nature may include miscarriage or tubal pregnancy, tumors in the pelvic cavity, bleeding disorders, cancer, pelvic inflammatory disease, uterine fibroids, or endometriosis. Further investigation should be undertaken for adolescents with menorrhagia and a hemoglobin value of less than 12 gm. It has been shown that 20% of adolescents with menorrhagia have underlying blood dyscrasias, such as von Willebrand's disease, leukemia, aplastic anemia, thalassemia major, or low platelets.

Treatment of menorrhagia includes dietary advice and iron and vitamin supplements. Oral contraceptives for a limited time may be advisable. An intrauterine device that contains the progestin levonorgestrel (Mirena) may be inserted into the uterus and left for 5 years to decrease the menstrual flow and provide contraception. Surgical options include endometrial ablation to destroy the uterine lining and hysterectomy.

MENOPAUSE

Menopause is a natural rite of passage that was taken for granted in previous times, but now there is an expectation that it must be "managed." Worse is the expectation that there are solutions that remove all menopausal symptoms—hot flashes, night sweats, vaginal dryness—while revving up the libido. If menopause has a defining symptom, it is the one-woman heat wave: the hot flash. African American women report more hot flashes than white and Hispanic women, and Asian women have the least hot flashes of all. Anxiety, smoking, and obesity increase symptoms. The influences of diet, caffeine, alcohol, and exercise are unclear. Subgroups of women may benefit from different interventions.

The most effective intervention for the control of hot flashes and other symptoms is estrogen replacement such as Premarin with or without progesterone or estradiol (Estrace). It is also the most reliable treatment to prevent osteoporosis. Transdermal estrogen patches that bypass the liver are available enabling a lower dose. Although clinicians are now advised to use the lowest dose of estrogen for the shortest duration of time, women's health groups are arguing that similar advice is not given to men who use testosterone supplements and erectile dysfunction products. The risk of side effects is much higher for these products, with much less publicity, than for the female hormonal supplements. This discussion will be ongoing.

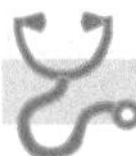

Clinical Implications

1. Female patients should be assessed for underlying causes when presenting with vague symptoms such as fatigue.
2. Female patients often may not report symptoms of depression because of cultural restraints.
3. The health care worker should be aware of depression as an underlying cause of many disorders.
4. Cardiac disease is often overlooked in women. They should be encouraged to undergo routine screening examinations.
5. Preventive measures against osteoporosis should begin in young women, with calcium and vitamin D supplements and attention to proper nutrition.
6. Careful history taking may be necessary to uncover cyclic disorders such as PMDD, menstrual migraine, or insomnia related to hormonal changes.
7. Every postpartum woman should be screened for depression.
8. Behavioral therapy and biofeedback may be useful adjuncts to treatment for menstrual migraine.
9. Insomnia is a common disorder in women and may be treated by various pharmacologic and herbal remedies.
10. Fibromyalgia is a complex disorder of women that may respond to various treatments.
11. Risk factors for women and heart disease include smoking, diabetes, hypertension, hyperlipidemia, family history of heart disease, lack of physical activity, and stress. Menopausal women have increased risk.
12. Stroke symptoms in women may include sudden numbness of any body part, sudden confusion or trouble speaking, visual problems or trouble focusing, sudden trouble walking or maintaining balance, and sudden severe headache.

CRITICAL THINKING QUESTIONS

1. A young married woman requests a pain medication for her back. She denies any other problems. Further questioning brings out the fact that she has a 6-week-old baby, her husband has resumed traveling, and she has been sleep deprived because of the baby's nighttime waking. What would be your course of action?
2. A patient states that she has felt very tired lately and requests a blood test to check for anemia and thyroid problems. You notice she has old slippers on her feet; she comments her shoes have been too tight for the past week or so. She comments that part of the reason she is tired is that she has to sleep in her recliner at night because she gets short of breath lying flat in her bed. What is the most likely diagnosis?
3. A teenage patient comments that she is in trouble in school because she has to stay home with a lot with severe headaches. She says the headaches seem to come if she eats chocolate and cheese, but she has not kept a record of when they occur or if there are any other food or allergy triggers. She says nothing but her mother's codeine medication will make them stop. She would like some of the codeine medicine for herself. How would you advise this patient?

REVIEW QUESTIONS

1. Drugs absolutely contraindicated during pregnancy are classified under which pregnancy category?
   a. A
   b. B
   c. C
   d. X

2. A medication that is useful in lowering cholesterol is:
   a. niacin.
   b. hylan.
   c. aspirin.
   d. ibuprofen.

3. For women, the daily dose of calcium salts beginning in young adulthood should be:
   a. 600 mg.
   b. 1200 mg.
   c. 1 gm.
   d. 1800 mg.

4. Which of the following is a possible secondary cause of osteoporosis?
   a. Excessive exercise
   b. Obesity
   c. Excessive weight loss
   d. High cholesterol

5. Serotonin reuptake inhibitors (SSRIs) may be used to treat:
   a. postpartum depression.
   b. PMDD.
   c. fibromyalgia.
   d. all of the above.

6. Insomnia in women may be caused by:
   a. chocolate.
   b. shift work.
   c. vitamin B_6
   d. all of the above.

7. Which disorder has the greatest mortality in women?
   a. Ovarian cancer
   b. Breast cancer
   c. Heart disease
   d. Obstetric complications

8. Triptans are pharmacologic agents that are useful in the treatment of:
   a. osteoporosis.
   b. postpartum depression.
   c. menstrual migraines.
   d. tension headaches.

9. What percentage of untreated postmenopausal women experience an osteoporotic fracture?
   a. 25%
   b. 50%
   c. 10%
   d. 75%

10. ACE inhibitors, angiotensin receptor blockers, and beta blockers are used to treat which medical condition?
    a. High blood pressure
    b. Menstrual cramps
    c. Osteoporosis
    d. Insomnia

Answers to the review questions can be found at the back of the book.

evolve Additional questions and activities can be found at *http://evolve.elsevier.com/asperheim/pharmacology*.

Drug Therapy in Older Adults

CHAPTER 24

Objectives

After completing this chapter, you should be able to do the following:

1. Define specific health problems seen in older adults.
2. Become aware of the differences in drug metabolism in older adults.
3. Become aware of nutritional problems in older adults and solutions.
4. Recognize health problems in older adults, such as hypothyroidism, that may be confused with senility.
5. Recognize structural changes in the aging body, particularly changes of the bone and connective tissue.
6. Recognize and assist in the solution of social problems of older adults when they are cared for in the home or a nursing facility.
7. Be aware that standard adult doses of many drugs may produce symptoms of a toxic overdose in older adults.
8. Be aware that many drug interactions and toxic effects are caused by the addition of drugs and herbal remedies that the older adult buys at the drugstore.
9. Recognize that complicated drug schedules are often the reason for noncompliance in older adult.

Key Terms

Dementia (dĭ-MĔN-shĕ), p. 234
Geriatric (JĔR-ē-ĂT-rĭk), p. 227
Metabolism (mĕ-TĂB-ĕ-LĬZ-ĕm), p. 228

About 6% of the world's population is 65 years old or older. In the United States, about 35 million people, or 13% of the total population, are in this age group. By 2030, an estimated 70 million persons, or about 20% of the population, will be 65 years old or older. As a result, **geriatric** medicine—medicine for older adults—has emerged as a vital and necessary health care discipline. The American Geriatrics Society was formed to increase the number of health care professionals trained in geriatrics and to expand and implement geriatric education and training for physicians, nurses, allied health personnel, and the general public.

Adults 65 years old and older consume one-third of all medications, and most take multiple prescribed and over-the-counter (OTC) drugs. Age-related physiologic changes and the presence of underlying disease, coupled with inappropriate prescribing and polypharmacy (the use of many different drugs), may predispose older patients to adverse drug reactions and drug-drug, drug-disease, or drug-food interactions (Box 24-1). To confuse the problem further, many older adults have several physicians prescribing different drugs for their health problems, which can account for many drug reactions.

Important advances in recent years have led to a better understanding of the effects of aging, how to distinguish these effects from other influences, and how they may be modified or alleviated in some way. Environmental changes and lifestyle factors such as diet, use of alcohol or drugs, smoking, and exercise all have an impact on a person's health status. A great deal of interest is focused in the areas of health promotion, disease prevention, and maintenance of good health and maximal independence as long as possible throughout the life span. Interactions of an older adult with society should be productive, satisfying, and rewarding for all involved. This chapter is focused on the treatment and specific health issues of older adults.

Box 24-1 Common Drug Interactions in Older Adults

DRUG-DRUG INTERACTIONS

- Digoxin and thiazide diuretics (hypokalemia causes digoxin toxicity)
- Cimetidine and warfarin (warfarin is potentiated)
- Cimetidine and phenytoin (phenytoin blood level is increased)
- Quinolone antibiotics and warfarin (warfarin is potentiated)
- NSAIDs and diuretics (decreased effectiveness of diuretics)
- NSAIDs and aspirin (increased erosion of stomach lining)
- ACE inhibitors and potassium-sparing diuretics (hyperkalemia)
- Warfarin and aspirin or NSAIDs (increased action of warfarin)
- Increased use of fiber or bulk laxatives (inhibits absorption of any drug)
- Antacid use (may inhibit absorption of many medications)
- Phenytoin and magnesium-based antacids (decreased absorption of phenytoin)

DRUG-FOOD INTERACTIONS

- Carbidopa/levodopa and food protein (decreased absorption of drug)
- Cyclosporine and grapefruit juice (increased serum level of cyclosporine)
- Tetracycline and dairy products (decreased absorption of tetracycline)
- Quinolone antibiotics and dairy products (decreased absorption of drugs)
- Monoamine oxidase inhibitors and wine, sausage, or cheese (causes severe hypertension)
- Sedatives and alcohol (increased sedation)
- Warfarin and psyllium (decreased absorption and decreased effectiveness of warfarin)
- Warfarin and vitamin E (increased effectiveness of warfarin)
- Iron tablets and tea, bran, or eggs (decreased absorption of iron)

DRUG-DISEASE INTERACTIONS

- Anticholinergic agents (urinary retention)
- Beta blockers (worsen asthma)

ACE inhibitors, angiotensin-converting enzyme inhibitors; *NSAIDs,* nonsteroidal anti-inflammatory drugs.

DRUG THERAPY IN OLDER ADULTS

Appropriate and effective drug therapy for older patients presents many challenges (Fig. 24-1). The following five points should be kept in mind when prescribing drugs for this age group:

1. *Obtain an accurate history.* The older patient should carry a list of current medications or preferably should bring all medicine bottles to each visit; this should include any OTC drugs the patient uses. The health care provider may discover that similar or interacting drugs have been prescribed by different physicians, or the patient may still be taking a drug that is no longer necessary.
2. *Dosages may need to be adjusted.* The usual adult dosage is based on the amount of drug needed for a healthy man weighing 150 lb. Age-related disorders may require a dosage that is 25% to 50% less than the usual adult dosage. The gastrointestinal tract may not have the "average" pH because of deficient acid production, the gastric emptying time may be slowed, and the gastric blood flow may be deficient. The distribution of a drug depends on body composition (amounts of lipid, water, and lean body mass), and these amounts change with age. Decreased levels of albumin resulting from suboptimal nutrition affect the binding and distribution of drugs. Drug **metabolism** (i.e., the sum of chemical changes that occurs as a drug is processed) in the liver depends on blood flow and the enzyme system; both may be altered. An age-related decline in renal function affects drug elimination from the body.
3. *Be vigilant about drug interactions.* Although it is impossible to remember every drug interaction and new interactions are frequently discovered, drug interactions should be checked for every drug combination. Drugs that have frequent interactions and are commonly used in older adults include warfarin, sedatives, antibiotics, and nonsteroidal anti-inflammatory drugs (NSAIDs) (see Box 24-1 for more interactions).
4. *Consider drug costs.* On average, older adults take 4.5 prescription drugs and 2.1 nonprescription medications. Use generic medications and less expensive alternatives whenever possible.
5. *Discontinue drugs whenever possible.* Older people sometimes tend to hoard drugs and resist change in their medications. Make an effort to design an efficient drug therapy plan, reducing the number of medications taken.

Medication compliance is also a factor that must be considered. If a patient has several different drugs that must be taken on different schedules—one taken before meals, one that must be taken 2 hours after meals, one taken four times a day, one taken three times a day, and so on—there are bound to be mistakes or forgotten doses. Whenever possible, simplify the regimen with once-a-day drugs, and avoid alternate-day therapy. Most importantly, the regimen must be reviewed at each visit and revised as needed. Medications that can be taken together should be reviewed and explained. A daily or weekly pillbox should be recommended and explained.

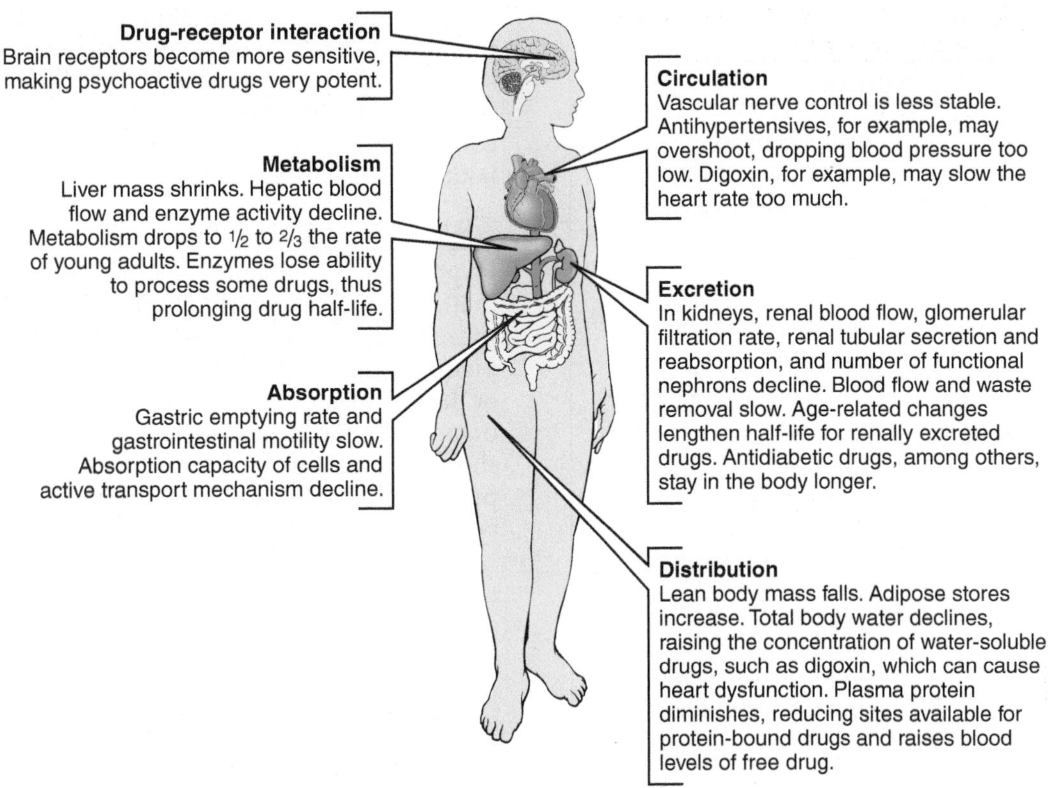

Drug-receptor interaction
Brain receptors become more sensitive, making psychoactive drugs very potent.
Metabolism
Liver mass shrinks. Hepatic blood flow and enzyme activity decline. Metabolism drops to 1/2 to 2/3 the rate of young adults. Enzymes lose ability to process some drugs, thus prolonging drug half-life.
Absorption
Gastric emptying rate and gastrointestinal motility slow. Absorption capacity of cells and active transport mechanism decline.
Circulation
Vascular nerve control is less stable. Antihypertensives, for example, may overshoot, dropping blood pressure too low. Digoxin, for example, may slow the heart rate too much.
Excretion
In kidneys, renal blood flow, glomerular filtration rate, renal tubular secretion and reabsorption, and number of functional nephrons decline. Blood flow and waste removal slow. Age-related changes lengthen half-life for renally excreted drugs. Antidiabetic drugs, among others, stay in the body longer.
Distribution
Lean body mass falls. Adipose stores increase. Total body water declines, raising the concentration of water-soluble drugs, such as digoxin, which can cause heart dysfunction. Plasma protein diminishes, reducing sites available for protein-bound drugs and raises blood levels of free drug.

FIGURE 24-1 Effects of aging on drug metabolism. (From Lewis SL, et al: *Medical-surgical nursing: assessment and management of clinical problems*, ed 8, St. Louis, 2011, Mosby.)

Patients must be counseled about illness and medications. Should they take certain medications if they are nauseated and not eating? Insulin dosage, for example, needs to be adjusted when illness occurs.

The patient's overall situation should be periodically assessed. Older adults often have many and chronic illnesses. Diminished liver or kidney function dramatically changes the effects of drug therapy. Changes in the patient's mental function, hearing, and vision must be evaluated periodically. The health care provider should not be hasty in attributing a new disability to "normal aging" because it may be a drug-induced effect (Box 24-2). All prescription bottles should be easy to open, and the patient must be able to read the labels on the bottles. A cursory examination should also be made to ensure the patient is able to read. Box 24-3 lists several factors that contribute to noncompliance in older adults.

NUTRITION IN OLDER ADULTS

An older adult who lives alone may become malnourished because of inattention to nutrition or an inability to obtain a sufficient supply of fresh food for a balanced diet. Depression and isolation are common problems that seem to increase as a person ages, and they are accompanied by a decreased ability for and interest in self-care and nutrition. Social programs, such as Meals-on-Wheels, have improved the lives of older patients because they address both their social isolation and their nutritional inadequacies.

Poorly fitting dentures or missing teeth create mechanical problems in chewing food. Dental needs may have to be addressed before nutrition deficits can be improved.

Many patients are on modified diets (e.g., a bland diet for ulcers, a low-fat or low-sodium diet, or a low-purine diet for the prevention of gout). Often older adults do not comprehend the instructions or simply do not know what they can eat. Patients often restrict their diets so much that they lose weight and become malnourished. Vitamin and mineral supplements are very beneficial, but they do not provide additional calories.

Dietary supplements are available that can enhance vitamin and mineral nutrition and provide additional calories. The supplement Enrich is a liquid nutritional supplement with fiber; an 8-oz serving contains 260 calories and 3.4 gm of dietary fiber. It is low in sodium and cholesterol and contains a complement of vitamins and minerals. The supplement Ensure provides nutritional and caloric enrichment; an 8-oz serving contains 250 calories. Similar to Enrich, Ensure is low in sodium and cholesterol. Ensure Plus is similar to Ensure but has 350 calories per 8-oz serving.

Box 24-2 Medications That Contribute to Cognitive Impairment in Older Adults

ANALGESICS
codeine
meperidine
morphine
NSAIDs
pentazocine

ANTICHOLINERGICS
oxybutynin
tolterodine

ANTIHISTAMINES
diphenhydramine
hydroxyzine

ANTIHYPERTENSIVE AGENTS
clonidine
diuretics
hydralazine
methyldopa
propranolol

ANTIMICROBIALS
gentamicin
isoniazid

ANTIPARKINSON AGENTS
amantadine
bromocriptine
carbidopa/levodopa

CARDIOVASCULAR DRUGS
atropine
digoxin
lidocaine
quinidine

HYPOGLYCEMICS
sulfonylureas

PSYCHOTROPICS
barbiturates
benzodiazepines
chlorpromazine
haloperidol
lithium
risperidone
SSRI antidepressants
tricyclic antidepressants

MISCELLANEOUS
cimetidine
corticosteroids
phenytoin

NSAIDs, nonsteroidal anti-inflammatory drugs; *SSRI*, selective serotonin reuptake inhibitor.

Box 24-3 Contributors to Noncompliance in Older Adults

- Complex treatment and dosing regimens
- High cost of drugs
- Inadequate understanding of therapy
- Physical disability (e.g., dysphagia)
- Medication side effects
- Cognitive impairment
- Inability to read drug label because of visual problems
- Poor communication

PREVENTIVE NUTRITION IN A PATIENT WITH A CHRONIC DISEASE

The diseases of aging—coronary heart disease, hypertension, cancer, glucose intolerance, and osteoporosis—are affected by many factors.

CORONARY ARTERY DISEASE

A diet including reduced fats, increased soluble fiber, vitamins with the trace elements copper and chromium, and a supplement of fish oil capsules has been found to be helpful in patients with coronary artery disease. Fish oil capsules reduce serum lipids and seem to decrease prostaglandin synthesis, which reduces inflammation. A patient can increase fish consumption to three to four times a week instead of taking the fish oil capsules.

HYPERTENSION

Hypertensive patients should decrease sodium intake and, particularly if diuretic medications are prescribed, increase potassium intake. Potassium supplements can be given, or the patient may increase his or her intake of foods high in potassium such as oranges, bananas, and raisins. Calcium and magnesium supplements or increased consumption of dairy products, beans, brown rice, broccoli, and fish may be in order.

CANCER

A diet high in fiber seems to be protective against colon and breast cancers. Fiber is provided naturally in fruits, vegetables, beans, and whole grains, or it can be added to the diet through the use of wheat bran or commercial fiber supplements. The antioxidant vitamins A, C, and E and the trace mineral selenium are being studied as protective against cancer. Antioxidants probably function as scavengers of "free radicals," products of tissue oxidation that cause cellular damage. Oranges and dark green vegetables also provide beta-carotene, as do many dietary supplements.

DIABETES

A diet with complex carbohydrates and 25 to 30 gm of dietary fiber daily has been shown to increase a patient's control of diabetes. A diet deficient in chromium has been associated with an increase in the incidence of type 2 diabetes; chromium supplements should be given. Food sources of chromium include brewer's yeast and nuts.

VISION PROBLEMS

Macular degeneration and cataracts may be slowed by administration of zinc supplements. Food sources of zinc include wheat germ, wheat bran, and oysters. Vitamins E and C supplements have been found to be beneficial in reducing the incidence of cataracts. Centrum Silver vitamins are advised for older adults because, in addition to being a well-rounded nutritional supplement, they provide a good source of lutein, which has been found to prevent macular degeneration.

OSTEOPOROSIS

Calcium, vitamin D supplements, and trace minerals such as magnesium and manganese have been used in the treatment of osteoporosis.

ARTHRITIS IN OLDER ADULTS

Many improvements have been made in the treatment of osteoarthritis, which is no longer looked on as a simple "wear-and-tear" disease. The articular cartilage has been found to be an active tissue that can undergo changes, rather than the unresponsive substance it was previously thought to be. Articular cartilage serves many important functions. It minimizes friction between joint surfaces, minimizing wear; it increases the contact area between bones within the joint, decreasing contact stress; it also helps dissipate energy and absorb shock. One of the earliest changes seen in osteoarthritis is an increase in the water content of cartilage. This change increases the porosity (the number of openings through which fluids can pass) of the cartilage and decreases its strength and load-carrying capacity.

NSAIDs have been shown to interrupt this inflammatory process and the subsequent thinning and breakdown of cartilage. Some NSAIDs have more effect on cartilage metabolism than others. Aspirin, ibuprofen (Motrin), and fenoprofen (Nalfon) have been shown to be the most beneficial in treating osteoarthritis. These agents are discussed in Chapter 15.

OSTEOPOROSIS IN OLDER ADULTS

As the life span increases, so do the long-term problems seen with osteoporosis in older women. The rates of illness and early death resulting from vertebral compression and fractures of various bones are very significant.

The most rapid bone loss in women occurs in the first 5 years after menopause. It has been shown that calcium supplements and exercise slow this process, but research has proven that the only true "treatment" is prevention in the form of supplemental hormone therapy. The vasomotor symptoms, or "hot flashes," of menopause are also reduced or eliminated with hormone therapy. The continued use of hormones in menopausal women is controversial at the present time. Annual physical examinations are necessary when hormone therapy is given to detect the early presence of hormone-dependent cancers such as breast or gynecologic cancer. Many commercially available estrogens can be given to prevent osteoporosis (see discussion in Chapter 18). Conjugated estrogen (Premarin) is most commonly prescribed.

When taking bisphosphonates, agents that prevent bone resorption, it is important that calcium supplements, 1000 to 1500 mg/day, be taken along with an adequate dose of vitamin D—1000 units daily in older patients at risk for osteoporosis. Hypocalcemia should be corrected before these drugs are administered. Adverse effects include esophagitis, esophageal ulcers, and perforations. The drug should be taken with a full glass of water to facilitate stomach emptying, and the individual should preferably stand for 30 minutes afterward. Lying down should be avoided for at least 30 minutes. No food should be taken for at least 30 minutes afterward, and waiting 1 hour or longer improves absorption. Generally, reconstructive dental work should be undertaken before these drugs are administered, or the drugs should be stopped for 4 months before visiting the dentist. Osteonecrosis and osteomyelitis of the jaw have been reported, but this risk is greater in patients with cancer who are taking these agents.

BISPHOSPHONATE MEDICATIONS USED IN THE PREVENTION OR TREATMENT OF OSTEOPOROSIS

alendronate (Fosamax). Alendronate is an agent that inhibits bone resorption. It has been shown to increase the mineral density of bone. It is used to prevent or treat osteoporosis.
Dosage: Adults only: (Oral) 5 to 10 mg in the morning once daily 30 minutes before the first food is eaten or 35 to 70 mg once weekly.

calcitonin (Calcimar, Miacalcin). Calcitonin may be administered by nasal spray or by injection to treat osteoporosis. It inhibits bone resorption.
Dosage: Adults only: (IM, Subcut) 100 international units daily; (Nasal Spray) 1 spray (200 international units) daily, alternating nostrils.

denosumab (Prolia). This agent is indicated when patients have failed on or been intolerant of other osteoporosis therapy. It is used for the treatment of osteoporosis when there is a history of fractures or a high risk for fracture.
Dosage: Adults only: (Subcut) 60 mg every 6 months.

etidronate disodium (Didronel). Etidronate is administered orally to treat Paget's disease and to treat osteoporosis sustained after corticosteroid therapy. Similar to the other agents in this class, it inhibits bone resorption.
Dosage: Adults only: (Oral) 5 mg/kg daily for no longer than 6 months.

ibandronate sodium (Boniva). The advantage of this agent is that it can be given orally daily or only once a month. IV administration is available as well.
Dosage: Adults only: (Oral) 2.5 mg once daily or 150 mg once monthly; (IV) 3 mg once every 3 months.

raloxifene hydrochloride (Evista). This agent is a selective estrogen receptor modulator. Its actions, similar to estrogen, are mediated through binding with estrogen receptors. In postmenopausal women, it preserves bone mass and increases bone mineral density. Compared with estrogen therapy, raloxifene seems to be associated with a lower risk of breast cancer in postmenopausal women.
Dosage: Adults only: (Oral) 60 mg daily.

risedronate sodium (Actonel). Risedronate inhibits bone resorption and modulates bone metabolism. It is used to treat Paget's disease of bone and osteoporosis.
Dosage: Adults only: (Oral) 5 mg daily or 35 mg once weekly.

zoledronic acid (Reclast, Zometa). In addition to preventing bone resorption in osteoporosis in elderly patients, zoledronic acid is used to treat hypercalcemia associated with malignancy and as an adjunct to the treatment of bone metastases of solid tumors and the osteolytic lesions of multiple myeloma.
Dosage: Adults only: (IV) For osteoporosis, 5 mg in an IV infusion once annually. Dosage schedules vary for the other indications.

PAIN AND AGING

Continual or recurrent pain resulting from malignancies, degenerative conditions, and other diseases is extremely common in older adults. Chronic pain causes physical and mental distress and has profound effects on the quality of life. Current estimates are that 80% of older adults have some illness or degenerative condition that predisposes them to chronic pain.

The painful manifestations of arthritis and osteoporosis have been discussed. Other causes of pain include atherosclerotic disease, angina, cancer, diabetic neuropathy, herpes zoster, and temporal arteritis. There is much evidence that pain in older adults continues to be underreported, underassessed, and undermanaged. The consequences of poorly controlled pain include impaired ambulation, reduced socialization, decreased independence in activities of daily living, and overall reduced quality of life. Pain and depression are strongly associated with each other, and each may exacerbate the other.

The potential for drug interactions and side effects is high when analgesic medications are administered; careful dosage adjustment should be made. The concern regarding addiction is not as great for older adults as for younger adults. Older patients take the analgesics until they get pain relief. Pain relief is their only concern; they normally have no separate underlying need for the drugs. It would be very rare for older patients to increase their use of opioids and exhibit the drug-seeking behaviors typical of a drug addict. These concerns should be put to rest when considering pain therapy. Long-acting and transdermal dosage forms may give the best results.

THE AGING THYROID AND HOW IT AFFECTS OLDER ADULTS

Changes in thyroid function occur as a natural consequence of aging. These changes are associated with a lowered rate of thyroid hormone secretion and clearance from the body or, less commonly, hyperthyroidism or carcinoma of the thyroid.

Hypothyroidism occurs commonly in older adults. It has been found that the pituitary secretion of thyroid-stimulating hormone (TSH) does not change with aging. When elevated levels of TSH are found in the blood, even if there are no recognizable signs of hypothyroidism, it is believed that the patient has subclinical hypothyroidism and should be given replacement therapy. When hypothyroidism occurs in older adults, it may differ greatly from the disorder in a younger person. The following clinical signs should increase the suspicion of hypothyroidism in an older adult:

- Unexplained elevations in plasma cholesterol or triglycerides
- Congestive heart failure
- Fecal impaction
- Macrocytic anemia
- Vague arthritic complaints
- Mild psychiatric disturbances
- The presence of a thyroidectomy scar
- A history of treatment with thyroid hormone
- Previous treatment with radioactive iodine
- Goiter

The treatment of hypothyroidism is replacement therapy with thyroid hormone; this can be given in the form of the natural gland (Armour Thyroid Tablets) or, more commonly, in the form of synthetic thyroxine (Synthroid). In most cases, the need for thyroid hormone replacement is permanent. The dosage is individualized according to the patient's needs and responses. These agents are discussed in Chapter 18.

When hyperthyroidism, or Graves' disease, occurs in older adults, the signs may be muted or masked. Congestive heart failure is the most common presenting symptom of hyperthyroidism. Weight loss, muscle weakness, palpitations, eyelid tremor, eyelid lag, exophthalmos (protruding eyeballs), and nervousness are also reported. The principal treatment for hyperthyroidism in older adults is radioactive iodine. The antithyroid drugs propylthiouracil and methimazole are used in younger patients, but they are less satisfactory in the older adult.

Thyroid cancer, or papillary carcinoma, is a more aggressive malignancy in older adults. The aggressiveness includes a more rapid rate of growth, metastases to distant sites, and recurrence after surgery. Surgery remains the treatment of choice, followed by antineoplastic drug therapy.

HYPERTENSION IN OLDER ADULTS

Hypertension in older adults must be treated more carefully than hypertension in younger patients. Older adults have slower sympathetic nervous system responsiveness and impaired autoregulation. Therapy should be slow and gradual, with avoidance of drugs such as prazosin that cause postural hypotension or drugs that may aggravate other medical problems the older patient may have.

It was thought previously that older adults needed to maintain a slightly higher systolic blood pressure for adequate passage of blood in the brain; however, this is no longer thought to be true. The blood pressure goal in older adults is less than 140/90 mm Hg. The diastolic pressure should not be allowed to decrease to less than 70 mm Hg.

Many home kits for monitoring blood pressure are available, and patients should be encouraged to use them. Lifestyle changes should be recommended, including weight loss; exercise; limiting alcohol consumption; and a diet low in fat, salt, and sugar. Drug therapy should be recommended when necessary. The patient's OTC medications should be monitored. NSAIDs, pseudoephedrine, caffeine preparations, and asthma inhalers all may increase blood pressure.

Diuretics may be used, although they are no longer the drugs of choice for older patients. Beta blockers should be used with caution. Calcium channel blockers are a good choice, as are angiotensin-converting enzyme inhibitors (ACE inhibitors) in certain patients. Long-acting dosage forms should be chosen whenever possible to keep the number of medication doses at a minimum.

ANTI-INFECTIVE THERAPY IN OLDER ADULTS

Older adults experience a higher incidence of vascular, metabolic, degenerative, and neoplastic disorders. They are also very susceptible to infectious complications of all these disorders. Antibiotic therapy can be challenging because the infection is sometimes well advanced before an older adult seeks treatment. Also, drug penetration into infected tissues may be inadequate because of atherosclerotic narrowing of the arteries, which limits the drug's access to the tissues. In addition, physiologic changes associated with aging result in an alteration of drug metabolism. Renal plasma flow declines with age; drugs dependent on "average" renal function for excretion may build up to toxic levels in the body. Congestive heart failure may slow circulation further.

Several categories of anti-infective drugs must be monitored in the older adult patient.

AMINOGLYCOSIDE ANTIBIOTICS

Gentamicin, tobramycin, amikacin, and kanamycin are used in older adults for infections caused by *Enterobacter* and *Pseudomonas* strains. Excretion of these agents is often delayed, however, and blood levels must be monitored carefully. Nephrotoxicity and ototoxicity are possible toxic effects.

PENICILLINS

Patients with impaired renal function may develop acute renal failure or hemolytic anemia when large doses of penicillin are given parenterally. Neurotoxic symptoms of muscle twitching, myoclonic jerking, and seizures have been reported as well. Large parenteral doses may be necessary for life-threatening, severe infections; choices may be limited.

CEPHALOSPORINS

Life-threatening hemorrhage may occur from wound sites or the gastrointestinal tract when cephalosporins are used to treat infection. The risk of hemorrhage is greatest in a poorly nourished patient who has cancer and who has undergone a surgical procedure. It has been theorized that cephalosporins interfere with intestinal production of vitamin K.

NITROFURANTOIN

Elderly patients who have been given nitrofurantoin for urinary tract infections have been reported to have an increased risk of agranulocytosis, hepatitis, and chronic pulmonary fibrosis. This agent should be used with caution, if at all, in older adults.

QUINOLONES

This class of antimicrobial agents has been shown to be highly favorable for use in older adults. Quinolones (norfloxacin, ciprofloxacin, levofloxacin, moxifloxacin, and ofloxacin) have a broad spectrum of activity, are active orally in twice-daily dosages, and can be prescribed for penicillin-sensitive patients. They should be used with caution in patients with seizure disorders. Because they are inactivated by the concurrent use of liquid antacids containing aluminum or magnesium, dosing of these agents should be separated by at least 2 hours. The drug interaction between quinolones and warfarin should be particularly noted. The effect of warfarin is enhanced when used with quinolones; careful monitoring and possible dosage adjustment may be necessary.

ANXIETY IN OLDER ADULTS

Anxiety is a prominent problem in older adults. An older patient is likely to have a wide array of medical illnesses that can produce symptoms that either mimic or trigger anxiety. These illnesses include cardiovascular disease; drug-related problems; endocrine, hematologic, immunologic, neurologic, or pulmonary problems; and some forms of cancer. In addition, older adults are often engaged in fewer productive activities and have more time to worry than do younger people.

Selective serotonin reuptake inhibitors (SSRIs) are effective in the treatment of anxiety in older adults. Buspirone (BuSpar) has been shown in studies to be well tolerated in this population. Buspirone is discussed in Chapter 14. Drugs such as the benzodiazepines (e.g., alprazolam, diazepam, and triazolam) are better avoided in older adults because these patients have a decreased ability to detoxify these agents, and impaired mental and motor function symptoms are intensified.

DRUGS USED TO TREAT ALZHEIMER'S DISEASE

Alzheimer's disease is the most common cause of **dementia**—progressive and permanent loss of cognitive and intellectual functions—in older adults. It is often underrecognized and undertreated. The prevalence of Alzheimer's disease doubles every 5 years after age 65 years, with an estimated 30% of people 85 years of age or older having some form of the disease. Impairment is cognitive, functional, and behavioral.

Screening for cognitive impairment can be performed with the Mini-Mental State Examination (MMSE). The MMSE is an easy-to-administer mental examination for preliminary and serial assessment of cognition (the ability to be aware, think, reason, and remember). A perfect score is 30; patients with dementia usually attain a score of 20 or less. More information on this examination can be found at www.minimental.com. Another test is the Alzheimer's Disease Assessment Scale–Cognitive Subscale (ADAS-Cog). Healthy nondemented patients score 0 to 1 on this test, whereas the scores of demented patients usually increase by 6 to 12 points per year. Neuroimaging using computed tomography, positron emission tomography, or magnetic resonance imaging can also help establish the diagnosis.

Drugs used to treat Alzheimer's disease (Table 24-1) are reversible inhibitors of the enzyme acetylcholinesterase, allowing an increase in the level of acetylcholine in the brain. The cholinergic system, which uses acetylcholine to transmit nerve impulses, is involved with memory and attention. Treatment results are often subjective and difficult to quantify; however, these drugs seem to cause improvement in symptoms compared with the administration of placebos. Side effects include bradycardia, increased gastric secretion and ulcers, and liver impairment.

Table 24-1 Drugs Used to Treat Alzheimer's Disease

Generic Name	Trade Name	Oral Dosage
donepezil hydrochloride	Aricept	5-10 mg/day
rivastigmine	Exelon	6 mg twice daily
tacrine hydrochloride	Cognex	10 mg four times daily
memantine hydrochloride	Namenda	5 mg daily

FAMILY CARE OF OLDER ADULTS AND CAREGIVER STRESS

When an older patient is living at home, a caregiver may be required. Meeting the needs of the older adult causes increased stress in the caregiver. There is often a sense of ambivalence because the son, daughter, or spouse who is the caregiver would otherwise be at a stage of life when most responsibilities are fulfilled, and this is the long-awaited free time for travel or other interests.

Parental care is different from child care. Child care is naturally expected to lessen as time goes on. The reverse is true with elder care. Adult children may begin with grocery shopping and transportation, add housecleaning and meal preparation, bathing and dressing, and, finally, feeding and coping with incontinence.

The apparent increasing incidence of elder abuse reflects emotional problems in the caregiver as normal coping mechanisms fail to relieve the stress of caring for an older adult. Health care personnel can play an important role in screening for elder abuse and offering appropriate support, education, advice, and intervention for the older adult and the caregiver. Caregiver stress can manifest as vague symptoms of fatigue, anxiety, depression, back strain, anger, guilt, frustration, social isolation, and a perception of poor health. Elements to screen for when interviewing the caregiver include a history of drug or alcohol abuse in the older adult or the caregiver, a family history of violence, a mention of "punishment" of the older adult by the caregiver, or a recent life stress for the caregiver.

Caregivers need specific advice. They must be encouraged to set realistic limitations on the amount of care they can give. Other family members should be encouraged to become involved and give relief to the primary caregiver. The use of adult day care centers for the older adult and temporary nursing home placement for time off should also be encouraged.

Self-help or support groups for caregivers are available in many communities. In addition, specific support groups are available for people dealing with patients with Alzheimer's disease. The health care worker should become familiar with local support groups and services for older adults so that suggestions for support and intervention can be given whenever necessary.

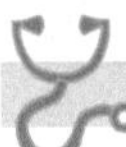

Clinical Implications

1. The metabolism of older adults differs significantly from the metabolism of younger adults. Older patients should be observed for signs of drug overdose.
2. Aging patients should not merely be considered as senile when behavior and abilities begin to change. A look for underlying diseases or drug reactions is always in order.
3. An older adult patient should be counseled thoroughly on the details of his or her special diet. Careful attention should be given to nutrition, with the recommendation of supplemental vitamins and minerals and dietary supplements.
4. Drug compliance is a problem in older adults. They should be counseled regarding the importance of taking the medications as prescribed. Long-acting medications and simplified drug dosage schedules should be used as much as possible.
5. Falling, confusion, and decreased cognitive abilities may be signs of overdosage of a sedative medication.
6. The use of OTC medications such as aspirin and ibuprofen can alleviate many of the symptoms of osteoarthritis.
7. Congestive heart failure may indicate thyroid abnormalities as well as specific problems with the myocardium of the heart.
8. The health care worker should be aware of problems with the caregiver of an older adult. Skilled counseling is possible only if the social problems are recognized.
9. Anxiety is a common problem of older adults. The use of anxiolytic agents can significantly relieve many of these symptoms.
10. Chronologic aging does not in itself mean a loss of function or a poor quality of life. Good medical care and the proper use of community services can provide many improvements for older adults.
11. Preventive nutrition may prevent or minimize some chronic illnesses in older adults.
12. Hypertension must be treated carefully to avoid conditions such as postural hypotension.
13. When infections become more numerous and severe, the tolerance to many antibiotics is decreased.
14. Drug interactions must be checked whenever a patient is receiving more than one medication.
15. Dementia should be assessed. If it is progressive, medications are available to alleviate the condition.

CRITICAL THINKING QUESTIONS

1. A patient came to the heart clinic today for her 6-month checkup. The chart shows a slow but steady weight loss for the past year. The patient says that she is so tired that it is hard to get to the grocery store, and mostly she just has toast and coffee for lunch and a sandwich for dinner. What may be some of her additional problems? How may they be improved?
2. A patient is admitted to the hospital for a broken hip. The physician ordered blood studies because of the large bruises over the patient's shoulder and upper back. The blood studies are normal. The patient's daughter says he "falls a lot." Should further investigation and studies be made?
3. A patient seems more and more confused each time she is seen in follow-up for hypertension. Her medications include digoxin, Lasix, Slow-K, Valium, and Dalmane. Should any of the medications be considered part of her problem?
4. A patient came to her physician for "burnout." She works full-time and has two teenage children, an elderly father with Alzheimer's disease, and a married daughter with a new baby. With no time for herself, her marriage is suffering, and she complains of sleep problems and anxiety. What suggestions may be made to improve her situation?

REVIEW QUESTIONS

1. A careful medication history should be taken from older adults because they:
   a. take very few medications.
   b. often combine herbal products with their medicines.
   c. are careful generally to see only one physician.
   d. have few underlying diseases.

2. When treating older adults, a great effort should be made to:
   a. get all medications on an every-4-hours schedule.
   b. make sure the patient has a medication for each illness.
   c. simplify the drug regimen as much as possible.
   d. get a specialist for each illness.

3. A symptom of osteoporosis may be:
   a. a swollen knee joint.
   b. painful hands in the morning.
   c. back pain and shortening of stature.
   d. weight gain.

4. Hypothyroidism in an older adult may have all the following symptoms *except:*
   a. goiter.
   b. fecal impaction.
   c. intolerance to heat.
   d. congestive heart failure.

5. A drug of choice for the treatment of anxiety in an older patient is:
   a. buspirone.
   b. phenobarbital.
   c. alprazolam.
   d. triazolam.

6. A side effect of donepezil may be:
   a. tachycardia.
   b. hypertension.
   c. bradycardia.
   d. increased renal output.

7. When giving medication to an older patient, the usual dose of a medication may need to be:
   a. increased.
   b. decreased.
   c. not changed.
   d. divided into two doses.

8. When prescribing various medications to an older patient, compliance with the drug schedule may be affected by:
   a. confusion.
   b. too many caregivers.
   c. osteoporosis.
   d. drug addiction.

9. Nitrofurantoin is a medication not recommended for older patients because of the risk of:
   a. agranulocytosis.
   b. pleocytosis.
   c. elevated white blood cell count.
   d. anemia.

10. The most common presenting sign of hyperthyroidism in older patients is:
    a. hypotension.
    b. intolerance to heat.
    c. slowed heart rate.
    d. congestive heart failure.

Answers to the review questions can be found at the back of the book.

evolve Additional questions and activities can be found at *http://evolve.elsevier.com/asperheim/pharmacology*.

Drug Therapy in Children

CHAPTER 25

Objectives

After completing this chapter, you should be able to do the following:

1. Understand that the scope of pediatrics covers more than treating illnesses.
2. Realize that growth, development, and overall health of a child often depend on environmental and social factors.
3. Understand the importance of referring to a drug manufacturer's recommendation on the dose of any medication for children.
4. Calculate a child's dose by applying the appropriate rule (Young's, Clark's, or Fried's) to the recommended adult dose.
5. Calculate a child's dose based on body surface area.

Key Terms

Clark's rule, p. 240
Fried's (FRE-DS) **rule,** p. 240
Young's rule, p. 240

The field of pediatrics is concerned with the fetus, the infant, and the child through adolescence. The care of a child is more all-encompassing than care of an adult. Health care professionals who care for children must consider that children are the most vulnerable in a society, and their needs require special attention. It is not sufficient merely to look for problems with the organ systems or biologic processes; the whole child must be considered at every step in his or her development and with regard to the treatment of his or her illness.

Proper nutrition of a growing child is crucial. Pediatricians carefully measure growth and developmental milestones because often a deviation from the previous growth curve may be the first sign of illness in a child. The genetic history is important because genetic aberrations are the cause of many diseases and developmental problems. Environmental and social situations contribute greatly to the health and well-being of the child. Increasing attention has been given to behavioral and social aspects of child health, ranging from many books written on child-rearing practices to the creation of major programs for the prevention and treatment of child abuse. Social programs are in place for the care of homeless children, children in poverty, children of migrant workers, and abandoned children.

A profound improvement in child health occurred after the development of vaccines, antibiotics, and disinfectants. Mortality rates decreased dramatically, and today's parents do not have to stand helplessly by while their children die of pneumonia, diphtheria, whooping cough, and influenza.

MEDICATIONS AND FETAL DEVELOPMENT

The first trimester of pregnancy is the most important in regard to organ development, and it is the time when the adverse effects of drugs are most prevalent. If possible, all maternal medications should be avoided during this period.

Teratogenic effects of drug exposure in utero may include gross malformations, as was the case of thalidomide, which caused limb deformities. Decreased growth and cognitive ability with behavioral defects have been commonly seen after maternal alcohol and illicit drug use. Transfer of human immunodeficiency virus (HIV) to the infant in utero and via lactation is well established. All prescription drugs are labeled for safety; the five categories of safety during pregnancy are defined in Chapter 23. In some cases, another category may be given for lactation. Generally, all drugs present in the mother's blood are equally present in the human milk. Infants may have side effects of maternal drugs (e.g., diarrhea from antibiotics). As mentioned, transfer of HIV has been shown to occur via human milk, and it is probable that other viruses are transferred as well.

MEDICATIONS USED TO TREAT CHILDREN

IMMUNIZATIONS

The health care professional should become acquainted with the immunization schedules for children and encourage the parents to stay on schedule. The current schedule is presented in Chapter 20.

ANTIBIOTICS

Parents may express a great deal of anxiety and even anger if a child's illness is not treated with antibiotics. The health care professional should be well versed in the futility of treating viruses with antibiotics and the increasing problems with microbial resistance to antibiotics and help counsel the parents with this information.

STIMULANTS FOR ATTENTION-DEFICIT/HYPERACTIVITY DISORDER

The stimulants used to treat attention-deficit/hyperactivity disorder are described in Chapter 12. Some parents insist on the "hyperactivity drugs" for 2-year-olds who are behaving within normal parameters. Social and environmental factors are important when deciding to prescribe these agents. In some cases, a child is unable to pay attention in school because he or she is worried about lack of food at home, domestic violence, parental substance abuse, or physical or sexual abuse. Counseling and listening to verbal and nonverbal cues are important.

DRUGS USED FOR ENURESIS

Enuresis is defined as voluntary or involuntary discharge of urine in bed after an age when bladder control would be expected. Most children with a mental age of 5 years have daytime and nighttime control of urine. Enuresis is diagnosed when urine is voided twice a week for at least 3 consecutive months. Enuresis is more common in boys; prevalence is 5% at age 7 years and 1% at age 18. In girls, the prevalence is 3% at age 7 years and extremely rare by age 18.

It is important to get the child's cooperation to treat the problem. The child should void before retiring, but awakening the child during the night and punishment for wetting are generally not useful. Various alarms are available that have variable success. Pharmacotherapy should be reserved for children in whom behavioral treatment is unsuccessful.

desmopressin acetate (DDAVP). This is a synthetic compound that is structurally related to the posterior pituitary antidiuretic hormone. It may be administered intranasally, orally, or parenterally to prevent or control polyuria and nocturia. Adult doses are provided because this agent may also be used in the management of diabetes insipidus.

Dosage: Adults and children: (Oral) 0.05 mg twice daily; dose may be adjusted to 0.9 mg/day in two divided doses.

Adults and children older than 12 years: (Intranasal) 5 to 40 mcg/day in two divided doses; (IV, Subcut) 2 to 4 mcg/day.

Children younger than 12 years: (Intranasal) 5 to 30 mcg/day in the evening.

imipramine hydrochloride (Tofranil). Imipramine is used to treat enuresis in children 6 years of age or older. It is an antidepressant, and there is a caution of increasing the risk of suicidal thinking and behavior. Most children take it without problems, however. The success rate is 50% after 6 months of treatment.

Dosage: Children older than 5 years: (Oral) 10 to 15 mg before bedtime, maximum dose 75 mg.

ANXIETY DISORDERS

Children have the same spectrum of anxiety disorders as adults, but anxiety is often not recognized early enough because of the child's inability to voice his or her concerns. Anxiety is strongly associated with common childhood worries such as fear of the dark, of storms, of separation, but it may progress to full-blown social phobias related to school or post-traumatic stress disorder after a traumatic experience. The problems are considered to be acute if they last less than 3 months and chronic if they last more than 3 months.

Medications used to treat anxiety are discussed in Chapter 14. Skilled child behavioral specialists are advised if the problem is severe.

CALCULATING CHILDREN'S DOSES

Children's doses of drugs need to be calculated in every case. There are several formulas for calculating dosage according to age and weight. Calculating

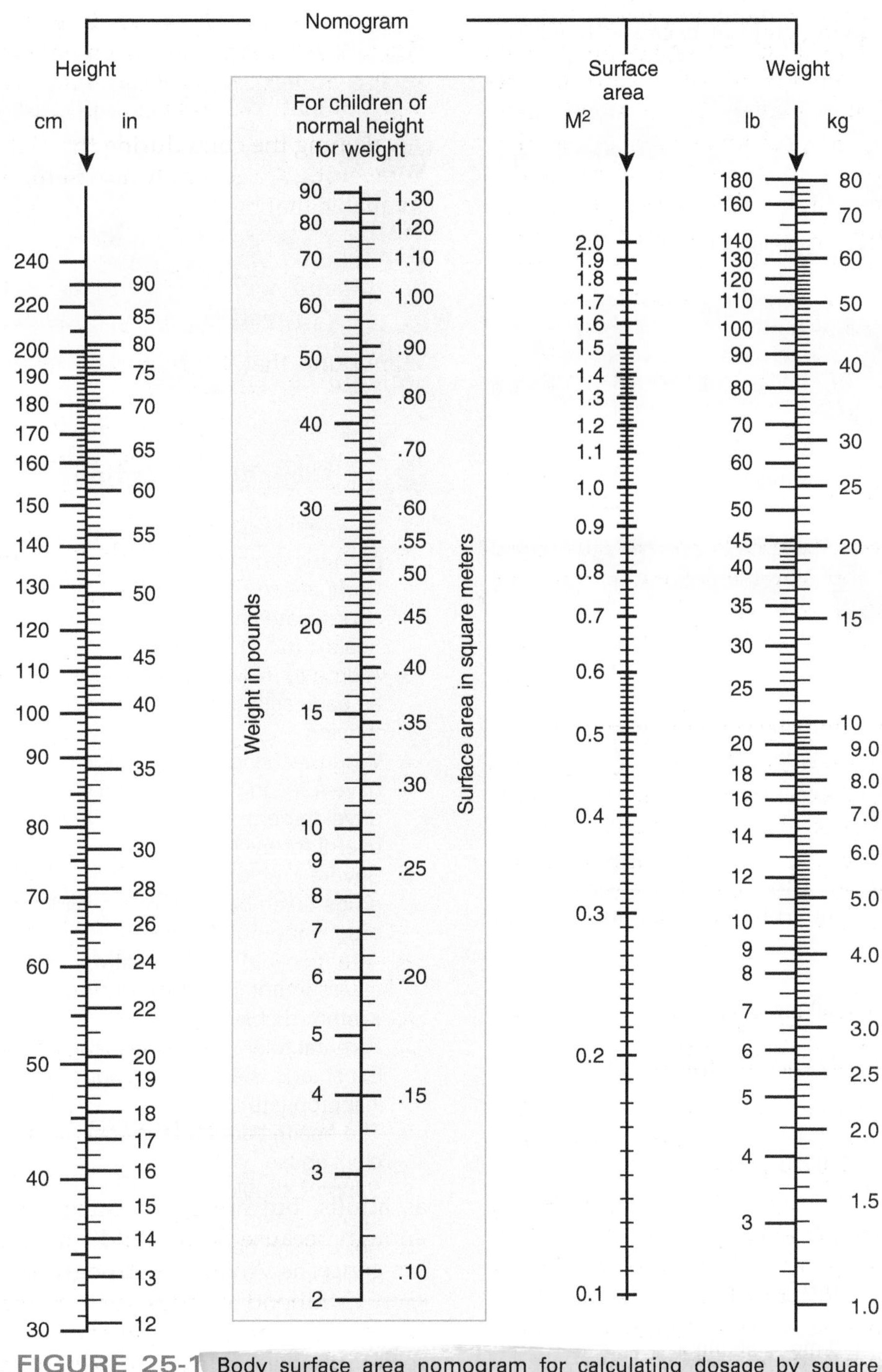

FIGURE 25-1 Body surface area nomogram for calculating dosage by square meter (m^2).

the recommended dosage per kilogram or pound of body weight is more accurate than calculating dosage according to age. Other factors besides age and weight also enter into determining dosages for children. For this reason, some physicians use the body surface area method to estimate the dosage for children. Charts are available to determine the body surface area in square meters according to height and weight.

It is generally not the responsibility of a health care professional other than the physician to calculate the dose of a drug for children, although the following formulas give the general method used. Drug manufacturers, after considerable research, give specific doses of drugs used for children, and these should always be carefully checked in the current drug literature or package insert. Many drugs are not advised for children because of the potential for harmful side effects on the growing child or because they have been insufficiently tested in children to give a recommended dosage range.

The following three formulas are useful in calculating dosage for infants and children. In **Young's rule,** the dosage is calculated as follows:

$$\frac{\text{Age of child in years}}{\text{Age of child (in years)} + 12} \times \text{average adult dose} = \text{child's dose}$$

Young's rule is not valid after 12 years of age. If the child is small enough to warrant a reduced dose after 12 years of age, the reduction should be calculated on the basis of **Clark's rule:**

$$\frac{\text{Weight of child (in pounds)}}{150} \times \text{average adult dose} = \text{child's dose}$$

Fried's rule, which is sometimes used in calculating dosages for infants younger than 2 years old, uses the following formula:

$$\frac{\text{Age in months}}{150} \times \text{average adult dose} = \text{child's dose}$$

Any unit of measure may be used in these formulas. The answer will be in the same units as used. If another unit is desired, conversion may be carried out as previously illustrated.

EXAMPLES

a. Find the dose of phenobarbital for a 4-year-old child (adult dose = 30 mg).

$$\frac{4}{4 + 12} \times 30 \text{ mg} = 7.5 \text{ mg}$$

b. Find the dose of cortisone for a 30-lb infant (adult dose = 100 mg).

$$\frac{30}{150} \times 100 \text{ mg} = 20 \text{ mg}$$

c. If the nurse draws 2 mL of acetaminophen 120 mg/5 mL into an oral dosing syringe, the dose contains _______ mg of acetaminophen.

$$\frac{2}{5} \times 120 \text{ mg} = 48 \text{ mg}$$

BODY SURFACE AREA NOMOGRAM

A body surface area nomogram is used for calculating pediatric doses by square meter of body surface (Fig. 25-1). The center enclosed box gives the square meters by weight in pounds only for children of normal height and weight. For children who are slender or obese, a straight line that connects the height and weight on the two outside scales can be used to read the square meters of body surface at the point where the line crosses the surface area scale in the center box.

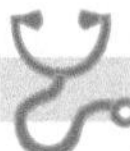

Clinical Implications

1. A careful family history is important when assessing a pediatric patient.
2. Comparison of the child's height and weight with the appropriate charts may give information about the child's health.
3. A drop to a lower percentile on the growth chart may be an early sign of illness in a child who was previously thriving.
4. When working with pediatric patients, it is important to have a feeling for the normal variants in growth and development. The Denver Developmental Screening is useful for evaluation.
5. Severe problems with the fetus may occur from drugs taken by the mother, particularly early in pregnancy.
6. Attention–deficit/hyperactivity disorder may be due to environmental problems as well as a true central nervous system problem.
7. Parental tolerance of behavioral issues varies greatly. Expectations about behavior of toddlers may be inappropriate.
8. The health care professional must be alert for signs of child abuse.
9. Support should be given to the parents to maintain the immunization schedule on time.
10. Anxiety and depression often begin in childhood. Signs of social anxiety should be observed.

CRITICAL THINKING QUESTIONS

1. A mother brings her 4-year-old son into the office because she is concerned that he is "hyperactive." She would like some sort of treatment to help calm him down. What would you tell the mother? What recommendations would you make?
2. Growth curves are used to measure the normal development of a child in regard to height and weight milestones. When a patient's height and weight fall below the growth curve, what could that indicate?

REVIEW QUESTIONS

1. When treating a child for an illness, it is important to focus on:
   a. the laboratory values as a representation of organ function.
   b. the signs and symptoms the child has.
   c. the development of the child.
   d. all of the above.

2. Teratogenic effects are commonly caused from drug exposure during which stage of life?
   a. In utero (during pregnancy)
   b. Neonate (birth to 1 month)
   c. Infant (1 month to 1 year)
   d. Child (1 to 12 years)

3. What is an appropriate treatment for a viral infection?
   a. Antibiotics
   b. Stimulants
   c. DDAVP
   d. Rest, fluids, and time

4. Enuresis is:
   a. an inability to pay attention in class.
   b. an overwhelming feeling of despair.
   c. nighttime wetting.
   d. a post-traumatic stress disorder.

5. Which of the following is *not* a recommended treatment for enuresis?
   a. Punishing the child (i.e., time-out)
   b. Imipramine hydrochloride
   c. Emptying the bladder before bedtime
   d. DDAVP

6. You have a 6-year-old patient who needs drug *X* (adult dose = 500 mg). Using Young's rule, calculate your patient's dose.
   a. 125 mg
   b. 166 mg
   c. 250 mg
   d. 375 mg

7. You have a 13-year-old patient who weighs 75 lb and who needs drug *X* (adult dose = 500 mg). Using Clark's equation, calculate your patient's dose.
   a. 125 mg
   b. 166 mg
   c. 250 mg
   d. 375 mg

8. You have a 15-month-old child who needs drug *X* (adult dose = 500 mg). Using Fried's rule, calculate your patient's dose.
   a. 25 mg
   b. 50 mg
   c. 100 mg
   d. 250 mg

9. A pharmacist draws up a 1.6-mL dose of acetaminophen concentrated drops 80 mg/0.8 mL into an oral dosing syringe. How many milligrams of acetaminophen are in the dose?
   a. 1.6 mg
   b. 16 mg
   c. 160 mg
   d. 1600 mg

10. What is the body surface area of a 50-lb child who is 3′4″ tall using the body surface area nomogram?
   a. 0.6 m^2
   b. 0.8 m^2
   c. 1.0 m^2
   d. 1.2 m^2

Answers to the review questions can be found at the back of the book.

evolve Additional questions and activities can be found at *http://evolve.elsevier.com/asperheim/pharmacology*.

CHAPTER 26

Home Health and End-of-Life Care

Objectives

After completing this chapter, you should be able to do the following:

1. Understand the necessity for and objectives of home health care.
2. Become aware of the different medications given in the home setting.
3. Appreciate the expanded role of the nurse and allied health professional in the home health field.
4. Assess the homebound patient and evaluate the environmental factors that affect the quality of the treatment.
5. Recognize side effects of medications administered.
6. Recognize factors that change the goals of drug therapy for a terminally ill patient.
7. Become familiar with the goals of palliative care.
8. Assist the patient and family with issues relating to the end of life.

Key Terms

Home health care, p. 242
Hospice (HŎS-pĭs), p. 244
Infusion (ĭn-FYŪ-zhĕn), p. 242
Prophylactic (PRŌ-fĭ-LĂK-tĭk) **therapy,** p. 243
Terminal illness, p. 244

Home health care is professional health care provided in the home, offering many services formerly available only in a hospital setting. Home health care has grown rapidly, and with it have grown opportunities for nurses and allied health care workers. Home care offers an acceptable, effective alternative to extended hospitalization. Cost-containment efforts by payers, newer techniques, and the increasing availability of sophisticated home health care providers have made all sectors in the health care field believe that this trend will increase in the future.

The home health care professional is a part of a collaborative team of nurse, physician, and other health care providers. Usually the home health worker is the only one of these individuals who sees a patient on a regular basis; he or she must be responsible for the assessment of the patient and must keep detailed records of these assessments, noting changes in the patient's condition, mental status, or blood pressure, so that the changes may be reported in a timely fashion.

The home health care worker must be acutely aware of the medications that the patient is taking and be knowledgeable about the effects, side effects, and potential toxic effect of each medication to avoid untoward effects. Appropriate corrective actions may be taken by other members of the team only if problems are reported.

A reassessment of theories and responsibilities of the health care provider must be made. The new role of home care in the health care system places more emphasis on responsibility and decision-making skills for nurses or other health care professionals. Some aspects of home health care are discussed in this chapter, but it is not all-inclusive.

HOME INFUSION THERAPY

Infusion is the introduction of a fluid, other than blood, into a vein. Home infusion can shorten or prevent hospitalization for certain patients in need of intravenous (IV) antibiotics, chemotherapy, hydration, pain management, immunoglobulins, transfusions, and parenteral nutrition. The main advantage of home infusion is that it offers the patient a more normal lifestyle with reduced medical costs. Home infusion is generally safe and effective. The following list includes many of the home infusion therapies now considered standard:

- Short-term and long-term antibiotics
- Antifungal and antiviral therapy
- Blood transfusions
- Total parenteral nutrition
- Pain management
- Chemotherapy
- Anticoagulation with heparin

Patients who are referred for home infusion often have no previous experience in this type of therapy. Before home infusion is offered to them, they must be screened for intellectual, psychological, social, and environmental factors that could negatively affect therapy. The patient should be medically stable after discharge from the hospital, with the exception of the need for IV therapy. Patients with hypotension, unexplained fevers, respiratory distress, active bleeding, recent emboli, or other conditions that render them medically unstable are poor risks for home health care. Medications that may cause allergic or severe adverse reactions should not be started in the home but may be continued by home therapy after initial doses are administered in a hospital setting.

Long-term central venous catheters are commonly used for home infusions. Blocked catheters may sometimes be reopened by infusing small amounts of acid or base solution, and clotted catheters may be opened by the infusion of urokinase. Pumps that can be programmed offer new alternatives for the administration of various medications at different times.

HOME INFUSION FOR CHILDREN

Home infusion therapy for children presents a different set of obstacles and opportunities. Hospitalization is a stressful and expensive event for a child and the family. The trend toward moving even high-technology care into the home is very beneficial. Particular problems occur with pediatric patients, however. Fear and its associated lack of cooperation and the limited intellectual ability and maturity of the child may cause problems. The maturity and cooperation of the parent or caregiver cannot be ensured either, and parents may be of limited intelligence or visually or physically handicapped themselves. Parents are not always dependable as allies in the care of the child.

Hematology and oncology patients are often candidates for home care. Blood and blood product administration, IV medication administration, and total parenteral nutrition are often done in the home.

Families should be encouraged to discuss the procedures with the home health caregiver, and the child's questions should be answered truthfully; the child should be given as much explanation as the situation warrants. Much of the anxiety and fear experienced by the child and the family are associated with a lack of information and a lack of comfort in their roles with regard to the infusion. Effective communication is essential.

HOME THERAPY FOR BONE MARROW TRANSPLANT PATIENTS

With the ability to treat malignant and nonmalignant diseases by means of bone marrow transplants comes the attendant problem of long-term therapy for these patients, often in a home setting. For a bone marrow transplant, the patient first has his or her bone marrow destroyed by myelosuppressive therapy and then receives a compatible marrow by infusion. After the bone marrow transplantation, immunosuppressive drugs are given to prevent rejection.

Prophylactic therapy—treatment that may prevent an illness or disorder—is aimed at preventing infections while a patient is in the immunocompromised state that follows transplantation. Antibiotics and antifungal and antiviral agents are used. Anemia is treated with whole blood transfusions or with packed cells, after these blood products are irradiated.

There is often general loss of the epithelium of the mouth and even the entire gastrointestinal tract. Pain control, oral hygiene, adequate nutrition, and fluid intake must be managed. Hepatic, renal, and pulmonary dysfunction can occur and must be managed appropriately. Pain associated with all the attendant problems must be managed within the guidelines of chronic pain management.

HOME CARE FOR DIABETIC PATIENTS

A patient with severe diabetes with secondary problems resulting from the disease often becomes a candidate for home health services. Diabetic retinopathy often leaves a patient severely visually compromised or totally blind. The patient cannot properly self-administer insulin injections or attend to personal hygiene, foot care, or skin care.

Syringes prefilled by a home health worker may facilitate continued partial self-sufficiency for the visually impaired patient. Continual observation of the patient for skin breakdown or infections and monitoring of blood glucose levels are necessary. Detailed inquiries about any diet management issues and assessment of the patient's level of skill in taking any other medications must be made.

PSYCHIATRIC HOME CARE

The move to decentralize health care and provide more services in the home has extended to psychiatric patients as well. Some patients may believe that discharge from the hospital means that "there is no more hope for me," rather than seeing it as a sign of improvement. At the other extreme, the patient's perception of being cured may prompt him or her to stop taking psychiatric medications altogether.

The home health care worker must be skilled in the assessment of the medication needs of the psychiatric patient and his or her compliance in taking them. An understanding of adverse side effects of the psychotropic drugs and recognition that the dosage may be too small or too large are important factors in providing home care.

Home health care workers who care for patients being treated for mental illness must be trained to collaborate with psychiatrists to provide adequate care. Assessing psychiatric issues requires that the health care provider be trained to listen; most assessment involves interviews and observation. When assessing a patient whose behavior indicates mental illness, the health care provider must ask himself or herself the following four questions:

1. Does the abnormal behavior reflect a new primary disorder, is it secondary to another disease, or is it a medication side effect?
2. Is the behavior precipitated by stress, or is it a sign that medication effects are different than predicted?
3. What is the level of aberrant behavior, and does it constitute a threat to the patient or to others?
4. How does the behavior relate to the culture and environment?

Imbalances of activity and rest, an inability to make appropriate food choices, poor self-care, and a deteriorating environment may be early signs that the patient's mental state is deteriorating.

END-OF-LIFE CARE

About the middle of the 20th century, care for the dying began to move out of the home and into the hospital. With the arrival of modern medicine and the techniques and procedures available in the hospital, more and more attempts to prolong life at any cost were made. As a result, death is often endured essentially alone, away from friends and family, in an intensive care unit, in the midst of painful and invasive procedures.

How do we know when a medical procedure is making the dying process unnatural and burdensome, or when it offers promise of cure or freedom from pain? How can we prepare for the death of a loved one and make the experience as meaningful and pain-free as possible? The hospice movement has led the way in answering these questions. A **hospice** is an institution that provides a centralized program of palliative and supportive care to dying persons and their families. This movement has taught us that letting a patient with **terminal illness** (a disease expected to cause death within a short period) die naturally does not mean stopping the patient's treatment or care.

Inadequate knowledge of health care professionals of pain management, symptom control, and other dimensions of terminal care have been cited as the major barrier to good end-of-life care. The issues and methods of pain management are discussed later in this chapter and in more depth in Chapter 13.

Although pain has been identified as the predominant symptom in a terminal illness, other critical symptoms and needs in the dying patient are being recognized through the practice of palliative care. For many people, fear of the unknown is at least as great as fear of death itself. Fear of uncontrollable pain, nausea, vomiting, embarrassment, and especially abandonment are very prominent in the patient's list of concerns. Presenting hospice as an option for treating a terminal illness can help with many of these unknowns. Good care of a dying person means making the body as comfortable as possible so that the patient can prepare for death mentally and spiritually. It means allowing the patient to live as fully as possible until the time he or she dies.

The needs of dying individuals have been described as follows:

- The need to be treated as a living human being
- The need to maintain a sense of hopefulness
- The need to be cared for by people who will help him or her maintain hopefulness
- The need to express feelings and emotions about death in one's own way
- The need to participate in decisions concerning one's care
- The need to be cared for by compassionate, sensitive, and knowledgeable people
- The need to expect continuing medical care, even though the goals may change
- The need to have all questions answered honestly and fully
- The need to seek spirituality
- The need to be free of physical pain
- The need to express feelings and emotions about pain in one's own way
- The need of children to participate in death
- The need to understand the process of death
- The need to die in peace and dignity
- The need to not die alone
- The need to expect that the sanctity of the body will be respected after death

There are many ways that the health care professional can assist the dying patient by dealing with the subject of death in a forthright manner in accordance with the patient's needs and wishes.

ISSUES TO RESOLVE IN END-OF-LIFE CARE

Delivering good palliative care requires a particular set of skills. These include knowledge of pain management and the ability to communicate about end-of-life issues such as advanced care planning, the use of cardiopulmonary resuscitation, and artificial life support. Other elective options include intubation, mechanical ventilation, surgery, dialysis, blood transfusions, artificial nutrition and hydration, antibiotics, and other medications and treatments as well as future admissions to the hospital or the intensive care unit. The treatment choices and the complexities increase as a patient's condition worsens. Many patients who initially choose a do-not-resuscitate (DNR) order make changes as time goes on. It is much better for all concerned to make these decisions well ahead of time.

The first step in palliative care is to establish goals. What is important to the patient and the family? This may be a continuing process because the goals may need to be adjusted as time passes. Preferences and understanding about death and the dying process vary widely, so they must be addressed. Specific issues that should be discussed with the patient and the family include the following:

- What do they know about the illness and the treatment options?
- How much information do they want to have?
- What decisions should be made by the patient, by the family, and by the health professional?
- What defines an acceptable quality of life for the patient?
- What roles will the physician and nurse play?
- Which family member will be the liaison between the patient and the health care team?
- Where would the patient like to die?
- Does the family have issues or preferences about being with the patient when he or she dies?

PAIN CONTROL

Pain control is a crucial subject for discussion with the patient. Patients need to know that most pain can be controlled with relatively simple therapies. The pain relief can be increased as the disease progresses. One question that patients should be asked is whether they are willing to trade full consciousness for pain relief because adequate control of pain may require sedation in some cases. In the final hours of life, the patient often experiences transient distress caused by dyspnea, agitation, and restlessness. Treatment for these symptoms also may require sedating medications.

Patients who cannot verbalize pain may still be experiencing it and are at risk for undertreatment; this is especially true for patients with dementia. In one study of patients who had been hospitalized for treatment of hip fracture, it was noted that patients with dementia received less than half the analgesic relief provided to patients with the same hip fracture but normal cognitive function. The health care worker should recognize that signs of restlessness, anxiety, or fearfulness in a patient who is unable to communicate may be a reaction to pain. An appropriate analgesic may be given to see whether the symptoms decrease.

DRUG SELECTION

There are many different drug choices for the various levels of pain that the patient may have. A general rule is that, as the pain progresses, a sustained-release form of a narcotic may be administered by mouth, and a short-acting "rescue" drug may be given for breakthrough pain between doses. Frequent use of the rescue drug (more than three to four times daily) may signal the need for an increase in the baseline long-acting drug. The usual dosage of the short-acting drug should be equivalent to 5% to 15% of the 24-hour baseline dosage of the long-acting drug. Pain control is discussed in more detail in Chapter 13, which also contains a list of oral and transdermal analgesic agents that are considered equivalent in potency to the effect of 10 mg of morphine administered intramuscularly (see Table 13-1).

TOLERANCE TO OPIOIDS

The use of opioids often raises fear of addiction in patients and health professionals. Such fear is almost always unwarranted. The risk of addiction is extremely small in patients with pain who have no history of substance abuse.

Severe pain allows patients to tolerate the sedative effects of opioids. Whether tolerance develops to the pain-relieving effects of opioids is a matter of controversy. Most of the data on opioid tolerance and physical dependence in humans come from studies involving subjects who were not in pain. Studies of patients with chronic pain who have taken opioids for a long time indicate that once the dosage required for pain relief is established, it generally remains stable unless the underlying disease progresses.

With long-term use of opioids, sudden withdrawal of the opioids or a significant reduction in dosage results in withdrawal symptoms such as sweating, nausea, diarrhea, and irritability. This type of physical dependence can also occur with other drugs such as antihypertensives and sedatives. Slowly tapering the dosage avoids the withdrawal symptoms.

When treating chronic pain, there is no ceiling or maximum opioid dose. Extremely large doses of morphine, such as several hundred milligrams every 4 hours, may be needed to relieve severe pain.

NUTRITION AND HYDRATION

Nutrition and hydration warrant special attention. There is perhaps no issue more common than concerns over the feeding of the dying patient. Very often the struggle over eating is really about fear of dying and losing a loved one. It is often easier for the patient than it is for the family to accept that the patient just cannot eat as much as he or she previously did.

Food is the way we energize our body. It is the means by which we keep our body moving and alive. In other words, we obviously eat to live. When a patient is preparing to die, it is perfectly natural that eating should stop. This is one of the hardest concepts for the family to accept. There is a gradual decrease in food consumption, with meats generally being refused first, then vegetables, followed by a preference for softer foods, and then liquids only. It must be remembered that it is okay not to eat. A different kind of energy is needed now—the spiritual energy to complete the task at hand.

Feeding tubes are often placed as a quick and easy solution to the time-consuming process of feeding a reluctant patient. Families may fear that the patient will "starve to death" rather than die of the disease. There is some evidence that artificial feeding may not lengthen the life of a patient but instead may just add to his or her problems by overloading a poorly functioning gastrointestinal tract. Removing the guilt and anxiety about this issue does everyone a service. The patient may be offered food and liquids and encouraged to take as much as desired without placing undue burdens or responsibilities on anyone.

HOSPICE CARE

GOALS

1. Patients can live at home. After all, this is where they are most comfortable. They have the opportunity to see friends and relatives and enjoy time with cherished pets and belongings.
2. They can stay as active as possible. Some limited trips with skilled assistance may be possible, or patients may help with daily living tasks as long as they are able.
3. Patients should be encouraged to express their feelings. The discussion of death and dying produces great anxiety in many family members in relation to their own fear of death. It is very important to patients that death be discussed, however. They may need to resolve old issues with family members or say goodbye, or they may wish to dispose of their possessions without relatives "shushing" them about talk of death.
4. Pain and other symptoms are relieved as much as is possible.
5. Hospice care should help people feel at peace. As the end of life approaches, it creates a loving environment where family members can say goodbye.

PALLIATIVE PERFORMANCE SCALE

The Palliative Performance Scale (PPS) is often used to evaluate the status of the patient. It gives a shortcut method of describing the patient's status (Table 26-1).

Table 26-1 Palliative Performance Scale

%	Ambulation	Activity and Evidence of Disease	Self-Care	Intake	Consciousness Level
100	Full	Normal activity, no sign of disease	Full	Normal	Full
90	Full	Normal activity, some sign of disease	Full	Normal	Full
80	Full	Normal activity with effort, some evidence of disease	Full	Normal/less	Full
70	Reduced	Unable to work normal job, some evidence of disease	Full	Normal/less	Full
60	Reduced	Unable to do hobby/housework, significant disease	Occasional help	Normal/less	Full/confusion
50	Mainly sit/lie	Unable to do any work, extensive disease	Considerable help	Normal/less	Full/confusion
40	Mainly in bed	Unable to do any work, extensive disease	Considerable help	Normal/less	Full/drowsy or confusion
30	Bed bound	Unable to do any work, extensive disease	Total care	Reduced	Full/drowsy or confusion
20	Bed bound	Unable to do any work, extensive disease	Total care	Minimal sips	Drowsy/coma
10	Bed bound	Unable to do any work, extensive disease	Total care	Mouth care only	Drowsy/coma
0	Death				

DRUGS USED FOR HOSPICE PATIENTS

Although effective pain management is paramount in the treatment of a hospice patient, other conditions may need attention and treatment as well. The agents used in the treatment of these other conditions are discussed elsewhere in this text; only a list is provided in Table 26-2, with some typical dosages given to hospice patients. Dosages of all of these agents may vary greatly depending on the patient and the circumstances of the illness.

Table 26-2 Drugs Used for Hospice Patients

Drug	Dosage
DRUGS FOR ANXIETY	
lorazepam (Ativan)	0.5-1 mg three times daily
alprazolam (Xanax)	0.25-0.5 mg three times daily
haloperidol (Haldol)	1-5 mg up to four times daily
diazepam (Valium)	10 mg four times daily
hydroxyzine (Atarax, Vistaril)	25 mg three times daily
chlorpromazine (Thorazine)	25-50 mg four times daily
DRUGS FOR SLEEPLESSNESS	
flurazepam (Dalmane)	15-30 mg at bedtime
temazepam (Restoril)	15-30 mg at bedtime
triazolam (Halcion)	0.25-0.5 mg at bedtime
DRUGS FOR DEPRESSION	
sertraline hydrochloride (Zoloft)	50-200 mg in the morning
paroxetine hydrochloride (Paxil)	20-50 mg in the morning
amitriptyline hydrochloride (Elavil)	50-150 mg at bedtime
desipramine hydrochloride (Norpramin)	10-150 mg at bedtime
DRUGS FOR NEUROPATHIC PAIN	
valproate sodium (Depakene)	250 mg three times daily
carbamazepine (Tegretol)	200 mg twice daily
gabapentin (Neurontin)	100 mg twice daily
divalproex (Depakote)	125 mg twice daily
phenytoin (Dilantin)	100 mg three times daily
DRUGS FOR NAUSEA OR VOMITING	
prochlorperazine (Compazine)	5-10 mg four times daily
promethazine hydrochloride (Phenergan)	25 mg three times daily
DRUGS FOR DIARRHEA	
diphenoxylate hydrochloride (Lomotil)	5 mg four times daily
DRUGS FOR CONSTIPATION	
Stool softeners	
Colace	5-150 mg twice daily
Peri-Colace	2 tablets twice daily
Senokot	2-4 tablets at bedtime
Dulcolax	1-3 tablets daily; (Rectal) 1 suppository daily
DRUGS FOR ABDOMINAL CRAMPING	
hyoscyamine (Levsin)	0.125 mg three times daily
scopolamine (Transderm Scop)	1-2 patches every 3 days
DRUGS FOR ORAL *CANDIDA*	
nystatin suspension (Mycostatin)	5 mL four times daily
clotrimazole (Mycelex)	10 mg troches five times daily
ketoconazole (Nizoral)	200 mg twice a day

Continued

Table 26-2 Drugs Used for Hospice Patients—cont'd

Drug	Dosage
DRUGS FOR VIRAL INFECTIONS	
acyclovir (Zovirax)	400 mg five times daily
DRUGS FOR REFLUX ESOPHAGITIS OR PEPTIC ULCERS	
cimetidine (Tagamet)	300 mg four times daily
famotidine (Pepcid)	20 mg twice daily
ranitidine (Zantac)	150 mg twice daily
DRUGS FOR MUSCLE SPASMS	
baclofen (Lioresal)	5 mg three times daily
diazepam (Valium)	5 mg three times daily
DRUGS FOR DYSPNEA	
Mild	
hydrocodone and acetaminophen (Vicodin or Lortab)	5 mg every 4 hr
Tylenol with codeine	30 mg four times a day
*Severe**	
morphine sulfate syrup	3-10 mg every 4 hr
hydromorphone hydrochloride (Dilaudid)	0.5-2 mg every 4 hr
Terminal	
midazolam hydrochloride (Versed)	0.25 mg/hr subcut, increased as necessary
DRUGS FOR PAIN CONTROL	
Mild Pain	
acetaminophen (Tylenol)	Up to 3-4 gm/day
aspirin	Up to 3-4 gm/day
ibuprofen (Motrin)	600-800 mg four times daily
indomethacin (Indocin)	25 mg three times daily
ketorolac tromethamine (Toradol)	10 mg four times daily
naproxen sodium (Naprosyn, Anaprox)	500 mg twice daily
Moderate Pain	
codeine sulfate (with aspirin or Tylenol)	130-200 mg every 3-4 hr
hydrocodone and acetaminophen (Vicodin)	30 mg every 3-4 hr
oxycodone hydrochloride (Percodan, Percocet)	30 mg every 3-4 hr
tramadol hydrochloride (Ultram)	50-100 mg every 4-6 hr (to 400 mg/day)
Severe Pain	
morphine sulfate	30-60 mg every 3-4 hr
morphine sulfate controlled-release (Oramorph SR, MS Contin)	90-120 mg every 12 hr
fentanyl citrate (Duragesic patch)	25-100 mcg/hr; (Parenteral) 0.1 mg/hr
hydromorphone hydrochloride (Dilaudid)	7.5 mg every 3-4 hr; (Parenteral) 1.5 mg every 3 hr
levorphanol tartrate (Levo-Dromoran)	3 mg four times daily; (Parenteral) 2 mg every 6 hr
meperidine hydrochloride (Demerol)	100-150 mg every 3-4 hr; (Parenteral) 100 mg every 3 hr
methadone hydrochloride (Dolophine)	20 mg every 6-8 hr; (Parenteral) 10 mg every 6 hr
oxymorphone hydrochloride (Numorphan)	(Parenteral) 1 mg every 3-4 hr

*The dosages for severe dyspnea can be increased by 50% every 4 to 12 hours until relief is obtained.

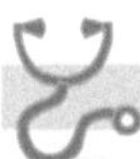

Clinical Implications

1. The role of a home health care provider places new responsibilities on the nurse or other health care provider.
2. Often the home health care worker is the only health care professional who sees the patient on a regular basis. It is important to remain alert for any changes in the patient's status.
3. Detailed records must be kept with regard to a patient's mental condition and personal hygiene as well as medical signs, such as blood pressure and pulse.
4. If there are signs that a patient is not medically stable, the medical provider should be notified immediately.
5. Pediatric patients may have excessive fears that interfere with therapy.
6. The abilities of the patient's home caregiver should be assessed.
7. Effective communication skills with the patient, family, and others on the health care team are essential.
8. New skills may need to be learned for infusions at the home site.
9. Pain management for a terminally ill patient has different goals than for an acutely ill patient.
10. Concerns regarding narcotic tolerance and habituation are not applicable when treating a terminally ill patient.
11. Skills in assessing patient compliance with medication are particularly important when visiting a psychiatric patient at home.
12. Clues from the home environment are often helpful when assessing a patient.
13. The dying process is natural, and death at home in a hospice environment has many advantages over death in a hospital, where frantic procedures may be done to prolong life at any cost.
14. Palliative care differs from therapeutic care in that a cure is no longer expected, but the patient is made as comfortable as possible.
15. A good quality of life may be experienced by the dying patient.
16. It is essential to be able to speak of death and dying with a terminally ill patient.
17. Much of the suffering of terminally ill patients has occurred because no one would let them speak of death or prepare themselves to die.
18. It is possible to relieve almost any level of pain with the medications available.
19. Patients who are not communicating well may be experiencing significant pain.
20. Anxiety and depression in a terminally ill patient may be masked as anger at the individuals around him or her.
21. Long-acting pain medication should be given routinely. The patient should not have to experience pain before each dose.
22. The dose and frequency of the rescue drug signifies when an increase in the long-acting analgesic is necessary.

CRITICAL THINKING QUESTIONS

1. A 67-year-old patient has been diagnosed with terminal colon cancer. He has had many surgical and radiation procedures and is now admitted to hospice care. The very anxious daughter who will be the primary caregiver states that she wants "everything possible" done for her father. How would you respond?
2. An 80-year-old patient who has cancer and Alzheimer's disease has refused to eat more than a spoonful at each meal for the last 3 days. Her husband is afraid she will starve to death and wants a feeding tube put in. How should this request be handled?
3. A 57-year-old patient has terminal metastatic breast cancer. She has just been admitted to hospice care. You are meeting with the patient, her husband, and her daughter for the first time. What will you say?
4. Every time a 74-year-old patient with terminal cancer wants to talk about death, his children quickly change the subject, telling him that he is going to get well and "not to talk like that." How could you help?
5. A patient has been an insulin-dependent diabetic for many years. Her blood glucose levels have been unstable lately, with several high or low readings. After visiting with her, she asks you to set her oven temperature because she is having trouble seeing the numbers. Would you have any recommendations for her care?
6. A patient with schizophrenia was stable on his psychiatric medication when discharged from the hospital. On your recent visit, you notice he is eating only bread, his appearance is becoming more disheveled, and he is obviously delusional. What would be your course of action?
7. A patient who is on IV medication for colon cancer reports more sores in his mouth today. What would you advise?

REVIEW QUESTIONS

1. Home infusion therapy may be used for all of the following *except:*
   a. antibiotic infusion.
   b. antiviral therapy.
   c. pain management.
   d. suspected pulmonary emboli.

2. Which of the following would be appropriate when working with a child undergoing home infusion?
   a. Tell the child, "Everything will be all right; don't worry."
   b. Discuss the procedures truthfully with the child, while reassuring him or her.
   c. Do not talk to the child at all; explain everything to the parent.
   d. Do not explain anything; just do your work.

3. Which would *not* be expected to be a problem with a diabetic home health patient?
   a. Visual problems limiting the ability to adjust the insulin dosage accurately
   b. Skin breakdown
   c. Confusion
   d. Strict adherence to an American Diabetes Association diet

4. An example of deficient end-of-life care would be:
   a. not using the newest experimental drug.
   b. talking about death with the patient if he or she wishes.
   c. inadequate pain control.
   d. maintaining hopefulness even with a terminal illness.

5. With a Palliative Performance Scale score of 50, a patient may be able to:
   a. continue to do light housework.
   b. mainly sit or lie quietly.
   c. do all personal hygiene tasks.
   d. enjoy reading novels.

6. A drug that may be used for anxiety is:
   a. morphine.
   b. promethazine.
   c. nystatin.
   d. lorazepam.

7. An agent useful for oral monilia is:
   a. hyoscyamine.
   b. nystatin.
   c. sertraline.
   d. desipramine.

8. The dose of codeine that would be equivalent to 40 mg of hydrocodone would be:
   a. 30 mg.
   b. 100 mg.
   c. 200 mg.
   d. 400 mg.

9. A terminally ill patient has been receiving morphine for about 4 months. Over this time, you would expect his dosage of morphine to have been:
   a. significantly increased.
   b. not changed.
   c. discontinued.
   d. significantly decreased.

10. The need to increase the dosage of an opioid to get the desired analgesia over time is called:
    a. addiction.
    b. habituation.
    c. tolerance.
    d. depression.

Answers to the review questions can be found at the back of the book.

evolve Additional questions and activities can be found at *http://evolve.elsevier.com/asperheim/pharmacology*.

Substance Abuse

CHAPTER 27

Objectives

After completing this chapter, you should be able to do the following:

1. Identify the risk factors that predispose patients to substance abuse.
2. Identify particular risk factors for substance abuse in teenagers.
3. Have an understanding of drug addiction and its symptoms.
4. Recognize withdrawal symptoms in drug dependence.
5. Recognize the symptoms shown by a patient under the influence of drugs.
6. Become familiar with the short and long-term effects of alcohol abuse.
7. Recognize drugs that are potentiated in their effects when taken with alcohol.
8. Identify the physical symptoms and dangerous sequelae of a drug overdose.
9. Identify drugs used to treat nicotine abuse.

Key Terms

Habit formation, p. 253
Psychoactive (SĪ-kō-ĂK-tĭv) **drug,** p. 251
Substance abuse, p. 251

Substance abuse, or *chemical abuse,* is the use or overuse of a chemical or substance in a way that leads to dependence and has adverse effects on the health and well-being of the user and others. It has become a national and international problem of gigantic proportions and affects all of us in some way. The use of **psychoactive drugs** (drugs possessing the ability to alter mood, behavior, or cognitive processes) by children and adolescents is no longer questioned. The most reasonable preventive effort is now focused on education. Rehabilitation programs have limited success but are increasing in numbers as the national problem persists.

According to a publication of the U.S. Department of Health and Human Services, more than 90% of adolescents in the United States are expected to use alcohol before graduating from high school, 50% are expected to use marijuana, 17% are expected to use cocaine, and 12% are expected to use hallucinogens. Of the 25,000 accidental deaths among youths annually, approximately 40% are alcohol-related.

The smoking of nicotine-containing cigarettes—long tolerated as a social function, a "bad habit" that was excused—is now also recognized as a chemical abuse and no longer tolerated in many public places. Second-hand smoke has been shown to be harmful to children and others in the environment. Various products and medications are available to treat nicotine addiction.

Studies have been done to try to determine the risk factors that predispose a child to substance abuse. The studies have shown that vulnerability to drug use is increased in children who have low self-esteem, a feeling of not belonging, a high need for social approval, inadequate bonding to family and society, inadequate communication and coping skills, an inability to defer gratification, and an inability to accept the consequences of their actions. A family history of alcoholism or substance abuse also greatly increases the risk.

A substance-abusing teenager may first come to medical attention as a result of trauma related to intoxication or secondary to an acute drug overdose.

The health care team should be responsible not only for treating the trauma but also for recognizing and assessing the substance abuse problem and, it is hoped, initiating some sort of remedial program. Most adolescents have three spheres of social interaction: school, family, and peers. Adolescents who are having difficulty in any one of these spheres may need referral for counseling and drug treatment. Convincing a patient and family members that a referral is needed is not always easy; there may be denial, a minimizing of the problem as a one-time occurrence, or a rejection of the values of society altogether.

During acute crises or overdoses in substance abusers, the health care professional is responsible for determining the type of drug taken, the method of administration, the time the drug was taken, and the previous pattern of substance abuse. This information can be obtained from the abuser, if responsive, or the family or friends. The health care professional is involved in the treatment and rehabilitation of the substance abuser at many levels, assisting the patient through the withdrawal period, observing the patient for other problems, and observing the effects of therapy and the patient's level of cooperation.

SEVEN SIGNS OF POSSIBLE DRUG INVOLVEMENT

1. Change in school or work attendance or performance (e.g., a student whose grades begin to fall or an employee whose absentee rate is a matter of concern)
2. Alteration of personal appearance (e.g., a person who was once neat now appears disheveled and disorderly)
3. Mood swings or attitude changes
4. Withdrawal from family contacts or from friends
5. Association with drug-using friends
6. Unusual patterns of behavior or mannerisms
7. Defensive attitude concerning drugs

DEPENDENCE ON NARCOTICS

Heroin is the narcotic of choice for most addicts in the United States. Although this drug is outlawed in the United States, illegal drug channels keep addicts supplied. Paregoric, morphine, oxycodone (OxyContin), and hydromorphone (Dilaudid) are often abused as well.

The desired sensation is euphoria (an exaggerated sense of physical and emotional well-being) after administration of the drug, usually intravenously. With continued use, a tolerance to the drug occurs, and higher doses are required for the euphoria. Over time, the addiction becomes so intense that the drug is taken for homeostasis and to prevent withdrawal symptoms. Accidental overdoses and death may occur inadvertently or in an attempt to obtain euphoria again.

Withdrawal symptoms from narcotics are severe and may be life-threatening. The first abstinence symptoms are malaise and weakness about 6 to 12 hours after the last dose. After 12 hours, yawning and perspiration occur, and the patient becomes anxious. After 24 hours, muscular contractions and pain, chills, increased rate and depth of respiration, blood pressure elevation, pupil dilation, and extreme agitation occur. Withdrawal symptoms peak in 48 hours and begin to subside in 72 hours. General symptoms of weakness and malaise may be present for several weeks.

Methadone maintenance programs have been developed to sustain narcotic addicts after withdrawal. Although methadone (Dolophine) is in itself an addicting narcotic, it produces little euphoria and allows the patient to function normally in society. Even with methadone, the percentage of addicts who are able to stop using narcotics is small.

methadone hydrochloride (Dolophine). Methadone may also be used to treat pain in nonaddicted patients. It has been a mainstay in the treatment of drug addicts who are legally maintained on methadone through clinics set up for this function. The dosage used for detoxification and maintenance is adjusted to control abstinence symptoms without causing respiratory depression or sedation. It is used orally only; a soluble tablet is dissolved in juice before being dispensed.

Dosage: Adults only: (Oral) Initial dosage should be based on the opiate tolerance of the patient. Initially 20 to 30 mg may be given. Stabilization of the maintenance dosage usually occurs at 80 to 120 mg/day.

SEDATIVE-HYPNOTIC ABUSE

Although sedative-hypnotic agents can be obtained through illegal channels, they are often obtained by prescription. Abusers may seek these prescriptions from many physicians simultaneously. These drugs become dangerous with overuse, particularly when combined with alcohol or other depressive drugs. Withdrawal is not as severe as with narcotic agents and is primarily characterized by insomnia, irritability, and anxiety-related symptoms.

MARIJUANA ABUSE

Marijuana is an intoxicant derived from the leaves and flowering tops of the *Cannabis* plant. It is generally smoked in cigarette form and produces a feeling of euphoria and a dreamy state. The length of the effect lasts 3 to 12 hours. Physical dependence can occur, although the question of true addiction is not settled. When a user exhibits a preference for the use of a chemical or substance but is not physiologically dependent, **habit formation** is said to have occurred. This term is generally used to refer to a less severe state than addiction.

Various disorders have been attributed to chronic use of marijuana, including chromosome breaks, personality and mental changes, cognitive problems, anxiety, and irritation when the drug is unavailable. Gynecomastia has been noted in males. Marijuana use can lead the dependent person to try other, more addicting substances for a greater euphoric effect.

MEDICINAL USES OF MARIJUANA (CANNABIS)

The medical use of cannabis has taken on a momentum of its own, often surging ahead of scientists' ability to measure the benefits of the drug accurately. Proponents claim cannabis provides relief from premenstrual syndrome, nausea and vomiting of chemotherapy, the physical wasting of acquired immunodeficiency syndrome (AIDS) and cancer, glaucoma, itching, insomnia, arthritis, depression, pain of childbirth, attention-deficit disorder, depression, bipolar disorder, post-traumatic stress disorder, peripheral neuropathy, Tourette's syndrome, epilepsy, and multiple sclerosis. Researchers are belatedly addressing this controversy to establish with scientific certainty whether such claims as pain relief, antinausea, and muscle relaxant effects have any medical validity.

Research is also needed to compare smoked marijuana and orally administered delta-9-tetrahydrocannabinol (THC), the most active ingredient. THC has been available for some time in a synthetic tablet form called dronabinol (Marinol). Theoretically, the smoked and oral forms of the drug should have the same effect, but most participants prefer the smoked form for better control of both the dosage and the onset of action. Marinol, when taken orally, requires about 2 hours to take effect, and then the ingested dose may be too high. When smoked, the chemicals in marijuana reach the bloodstream in seconds and reach the brain soon thereafter. Users can regulate the effect puff by puff. It has been found to bind to a protein that is on the surface of nerve cells.

It is believed by some health care experts that marijuana has too many effects on the body to be readily controlled as a therapeutic drug. Some of its actions are readily apparent to those who have tried it: It produces a sense of well-being, a ravenous appetite, altered time and distance perception, and talkativeness. Users also experience a disruption of short-term memory and suppressed immune defenses. Research will undoubtedly shed light on this matter in the coming years. At the present time, there are licensed and certified growers of marijuana for medical use.

dronabinol (Marinol). Dronabinol is a synthetic cannabinoid. It has been prescribed for anorexia and weight loss in AIDS patients and for chemotherapy-induced nausea and vomiting. No other conditions have been approved for treatment.
Dosage: Adults only: (Oral) Appetite stimulation—2.5 mg twice daily before lunch and supper; nausea and vomiting—5 mg/m^2 1 to 3 hours before chemotherapy and repeated every 2 to 4 hours for up to 6 doses daily.

Sativex spray. Currently approved in Canada only, this is a spray of synthetic cannabinoids that can be administered under the tongue for rapid absorption. It has been used for nausea and vomiting and is said to relieve the symptoms of multiple sclerosis.
Dosage: Adults only: (Oral Spray) 1 spray under the tongue three times daily.

COCAINE ABUSE

Although cocaine was previously thought to be a relatively "safe" recreational drug, it is now considered one of the most potent of all the addictive drugs. In 1984, the highly potent, highly addictive "crack" form of cocaine was introduced, and its availability, along with its relatively inexpensive price, has greatly increased the number of addicts. It is believed that even one use of crack cocaine makes the first-time user an addict because the urge for another "high" is so intense.

When applied locally, cocaine is a very effective anesthetic. When given systemically, cocaine is a central nervous system (CNS) stimulant with effects that are similar to those of amphetamine. It produces a strong stimulant and euphoric effect and increases pulse rate, blood pressure, and respiratory rate. Many reports have documented cocaine-related myocardial ischemic events after systemic administration of cocaine. The risk of an acute myocardial infarction is increased by a factor of 24 during the 60 minutes after the use of cocaine. Cigarette smoking after taking cocaine induces vasoconstriction of the coronary arteries and increases the risk of myocardial events. The increase in systemic arterial pressure induced by cocaine has been implicated as a cause of aortic dissection or rupture.

The user feels a heightened sense of self-confidence, clarity of thought, and alertness and increased energy and well-being. Reductions in the need for sleep and food are common. The intoxicated individual may have tremulousness, dysphoria, delirium, delusional thinking, and assaultive behavior. Withdrawal symptoms include deep depression and profound exhaustion. Suicidal behavior is common during withdrawal. Medications are now used to treat cocaine addicts and to assist in the withdrawal with replacement drugs. These include antidepressants such as desipramine, imipramine, protriptyline, and trazodone. Lithium, usually prescribed for manic-depressive disorder, has been effective, especially if combined with an antidepressant. Amino acid supplements containing tyrosine and tryptophan, when combined with an antidepressant, seem to block the cocaine high.

ALCOHOL ABUSE

Alcohol, the most common "street drug" today, is losing much of its social acceptability as the effects of its abuse become recognized. However, in contrast to other abused agents, alcohol does have some beneficial effects when used in moderation. It has been shown to increase the level of high-density lipoproteins (the "good" type of cholesterol) and reduce the risk of coronary disease. Its effect on behavior is well known, ranging from a sense of relaxation in small doses to abnormal behavior, a loss of sensorimotor control, or even coma in overdose.

As intake progresses, the abuser loses the ability to perform fine motor movements, memory and discrimination become dulled, and nausea and vomiting result. It is believed that the cumulative effects on the CNS and liver progress with each dose.

Infants born to alcohol abusers have a cluster of birth defects known as fetal alcohol syndrome. This condition is typified by a characteristic elfin facies and mental retardation. Some researchers believe that even small doses of alcohol during pregnancy may harm the fetus.

Many prescription drugs are potentiated by even small amounts of alcohol (Table 27-1). These are generally agents that have sedation as a side effect and include antihistamines, tranquilizers, some antidepressants, sleeping medications, and many muscle relaxants. Alcohol generally should be avoided when taking any prescription medication.

Table 27-1 Prescription Drugs Affected by Alcohol

Alcohol Combined With	May Cause
Sleeping medication	Rapid intoxication with small amounts of alcohol
Tranquilizers	Increased sedation
Antidepressants	Excessive drowsiness
Motion sickness medication	Mental confusion
Pain relievers	Increased sedation
Muscle relaxants	Increased sedation
Antihistamines	Increased sedation
Allergy medicine	Increased sedation
Antiangina medication	Dizziness, fainting
Antihypertensives	Lack of muscle coordination, falling
Aspirin	Increase in gastric irritation and bleeding
NSAIDs	Increased gastric pain
Potassium tablets	Increased gastric pain
Anticoagulants	Effectiveness decreased with alcohol
Metronidazole (Flagyl)	Severe reaction, similar to that of disulfiram (Antabuse)—nausea, tachycardia, dyspnea
Oral hypoglycemic agents	Increased hypoglycemia
Certain antibiotics	Efficiency decreased
Anticoagulants	Changes in the effectiveness of the drug controlling the condition
Oral hypoglycemic agents	Increased hypoglycemia
Seizure medications	Increased sedation

NSAIDs, Nonsteroidal anti-inflammatory drugs.

NICOTINE ABUSE

Cigarette smoking remains a leading cause of preventable disease and premature death in many countries of the world. Inhalation of smoke distills nicotine from the tobacco, and smoke particles carry the nicotine into the lungs where it is rapidly absorbed into the pulmonary venous circulation. Nicotine enters the arterial circulation and moves quickly from the lungs to the brain where it binds to nicotinic cholinergic receptors. Neurotransmitters subsequently are released that produce psychoactive effects that are rewarding. One of them, dopamine, signals a pleasurable experience and is critical for the reinforcement effects. As use continues, tolerance develops. The rewarding effects are diminished, and physical dependence is induced. Withdrawal symptoms occur when nicotine is withdrawn.

When a person who is addicted to nicotine stops, the urge to resume is recurrent and persists long after the withdrawal symptoms abate. With regular smoking, the smoker has "cues" for smoking, associating specific moods, situations, or environmental factors with smoking, and these can trigger relapse. Nicotine patches and gum are available over-the-counter (OTC) for self-monitored use. Other agents are available for the treatment of nicotine abuse as well.

bupropion hydrochloride (Zyban). Bupropion is also used as an antidepressant under the trade name Wellbutrin. Zyban is available as a 60-tablet packet that controls the dosage for nicotine withdrawal. Patients should begin bupropion while still smoking because effective blood levels are not attained for 1 week. A

Table 27-2 Comparative Symptoms of Drug Use

Drug	Physical Symptoms	Signs to Look for	Dangerous Effects
Inhalants (gas, aerosols)	Nausea, dizziness, headaches, lack of coordination	Odor of substance on breath, intoxication symptoms	Unconsciousness, brain damage, sudden death
Heroin, narcotics	Euphoria, drowsiness, nausea, vomiting	Pinpoint pupils, needle tracks on arms	Death from overdose, AIDS, hepatitis from needles
Cocaine, amphetamine	Talkativeness, hyperalert state, increased blood pressure	History of weight loss, hyperactivity, ulcers in nasal mucosa	Sudden death, hallucinations, paranoia
Barbiturates, alcohol, tranquilizers	Intoxication, slowed heart and respiratory rates	Capsules and pills, history of seeing more than one physician, slurred speech	Death from overdose, especially in combinations with alcohol
Hallucinogens (LSD, PCP)	Altered mood, panic, focus on detail	Capsules, blotter squares	Unpredictable and violent behavior
Marijuana	Altered perceptions, euphoria, laughing, red eyes, dry mouth	Cigarette papers, odor of burnt rope	Panic reaction, impaired memory

AIDS, acquired immunodeficiency syndrome; *LSD*, lysergic acid diethylamide; *PCP*, phencyclidine hydrochloride.

day to quit should be scheduled within the first 2 weeks of therapy. Counseling is strongly advised as well. Treatment is generally for 7 to 9 weeks and may be combined with nicotine supplements.
Dosage: Adults and adolescents: (Oral) 150 to 300 mg daily.

nicotine, inhaled (Nicotrol). This product comes as cartridges that resemble cigarettes. There seems to be some clinical improvement with the hand-to-mouth motion allowed. Each cartridge has 4 mg of nicotine, but only 2 mg is absorbed. Patients experienced less craving by day 3. The cartridges are to be used for 6 to 12 weeks, then gradually tapered over another 6- to 12-week period.
Dosage: Adults only: (Inhalation) 6 to 16 cartridges per day.

varenicline (Chantix). Patients should be instructed to set a date to quit smoking and begin varenicline 1 week before that date. Patients titrate the dosage themselves during the course of the treatment. Side effects include nausea, sleep disturbance and abnormal dreams, constipation, flatulence, and vomiting.
Dosage: Adults only: (Oral) Begin with 0.5 mg once daily; titrate up to 1 mg twice daily for about 11 weeks.

SYMPTOMS OF DRUG ABUSE

Table 27-2 presents a general method for determining the most likely agent of abuse when a patient presents with abnormal drug-induced behavior. Substance abusers may not have taken only a single substance. Drugs are often taken in combination, and they are often combined with alcohol.

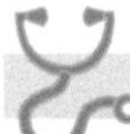

Clinical Implications

1. Drug abuse among adolescents is very common. Assessment of the patient should include questions about substance and alcohol abuse.
2. A vigorous denial of drug use should not be accepted at face value if the adolescent has risk factors for substance abuse.
3. The withdrawal symptoms from drug usage are unpleasant and may be severe and life-threatening. Many interventions can be used to ease some of the discomfort and prevent adverse outcomes.
4. After acute drug withdrawal, the addiction problem remains. Subsequent follow-up is crucial, and abstinence must be reinforced and encouraged.
5. Substance abuse can develop using only prescription medications. Questioning a patient about drug compliance and about the use of several physicians as prescription drug sources can uncover this problem.
6. There is no "safe" recreational drug.
7. The most commonly abused substance is alcohol. Society provides many situations in which alcohol abuse is approved or tolerated. Societal norms are now found to be detrimental when attempting to control alcohol abuse.
8. Cocaine is a dangerous and extremely addicting drug, particularly in the "crack" form.
9. Many drugs are useful in the treatment of cocaine and heroin addiction. These agents both reduce the craving for the drug and help prevent recurrence of the addictive pattern.
10. The symptoms of drug abuse, although not explicit in many cases, can enable the health care provider to identify patients who may be under the influence of drugs.

CRITICAL THINKING QUESTIONS

1. A patient has been brought to the emergency department after a car accident. She has a broken wrist and multiple bruises. Although you expect to find her worried and in pain, she is bright, cheerful, talkative, and alert. What other assessment may be made on this patient?
2. A patient is brought in for psychological testing by his parents. In grade school, he was an excellent student. He seems to have adjustment problems in high school, however. His grades are barely passing, he seems to have no friends, and his clothes are disheveled and dirty. What line of questioning may be appropriate here?
3. A patient calls the clinic to say she needs a new prescription for Valium. Her entire bottle of tablets was accidently thrown out with the trash. You notice on her chart that her purse was stolen just 2 weeks ago, necessitating a new prescription. She also has headaches that require numerous pain medications, and requests are often called in just before the office closes. The physicians sharing night call report numerous requests for prescription refills. What additional problems may need to be pursued?

REVIEW QUESTIONS

1. A symptom of heroin withdrawal may be:
   a. sedation.
   b. tolerance.
   c. hypertension.
   d. pupil constriction.
2. A drug frequently used in maintenance programs for narcotic addicts is:
   a. heroin.
   b. morphine.
   c. hydrocodone.
   d. methadone.
3. A commonly abused drug that is a CNS stimulant is:
   a. cocaine.
   b. procaine.
   c. Marcaine.
   d. heroin.
4. For an opioid addict, the desired sensation after taking a drug is:
   a. sedation.
   b. euphoria.
   c. hypotension.
   d. enhanced school or work performance.
5. The dreamy state after smoking marijuana may last:
   a. 30 minutes.
   b. 2 hours.
   c. 3 to 12 hours.
   d. 2 weeks.
6. A beneficial effect of alcohol when consumed in moderation is:
   a. increased blood count.
   b. decreased blood count.
   c. decreased low-density lipoproteins.
   d. increased high-density lipoproteins.
7. The most commonly abused substance is:
   a. crack cocaine.
   b. heroin.
   c. prescription drugs.
   d. alcohol.
8. Which of the following signs may occur in a person secretly abusing drugs?
   a. A calm, reflective demeanor
   b. Withdrawal from family contacts
   c. A very neat appearance
   d. Improved school or work performance
9. When an addict does not take the drug of abuse, he or she is likely to experience:
   a. tolerance.
   b. increased level of addiction.
   c. lessening of tolerance.
   d. withdrawal symptoms.
10. Alcohol can potentiate the effects of all of the following prescription drugs *except:*
    a. tranquilizers.
    b. sleeping pills.
    c. muscle relaxants.
    d. oral contraceptives.

Answers to the review questions can be found at the back of the book.

evolve Additional questions and activities can be found at *http://evolve.elsevier.com/asperheim/pharmacology.*

Herbal Therapies and Drug-Herb Interactions

CHAPTER 28

Objectives

After completing this chapter, you should be able to do the following:

1. Identify common herbal medicines and their therapeutic actions.
2. Recognize prescription drugs that commonly interact with herbal products.
3. Recognize symptoms that may indicate a patient is taking herbal medicines.
4. Understand the different ways herbs react with other drugs.
5. Assist the patient in choosing appropriate herbal remedies.

Key Terms

Health food products, p. 257
Herb, p. 257
Interaction, p. 257
Natural remedy, p. 257
Pharmacodynamic (FĂR-mĕ-kō-dī-NĂM-ĭk), p. 263
Pharmacokinetic (FĂR-mĕ-kō-kī-NĔT-ĭk), p. 263

Herbal remedies are available in any drugstore or health food store and are popular with consumers. **Health food products**—goods manufactured to supplement an individual's nutrition or wellness—seem to proliferate daily.

Historically, many of the first drugs came from plants. The word "drug" comes from the French word *drogue,* meaning herb. Aspirin, morphine, quinine, and digitalis, to mention a few currently used medications, are derived from plant sources. As skills in the laboratory have advanced, scientists have been able to extract only the active ingredients of plant sources, standardizing the dosage and reliably obtaining predictable results from each dose. In earlier forms of drugs, such as digitalis leaf, the entire leaf was pulverized and formed into a tablet. Early thyroid preparations were merely pulverized thyroid glands. In these forms, it was more difficult to determine the strength and potency of each preparation. This difficulty persists with the use of nonstandardized herbal remedies.

One of the many problems with these products used for self-healing is that consumers may waste their money because there is often no scientific basis for the sometimes outrageous claims made for these products; a more serious concern is that the products may be harmful to people with certain medical conditions. To an increasingly alarming degree, these products have been found to interfere with or alter the metabolism of many prescription drugs. The altered effect that occurs when two or more drugs and herbs are taken together is referred to as an **interaction,** and the results of such an interaction can be disastrous.

In the United States, at least five times as many people use medicinal herbs at the present time compared with at the start of the 1990s. The term **natural remedy** is used to refer to any treatment that can be used by nonprofessionals to alter a condition. The term **herb** is used to refer to any plant or plant part valued for its medicinal, savory, or aromatic qualities. Some surveys show that 35% to 48% of people surveyed had taken a natural remedy within the past year, and about one-third took them every day. Many patients do not admit to using alternative therapies because of embarrassment or fear of censure. It is very important to

Box 28-1 Rules of Thumb When Taking Herbal Therapies

- Avoid products containing multiple herbs.
- Stop all supplements 3 weeks before surgery.
- Buy from a reliable source.
- Tell the physician and pharmacist about herbs being taken.
- Children, pregnant women, and nursing mothers should not take herbs unless medically advised.
- Persons under a physician's care for any disease or taking prescription medications should not take herbs unless medically advised.

assess the use of herbal remedies as a part of any medical history (Box 28-1).

The difficulty in determining potency, pharmacologic activity, and standardization of doses in the products of the health food industry presents obvious problems. No regulatory agency such as the U.S. Food and Drug Administration (FDA) oversees herbal products. When a manufacturer or health food store claims that a natural remedy may be "good" for migraine headaches, jittery nerves, sleep, memory enhancement, colds, and so forth, there is no guarantee that the product will do what the label advertises.

The safety issues related to herbal medications are complex. There is the possibility of toxicity of the herbal constituents, the possibility of contaminants or adulterants, and the potential for interactions between herbs and prescription medications. Generalizations about the efficacy of herbal medicines are impossible. Some herbal products have shown efficacy for certain conditions, whereas others have shown no efficacy. Some manufacturers have inflated their claims, whereas others ignore the potential dangers of the substances.

With these disclaimers in mind, this chapter sorts out some of the literature and discusses common herbal and natural remedies, their side effects, and the interactions that may occur with prescription drugs. Common herbs are included; herbs with no proven medicinal value and herbs with less common usage have been omitted. When a proven therapeutic dosage is available, it is provided; in most cases, a simple list of the forms that are commercially available is provided.

HERBAL THERAPIES

aloe. Gel from the cactuslike leaves of the aloe plant has been used since prehistoric times. Rubbing aloe on skin to soothe minor burns, treat infections, and moisturize dry patches of skin is an accepted remedy. Its topical use to treat psoriasis is new and unproven, but it seems to work better than a placebo. It has been taken internally as a cathartic; this is not generally recommended because of adverse effects when aloe is taken orally, including heart arrhythmias, edema, and nephropathies.

How supplied: Capsule: 250 mg, 470 mg.
Gel: 72%, 99%.

angelica. The medicinal parts of angelica are the seeds, whole herb, and root. According to legend, angelica was revealed to a monk by an angel as a cure for plague. Although its effect on plague is unknown, it has been shown to promote circulation to the extremities and produce a warming effect on the body. Women have found it useful in the treatment of menstrual cramps. Applied externally, it gives some relief to arthritic joints. It is also useful in the local treatment of lice and has been used in folk remedies as a treatment for respiratory infections.

How supplied: Comminuted (broken or crushed into small pieces) root in a daily dose of 4.5 gm.
Tincture: 1:5 solution for internal or external use.

arnica. The medicinal parts of the arnica plant include the dried flowers, the leaves, and the dried rhizome and roots. Taken internally, it has been used to treat respiratory infections. Externally, it has been shown to be effective as an antiseptic and an analgesic. It relieves muscle spasms and joint pain when applied topically.

How supplied: Whole herb.
Tincture: 1:10 using 70% ethanol.
Ointment: 15% arnica in a neutral base.

asafetida. The oily gum-resin is the active ingredient of this plant. It has a mild intestinal disinfectant effect and has been used to treat dyspepsia and irritable bowel syndrome. Its effectiveness as a sedative is less certain. It has a putrid odor and a bitter taste—hence its nickname "devil's dung."

How supplied: Tincture: 1:5 solution; recommended dose, 20 drops orally.

black cohosh. The roots and dark-colored rhizomes of black cohosh are used to treat premenstrual tension, dysmenorrhea, and the hot flashes of menopause. The old-time remedy "Lydia Pinkham's Vegetable Compound" contained many natural ingredients, including black cohosh. It appears that at least three fractions of the herb suppress luteinizing hormone and bind to estrogen receptors. It is contraindicated during pregnancy because it is associated with an increased risk of spontaneous abortion.

How supplied: Capsule: Strengths range from 60 to 545 mg.

black root. Also known as Beaumont root and Culver root, black root is native to North America but is now cultivated worldwide. The dried rhizome and roots are used in folk medicine as a purgative and emetic. By inducing vomiting and diarrhea, it was believed to clean the blood. It is used as an antiflatulent, laxative, and bowel evacuant.
How supplied: Powder: Place 1 teaspoon of the powdered root in 1 cup of boiling water. Steep 30 minutes to make a tea. Ingest 2 to 3 oz of the tea before each meal.

blackthorn. Also known as sloe and wild plum, the flower and the berry of blackthorn are used for medicinal purposes. It is used orally to treat bloating, common cold symptoms, and upset stomach. Berry extracts have been used locally in the mouth as a gargle for throat inflammation. The berry marmalade has been used to treat upset stomach.
How supplied: Powder: Place 1 to 2 gm of the dried berries in 150 mL of boiling water; steep 10 minutes, then strain. Allow to cool, then use as a gargle twice daily.

chamomile. A cup of chamomile tea made from the flowers of the plant typically was used to relieve female anxiety. It is still a popular remedy for nervous stomach and is known for its calming effect on smooth muscle of the intestinal tract. Used externally, it relieves skin irritations and hemorrhoids. When used as a mouthwash, it may relieve the pain of toothache.
How supplied: Capsule: Strengths range from 125 to 354 mg.

Liquid: 1:4 dilution.

Tea: 3 gm of the herb in 1 cup of hot water; steep for 5 to 10 minutes, then strain.

cayenne (capsicum). Hot, spicy food may be good for your health. When taken orally, cayenne is a digestive aid. It stimulates the production of gastric juices and helps relieve gas. In addition, peppers contain vitamin C, iron, calcium, phosphorus, and B-complex vitamins. Biting into a chili pepper triggers the release of endorphins in the brain, and this mechanism is known to relieve pain. Various antimicrobial effects have been shown after administration of cayenne pepper. Capsaicin, the active ingredient of the pepper, can be applied topically to relieve the pain of diabetic neuropathy and for the topical treatment of muscle and joint disorders. It is a common ingredient in self-defense sprays. When sprayed into an attacker's eyes, it causes immediate blindness and irritation for up to 30 minutes, with no permanent effect.
How supplied: Capsule: Strengths range from 400 to 500 mg.

Cream: 0.25% and 0.75% in a neutral base.

chaparral. The chaparrals are a group of related shrubs found in the southwestern United States and in Mexico. The leaflets and twigs are used medicinally to make tea. Chaparral has long been used by Native Americans to treat respiratory infections and painful conditions such as arthritis and abdominal pain. Cancer patients have reportedly benefited from the use of chaparral tea, and this effect is still being studied. Chaparral is known to contain potent antioxidants.
How supplied: Powdered leaflets.

chondroitin sulfate. Chondroitin sulfate is a naturally occurring substance found in most mammalian cartilage. Its main use as a supplement is for relieving symptoms of arthritis. It is often combined with glucosamine in a daily supplement.
How supplied: 800 to 1200 mg orally daily alone or in combination.

comfrey. The fresh root and leaves of comfrey are used medicinally. The healing effects of this plant are attributed to its active ingredient, allantoin, an agent that promotes cell proliferation. Poultices and ointments made from comfrey have been shown to have healing and anti-inflammatory effects when applied topically. It has been taken internally for the treatment of gastritis and peptic ulcers and for inflammatory conditions. It is hepatotoxic; long-term oral use is not advisable.
How supplied: Comminuted herb.

Tea: 5 to 10 gm in 1 cup of boiling water; steep for 10 to 15 minutes.

echinacea. Extracts made from this root were favorite cold remedies before antibiotics. Laboratory studies have shown that some of the many types of echinacea available boost the immune system. Herbalists tend to prefer liquid tinctures made with alcohol because direct contact with the throat may enhance echinacea's effect. It may be taken prophylactically to prevent colds or be taken early in the course of the infection.
How supplied: Capsule: Strengths range from 100 to 500 mg.

Liquid: 120 mg/5 mL.

Tea: 1 teaspoon of the ground root in 1 cup of boiling water; steep for 10 minutes, then strain.

ephedra (ma-huang). The young canes and the dried rhizomes of this plant are the medicinal parts. It has been used for many centuries, particularly in Asia, to treat colds, asthma, and other respiratory symptoms. The use of the standardized ephedrine/pseudoephedrine has now largely supplanted use of the crude drug for respiratory diseases. It has been used in the past in proprietary diet preparations; however, these have

been removed from the market owing to the number of untoward side effects. When taken orally, there is an increased heart rate, increased blood pressure, a perceived increased energy, nasal decongestion, and bronchodilation. Toxic psychosis can be induced by this drug, as can life-threatening seizures, tachycardia, hypertension, and heart failure. Life-threatening poisonings are seen with very high dosages of the drug.
How supplied: Powdered herb.

Tea: 1 to 4 gm in 1 cup of hot water.

Tincture: 1 part drug to 4 parts alcohol/water mixture; recommended dosage 6 to 8 mL.

feverfew. Much interest has been focused on the activity of feverfew leaves in the prevention of migraine headaches, and some newer studies seem to confirm its effectiveness for this purpose. However, its effectiveness has not been confirmed when used as a digestive aid; when used to treat intestinal parasites, arthritis, and menstrual cramps; or when used as a local anesthetic. An increase in mouth ulcers has been reported with chronic use. It has been combined with ginger to stave off migraine headaches or lessen their severity.
Recommended dosage for migraine prevention: 0.2 to 0.5 mg of parthenolide (the active ingredient) daily, in fresh or dry powdered leaves.
How supplied: Capsule: Strengths range from 80 to 1000 mg.

Tea: 2 teaspoons of the herb in 1 cup of hot water; steep for 25 minutes.

garlic. Garlic has long been a staple of both medicine and cuisine the world over. In ancient times, garlic was used in poultices as an effective antibacterial. It has shown some effectiveness in decreasing cholesterol and triglyceride levels while increasing high-density lipoprotein levels. It interferes with platelet adhesiveness and reduces blood glucose levels, but studies have not shown a lowering of blood pressure, as claimed. The benefits of garlic seem to come from a compound called allicin, which breaks down into many other compounds. For the full benefit, it should be eaten raw.
How supplied: Fresh garlic bulb, dried powder, oil, and aqueous extracts.

Capsule: Strengths range from 3 to 5000 mg.

ginger. The ginger root has been used for centuries for various ailments. It is taken for heartburn, as an antiemetic, and as an anti-inflammatory. It also increases the tone and peristalsis of the intestine. It has been compared favorably with scopolamine and dimenhydrinate when used to prevent motion sickness. It may be taken in moderation for the treatment of morning sickness in pregnant women. When combined with feverfew, it has been reported to stave off migraines or lessen their severity. There are reports that the cookie called a ginger snap works almost as well as the herb itself.
How supplied: Powdered or fresh herb.

Capsule: Strengths range from 100 to 1000 mg.

Tea: 0.5 to 1 gm in 1 cup of boiling water; steep 5 minutes.

Ginkgo biloba. Studies have shown that seeds and leaves of the ginkgo tree can relieve the symptoms of intermittent claudication, increase walking performance, and diminish lower extremity pain. It has been studied in the treatment of Alzheimer's disease, and there are significant, if modest, benefits from the herb. It is known for its antioxidant effect as well. An increase in bleeding time and subdural hematomas has been observed after prolonged use, however, and it should not be taken with warfarin because it enhances the anticoagulant effect.
How supplied: Capsule: Strengths range from 30 to 500 mg.

Pulverized leaves: 3 to 6 gm as an infusion in 1 cup of hot water.

ginseng. In Chinese, *gin* means "man," and *seng* means "essence," a reflection of the root's humanlike appearance and its supposed ability to cure just about everything. It has been used as a stimulant, as a tonic, and as a treatment for menopausal hot flashes. It has been claimed to enhance cognitive function, but this has not been substantiated. It is currently used for the treatment of a subjective "lack of stamina." It should not be used with warfarin or nonsteroidal anti-inflammatory drugs (NSAIDs) because it enhances the anticoagulant effect of these agents.
How supplied: Comminuted root.

Capsule: Strengths range from 100 to 1250 mg.

glucosamine. Glucosamine is a naturally occurring aminosaccharide that is necessary for the lubricating fluids in the body and construction and maintenance of all connective tissues. Supplements are generally taken to reduce pain and immobility associated with osteoarthritis, especially in the knee joint. It is often combined with chondroitin in tablet form.
How supplied: Tablet: 1500 mg daily alone or in combination.

goldenseal. The medicinal parts of goldenseal are the air-dried rhizome and root fibers, which contain the active alkaloids hydrastine, berberine, and canadine. It is

poorly absorbed when given orally but has shown some effectiveness in the treatment of bacterial infections, notably with *Salmonella, Shigella,* and *Klebsiella* species, as well as in vitro activity against the intestinal parasites *Giardia lamblia, Trichomonas,* and *Entamoeba histolytica*. It has been used in the past to treat eye infections, notably trachoma. It also has hypotensive, antisecretory, antitumor, and sedative properties. Prolonged use can cause digestive disorders and constipation, mucous membrane irritation, and occasionally hallucinations. It has an antagonistic effect on the anticoagulant activity of heparin.
How supplied: Capsule: Strengths range from 500 to 1000 mg.

Extract: 5% hydrastine.

gotu kola. The fresh and dried leaves of this plant may be taken orally to relieve anxiety, depression, and fatigue. It is believed to bind with gamma-aminobutyric acid (GABA), which is a neurotransmitter in the brain. When applied topically, it appears to speed up wound healing and has an anti-inflammatory effect.
How supplied: Capsule: 60 mg of the extract two to three times daily.

Topical: 1% cream.

grapeseed extract. This product is obtained as a byproduct of wine manufacturing. Its components are members of a group called flavinoids. These substances are claimed to have antioxidant, vasodilatory, and antiplatelet aggregation properties. Grapeseed extract is generally taken to treat venous and capillary disorders such as retinopathies, venous insufficiency, and vascular fragility. It is used in folk medicine for preventing cardiovascular diseases and for the neuropathy of diabetes.
How supplied: Capsule: 150 to 300 mg daily.

green tea. The tea plant has leathery, dark, green leaves that have been used medicinally for more than 5000 years to promote digestion, improve mental faculties, decrease flatulence, and regulate body temperature. When the leaves are fermented and oxidized, black and oolong teas are made. Green tea has six times the antioxidant activity as the black teas. The improvement in mental facilities is due to the caffeine content.
How supplied: One teaspoon steeped in 1 cup of hot water.

hops. This perennial plant has male and female flowers. The female, conelike flowering parts are used medicinally. It has been used as an appetite stimulant, as treatment of neuropathies and headaches, and as a sedative. Its most common use is in the commercial preparation of beer, to which it imparts the characteristic flavor.
How supplied: Comminuted herb.

Liquid extract: 1:1 in 45% ethanol.

Tea: 1 teaspoon in 1 cup of boiling water; steep for 10 to 15 minutes.

horse chestnut. The seeds and leaves of the horse chestnut are used medicinally. When taken internally, horse chestnut has been noted to reduce vascular permeability and exert a vascular tightening effect. It is used to treat lower extremity edema caused by venous insufficiency. Horse chestnut has a coumarin component; it enhances the effect of coumarin given therapeutically. Long-term use is not advisable because of the side effects of liver and kidney toxicity. It may be used topically for the treatment of hemorrhoids.
How supplied: Capsule: Strengths range from 250 to 485 mg.

Tincture: 1:1 in 75% ethanol.

juniper. The berry cones of juniper, when administered orally, act as a diuretic. It also has an antihypertensive effect. The most common uses are as a flavoring for gin and as an ingredient in bath salts. Prolonged oral administration may result in nephrotoxicity.
How supplied: Comminuted berries.

Capsule: 515 mg.

Tea: 0.5 gm in 1 cup of boiling water; steep for 10 to 15 minutes.

kava kava. South Pacific islanders have made a relaxing drink from the dried rhizome and roots of the kava plant for centuries. Ceremonial use has documented euphoria, muscle weakness, and, in higher doses, deep sleep. Several more recent, well-documented studies have shown that kava kava can relieve anxiety and stress. When chewed, it causes numbness in the mouth. Several cases of acute liver failure and cirrhosis have occurred following regular use. It should not be used by persons with underlying liver problems or persons who frequently drink alcoholic beverages.
How supplied: Capsule: Strengths range from 100 to 500 mg.

milk thistle. The active ingredients of the milk thistle seed are silymarin and silybin. In vivo tests have shown that there is increased protein synthesis in the liver cells after taking this agent owing to increased activity of ribosomal RNA. This increased protein synthesis reportedly activates the regenerative capacity of the liver through cell development. Hepatic protection may also be attributed to its

antioxidant properties and its alteration of the liver cell membrane, preventing the entrance of toxins into the cell. It is used as an adjunct in the treatment of alcoholic cirrhosis and hepatitis. It has been used in the treatment of *Amanita* mushroom poisoning. There is no evidence that it has a direct antiviral effect on the hepatitis virus; hepatitis B surface antigen levels remain unchanged. It is believed to aid in restoring hepatic function after viral or other damage.
Dosage: 140 mg of silymarin (active ingredient) three times daily.
How supplied: Capsule: Strengths range from 70 to 1050 mg.

red clover. The dried flower heads of the clover may be taken internally to treat coughs and respiratory conditions. It is used externally to treat chronic skin conditions such as psoriasis and eczema. It has been used with other herbs as the "red clover combination" for the treatment of cancer. Its usefulness as an antineoplastic has not been proved. Red clover produces a coumarinlike anticoagulant effect, causing an additive effect with warfarin. It also enhances the antiplatelet effect of NSAIDs.
How supplied: Comminuted herb.
Liquid extract: 1:1 prepared in 25% ethanol.
Tea: 4 gm in 1 cup of boiling water; steep for 10 to 15 minutes.

red yeast rice extract. These yeast cells grow on the surfaces of regular, refined white rice grains, where they thrive, causing the rice to attain a deep red shade. The yeast cells are then killed so the rice can be pulverized into a uniform powder. Red yeast rice extract has been used in wine making and to block cholesterol production in the body, particularly the low-density lipoprotein component; it reduces triglycerides as well. It should not be taken in the presence of liver disease, and it is contraindicated in pregnancy.
How supplied: Capsule: Two 600 mg capsules orally daily.

saffron. Saffron has been taken to stimulate the gastric juice and to treat headaches, vomiting, and fever. It has been studied more recently for its effect on depression when taken twice daily, usually added to rice.
How supplied: Powder: ½ teaspoon added to rice twice daily.

saw palmetto. The berries of the saw palmetto, a type of palm tree native to Florida, are the active parts of this plant. The mechanism of action for the effect of saw palmetto in suppression of the symptoms of benign prostatic hypertrophy is poorly understood. It is believed to inhibit testosterone reductase, an enzyme that converts testosterone to 5-alpha-testosterone in the prostate. It reduces the symptoms of benign prostatic hypertrophy, including urinary hesitancy, nocturia, and frequent urination. It also has been shown to reduce blood levels of prostate-specific antigen. Concomitant prostate carcinoma should always be considered and ruled out when symptoms of prostate obstruction are present.
How supplied: Capsule: Strengths range from 80 to 1000 mg.

slippery elm. The dried inner rind of the bark of slippery elm is used medicinally by many native peoples. The active ingredient is the mucilage that is derived from the inner bark when it is soaked in water. This substance may be used locally as a demulcent to treat many topical conditions, including ulcers, wounds, abscesses, and toothaches. Taken internally, it is a soothing drink that relieves irritations of the mucous membrane.
How supplied: Comminuted herb.
Capsule: 370 mg.

St. John's wort. The medicinal parts of St. John's wort include the fresh buds and flowers, but all aboveground parts of the plant may be used. In studies completed in Germany, it has been shown to treat mild to moderate depression effectively. It is now a component of various herbal remedies for the treatment of anxiety and depression. Its use in combination with selective serotonin reuptake inhibitors and tricyclic antidepressants is being studied.
How supplied: Capsule: Strengths range from 125 to 1000 mg.
Tea: 2 to 3 gm of dried herb in 1 cup of hot water.
Liquid: 300 mg/5 mL.
Transdermal: 900 mg/24 hr.

tea tree oil. This oil comes from the leaves of the Australian tree *Melaleuca alternifolia*. It is available as a pure oil and is an ingredient in skin creams and gels, toothpaste, dental floss, mouthwash, deodorant, shampoos, and toothpicks. It is a topical antifungal and antibiotic for infections of the skin and mucous membranes. Tea tree oil is used as a topical treatment for acne, tinea pedis, head lice, cradle cap, gingivitis, canker sores, warts, and scabies, and in a douche for nonspecific vaginitis.
How supplied: For toenail onychomycosis (a fungal disease of the nails)—100% oil applied to toenails twice daily. For acne or other topical conditions—5% to 15% oil preparations three or four times daily.

turmeric. Turmeric is grown naturally in India and is often used as a seasoning for curry. It has been observed that the incidence of Alzheimer's disease in India is the lowest of any country and is less than one-fourth the incidence in the United States. Some studies have found that turmeric breaks up amyloid deposits in the brain, the abnormal protein that builds up in Alzheimer's disease. It also has antihyperlipidemic, anti-inflammatory, and antioxidative activity. Stomach complaints can occur with regular use. Topically, it may be used for skin ulcers and pruritic rashes.

How supplied: Powder: 0.5 to 1 gm of powder in boiling water for tea. May be added to curry or applied topically. Usual dose is 1.5 to 3 gm daily.

valerian. Hippocrates and Galen both used the root of the valerian plant as a sedative to treat insomnia; it is still used effectively for this purpose today. Its main disadvantage seems to be its disagreeable smell. It is often combined with hops or St. John's wort in commercial products.

Recommended dosage for insomnia: 300 to 600 mg 2 hours before bedtime.

How supplied: Capsule: Strengths range from 100 to 1000 mg.

Tea: 1 teaspoon (3 to 5 gm) of powdered root in 1 cup of hot water; steep for 10 to 15 minutes, then strain.

white willow. The bark of young (2- to 3-year-old) willow branches is harvested for medicinal use during early spring. The active ingredient is salicin, the precursor of salicylic acid, which is itself the precursor of acetylsalicylic acid (aspirin). It has antirheumatic, anti-inflammatory, and antipyretic effects. The tannin component of the bark has astringent properties on mucous membranes. White willow also reduces platelet aggregation similar to aspirin. It should not be taken with warfarin or NSAIDs.

How supplied: Comminuted herb.

Tea: 2 to 3 gm in cold water; bring to a boil, then steep for 5 minutes.

DRUG-HERB INTERACTIONS

It is essential that health care professionals know what herbal preparations a patient is taking. Queries about the use of over-the-counter (OTC) or proprietary drugs should be part of every medical history. If the patient senses that the health care worker is judgmental, a full and accurate history may not be obtained.

Herbal medicines interact with drugs in two general ways: pharmacokinetically and pharmacodynamically. **Pharmacokinetic** effects include alterations in drug absorption, distribution, metabolism, or excretion. These biologic changes may act to increase or decrease the amount of drug available to have the desired effect. **Pharmacodynamic** interactions change the way a drug affects a tissue or organ system; this may result in increased or decreased effect on the targeted end organ for the drug. Table 28-1 lists some known drug-herb interactions.

It is important to ask the right questions when interviewing a patient about the use of drugs and herbal remedies to avoid possible drug-herb interactions. To obtain the necessary information, the health care provider may include the following topics in the patient interview:

- Remember to inquire about lifestyle, such as smoking. Smoking may alter the metabolism of certain drugs such as theophylline.
- Ask about diet, including specific types of food the patient eats and the quantity. Diets with excessive amounts of green leafy vegetables may have sufficient amounts of vitamin K to interfere with the effects of warfarin (Coumadin). Diet is also important for patients taking monoamine oxidase inhibitors because of their need to avoid foods with high tyramine content, such as cheese and wine.
- Ask to see all of the prescription medications that a patient is taking. Patients can often remember only part of a list of medications.
- Ask what the patient may take when he or she has a headache, indigestion, pain, or the need for a laxative. Ask specifically about herbs or natural remedies.
- Ask about alcohol consumption in a nonthreatening manner. The physician should be notified if the patient consumes more than four alcoholic drinks per day.
- Medication compliance is an issue, particularly for older patients. The spouse or caregiver should be questioned about the reliability of the patient managing her or his own medications.

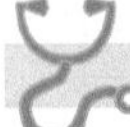

Clinical Implications

1. Herbal remedies should not be disregarded as useless; many have significant pharmacologic actions.
2. A careful history should be taken to ascertain whether a patient is taking any herbal or other proprietary remedies. Patients may not answer questions truthfully if they think the health care provider is being judgmental about herbal remedies.
3. Plants have been the source of many commonly used pharmacologic agents as well as herbal remedies.
4. The health care provider should be particularly aware of the many herbal remedies that may cause bleeding problems when the patient is taking warfarin or NSAIDs.
5. Herbal remedies may have active ingredients that are similar to commonly used drugs.
6. Many herbs alter the metabolism of another drug in the body. This alteration may be an increase or a decrease in the potency of the other drug.

Table 28-1 Drug-Herb Interactions

Herb	Reduces Effect	Enhances Effect	Avoid Use with
aloe		Potassium loss of diuretics	
black cohosh		Antihypertensives, diuretics, antiplatelet action of NSAIDs, warfarin	Pregnancy
capsicum		Antihypertensives	
chamomile		Sedatives, warfarin, antiplatelet action of NSAIDs	
comfrey			Preexisting liver disease
echinacea	Immunosuppressants, cyclosporine, azathioprine		Autoimmune disorders, multiple sclerosis
ephedra	Antihypertensives, phenothiazines	Theophylline, epinephrine, caffeine, decongestants, stimulants	Hypertension, diabetes, psychiatric disorders, cardiac arrhythmias, MAO inhibitors
feverfew		Antiplatelet action of NSAIDs, warfarin	Pregnancy, lactation
garlic		Antiplatelet action of NSAIDs, warfarin	
Ginkgo biloba		Antiplatelet action of NSAIDs, warfarin	Tricyclic antidepressants
ginger		Antiplatelet action of NSAIDs, warfarin, digitalis	Gallstones, bleeding disorders
ginseng		Antiplatelet action of NSAIDs, warfarin, phenelzine	Diabetes, MAO inhibitors
goldenseal	Heparin	Antihypertensives, sedatives	G6PD deficiency
hawthorn		Digitalis, antihypertensives	Pregnancy, lactation
horse chestnut		Antiplatelet action of NSAIDs, warfarin	
juniper berries		Lithium, diuretics	Preexisting liver disease
kava kava	Levodopa and other anti-Parkinson drugs	Sedatives, hypnotics, antihistamines, alcohol, alprazolam	Depressive disorders; pregnancy, lactation
red clover		Antiplatelet action of NSAIDs, warfarin	
saw palmetto	Estrogens, androgens, adrenergic drugs, oral contraceptives		Pregnancy, lactation
St. John's wort	Theophylline, coumarin, digoxin, indinavir, cyclosporine, oral contraceptives	SSRIs, tricyclic antidepressants	MAO inhibitors
valerian		Sedatives, hypnotics, antihistamines, benzodiazepines	Pregnancy, lactation
white willow	probenecid	Antiplatelet action of NSAIDs, warfarin, phenytoin, methotrexate	Preexisting bleeding tendencies

G6PD, glucose-6-phosphate dehydrogenase; *MAO,* monoamine oxidase; *NSAIDs,* nonsteroidal anti-inflammatory drugs; *SSRIs,* selective serotonin reuptake inhibitors.

7. Herbal remedies may affect many diseases such as hypertension, diabetes, and immune disorders. The health care provider needs to advise patients with these diseases not to take herbal remedies without medical advice.
8. There is often an enhanced feeling of well-being when a person is taking proprietary medications. These should not be discouraged unless there is evidence that a combination may be harmful.
9. Many herbal remedies do not exert their advertised effect. There is no regulation to determine truth in advertising with regard to herbs.
10. The health care provider should become familiar with common herbal formulations and advise patients regarding which may be helpful and which to avoid.

CRITICAL THINKING QUESTIONS

1. A patient arrives at the physician's office to have his rash treated. You notice dark red patches on his forearms. He has a previous history of thromboembolic disorders and has been maintained for 9 months on a low dose of warfarin without any previous changes in his international normalized ratios, which have always been maintained in the optimal range of 2.5 to 3.5. What could be the cause of the rash? What questions would you ask the patient?
2. A patient arrives with some new herbal remedies he has begun taking. These are hawthorn, goldenseal, and angelica. You notice his regular medicines are verapamil (Calan SR), hydrochlorothiazide (HydroDIURIL), and Colace. Would there be any conflicts here? What do you advise?
3. A generally healthy older patient who takes no medications except calcium and vitamins complains of chronic insomnia. She does not want to take any prescription sedatives, fearing that they may be habit-forming. What herbal remedies may be recommended?

REVIEW QUESTIONS

1. The term *herb* may be applied to:
   - **a.** any drug.
   - **b.** any plant part used in medicine.
   - **c.** any plant.
   - **d.** a drug considered for prescription use.
2. A claim made about the intended use of an herbal product may:
   - **a.** not be trusted at all.
   - **b.** not be proven by established medical standards.
   - **c.** be believed in its entirety.
   - **d.** be considered safe because the herbal product is a natural drug.
3. A product used to relieve the symptoms of menopause is:
   - **a.** asafetida.
   - **b.** cayenne.
   - **c.** black cohosh.
   - **d.** angelica.
4. Garlic has been shown to:
   - **a.** lower cholesterol levels.
   - **b.** treat pain.
   - **c.** treat heartburn.
   - **d.** help with weight loss.
5. An herb used as a cold remedy is:
   - **a.** ginger.
   - **b.** chaparral.
   - **c.** echinacea.
   - **d.** feverfew.
6. A sedative drink can be made from:
   - **a.** *Ginkgo biloba.*
   - **b.** kava kava.
   - **c.** tea tree oil.
   - **d.** saw palmetto.
7. Which herb is thought to relieve prostatic hypertrophy?
   - **a.** Kava kava
   - **b.** Slippery elm
   - **c.** Red clover
   - **d.** Saw palmetto
8. Which herb was a precursor of aspirin?
   - **a.** White willow
   - **b.** Valerian
   - **c.** Asafetida
   - **d.** Cayenne
9. Which herb should *not* be taken with warfarin?
   - **a.** Valerian
   - **b.** Aloe
   - **c.** White willow
   - **d.** Kava kava
10. When a patient is scheduled for surgery, all herbs should be discontinued:
    - **a.** 1 day before surgery.
    - **b.** 7 days before surgery.
    - **c.** 3 weeks before surgery.
    - **d.** not at all.

Answers to the review questions can be found at the back of the book.

evolve Additional questions and activities can be found at *http://evolve.elsevier.com/asperheim/pharmacology.*

CHAPTER 29

Interactions

Objectives

After completing this chapter, you should be able to do the following:

1. Name the different types of drug interactions.
2. Advise patients about the various over-the-counter (OTC) medications and how they may affect prescription drugs.
3. Realize that herbs and other natural products may be harmful when combined with various medications.
4. Make older adults aware of multiple-drug adverse reactions.
5. Realize that vague or unusual symptoms may be due to drug toxicity.

Key Terms

Drug-condition interactions, p. 267
Drug-drug (or drug-herb) interaction, p. 266
Drug-food (or beverage) interaction, p. 267
Drug toxicity, p. 266

Drug toxicity is a common and increasingly significant health problem. This problem often goes unrecognized by both physicians and patients who do not suspect it as the cause of new symptoms such as disorientation, blurred vision, memory loss, syncope, and falls. These symptoms may be attributed to a new medical condition, which, predictably, may result in more tests and more medications.

The complaint of "I just don't feel well" may be due to confusion or dehydration, a viral illness, changes in blood pressure, or changes in mental ability. Drug toxicity should always be kept in mind, especially if the patient is taking multiple medications. **Drug toxicity** refers to adverse reactions that may result when a medication dose is too high or when something happens to interfere with the person's ability to metabolize the drug. The more drugs a patient takes, the more likely one of the drugs will build up to a toxic level.

Patients may see multiple physicians and use multiple pharmacies. Changing this situation by collecting all specialists' records in one place and instructing the patient to the use one pharmacy only may reveal some previously unforeseen problems. Most pharmacies have computer programs that alert the pharmacist to drug incompatibilities or issue warnings based on the groups of drugs a patient is taking.

Most drugs are metabolized by the liver and excreted by the kidney. In an older patient, the ability of these organs to process drugs progressively declines, and a drug that had been handled well in the past may begin to cause problems. Specific interactions are discussed with the individual classes of drugs. These should be examined carefully when the drugs are discussed.

THREE BROAD CLASSES OF INTERACTIONS

DRUG-DRUG (OR DRUG-HERB) INTERACTIONS

A **drug-drug (or drug-herb) interaction** occurs when one drug modifies the effectiveness of another drug by interfering with an enzyme reaction. An example of a drug-drug interaction is fluoxetine inhibiting the cancer suppressive effect of tamoxifen. Omeprazole has been shown to interfere with the antiplatelet agent clopidogrel.

Drug-drug interactions can also show additive effects of drugs. This may be an additive effect for an unwanted side effect (i.e., aspirin and ibuprofen may be additive for gastric irritation and ulcer formation).

The additive effect may be on the desired effect of the drug (i.e., aspirin taken with coumarin causes increased bleeding problems). Alcohol is additive with sedatives or narcotic pain medications. Sedation may increase to respiratory depression in high doses.

Another way drug-drug interactions occur is through excretory interference. The ability of the body to excrete one drug may be inhibited by another agent. Examples of drug interactions are presented in boxes and tables throughout this text. Following is a list of the boxes and tables for easy reference:

Box 7-1: Related Drugs That May Cross-React with Sulfonamides, p. 57
Box 11-1: Drugs That Interact with Coumarin, p. 99
Table 14-1: Drug Interactions with Lithium, p. 132
Table 14-3: Drug Interactions with the Selective Serotonin Reuptake Inhibitors (SSRIs), p. 134
Box 24-1: Common Drug Interactions in Older Adults, p. 228
Table 27-1: Prescription Drugs Affected by Alcohol, p. 254
Table 28-1: Drug-Herb Interactions, p. 264

DRUG-FOOD (OR BEVERAGE) INTERACTIONS

Food and beverages can also change the effectiveness of a drug. A **drug-food (or beverage) interaction** occurs when some drugs and certain foods or beverages are taken at the same time. Grapefruit or grapefruit juice may interfere with the action of calcium channel blocker antihypertensives. Milk and milk products inactivate the antibiotic tetracycline. A full stomach inhibits absorption of many oral antibiotics.

DRUG-CONDITION INTERACTIONS

A **drug-condition interaction** occurs when a preexisting health condition is made worse when taking a drug. A drug that must be metabolized by the liver may increase to toxic amounts if the patient has liver disease caused by alcoholic cirrhosis, hepatitis, or some general anesthetics. Elevation in liver enzymes should raise awareness for liver damage. Similarly, severe kidney disease from diabetes or other causes may interfere with excretion of many drugs. Serum elevation of blood urea nitrogen or creatinine should alert the health care provider to this possibility.

Drug sensitivity often is caused by certain body conditions (i.e., pregnancy or older age). Many cancer drugs would be harmful to a fetus and cannot be prescribed to a pregnant woman. An older adult can be very sensitive to sedatives, which may cause disorientation and falls, even in customary adult doses.

DRUGS WITH THE HIGHEST POTENTIAL FOR HARM

Three classes of medications account for almost half of emergency department visits for adverse drug reactions: (1) anticoagulants (clopidogrel, warfarin); (2) antidiabetic agents (glipizide, insulin, metformin); and (3) so-called narrow therapeutic agents (digoxin, lithium, phenytoin, theophylline, valproic acid). Other medications that may cause problems, particularly in older adults, include sedatives, tranquilizers, aspirin, nonsteroidal anti-inflammatory drugs, and pain medications.

HOW TO AVOID DRUG TOXICITY REACTIONS

1. Patients should know all the medications they are taking. A list of all medications can be carried in a purse or wallet for quick reference.
2. Patients should never take any herb or over-the-counter (OTC) drug without first discussing it with the physician. Some OTC medications and information about their interactions are presented in Table 29-1.

Table 29-1 Over-the-Counter Drug Categories with Cautions for Patients

Category	Drug Interaction Cautions for Patients
Caffeine stimulants	Limit foods and beverages that also have caffeine; nervousness, irritability, tachycardia, and sleeplessness may result
Cough medicine	Additive with sedatives and tranquilizers; check with physician if you have glaucoma or prostate urinary retention
Bronchodilators	Check with physician if you have heart disease, hypertension, or thyroid problems, or are receiving prescription medications for asthma
Laxatives	Do not use with abdominal pain; phosphates are dangerous for kidney disease
Nasal decongestants	May aggravate heart disease, thyroid disease, hypertension, or urinary retention
Nicotine replacement, gum, or patches	Do not use if you continue to smoke or take prescription drugs to stop smoking; dosages of medications for depression, asthma, hypertension, or heart disease may need adjustment
Nighttime sleep aids	Additive with sedatives and tranquilizers; check with physician if you have emphysema, glaucoma, or urinary retention; avoid alcoholic beverages
Pain relievers	Avoid alcoholic beverages; read label to avoid overdose
Topical acne products	Check with physician if you are also using prescription medications for acne; dry or irritated skin may result

3. Patients should always read the package insert that comes with OTC medication *before* taking it. Labels or package inserts have information on the active ingredients, use of the drug, warnings about when the drug should not be used, and directions about the length of time the drug should be taken and the amount of drug that may be safely used.
4. Patients should get blood tests to detect drug serum levels when drug toxicity is suspected.

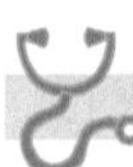

Clinical Implications

1. Older adults may have declining organ function and may be particularly susceptible to adverse drug reactions.
2. All patients should be asked about the OTC drugs they take, and a complete list should be made of their medications.
3. Just because a product is "natural" does not mean it is harmless to all people.
4. All patients taking prescription medications should carry a list of the medications and dosages with them at all times.
5. Cognitive impairment or new symptoms such as an impaired gait may be due to an adverse reaction to a drug.
6. Blood tests for liver and kidney function should be documented for all patients.
7. If blood tests for liver and kidney function are abnormal, the list of medications the patient is taking should be carefully evaluated.
8. Even small or moderate amounts of alcohol may adversely affect patients receiving many medications.
9. Children have been harmed by giving overdoses of OTC medications. All labels and dosages should be observed, including the length of time a medication may be taken before seeking medical advice.
10. The first trimester of pregnancy is the most critical time for adverse effects on the fetus.

CRITICAL THINKING QUESTIONS

1. An older adult presents to the clinic with many bruises on his body caused by some recent falls. He states his medication has not changed recently. He is taking lisinopril, atorvastatin, and oxybutynin. When questioned, he says he has taken an OTC sleeping pill for insomnia since his wife died. What advice should be given, and what tests may be ordered?
2. A patient is admitted to the hospital with a swollen warm knee and multiple purple ecchymoses on his extremities. He is taking coumarin, digoxin, losartan, and hydrochlorothiazide. He said sometimes he takes Advil for his arthritis pain, and the knee seems to be getting worse.
3. A patient who is a heavy smoker wants medication to help him stop smoking. He has heard that you get "bad dreams" from Chantix, and he wants a strong sleeping pill so he does not have to worry about that. What advice should be given?

REVIEW QUESTIONS

1. Toxicity from a drug can cause:
   a. blurred vision.
   b. disorientation.
   c. a complaint of "I don't feel well" from the patient.
   d. all of the above.

2. Consumption of spinach can decrease the effectiveness of warfarin (Coumadin). What type of drug interaction does this represent?
   a. Drug-drug
   b. Drug-herb
   c. Drug-food
   d. Drug-condition

3. Acetaminophen is known to have adverse effects on the liver even at normal doses. A patient who has liver disease needs to be cautious when taking acetaminophen because of what type of drug interaction?
   a. Drug-drug
   b. Drug-herb
   c. Drug-food
   d. Drug-condition

4. Which of the following classes of medications have the lowest potential to cause harm?
   a. Anticoagulants
   b. Antibiotics
   c. Antidiabetics
   d. Narrow therapeutic agents

5. To avoid drug toxicities, a patient should:
   a. get prescriptions filled at many different pharmacies.
   b. see many different prescribers.
   c. self-treat with OTC and herbal preparations.
   d. have a current drug list that is shared with all health care providers.

6. An example of a patient who is at a low risk of having an adverse drug reaction is:
   a. a 21-year-old patient who frequently mixes alcohol with cough and cold medications.
   b. an 89-year-old woman who is taking 10 medications and has memory problems.
   c. a 35-year-old man who is in good health and reviews his prescription and OTC medications with his physician and pharmacist.
   d. a 24-month-old child who is given a larger than recommended dose of Tylenol.

7. A nasal decongestant may adversely affect all of the following diseases *except:*
   a. osteoarthritis.
   b. hypertension.
   c. heart disease.
   d. thyroid disease.

8. Which of the following agents is most likely to cause dry or irritated skin?
   a. acetaminophen (pain reliever)
   b. diphenhydramine (sleep aid)
   c. benzoyl peroxide (topical acne product)
   d. docusate (laxative)

9. Which of the following agents is most likely to cause drowsiness?
   a. acetaminophen (pain reliever)
   b. diphenhydramine (sleep aid)
   c. benzoyl peroxide (topical acne product)
   d. docusate (laxative)

10. Which of the following agents is most likely to cause abdominal pain?
    a. acetaminophen (pain reliever)
    b. diphenhydramine (sleep aid)
    c. benzoyl peroxide (topical acne product)
    d. docusate (laxative)

Answers to the review questions can be found at the back of the book.

evolve Additional questions and activities can be found at *http://evolve.elsevier.com/asperheim/pharmacology.*

Glossary

A

abortifacient Agent that induces abortion.

ACE inhibitor Agent that inhibits angiotensin-converting enzyme (ACE).

acetylcholine (ăs-ĕ-tĭl-KŌ-lēn) Neurotransmitter agent widely distributed in body tissues, with a primary function of mediating synaptic activity of the nervous system and skeletal muscles.

achlorhydria (Ā-klŏr-HĪ-drē-ĕ) Absence of hydrochloric acid in the stomach.

acidosis (ĂS-ĭ-DŌ-sĭs) Decrease in the alkali reserve of the blood, notably in the bicarbonates, with lowering of the blood pH.

acne Inflammatory eruption of the skin.

active immunity Production of natural antibodies against an antigen, or attenuated microorganism, injected into the body.

addiction State in which the use of drugs is compulsive; withdrawal symptoms occur if the drug is withdrawn.

Addison's disease Adrenal insufficiency, which is fatal if not treated with corticosteroid hormones. Symptoms include bronzing of the skin, emaciation, and anemia.

additive effect Combined effect of two drugs that is equal to the sum of the effects of each drug taken alone.

adjunct Additional drug or chemical substance used to increase the efficacy or safety of a primary drug or to facilitate its action.

adrenergic (ĂD-rĭ-NŪR-jĭk) Agent that produces stimulating effects on the sympathetic nervous system (adrenaline-like effects).

adrenergic blocking agent Drug that interferes with adrenergic, or sympathetic nervous system, actions.

adverse or untoward effect Action, usually negative, that is different from the planned effect.

aerosols Active pharmaceutical agents in a pressurized container.

agranulocytosis (ā-GRĂN-yū-lō-sī-TŌ-sĭs) Toxic condition often caused by reactions to drug therapy in which a certain type of white blood cell—cells with very small granules in the cell body—is deficient or absent.

AIDS Acquired immunodeficiency syndrome.

alkaloid (ĂL-kĕ-loĭd) Organic substance, basic in reaction, often the active ingredient of plant medicinals.

alkalosis Increase in the bicarbonate content of the blood, with a subsequent increase in the blood pH.

alkylating (ĂL-kĭ-LĀ-tĭng) **agent** Any substance that contains an alkyl radical and is capable of replacing a free hydrogen atom in an organic compound.

allergen Substance capable of producing an allergic reaction.

allergic reaction Untoward reaction that develops after an individual has taken a drug.

allergy Hypersensitivity reaction provoked by a sensitizing agent, or allergen.

alopecia Baldness or loss of hair.

amide Substance derived from ammonia.

amino acid Organic acid composed of carbon, hydrogen, and nitrogen. Amino acids are components of protein molecules.

analgesia (ăn-ăl-JĒ-zē-ă) The relief of pain.

analgesic Substance used to relieve pain.

analog Substance structurally or chemically similar to another related drug or chemical but that has different effects.

anaphylaxis (ĂN-ĕ-fĭ-LĂK-sĭs) Severe, life-threatening allergic reaction accompanied by vasodilation, lowered blood pressure, and shock.

androgen (ĂN-drĕ-jĭn) Any steroid hormone that increases male characteristics.

anemia Reduction in the hemoglobin content or number of red blood cells.

anesthesia (ăn-ĕs-THĒ-zē-ă) Loss of sensation resulting from pharmacologic depression of the central nervous system.

anesthetic (ăn-ĕs-THĔ-tĭk), **general** Agent that induces analgesia, then unconsciousness.

anesthetic, local Agent, usually injected, that interferes with local nerve transmission and produces deadening, or anesthesia, of a small area of the body.

angina pectoris (ăn-JĪ-nĕ PĔK-tĕr-ĭs) Severe chest pain resulting from ischemia of the cardiac muscle; it may radiate to other locations, notably the left shoulder or arm.

animal products Primarily glandular products that are currently obtained from animal sources (e.g., thyroid hormone, insulin).

anorexia (ĂN-ō-RĔK-sē-ă) Loss of appetite.

anorexia nervosa Eating disorder in which there is an aberration of eating patterns, severe weight loss, and malnutrition.

antacid Agent that destroys gastric acids, either in whole or in part, by neutralizing or adsorbing them and rendering them inactive.

antagonism Combined effect of two drugs that is less than the effect of either drug taken alone.

antagonist Drug that opposes a bodily system or expected effect.

antibiotic Agent that kills or inhibits microorganisms.

antibody Substance produced by the body as a reaction to the intrusion of a foreign compound, or antigen; the antibody is designed to counteract or neutralize the offending antigen.

anticoagulant (ăn-tĭ-kō-ĂG-ū-lănt) Substance used to delay blood clotting.

anticonvulsant (ăn-tĭ-kŏn-VŬL-sănt) Substance used to prevent or treat seizures.

antidepressant (ăn-tĭ-dĕ-PRĔS-ănt) Drug used to produce mood elevation or mild central nervous system stimulation.
antidote (ĂN-tĭ-dōt) Agent that neutralizes a substance or counteracts its effects.
antiemetic (ĂN-tĭ-ĭ-MĔT-ĭk) Agent that prevents vomiting.
antigen Any substance that stimulates the production of antibodies in the body or any substance that reacts with previously formed antibodies.
antihistamine (ĂN-tĭ-HĬS-tă-mĭn) Agent that prevents or diminishes the pharmacologic effects of histamine, used in the treatment of allergy-type syndromes.
antihypertensive (ăn-tĭ-hī-pĕr-TĔN-sĭv) **drug** Agent used in the treatment of high blood pressure.
antilipidemic (ĂN-tĭ-LĬP-ĭ-DĒ-mĭk) **drug** Drug that reduces the amount of lipids in the serum.
antimetabolite (ăn-tĭ-mĕ-TĂB-ĕ-līt) Substance that competes with, replaces, or antagonizes a bodily function.
antineoplastic (ĂN-tĭ-NĒ-ō-PLĂS-tĭk) **drug** Agent used in the treatment of cancer.
antioxidant (ĂN-tĭ-ŎK-sĭ-dĕnt) Agent that inhibits oxidation and neutralizes the effects of free radicals.
antiplatelet (ăn-tĭ-PLĀ T-lĭt) **agent** Agent that destroys platelets or inhibits their function.
antiprostaglandin (ăn-tĭ-PRŎS-tă-GLĂN-dĭn) Agent that counteracts the effect of a prostaglandin on a specific tissue.
antipyretic (ĂN-tĭ-pī-RĔT-ĭk) Substance used to lower body temperature.
antiseptic Substance that inhibits the growth of microorganisms.
antispasmodic Agent used to decrease peristaltic activity of the gastrointestinal tract.
anxiolytic (ĀNGK-sē-ō-LĬT-ĭk) **agent** Agent that is used to relieve anxiety.
aplastic anemia Dysfunction of the bone marrow, often occurring as a reaction to drug therapy, in which there is a severe decrease in the production of erythrocytes and white blood cells.
Arabic (ĂR-é-bîk) **numeral system** System that uses symbols and decimal places to express numbers.
arachnoiditis Inflammation of the arachnoid membrane covering the brain.
arthritis Inflammation of joints.
ascites (ĕ-SĪ-tēz) Presence of large amounts of fluid in the abdominal cavity.
asphyxia (ăs-FĬK-sē-ĕ) Suffocation.
asthma (ĂS-mĕ) Condition in which there is constriction of the lung bronchioles in response to allergic or emotional phenomena, producing symptoms of dyspnea, constriction in the chest, coughing, and expiratory wheezing.
astringents (ĕ-STRĬN-jĕnts) Substances that cause tissues to contract, helping to reduce secretions.
ataxia (ĕ-TĂK-sē-ĕ) Muscular incoordination, with staggering gait.
atherosclerosis (ĂTH-ĕ-RŌ-sklĕ-RŌ-sĭs) Deposition of fatty material in the walls of the blood vessels.
athetosis (ĂTH-ĕ-TŌ-sĭs) Recurrent, slow, and continual body movements, usually the result of a brain lesion.
atrium (*pl.* **atria**) One of the upper chambers of the heart.
automatic stop policy Institutional policy that discontinues a drug order or prescription after a specified time.
autonomic (ăw-tō-NŌM-ĭk) **nervous system** Nervous system that controls many body organ systems automatically or involuntarily; composed of nerves leading from the central nervous system that innervate and control smooth muscle, cardiac muscle, and glands.
Avoirdupois (ăv-ĕr-dĕ-POIZ) **system** System used for common household measurements, including teaspoon, tablespoon, cup, pint, and quart.
avitaminosis Condition that develops from a lack of vitamins.

B

bacteremia (BĂK-tĭ-RĒ-mē-ĕ) Presence of microorganisms in the bloodstream.
bactericide Substance that kills bacteria.
bacteriostatic Substance that inhibits the growth of bacteria.
barbiturates (băr-BĬCH-ū-rătĕs) Drugs derived from barbituric acid that act as sedatives or hypnotics; phenobarbital and secobarbital are examples.
beriberi Condition caused by a nutritional deficiency of thiamine (vitamin B_1), with symptoms and neurologic involvement such as weakness, paralysis, edema, and mental deterioration.
beta blockers Class of drugs so named for blocking beta-adrenergic receptors in the sympathetic nervous system; used in the treatment of cardiac arrhythmias and after myocardial infarction.
beta-lactam antibiotics Cephalosporin group, named by an element of their chemical structure.
biosynthesis Formation of a chemical compound by enzymes either within an organism (in vivo) or in the laboratory (in vitro) by fragmentation of cells.
biotechnology Field of pharmacology that involves using living cells, usually altered cultures of *Escherichia coli,* to manufacture drugs.
bladder Membranous sac that collects urine produced by the kidneys.
blood dyscrasia (dĭs-KRĀ-zhĕ) Any abnormal condition in the type or number of the formed elements (cells) of the blood.
Bowman's capsule Renal glomerular capsule.
bradycardia (BRĂD-ē-KĂR-dē-ĕ) Slowing of the heartbeat.
broad-spectrum antibiotic Antibiotic that is effective against a wide range of infectious microorganisms.
bronchiole (BRŎNG-kē-ōl) Tiny, thin-walled lung tubules near the alveoli.
bronchoconstrictor Agent that causes tightening or narrowing of the lung bronchioles.
bronchoconstriction Narrowing of the bronchial airways.
bronchodilator Agent that causes relaxation and enlargement of the bronchi.

C

calibration Measurement of an intravenous solution delivered "per drop."
cancer Tumor or unnatural growth in the body.
Candida albicans (KĂN-dĭ-dĕĂL-bĕ-kănz) Yeastlike organism that produces cutaneous or mucous membrane infections.
candidiasis (KĂN-dĭ-DĪ-ĕ-sĭs) Superinfection with the fungus *Candida albicans;* may be in the form of diaper rash, oral mucous membrane involvement (thrush), vaginitis, or infection of the skin or nails. If superinfection occurs in the gastrointestinal tract, diarrhea commonly results.
capsules Powdered or liquid drugs placed in soft gelatin capsules (e.g., cod liver oil capsules, Benadryl capsules).
carcinogen Agent that produces cancer.
carcinoma (KĂR-sĭ-NŌ-mĕ) Malignant neoplasm caused by excessive cellular proliferation; also known as cancer.
carminative (kär-MĬN-ĕ-tĭv) Agent used to expel gas from the gastrointestinal tract.

catalyst (KĂT-ĕ-lĭst) Substance that increases the speed of a chemical reaction but is not used up or permanently changed in any way by the reaction.
cathartic (kĕ-THĂR-tĭk) Strong laxative that produces frequent, watery stools.
CD4 cells Subpopulation of lymphocytes referred to as the helper T cells. The CD4 cell count corresponds to the severity of HIV infection.
Celsius (SĔL-sē-ĕs) **scale** Scale commonly used to measure temperature; also called centigrade scale.
cephalosporin (SĔF-ĕ-lō-SPŎ-rĭn) Antibiotic derived from the microorganism *Cephalosporium falciforme* and similar to penicillin; cephalexin and cefdinir are examples.
cerebral palsy Nonspecific term for motor, speech, and mental dysfunctions resulting from brain damage, usually at birth.
chancroid (SHĂNG-krŏĭd) Venereal infection, with lesions involving the genitalia and enlarged, painful inguinal lymph nodes.
chemical substances Agents that may be made synthetically (e.g., sulfonamides, aspirin, sodium bicarbonate).
chimeric antibody Antibody in which the antigen-binding part of a mouse antibody is fused to the part of a human antibody that controls its function; produced by genetic engineering.
cholinergic (KŌ-lēn-ŬR-jĭk) Agent that produces the effects of stimulation of the parasympathetic nervous system (acetylcholinelike effects).
cholinergic blocking agent Agent that interferes with the cholinergic, or parasympathetic nervous system, functions.
Clark's rule Formula used for calculating dosage for infants and children.

$$\frac{\text{Weight of child (in pounds)}}{150} \times \text{average adult dose} = \text{child's dose}$$

coanalgesic (KŌ-ăn-ăl-JĒ-sĭk) Drug that may be used to potentiate pain relief.
colitis Inflammation of the colon with accompanying diarrhea, often associated with mucus or blood.
complex fraction Fraction in which either the numerator or the denominator is also in fraction form.
congestive heart failure Condition in which the heart is unable to circulate blood satisfactorily.
constipation Condition in which bowel movements are infrequent or incomplete.
contraceptive Agent that prevents conception.
Controlled Substances Act Law (effective May 1, 1971) that requires that every person who manufactures, dispenses, prescribes, or administers any controlled substance be registered annually with the Attorney General, under the direction of the Drug Enforcement Administration (DEA).
convulsion (seizure) Involuntary muscle contractions, either focal or generalized, usually occurring as a result of brain dysfunction.
corticosteroid (KŎR-tĭ-kō-STĬR-ŏyd) Any of the hormones produced by the adrenal cortex (other than sex hormones) that influence or control key processes of the body.
cortisone Glucocorticoid not normally secreted in significant amounts by the adrenal cortex. It exhibits no biologic activity until converted to hydrocortisone.
coryza Engorgement of the nasal mucous membranes, accompanied by increased nasal discharge and often sneezing.
COX-2 inhibitor Class of NSAIDs that preferentially inhibit cyclooxygenase-2 over cyclooxygenase-1, to reduce side effects of the medication.
cretin (KRĒ-tĭn) Person with congenital hypothyroidism that results in mental retardation and stunted physical growth.
crystalluria (KRĬS-tĕ-LŪR-ē-ĕ) Crystals in the urine.
Cushing's disease (or syndrome) Condition caused by overactivity of the adrenal gland, causing florid facies, edema, striae, demineralization of bone, and other effects.
cyanosis (SĪ-ĕ-NŌ-sĭs) Bluish tinge of the skin and mucous membranes, usually caused by excessive amounts of deoxygenated hemoglobin in the blood.
cyclooxygenase-2 (COX-2) Enzyme in the body that is involved in the inflammatory process.
cystitis (sĭs-TĪ-tĭs) Inflammation of the urinary bladder.
cytokine Protein secreted by certain cells that regulates immune response.

D

DEA Drug Enforcement Administration.
decimal A fraction whose denominator is 10 or any multiple of 10, which is expressed by proper placement of the decimal point rather than a written denominator.
dementia (dĭ-MĔN-shĕ) Loss of cognitive and intellectual functions.
demulcent (dĭ-MŬL-sĕnt) Substance used to soothe or reduce irritation of a surface.
denominator The lower number of a fraction below the vinculum ("divide by" line); indicates how equal parts are in the whole object.
deoxyribonucleic acid *See* DNA.
dependence Severe attachment to a drug or agent; an addiction.
depressant Agent that causes reduction in activity of a bodily system.
depression (1) Decrease in activity of cells caused by the action of a drug. (2) Unnatural state of lethargy, inactivity, and sadness.
dermatitis Inflammatory condition of the skin.
diabetes insipidus Disease caused by a decrease in the hormone vasopressin, permitting large amounts of very dilute urine to be passed regardless of the body fluid status. The condition is accompanied by extreme thirst and dehydration.
diabetes mellitus Condition brought about by a deficiency of functional insulin from the pancreas, interfering with the ability of the body to metabolize glucose. Hyperglycemia, glycosuria, atherosclerosis, decreased resistance to infection, retinal hemorrhages, and kidney damage are manifestations of the disease.
diagnostic Pertaining to the art or act of determining the nature of a patient's disease.
diarrhea Abnormally frequent bowel discharges.
Dietary Reference Intakes (DRI) Guidelines established by the U.S. Department of Agriculture listing the nutrients necessary for good health.
digestant Drug that promotes the process of digestion in the gastrointestinal tract and constitutes a type of replacement therapy in deficiency states.
digestion Mechanical, chemical, and enzymatic processes whereby food is converted to material suitable for use in the body.
disinfectant (germicide) Substance that destroys microorganisms on objects; usually too irritating to be used on human tissue.
diuresis (dī-ūr-RĒ-sĭs) The formation of urine.
diuretic Substance used to increase the output of urine.

DNA Deoxyribonucleic acid; the component of genes that carries information.

dosage Size amount, frequency, and number of doses of a therapeutic agent to be administered to a patient.

dosage forms Systems used to deliver drugs.

dose Amount of a drug or other substance to be administered at one time.

double helix The twin coil structure of DNA.

drug Any substance used as medicine (e.g., used to diagnose, cure, mitigate, treat, or prevent disease).

drug allergy Reaction resulting from hypersensitivity to a drug.

drug order Consists of the name of the drug, the dosage, when the drug is to be given, how it is to be given, how many times it is to be given, the date of the order, and the signature of the physician who wrote the order.

drug standards Published lists of the known value, strength, quality, and ingredients of various drugs.

dyscrasia (dĭs-KRĀ-zhĕ) Abnormal state.

dysmenorrheal (DĬS-mĕn-ĕ-RĒ-ĕ) Painful menstruation.

dyspnea Difficulty breathing.

E

ED Erectile dysfunction.

edema (ĭ-DĒ-mĕ) Excessive accumulation of fluid in the tissue spaces.

elixirs Solutions containing alcohol, sugar, and water. They may or may not be aromatic and may or may not have active medicinals. Most frequently, they are used as flavoring agents or solvents (e.g., terpin hydrate elixir, phenobarbital elixir).

embolus (*pl.* emboli) (ĔM-bĕ-lĕs) Blood clot, or portion of a clot, that has broken away from its site of formation and traveled via the bloodstream to another site within the body.

emesis (ĔM-ĕ-sĭs) Vomiting.

emetic (ĭ-MĔT-ĭk) Substance used to induce vomiting.

emollient (ĭ-MŎL-yĕnt) Substance that softens tissue, particularly skin and mucous membranes.

emulsions Suspensions of fat globules in water (or water globules in fat) with an emulsifying agent (e.g., Haley's M-O, Petrogalar). (Homogenized milk is also an emulsion.)

endocrine gland Ductless gland that secretes internally.

enuresis (ĕn-ū-RĒ-sĭs) Involuntary discharge of urine.

enzyme Substance formed by living cells that promotes or enhances a particular chemical reaction in the body by functioning as a catalyst.

epilepsy Brain dysfunction in which abnormal electrical discharges occur at intervals, causing motor seizures or psychic phenomena.

epileptic equivalents Disorders that resemble epilepsy but are caused by other conditions.

epinephrine Natural adrenal medulla hormone.

equivalent (ĭ-kwĬV-ĕ-lĕnt) **fractions** Fractions whose terms are different but that may be reduced to the same fraction.

erythema (ĔR-ĭ-THĒ-mĕ) Reddening of the skin.

erythrocyte (ĕ-RĬTH-rĕ-SĪT) Red blood cell; contains hemoglobin, which is responsible for carrying oxygen to body tissues.

essential fatty acids Molecules found within fats that are not produced by the body but are necessary for proper functioning.

estrogens (ĔS-trŏ-jĭns) One of a group of hormonal steroids that promote the development of female sex characteristics.

exocrine gland Gland with a duct, which secretes outwardly or onto a luminal surface.

extravasation Forcing of a substance (e.g., a drug, blood) from its proper or intended vessel into surrounding tissue.

extremes The first and fourth terms of a proportion; the product of the extremes equals the product of the means.

F

Fahrenheit (FĂR-ĕn-HĪT) **scale** Scale commonly used to measure temperature on most clinical thermometers in the United States.

fiber Food substance found only in plants that is not digested by gastrointestinal enzymes.

fibrillation Quivering of cardiac muscle fibers, rendering the heart unable to contract with sufficient force to circulate blood effectively.

fibromyalgia Disorder characterized by a complex set of painful signs and symptoms; widespread pain, fatigue, and poor sleep are common symptoms.

fluid extract Alcoholic liquid extract of a drug made by percolation so that 1 mL of the fluid extract contains 1 gm of the drug. Only vegetable-based drugs are used (e.g., glycyrrhiza fluid extract).

follicle-stimulating hormone (FSH) Hormone that stimulates the maturation of the graafian follicles in the ovary.

fraction Mathematical term indicating division; expresses the number of equal parts into which a whole is divided.

Fried's (FRĒDS) **rule** A formula used to calculate dosage for infants and children.

$$\frac{\text{Age in months}}{150} \times \text{average adult dose} = \text{child's dose}$$

fungus General term for a group of microorganisms that includes yeasts and molds.

G

ganglion (GĂNG-glē-ŏn) A group of nerve cell bodies.

gels Aqueous suspensions of insoluble drugs in hydrated form; aluminum hydroxide gel, USP-NF is an example.

gene Functional unit of heredity that occupies a specific place on a chromosome.

gene therapy Application of genetic principles to the treatment of human disease.

genome (JĒ-nōm) A complete set of chromosomes.

geriatric (JĔR-ē-ĂT-rĭk) Pertaining to old age or elderly people.

gland Organized aggregation of cells that functions as a secretory or excretory organ.

glaucoma (glô-KŌ-mĕ) Serious eye disorder in which normal drainage of intraocular fluid is impaired, causing increased intraocular pressure. Blindness results if treatment is delayed.

glomerulus (glō-MĔR-yū-lĕs) Tuft of capillaries projecting into the glomerular capsule. The capillaries allow filtration of water, salt, and impurities from the blood and are responsible for the first stage in urine formation.

glycosuria (GLĪ-kō-SŎŎR-ē-ĕ) Glucose in the urine.

goiter (GŎY-tĕr) Enlargement of the thyroid gland; may occur with either hypothyroidism or hyperthyroidism.

gram Unit of weight used within the metric system.

gynecomastia Abnormal enlargement of one or both breasts in a boy or man.

H

habit formation Condition in which drugs are routinely taken as a matter of course, not as a matter of necessity. Withdrawal symptoms are not seen on cessation of the habit.

health food products Goods manufactured to supplement a person's nutrition or wellness.

hematinic (HĔM-ĕ-TĬN-ĭk) Agent that increases the number of erythrocytes or the hemoglobin concentration of the blood; examples are iron and B vitamins.

hemoglobin Red pigment in erythrocytes that reversibly combines with oxygen, transporting it to tissues.

hemosiderosis (HĒ-mō-SĬD-ĕ-RŌ-sĭs) Condition in which there is an excessive deposition of iron in the tissues, particularly in the liver, causing cirrhosis, and in the pancreas, causing diabetes mellitus.

hepatitis Inflammation of the liver.

hepatotoxicity Producing adverse effects or damage to the liver.

herb Any plant or plant part valued for its medicinal, savory, or aromatic qualities.

herbal remedy Drug derived from a plant, generally available without a prescription.

hirsutism (HŬR-sū-TĬZ-ĕm) Excessive growth of facial or body hair.

histamine (HĬS-tă-mĭn) Amino acid that, when released in the body, produces the symptoms of allergic reactions; nasal secretions are increased, engorgement of capillary beds occurs, visceral muscles are stimulated, and lung bronchioles are constricted.

HIV Human immunodeficiency virus.

Hodgkin's disease Form of lymphoma characterized by enlargement and malignant degeneration of the lymph nodes, eventually spreading to involve the liver, spleen, and other internal organs.

home health care Professional health care providing many services in the home environment that were formerly available only in a hospital setting.

hormone Agent secreted by the endocrine glands into the bloodstream that produces or alters bodily functions.

hormone replacement therapy (HRT) Administration of hormones, often estrogen and progestin, to reduce the symptoms of menopause and decrease the possibility of osteoporosis in women after menopause.

hospice (HŎS-pĭs) Institution that provides a centralized program of palliative and supportive care to dying patients and their families.

hydrocortisone Glucocorticoid hormone secreted by the adrenal cortex.

hypertension Blood pressure persistently exceeding 140/90 mm Hg.

hypertensive Agent used to elevate blood pressure therapeutically.

hyperthyroidism (HĪ-pĕr-THĪ-rŏy-DĬZ-ĕm) Condition caused by excessive activity of the thyroid gland, with accompanying hypertension, nervousness, tachycardia, and exophthalmos. Also known as Graves' disease.

hyperuricemia (HĪ-pĕr-ū-rē-SĒ-mē-ă) Increased uric acid levels in the blood, often associated with gout or gouty arthritis.

hypervitaminosis Condition that develops as a result of an overdose of vitamins.

hypnotic Agent used to induce sleep.

hypochlorhydria (HĪ-pō-klō-RHĬD-rē-ĕ) Decrease in the amount of gastric hydrochloric acid.

hypoglycemia Deficiency of glucose in the blood.

hypotension Lowered blood pressure.

hypotensive Agent used to decrease blood pressure.

hypothyroidism Decreased functioning of the thyroid gland, with subsequent slowing down of mental and motor functions.

I

idiosyncrasy (ĬD-ē-ō-SĬN-krĕ-sē) Abnormal sensitivity to a drug, or a reaction not intended.

immunity State in which an individual is not susceptible to a certain disease.

immunizing agent Biologic preparation injected to produce immunity to disease.

immunosuppression (ĬM-yĕ-nō-sĕ-PRĔSH-ĕn) Interference with the development of antibody response to a disease.

immunosuppressive Agent that interferes with the body systems that resist infection and foreign materials.

immunotherapy (ĬM-yĕ-nō-THĔR-ĕ-pē) Treatment of conditions by enhancing or altering the immune system of the body.

improper fraction Fraction in which the numerator is larger than the denominator.

incontinence (ĭn-KŎN-tĭ-nĕns) Inability to control the discharge of excretions, urine, or feces.

inflammation (ĬN-flĕ-MĀ-shŭn) Pathologic reaction by the body in response to an injury or abnormal stimulation by an agent.

infusion (ĭn-FYŪ-zhĕn) Introduction of fluid other than blood into a vein.

inhaled administration Introduction of a drug or substance to the body via breathing or inhaling.

inotropic (ĬN-ō-TRŎP-ĭk) **drug** Agent that increases myocardial contractility.

INR International normalized ratio.

inscription Part of the prescription that states the name and quantities of the ingredients.

insulin Pancreatic hormone that aids in the use of glucose as energy, stores excess glucose as glycogen in the liver, and is responsible for the conversion of glucose to fat.

insulin syringe Syringe specifically used for insulin dosing, calibrated in units per milliliter.

interaction Altered effect that occurs when two or more drugs or herbs are taken together.

International Normalized Ratio (INR) Standardized format for reporting thromboplastin values. It is used to adjust the dose of anticoagulant medications.

intra-arterial injection Insertion of a needle into an artery to administer a drug or other substance.

intradermal injection Insertion of a needle into the dermis of the skin to administer a drug or other substance.

intramuscular (IM) injection Insertion of a needle into a muscle to administer a drug or other substance.

intravenous (IV) injection Insertion of a needle into a vein to administer a drug or other substance.

intrinsic factor Substance in the gastric wall that is necessary for vitamin B_{12} absorption.

J

jaundice Yellow pigmentation noticeable in the skin and mucous membranes that is caused by an increase in the amount of serum bilirubin, usually as a result of a liver disorder.

L

laxative Cathartic agent that evacuates the bowel by a mild action.

leukemia Condition characterized by uncontrolled proliferation of leukocytes, or white blood cells.

leukocyte (LŪ-kĕ-sīt) White blood cell; responsible for antibody production and defense against infectious agents in the body.

leukopenia (LŪ-kō-PĒ-nē-ĕ) Decrease in the number of white blood cells in the blood.

liniment Mixture of drugs with oil, soap, water, or alcohol intended for external application with rubbing (e.g., camphor liniment, chloroform liniment).

liter Unit of volume used within the metric system.

local effects Effects limited to the site of application.

long-acting or sustained-release dosage forms Active pharmaceutical agents that are either layered in tablet form for release over several hours or placed in pellets within a capsule. The pellets are of varying size and disintegrate over 8 to 24 hours. These dosage forms must not be broken or crushed because their efficacy depends on release of the various layers over time.

lotions Aqueous preparations containing suspended materials intended for soothing, local application. Most are patted on rather than rubbed (e.g., calamine lotion, Caladryl lotion).

lowest common denominator Lowest possible number that is divisible by the denominators of two or more fractions.

luteinizing hormone Hormone that stimulates development of the corpus luteum.

lymphocyte (LĬM-fĕ-sīt) White blood cell, formed in the lymph tissues of the body, such as the spleen, lymph nodes, and tonsils. Cells are active in antibody formation to counteract infection.

lymphoma (lĭm-FŌ-mĕ) Any of a group of malignant conditions involving lymphoid tissue.

lymphosarcoma (lĭm-FŌ-săr-KŌ-mĕ) Tumor of the lymph nodes in which the nodes contain masses of rounded malignant cells that resemble lymphocytes.

M

macrolide (MĂ-krō-līd) **antibiotics** Chemical class of antibiotics that includes erythromycin, azithromycin, clarithromycin, and dirithromycin.

malaise (mă-LĀZ) Generalized, nonspecific discomfort or unease.

means The second and third terms of a proportion; the product of the means equals the product of the extremes.

meningitis (MĬN-ĭn-JĪ-tĭs) Infection of the meninges, the lining of the brain and the spinal cord.

menopause (MĔN-ĕ-pŏz) The time at which fertility and menstruation cease in a woman.

menorrhagia (MĔN-ĕ-RĀ-jē-ĕ) Excessive menstrual flow.

menstrual migraines Headaches of moderate to severe intensity that occur around the time of menstruation in a woman.

metabolism (mĕ-TĂB-ĕ-LĬZ-ĕm) Chemical changes in living organisms by which energy is produced and tissue repairs are affected.

meter Unit of distance or length used within the metric system.

metric system System of weights and measures used in medicine.

migraine Paroxysmal, intensely painful headache caused by vasomotor disturbances in a scalp artery, often accompanied by psychic phenomena, nausea, and vomiting.

mineral Naturally occurring, inorganic substance that is necessary to body function.

miosis (mī-Ō-sĭs) Pupil constriction.

mixed number Number consisting of a whole number and a fraction.

moniliasis (MŌ-nĕ-LĪ-ĕ-sĭs) Superinfection with the fungus *Candida albicans* (*see* Candidiasis).

monoamine oxidase inhibitors (MAOIs) Agents that inhibit monoamine oxidase, a naturally occurring hormone that is involved in the breakdown of several neurotransmitters in the brain, including epinephrine, dopamine, and serotonin.

monoclonal (MŎN-ĕ-KLŌ-nĕl) **antibody** Very specific antibody that binds to one receptor only.

multiple myeloma Malignant disease of the bone marrow characterized by bone destruction, often with pathologic fractures, anemia, hyperglobulinemia, hypercalcemia, and increased numbers of immature cells in the bone marrow.

mycosis fungoides (mī-KŌ-sĭs fŭng-GŎY-dēz) Form of lymphoma that has numerous cutaneous manifestations, such as eczema, nodules, tumors, infiltrations, and ulcerations.

mydriasis (mĭ-DRĪ-ĕ-sĭs) Dilation of the pupil.

myxedema (MĬK-sĕ-DĒ-mĕ) Hypothyroidism, with onset usually in late childhood or adulthood, characterized by puffiness of the skin and a slowing of mental and motor functions.

N

narcotic (năr-KŎT-ĭk) Any drug derived from opium or its synthetic equivalents.

narrow-spectrum antibiotic Antibiotic that is effective against only a few microorganisms.

natural remedy Any treatment that can be used by nonprofessionals to alter a condition.

neoplasm (NĒ-ō-PLĂZ-ĕm) Unnatural growth or tumor in the body; a cancer.

nephritis (nĕ-FRĪ-tĭs) Inflammation of the kidney.

nephron (NĔF-rŏn) Functional unit of the kidney, consisting of the glomerulus, the glomerular capsule, and the collecting tubules.

neuron (NŪR-ŏn) One cell of the nervous system, the functional unit.

neurosis (nū-RŌ-sĭs) Emotional disorder characterized by anxiety or depressive reaction but in which the patient has not lost contact with reality.

neutropenia (NŪ-trō-PĒ-nē-ĕ) Decrease in the number of neutrophils (a type of white blood cell) in the blood.

nocardiosis (nō-KĂR-dē-Ō-sĭs) Systemic fungus infection, often with granuloma formation in various organs.

nocturia (nŏk-TŪR-ē-ĕ) Frequent urination during the night.

norepinephrine Hormone secreted by the adrenal medulla, released with epinephrine in response to stress.

NSAID Nonsteroidal anti-inflammatory drug; a drug that prevents the synthesis of prostaglandins at the site of inflammation.

numerator The upper number of a fraction above the vinculum ("divide by" line); indicates how many parts are in the fraction.

nystagmus Involuntary, rapid rhythmic movement of the eyeball.

O

ointments Mixtures of drugs with a fatty base for external application, usually by rubbing (e.g., zinc oxide ointment, Ben-Gay ointment).

opiates Drugs derived from opium.

opioid (Ō-pē-ŏĭd) Agent, natural or synthetic, that is similar in structure and effect to opium derivatives.

opisthotonos (Ō-pĭs-THŎT-ĕ-nĕs) Tetanic muscle spasm characterized by arching of the back, inability to speak, and loss of muscle control; the patient is usually conscious. Occurs as a rare drug hypersensitivity reaction.

oral administration Introduction of a substance to the body via the mouth.

orthopnea Difficulty breathing when lying down, which is relieved on sitting up.

osmosis Process in which water travels through a semipermeable membrane to equalize concentrations of fluid on either side of the membrane.

osteoarthritis Condition caused by erosion of articular cartilage.

osteomalacia (ŎS-tē-Ō-mĕ-LĀ-shĕ) Softening of the bones, resulting from interference with calcium deposits in bony tissue.

osteoporosis Thinning and increased porosity of the bone, with resultant deformities or fractures; common in postmenopausal women.

ototoxic Producing adverse effects on the organs or nerves involved in hearing.

oxytocic (ŎK-sĭ-TŌ-sĭk) **agent** Drug used to produce effects similar to oxytocin, especially stimulation of uterine contractions.

P

palliation Treatment that improves the comfort or well-being of a patient but is not curative.

palliative Agent or measure that relieves symptoms.

pancytopenia (PĂN-sī-tē-PĒ-nē-ē) Condition in which there are decreased numbers of all blood cells.

Para-aminobenzoic acid (PABA) Substance needed to synthesize folic acid, an essential enzyme.

paralysis Inability to move an affected body part.

parasympathetic (păr-ă-sĭm-pă-THĔT-ĭk) **nervous system** Part of the autonomic nervous system that functions, through the use of acetylcholine, in actions of normal body maintenance.

parasympatholytic Agent that counteracts the effects of the parasympathetic nervous system.

parasympathomimetic (PĔR-ĕ-SĬM-pĕ-THŌ-mĭ-MĔT-ĭk) Agent that produces stimulating effects on the parasympathetic nervous system.

parenteral administration Introduction of a drug or other substance to the body via injection.

paresis (pĕ-RĒ-sĭs) Weakness of an affected body part.

paresthesia (PĔR-ĕs-THĒ-zhĕ) Abnormal skin sensation of crawling, burning, or tingling, not caused by surface stimuli.

Parkinson's disease Progressive condition resulting primarily from deterioration of certain brain nuclei; characterized by rigidity, tremors, akinesia, and loss of spontaneous or automatic movement.

parkinsonism Syndrome resembling Parkinson's disease but occurring instead as a side effect of certain drugs, notably tranquilizers, and reversible after withdrawal of the drug.

passive immunity Injection of previously formed antibodies into the body.

penicillin Any of the group of antibiotics derived from cultures of species of the fungus *Penicillium*.

peptic Relates to the stomach, to gastric digestion, or to pepsin.

peptide Group of two or more amino acids.

percent Fraction whose numerator is expressed and whose denominator is understood to be 100; usually indicated by the percent symbol, %.

perimenopausal Relating to the period around the onset of menopause.

peristalsis (PĔR-ē-STĂL-sĭs) Automatic contractions of the gastrointestinal tract.

pharmacodynamics (FĂR-mĕ-kō-dī-NĂM-ĭks) Study of how a drug acts on a living organism.

Pharmacokinetics (FĂR-mĕ-kō-kĭ-NĔT-ĭks) Study of the body's actions on a drug, including the mechanisms of absorption, distribution, metabolism, and excretion.

pharmacology Broad term that includes the study of drugs and their actions in the body.

pharmacy Art of preparing, compounding, and dispensing drugs for medicinal use.

pheochromocytoma (FĒ-ō-KRŌ-mō-sī-TŌ-mĕ) Tumor of the sympathetic nervous system, usually located in the adrenal medulla, that may cause severe, intermittent, or persistent hypertension.

photosensitizer (FŌ-tō-SĔN-sĭ-TĪZ-ĕr) Agent that makes the skin more susceptible to burning and sun damage.

physical dependence Condition in which continuous use of a drug is required for proper functioning, and the user would experience withdrawal symptoms if the drug is discontinued.

pills Single-dose units made by mixing a powdered form of a drug with a liquid such as syrup and rolling it into a round or oval shape (e.g., Hinkle's pills). These are largely replaced by other dosage forms today.

place value Value of a digit based on its position relative to the decimal point.

plant parts or products Crude drugs that may be obtained from any part of various plants and used medicinally (e.g., ergot, digitalis, opium). Leaves, bark, fruit, roots, rhizomes, resin, and other parts may be used.

polycythemia (PŎL-ē-sī-THĒ-mē-ē) **vera** Condition characterized by increased numbers of red blood cells in the blood. Occasionally occurs as a premalignant disorder before the onset of leukemia. Common in individuals living at high altitudes for prolonged periods.

postpartum depression Depression occurring in a mother following the birth of her child.

potentiation Effect that occurs when a drug increases or prolongs the action of another drug, the total effect being greater than the sum of the effects of each drug used alone.

powders Single-dose quantities of a drug or mixture of drugs in powdered form wrapped separately in powder papers (e.g., Seidlitz powder).

premenstrual dysphoric disorder Mood disorder occurring in women before or during menstruation; symptoms include anxiety, irritability, and emotional sensitivity.

prescription Order for medication, therapy, or a therapeutic device given by a properly authorized person.

progesterone Hormone that prepares the uterus for reception of the ovum.

proper fraction Fraction in which the numerator is smaller than the denominator; designates less than one whole unit.

prophylactic (PRŌ-fĭ-LĂK-tĭk) Agent or device used to prevent an undesired effect or disease.

prophylactic (PRŌ-fĭ-LĂK-tĭk) **therapy** Treatment used for the prevention of an effect or disease.

proportion Mathematical expression showing the relationship between two equal ratios.

prostaglandin inhibitors Agents that interfere with the effects of prostaglandins.

prostaglandins (PRŎS-tĕ-GLĂN-dĭn) Short-acting hormones that perform many functions in the body and exert their effect close to the site of production.

prothrombin Protein produced by the liver, necessary for normal blood clotting.

prothrombin time (PT) Measurement of the prothrombin level in the blood. Measurement is performed routinely to assess the effectiveness of anticoagulant therapy.

pruritus (prū-RĪ-tĕs) Itching sensation of the skin.

pseudoaddiction (SŪ-dō-ăd-DĬK-shŭn) Drug-seeking behaviors that may occur when a patient's pain is undertreated.

psychoactive (SĪ-kō-ĂK-tĭv) **drug** Agent possessing the ability to alter mood, behavior, or cognitive processes.

psychosis Severe mental disease in which the patient's contact with reality is diminished or lost.

PT Prothrombin time.

purpura (PŬR-pĕr-ĕ) Multiple small hemorrhagic areas in the skin or mucous membranes.

pyelitis (PĪ-ĕ-LĪ-tĭs) Inflammation of the renal pelvis.

pyelonephritis (PĪ-ĕ-lō-nĕ-FRĪ-tĭs) Inflammation of the pelvis and glomerular tissues of the kidney.

Q

quinolones (KWĬN-ĕ-lōns) Group of synthetic antibiotics structurally related by having the same (quinolone) nucleus.

R

recombinant (rē-KŎM-bĭ-nĕnt) Cell or organism that has received genes from different parental strains.

Recommended Daily Allowance (RDA) Value established by the U.S. Department of Agriculture to be the average daily dietary intake sufficient to meet the nutrition requirement of 97% to 98% of healthy individuals.

reduced fraction Fraction at its lowest terms in which the numerator and denominator cannot be divided exactly by the same number, with the exception of 1.

respiration Process of exchanging oxygen and carbon dioxide via the respiratory system.

retinopathy Disorder of the retina that may cause blindness (e.g., diabetic retinopathy).

Reye's syndrome Disease of the brain characterized by fever, vomiting, and swelling of the kidneys and brain; may be linked to aspirin intake in children.

rheumatoid arthritis Generalized connective tissue disease that inflames many joints.

rickets Condition caused by a deficiency of vitamin D. Calcium and phosphorus imbalances cause softening of the bones and characteristic deformations, such as bowed legs and rachitic "rosary" on the costochondral junctions.

ringworm Topical fungal infection of the skin, hair, or nails, often circular in appearance and spreading peripherally.

RNA Component of the cell nucleus or cytoplasm that carries genetic information and aids in the correct assembly of DNA and proteins.

Roman numeral system System that uses letters to designate numbers; lower case Roman numerals are occasionally used in prescriptions.

S

schedules of controlled substances Classification system that categorizes drugs by their potential for abuse.

schizophrenia Type of psychosis in which the patient typically withdraws from reality, exhibiting unpredictable moods, disturbances in the stream of thought, and regressive tendencies to the point of deterioration, often with hallucinations and delusions.

scurvy Vitamin C deficiency characterized by weakness, gum hemorrhages, loosening of the teeth, and subcutaneous hemorrhages.

sedative Agent used to quiet a patient without inducing sleep.

seizure *See* Convulsion.

selective serotonin reuptake (SĔR-ĕ-TŌ-nĭn rē-ŬP-tāk) **inhibitors (SSRIs)** Drugs that increase serotonin availability in the central nervous system, which is believed to produce an antidepressant effect.

senility Term that relates to various organic physical and mental disorders that occur in old age.

serotonin Powerful neurotransmitter that produces vasoconstriction, inhibits gastric secretion, and stimulates smooth muscles.

shock Sudden decrease in blood pressure as a result of an injury or blood loss.

side effect Unpredictable effect that is not related to the main action of the drug.

signatura (Sig) Part of the prescription that gives directions to the patient.

solutions Aqueous liquid preparations containing one or more substances that are completely dissolved. Every solution has two parts: the solute (the dissolved substance) and the solvent (the substance, usually a liquid, in which the solute is dissolved).

spirits Alcoholic solutions of volatile substances (e.g., camphor spirit). These are also known as essences (e.g., essence of peppermint).

SSRI Selective serotonin reuptake inhibitor.

status asthmaticus Prolonged attack of asthma; poorly responsive to drug therapy and lasting several days.

status epilepticus Rapid succession of epileptic seizures in which the patient does not regain consciousness between seizures.

stem cells Cells that are totipotent, or able to give rise to all the cells of the body.

steroid (STĬR-ŏyd) **antagonists** Diuretics that act by inhibiting aldosterone, an adrenal hormone that promotes the retention of sodium and the excretion of potassium.

Stevens-Johnson syndrome Severe, life-threatening allergic drug reaction. Excoriations of the skin, mucous membranes, and cornea and inflammation of the internal organs occur. Decreased blood pressure may bring about shock and death.

stimulant Agent that promotes or enhances the activity of a body organ or tissue.

stimulation Increase in the activity of cells produced by drugs.

subcutaneous (subcut) injection Insertion of a needle beneath the skin into the fat or connective tissue just underlying the dermis layer.

sublingual administration Placing medication under the patient's tongue, where it must be retained until it is dissolved or absorbed.

subscription Part of the prescription that gives directions to the pharmacist.

substance abuse Use or overuse of a chemical or substance in a way that leads to dependence and has adverse effects on the health and well-being of the user and others.

sulfonamides (sĕl-FŎN-ĕ-mīd) Anti-infective agents modeled after PABA; also known as "sulfa drugs."

suppositories Mixtures of drugs with some firm base such as cocoa butter, which can be molded into shape for insertion into a body orifice. Rectal, vaginal, and urethral suppositories are the most common types (e.g., Furacin vaginal suppositories, Dulcolax suppositories), but nasal or otic suppositories may be made.

sympathetic (sĭm-pă-THĔT-ĭk) **nervous system** Part of the autonomic nervous system that prepares the body for immediate action in a stressful or emergent situation (i.e., "fight or flight" response).

sympatholytic Agent that counteracts the effects of the sympathetic nervous system.

sympathomimetic (SĬM-pĕ-THŌ-mĭ-MĔT-ĭk) Agent that produces stimulating effects on the sympathetic nervous system.

synapse (SĬN-ăps) Connection between two or more neurons.

synergism (SĬN-ĕr-JĬSM) Joint action of agents in which their combined effect is more intense or longer in duration than the sum of their individual effects.

syrups Aqueous solutions of a sugar. These may or may not have medicinal substances added (e.g., simple syrup, ipecac syrup).

systemic effects General effects caused by a drug being absorbed into the blood and carried to one or more tissues in the body.

T

tablets Single-dose units made by compressing powdered drugs in a suitable mold (e.g., aspirin tablets). Special forms of tablets include sublingual tablets (to be held under the tongue until dissolved) and enteric-coated tablets (with a coating that prevents their absorption until they reach the intestinal tract).

tachycardia (TĂK-ē-KĂR-dē-ĕ) Increased heart rate.

targeted therapy Treatment directed specifically at an abnormal or missing site in the body.

terminal illness Disease expected to cause death within a short time.

testosterone Hormone responsible for development of the male reproductive tract and maintenance of male secondary sex characteristics.

tetany (TĔT-ĕ-nē) Condition caused by a decreased concentration of ionized calcium in the blood, leading to increased irritability of muscles and painful tonic muscle spasms.

tetracycline (TĔT-rĕ-SĪ-klēn) Broad-spectrum antibiotic.

therapeutic Pertaining to treatment of disease.

thiazide diuretics Diuretics that act partly by inhibiting carbonic anhydrase; partly by acting directly on the collecting tubules; and partly by promoting excretion of sodium, potassium, chloride, and bicarbonate along with water.

thrombocytopenia Decreased number of platelets.

thrombolysis (thrŏm-BŎL-ĭ-sĭs) Process of dissolving a blood clot.

thrombolytic (THRŎM-bō-LĬT-ĭk) **therapy** Drug therapy used to dissolve blood clots.

thrombophlebitis (THRŎM-bō-flĕ-BĪ-tĭs) Inflammation of the walls of a vein, with resultant clotting of blood at the site.

thrombus A blood clot in the heart or blood vessels that remains attached at the site of formation.

thrush *Candida albicans* infection of the oral mucous membranes, typically in the form of small, white macular spots.

tinctures Alcoholic or hydroalcoholic solutions prepared from drugs (e.g., iodine tincture, digitalis tincture).

tolerance Increasing resistance to the usual effects of an established dosage of a drug as a result of continued use.

toxicology Science that deals with poisons—their detection and the symptoms, diagnosis, and treatment of conditions caused by them.

toxin Poisonous substance released by microorganisms.

toxoid Altered form of toxin that may be injected to produce immunity to a specific disease or microorganism.

toxoplasmosis (TŎK-sō-plăz-MŌ-sĭs) Disease caused by infection with the protozoan *Toxoplasma*. May take the form of a respiratory infection, encephalomyelitis, or a dermatitis.

trachoma (trĕ-KŌ-mĕ) Inflammatory disease of the eye involving the conjunctiva and cornea, producing photophobia, pain, and excessive lacrimation. If not treated, it may lead to blindness through vascularization of the cornea.

tranquilizer (TRĂNG-kwĕ-LĪZ-ĕr) Agent used to calm anxiety or agitation during waking hours.

transgene A transplanted gene.

troches (TRŌ-kēs) Flat, round, or rectangular preparations that are held in the mouth until they dissolve; also called lozenges.

tuberculin syringe Type of syringe; may be used in place of an insulin syringe in insulin dosing, but unit dosage must be converted to the equivalent number of milliliters before administration.

tumor Unnatural growth in the body.

U

ulcer Lesion through skin or mucous membrane resulting in loss of tissue, usually with inflammation.

units per milliliter Unit of measurement for insulin dosing.

ureter Tube that carries urine from the kidney to the bladder.

urethra Tube that carries urine from the bladder to the exterior of the body.

urticaria (ŬR-tĭ-KĔR-ē-ĕ) Condition in which pruritic wheals or welts appear on the skin, usually as a response to an allergic phenomenon; also known as hives.

V

vaccine Any preparation intended for use to produce active immunologic prevention of a disease.

vasoconstrictor (văs-ō-kŏn-STRĬK-tŏr) Agent that causes narrowing of the blood vessels.

vasodilator (văs-ō-DĪ-lā-tŏr) Agent that causes blood vessels to relax or increase in diameter.

vector A carrier of disease.

ventricle One of the lower chambers of the heart.

vertigo Dizziness.

virus Minute parasitic microorganism that is able to replicate only within a cell of a living plant or animal host.

vitamin Organic compound that cannot be synthesized in the human body but is present in minute amounts in foodstuffs. It is required for normal growth, development, and well-being.

W

waters Saturated solutions of volatile oils (e.g., peppermint water, camphor water).

withdrawal Syndrome that occurs when a drug-dependent person discontinues the drug suddenly; characterized by anxiety, insomnia, irritability, and often physical illness that may be severe.

withdrawal symptoms Unpleasant or life-threatening symptoms that occur when an addict does not take the substance to which he or she is addicted.

Y

Young's rule Formula used in calculating dosage for infants and children. Young's rule is not valid for use in children older than 12 years of age.

$$\frac{\text{Age of child (in years)}}{\text{Age of child (in years)} + 12} \times \text{average adult dose} = \text{child's dose}$$

Answers to Exercises and Review Questions

CHAPTER 1

Roman Numerals

(p. 2)

A.

1. XXXV
2. LXXXIX
3. LXXII
4. LV
5. CI
6. XCII
7. CXXXV
8. MDLXXX
9. CCCXLI
10. DCCXXIX

B.

1. 1211
2. 720
3. 166
4. 529
5. 3006
6. 800
7. 56
8. 75
9. 2673
10. 61

Fractions

(p. 3–4)

A.

1. $1\frac{1}{2}$
2. $1\frac{2}{5}$
3. 2
4. 3
5. $1\frac{8}{9}$
6. $3\frac{1}{8}$
7. $15\frac{4}{5}$
8. $7\frac{1}{9}$
9. $8\frac{2}{3}$
10. $4\frac{1}{10}$

B.

1. $\frac{4}{3}$
2. $\frac{9}{2}$
3. $\frac{703}{7}$
4. $\frac{73}{8}$
5. $\frac{54}{5}$
6. $\frac{34}{5}$
7. $\frac{17}{8}$
8. $\frac{69}{4}$
9. $\frac{965}{12}$
10. $\frac{441}{4}$

(p. 4)

1. $\frac{5}{20}$
2. $\frac{18}{39}$
3. $\frac{24}{60}$
4. $\frac{14}{36}$
5. $\frac{40}{32}$
6. $\frac{24}{51}$
7. $\frac{49}{63}$
8. $\frac{18}{16}$
9. $\frac{18}{21}$
10. $\frac{21}{10}$

(p. 5)

1. $\frac{7}{12}$ and $\frac{6}{12}$
2. $\frac{18}{21}$ and $\frac{14}{21}$
3. $\frac{3}{9}$ and $\frac{2}{9}$
4. $\frac{8}{20}$ and $\frac{8}{20}$
5. $\frac{3}{24}$ and $\frac{8}{24}$
6. $\frac{15}{60}$, $\frac{12}{60}$, $\frac{10}{60}$
7. $\frac{8}{12}$, $\frac{6}{12}$, $\frac{9}{12}$
8. $\frac{18}{24}$, $\frac{20}{24}$, $\frac{21}{24}$
9. $\frac{80}{90}$, $\frac{81}{90}$, $\frac{30}{90}$
10. $\frac{20}{75}$, $\frac{45}{75}$, $\frac{12}{75}$
11. $\frac{16}{12}$, $\frac{6}{12}$, $\frac{3}{12}$
12. $\frac{18}{30}$, $\frac{20}{30}$, $\frac{12}{30}$

(p. 5)

1. $1\frac{7}{36}$
2. $1\frac{2}{3}$
3. $6\frac{11}{24}$
4. $18\ \frac{1}{3}$
5. $1\frac{5}{12}$
6. $11\frac{1}{5}$
7. $5\ \frac{7}{12}$
8. $6\ \frac{5}{6}$
9. $37\frac{33}{56}$
10. $10\frac{1}{8}$

(p. 6)

1. $\frac{5}{18}$
2. $\frac{1}{21}$
3. $\frac{5}{8}$
4. $1\frac{3}{7}$
5. $1\frac{3}{8}$
6. $3\frac{1}{5}$
7. $3\frac{1}{3}$
8. $14\frac{4}{5}$
9. $3\frac{1}{12}$
10. $3\frac{1}{6}$

(p. 6)

1. $\frac{1}{12}$
2. $\frac{35}{72}$
3. 4
4. $1\frac{17}{75}$
5. $14\frac{1}{6}$
6. 33
7. 4
8. 20
9. $\frac{2}{27}$
10. $\frac{1}{25}$

(p. 7)

1. $\frac{24}{35}$
2. $\frac{1}{4}$
3. $\frac{14}{15}$
4. $\frac{1}{6}$
5. 6
6. $1\frac{1}{8}$
7. 2
8. $\frac{7}{8}$
9. $1\frac{1}{5}$
10. $\frac{41}{100}$

(p. 7)

1. $\frac{1}{3}$
2. $\frac{5}{7}$
3. $\frac{1}{500}$
4. $\frac{1}{9}$
5. $\frac{42}{83}$
6. $\frac{2}{17}$
7. $\frac{1}{8}$
8. $\frac{1}{11}$
9. $\frac{1}{75}$
10. $\frac{4}{9}$

Decimals

(p. 8)

A.

1. Three hundredths
2. Eighty-nine thousandths
3. Twenty-three and five tenths
4. Five and twenty-one hundredths
5. Twenty-nine ten-thousandths
6. Two hundred and nine hundredths
7. Thirty-seven and two hundred eighty-two thousandths
8. Four thousand two hundred fifty-six and three hundred fifty-three thousandths
9. Two hundred fifty-six and one hundredth
10. Eight ten-thousandths

B.

1. 0.004
2. 0.26
3. 5.000003
4. 0.07
5. 3.1
6. 0.088
7. 233.000057
8. 2.3
9. 8.04
10. 25.003

(p. 8)

1. 10.898
2. 49.59
3. 12.42
4. 6.53
5. 302.76
6. 1.783
7. 6.09
8. 7.045
9. 77.68
10. 2.47

(p. 9)

1. 0.646
2. 0.04
3. 41.28
4. 728.697
5. 0.018
6. 3.22
7. 4.7
8. 34.5
9. 2.837
10. 105.71

(p. 9)

1. 3.2
2. 0.011

3. 0.0945
4. 140
5. 0.8907
6. 240
7. 0.00009
8. 99.446
9. 120
10. 11.24508

(p. 9–10)
1. 60.000
2. 2.338
3. 133.462
4. 6.195
5. 20.000
6. 3.650
7. 20.000
8. 8.456
9. 3.435
10. 0.085

(p. 10)
A.
1. 0.8
2. 0.167
3. 0.22
4. 0.867
5. 4.4
6. 7.125
7. 0.704
8. 0.6754
9. 4.719
10. 2.611

B.
1. $^{28}/_{100}$ reduced to $^{7}/_{25}$
2. $5^{7}/_{100}$
3. $^{22}/_{10,000}$ reduced to $^{11}/_{5000}$
4. $1^{28}/_{100}$ reduced to $1^{7}/_{25}$
5. $3^{4}/_{100}$ reduced to $3^{1}/_{25}$
6. $^{575}/_{1000}$ reduced to $^{23}/_{40}$
7. $^{76}/_{100}$ reduced to $^{19}/_{25}$
8. $^{15,325}/_{100,000}$ reduced to $^{613}/_{4000}$
9. $6^{9}/_{100}$
10. $^{1}/_{100}$

Percentage
(p. 11)

	Fraction	Decimal	Percent
1.	—	0.25	25%
2.	$1^{25}/_{100}$	—	125%
3.	$^{5}/_{1000}$	0.005	—
4.	—	0.125	12.5%
5.	$^{14}/_{25}$	—	56%
6.	—	0.006	0.6%
7.	$^{3}/_{50}$	0.06	—
8.	$^{3}/_{4}$	—	75%
9.	$^{1}/_{5}$	0.2	—
10.	$^{3}/_{25}$	0.12	—
11.	$^{1}/_{20}$	—	5%
12.	$^{18}/_{25}$	0.72	—

(p. 11)
1. 18
2. 4.2
3. 0.75
4. 216
5. 13.4
6. 0.02
7. 37.5
8. 6
9. 1.2
10. 50.544
11. 137.5
12. 3.238

(p. 11)
1. 10%
2. 40%
3. 17.6%
4. 31.3%
5. 60%
6. 56.3%
7. 17.6%
8. 200%
9. 400%
10. 20%
11. 20%
12. 200%

Proportion
(p. 12)
1. 4
2. 400
3. 20
4. 10
5. 5000
6. 48
7. 3
8. 5
9. 36
10. 56
11. 90
12. 14
13. 28
14. 1.04
15. 25

Fahrenheit and Celsius
(p. 13)
1. 68° F
2. 140° F
3. 215.6° F
4. 95° F
5. 104° F
6. 38.3° C
7. 21.1° C
8. 48.9° C
9. 40° C
10. 36° C

Systems of Measurement
(p. 14)
1. 1 gm
2. 0.5 gm
3. 2 L
4. 1.5 gm
5. 100 mL
6. 0.75 gm
7. 1000 gm
8. 5000 mL
9. 0.004 gm
10. 0.1 kg
11. 250 mL
12. 6 mg
13. 0.25 gm
14. 2500 mL
15. 50 mg

(p. 14–15)
A.
1. 2 teaspoons
2. 16 ounces
3. 4.5 kg
4. 2 ounces
5. 10 kg
6. 90 gm
7. 12 teaspoons
8. 1 fluid ounce
9. 18 teaspoons
10. 154 pounds

B.
1. 500 mL
2. 4 cc
3. 15 mg
4. 100 mg
5. 1 pint
6. 15 mL
7. 13.6 kg
8. 6 teaspoons
9. 1.5 gm
10. 60 gm
11. 75 mL
12. $2^{1}/_{2}$ ounces
13. 1000 mg
14. 2 teaspoons
15. $^{1}/_{2}$ ounce
16. 2500 mL
17. 1 ounce
18. 6.6 pounds
19. 75 kg
20. $1^{1}/_{2}$ quarts

CHAPTER 2
1. c
2. a
3. d
4. a
5. a
6. b
7. c
8. c
9. d
10. d

CHAPTER 3
1. d
2. b
3. b
4. d
5. d
6. a
7. a
8. a
9. d
10. d

CHAPTER 4
1. d
2. c
3. b
4. c
5. c
6. c
7. d
8. d
9. a
10. b

CHAPTER 5
1. c
2. a
3. d
4. c
5. b
6. a
7. c
8. a
9. c
10. a

CHAPTER 6
1. c
2. c
3. d
4. b
5. c
6. d
7. c
8. b
9. b
10. c

CHAPTER 7
1. a
2. c
3. c
4. c
5. d
6. c
7. c
8. a
9. b
10. d

CHAPTER 8
1. d
2. b
3. a
4. d
5. c
6. a
7. a
8. b
9. c
10. d

CHAPTER 9
1. d
2. a
3. b

4. d
5. b
6. c
7. a
8. c
9. d
10. c

CHAPTER 10
1. b
2. d
3. b
4. d
5. a
6. d
7. a
8. c
9. d
10. d

CHAPTER 11
1. c
2. a
3. c
4. a
5. d
6. d
7. c
8. b
9. d
10. b

CHAPTER 12
1. a
2. d
3. d
4. c
5. d
6. a
7. d
8. d
9. a
10. c

CHAPTER 13
1. c
2. b
3. c
4. d
5. c
6. d
7. d
8. a
9. b
10. a

CHAPTER 14
1. b
2. c
3. d
4. b
5. a
6. b
7. d
8. d
9. b
10. b

CHAPTER 15
1. b
2. d
3. a
4. c
5. c
6. b
7. c
8. a
9. c
10. c

CHAPTER 16
1. b
2. a
3. c
4. b
5. c
6. d
7. c
8. a
9. a
10. c

CHAPTER 17
1. d
2. c
3. b
4. c
5. b
6. d
7. c
8. b
9. b
10. a

CHAPTER 18
1. a
2. b
3. a
4. a
5. b
6. c
7. c
8. d
9. a
10. d

CHAPTER 19
1. a
2. c
3. c
4. c
5. d
6. a
7. b
8. d
9. c
10. b

CHAPTER 20
1. b
2. c
3. c
4. b
5. d
6. c
7. c
8. b
9. a
10. a

CHAPTER 21
1. b
2. c
3. c
4. a
5. c
6. b
7. a
8. d
9. d
10. d

CHAPTER 22
1. a
2. c
3. c
4. d
5. a
6. b
7. c
8. a
9. c
10. d

CHAPTER 23
1. d
2. a
3. b
4. c
5. d
6. b
7. c
8. c
9. b
10. a

CHAPTER 24
1. b
2. c
3. c
4. c
5. a
6. c
7. b
8. a
9. a
10. d

CHAPTER 25
1. d
2. a
3. d
4. c
5. a
6. b
7. c
8. b
9. c
10. b

CHAPTER 26
1. d
2. b
3. d
4. c
5. b
6. d
7. b
8. c
9. a
10. c

CHAPTER 27
1. c
2. d
3. a
4. b
5. c
6. d
7. d
8. b
9. d
10. d

CHAPTER 28
1. b
2. b
3. c
4. a
5. c
6. b
7. d
8. a
9. c
10. c

CHAPTER 29
1. d
2. c
3. d
4. b
5. d
6. c
7. a
8. c
9. b
10. d

Therapeutic Index

Note: Page numbers followed by *b* indicate boxes, *f* indicate figures, and *t* indicate tables.

A

Acne, treatment of
 antiinflammatory and peeling agents, 76–77
 cleansing agents, 76
 topical antibiotics, 76–77
Acquired immune deficiency syndrome (AIDS) therapy
 fusion inhibitors, 61–62
 NNRTIs, 60–61
 NRTIs, 60
 protease inhibitors, 61, 130*b*
Allergic disorders, asthma, 83, 83*b*
 bronchodilators, 83–85, 84*b*
 environmental control, 83
 inhaled agents, 84–85
 preventive medications, 85–86
Alternative medicine, herbal remedies, 257–265, 258*b*, 263*b*
Alzheimer's disease management, 234, 234*t*
Appetite disorders, 157

C

Cancer, drugs used to treat
 alkylating agents, 199–200
 antimetabolites, 199–202
 antitumor antibiotics, 199, 204–205
 enzyme inhibitors, 199, 205
 hormones, 199, 202–204
  androgens, 202
  antiandrogens, 202
  antiestrogens, 202–203
  estrogens, 202
 immunomodulating agents, 199, 205–206
 miscellaneous agents, 207–208, 207*t*
 molecular medicine, 199, 206, 212, 214–215
 platinum-containing agents, 199, 206
 supportive agents, 208–209
 targeted therapies, 199, 206, 212
Constipation, drugs used to treat, 159–161

D

Depression, drugs used to treat, 133–136, 133*b*
 MAOIs, 134–135
 SSRIs, 133–134, 134*b*, 134*t*
 tricyclic antidepressants, 135
Diabetes mellitus, drugs used to treat, 168–172
 insulin, 168–170, 168*t*, 169*t*
 oral hypoglycemic agents, 170–172
Diarrhea, drugs used to treat, 161–162

E

Enuresis, drugs used to treat, 184–185, 238
Epilepsy, drugs used to treat, 113–115
Erectile dysfunction, drugs used to treat, 140, 186

F

Fungal infection, treatment of, 57, 57*t*, 72–73, 73*f*, 73*t*

H

Head lice, treatment of, 62–63
Heart failure, drugs used to treat, 89
 ACE inhibitors, 90–91
 beta blockers, 91
 inotropic drugs, 89–90, 90*b*
Hepatitis, treatment of, 58*t*, 59
Herpesvirus infections, drugs used to treat, 58*t*, 59
 genital herpes, 58*t*, 59
 herpes simplex, 58*t*, 59
Hypertension, drugs used to treat, 94–97
 ACE inhibitors, 90–91
 aldosterone inhibitors, 92
 alpha blockers, 95–96
 ARBs, 91–92
 beta blockers, 91
 calcium channel blockers, 96–97, 96*b*
 central alpha agonists, 95
 diuretics, 89

I

Immune disorders, immunosuppressives, 192–193, 192*b*
Impotence therapy, 140, 186
Infections, treatment of
 antibiotics, 49–55, 49*b*, 51*t*, 52*t*, 53*t*, 54*t*, 62*b*
 antifungal agents, 57, 57*t*
 antiparasitic agents, 62–63, 62*b*
 antiviral agents, 58–62, 58*t*
 sulfonamides, 55–57, 57*b*
Inflammatory conditions, treatment of
 corticosteroids, 167–168, 192
 COX-2 inhibitors, 142, 142*b*
 NSAIDs, 140–142, 141*b*, 142*b*
Influenza, drugs used to treat, 58, 58*t*

L

Lice, drugs used to treat, 62–63

M

Migraine headaches, drugs used to treat
 analgesics, 109–111, 123–124, 123*t*
 analgesics, nonnarcotic, 111
 triptans, 111–112, 112*b*
Multiple sclerosis, drugs used to treat, 193–194

N

Nausea, drugs used to treat, 158–159, 158*b*

O

Obesity, drugs used to treat, 157–158, 158*b*
Osteoporosis, drugs used to treat, 44, 220, 230–232

P

Painful conditions
 analgesics, narcotic, 109–111, 123–124, 123*t*
 analgesics, nonnarcotic, 111
 in end-of-life care, 244–246, 248*t*
 transdermal dosage forms, 110
Parkinsonism, drugs used to treat, 115–116, 116*b*, 116*t*
Parkinson's disease, drugs used to treat, 115–116, 116*b*, 116*t*
Peptic ulcer disease, drugs used to treat
 antacids, 156–157, 156*b*
 antisecretory agents, 155–156, 155*b*, 156*b*
 Helicobacter pylori, drugs used to treat, 154–155
Prostatic hypertrophy, drugs used to treat, 185–186, 185*b*
Psychiatric disease, drugs used to treat
 anxiety/nervousness, 130–131, 130*b*, 136–137, 136*b*
 psychoses, 131–132

R

Rheumatic disorders, drugs used to treat, 214
 immune suppressive agents, 213
 monoclonal antibodies, 212–213
 NSAIDs, 140–142, 141*b*, 142*b*

S

Scabies, treatment of, 62–63
Seizures, drugs used to treat, 113–115

T

Thyroid disorders, drugs used to treat
 hyperthyroidism (Graves' disease), 165–166, 166*b*
 hypothyroidism, 165–166, 166*t*

U

Urinary tract infections, drugs used to treat
 sulfonamides, 55–57, 57*b*
 urinary antiseptics, 183–184

V

Varicella zoster (shingles), drugs used to treat, 58*t*, 59
Vitamin deficiencies, drugs used to treat, 41–43, 43*b*

W

Warts, 77–78, 78*f*
Weight loss aids, 157–158, 158*b*
Worms, intestinal, treatment of, 62

General Index

Note: Page numbers followed by *b* indicate boxes, *f* indicate figures, and *t* indicate tables.

A
Aarane, 86
Abacavir, 60
Abatacept, 214
Abbokinase, 99
Abciximab, 100, 213, 215
Abilify, 131
Abraxane, 208
Absorption inhibitors, 157–158, 158*b*
Acacia, 71–72, 161
Acarbose, 171
Accolate, 86
AccuNeb, 84
Accupril, 91
Accutane, 77
ACE inhibitors. *See* Angiotensin-converting enzyme inhibitors
Aceon, 91
Acetaminophen, 69, 111, 121–122, 143*b*, 220–221, 248*t*
Acetazolamide, 57*b*, 76*b*
Acetohexamide, 57*b*, 76*b*
Acetylcholine, 146
Acetylcholinesterase, 146, 149, 234
Acetylcholinesterase inhibitors, 149
Acetylcysteine, 86
Acetylsalicylic acid, 141, 141*b*
Aclovate, 78*t*
Acne, treatment of, 76–77
Acquired immune deficiency syndrome (AIDS), 59–62
  fungal infection with, 57
  fusion inhibitors for, 61–62
  NNRTIs for, 60–61
  NRTIs for, 60
  protease inhibitors for, 61, 130*b*
Acrivastine, 69
ActHIB, 189
Acticin, 63
Actinomycin D, 204
Actiq, 122
Activase, 99
Actonel, 220, 232
Actos, 171
Acyclovir sodium, 58*t*, 59, 248*t*
Adacel, 191
Adalat, 96
Adalimumab, 214
Adapalene solution, 76
Adapin, 135
ADD. *See* Attention-deficit disorder
Adderall, 105
Addiction
  barbiturates, 108
  narcotic, 109
Addison's disease, 167
ADHD. *See* Attention-deficit/hyperactivity disorder
Adipex-P, 106
Administration of medications. *See* Drug administration
Adrenal glands, 167–168
Adrenalin, 84, 94, 146–147, 147*f*
Adrenergic agents, 146–147, 147*f*, 264*t*
Adrenergic blocking agents, 147–149
Adrenocorticotropic hormone, 164, 165*f*, 167
Adriamycin, 204
Adsorbents, 161
Advair Diskus, 85
Advicor, 101
Advil, 122, 141
AeroBid, 85
Aerosporin, 54*t*
Afinitor, 207*t*
Agar, 159
Aggrastat, 100
Aggrenox, 100
AIDS. *See* Acquired immune deficiency syndrome
Albendazole, 62
Albenza, 62
Albuterol, 84
Alclometasone dipropionate, 78*t*
Alcohol, 116*b*, 228*b*
  abuse of, 251, 254, 254*t*, 255*b*, 255*t*
  interactions with, 254*t*, 264*t*, 266–267, 267*t*
  sedative uses of, 72, 112–113
  topical use of, 74–75
Aldactazide, 182
Aldactone, 92, 182, 219
Aldara, 77–78
Aldesleukin, 206, 214
Aldomet, 95, 148
Aldoril, 148
Aldosterone, 167
Aldosterone inhibitors, 92, 182, 219
Alemtuzumab, 214–215
Alendronate, 220, 231
Aleve, 142
Alferon N, 206
Alfuzosin hydrochloride, 185
Alimta, 201, 207*t*
Aliskiren, 219
Aliskiren and valsartan, 92
Aliskiren hemifumarate, 92
Alkeran, 199
Alkylating agents, 199–200
Allegra, 68
Allegra-D, 68
Allerest, 69
Allergic disorders, asthma, 83, 83*b*
  bronchodilators for, 83–85, 84*b*
  environmental control for, 83
  inhaled agents for, 84–85
  preventive medications, 85–86
Allergic reactions, 65–66, 69*b*
  causes of, 66
  drugs causing, 66
  immunotherapy for, 69
  prostaglandins and, 140
  treatment of, 67–69, 67*b*, 69*b*
Allopurinol, 142
Almotriptan malate, 111–112
Aloe, 75*b*, 258–263, 264*t*
Alosetron hydrochloride, 161
Aloxi, 209
Alpha blockers, 95–96, 147, 186
Alpha-tocopherol (E), 42, 228*b*
Alprazolam, 116*b*, 130, 134*t*, 155, 234, 248*t*, 264*t*
Alprostadil, 140
Alprostadil sterile solution, 140
Altace, 91
Alteplase, 99
Alternative medicine, herbal remedies, 257–265, 258*b*, 263*b*
Altretamine, 207*t*
Aluminum hydroxide gel, 156
Aluminum salts, 72
Alvesco, 85
Alzheimer's disease, 234, 234*t*
Amantadine hydrochloride, 58*t*, 76*b*, 230*b*
Amaryl, 171
Ambien, 108
Amcinonide, 78*t*
Amerge, 112
Amethopterin, 201
Amikacin sulfate, 54*t*, 233
Amikin, 54*t*
Amiloride, 76*b*
Amiloride hydrochloride, 183
Aminoglycosides, 55*b*, 233
Aminophylline, 84
Amiodarone hydrochloride, 92, 186
Amitiza, 161
Amitriptyline, 76*b*, 125, 136, 221
Amitriptyline hydrochloride, 135, 248*t*
Amlodipine besylate, 96
Amoxicillin, 51*t*, 155
Amoxicillin and clavulanic acid, 51*t*
Amoxil, 51*t*, 155
Amphetamine, 255*t*
Amphetamine salts, 105
Amphojel, 156
Amphotericin B, 57*t*
Ampicillin, 51*t*
Ampicillin sodium and sulbactam, 51*t*
Amyl nitrite, 94
Anakinra, 214
Analgesics, 221, 230*b*. *See also* Nonsteroidal anti-inflammatory drugs
  antimigraine agents, 111–112, 112*b*, 223
  co-, 124–125
  in end-of-life care, 245–246, 248*t*
  for mild pain, 121–122
  for moderate pain, 122
  narcotic, 109–111, 117*b*, 123–124, 123*t*, 127*b*, 245–246, 252, 255*t*, 266–267
  non-narcotic, 111
  for older adults, 232
  opioid, 109–111, 117*b*, 123–124, 123*t*, 127*b*, 221, 223, 245–246
  for severe pain, 122–123
Anaphylaxis, 65
Anaprox, 122, 142, 248*t*
Anastrozole, 203
Ancobon, 57*t*
Androderm, 177–178
AndroGel, 177
Androgens, 202, 264*t*
Anectine, 150
Anemia, 39–40, 42–44
Anesthetics
  general, 106–107, 106*t*, 107*t*, 117*b*
  local, 72, 107, 107*t*, 117*b*, 125
  volatile, 106*t*
Angelica, 258
Angina pectoris, 91, 94, 96
Angiomax, 98
Angiotensin I, 90
Angiotensin II, 90
Angiotensin receptor blockers (ARBs), 91–92, 219
Angiotensin-converting enzyme (ACE) inhibitors, 90–91, 132*t*, 169, 219, 228*b*, 233
Anidulafungin, 57*t*
Anorexia, 157
Ansaid, 141
Antacids, 156–157, 156*b*, 162*b*, 228*b*, 233–234
Antiandrogens, 202
Antibiotics, 49–55, 49*b*, 54*t*, 55*b*, 63*b*, 228, 230*b*, 233–234, 254*t*, 267. *See also* Antitumor antibiotics
  beta-lactams, 51–52, 52*t*
  for children, 49*b*, 55*b*, 238

Antibiotics (*Continued*)
dosage of, 25–26
macrolides, 53, 53*t*, 130*b*
penicillins, 50, 51*t*, 233
quinolones, 54, 54*t*, 228*b*, 233–234
tetracyclines, 53, 53*t*
Anticholinergic agents, 150, 150*b*, 228*b*, 230*b*
Anticoagulants, 97–99, 99*b*, 102*b*, 254*t*, 267
Anticonvulsants, 113–115, 124, 223–224
in anxiety disorders, 136–137
Antidepressants, 99*b*, 105*b*, 124–125, 130*b*, 133–136, 133*b*, 134*b*, 134*t*, 137*b*, 221, 253–254, 264*t*
alcohol and, 254, 254*t*
nonpsychiatric uses of, 136
Antidiarrheals, 161–162, 162*b*
Antiemetics, 158–159, 158*b*, 162*b*, 208–209
Antiestrogens, 202–203
Antifungal agents, 57, 57*t*, 63*b*
topical use of, 72–73, 73*f*, 73*t*
Antihelmintic drugs, 62
Antihistamines, 65–69, 67*b*, 69*b*, 108*b*, 116*b*, 124, 230*b*, 254, 254*t*, 264*t*
combinations of, 69
intranasal, 68
nonsedating, 68
traditional (sedating), 67–68
Antihypertensive agents, 94–97, 95*b*, 96*b*, 174*b*, 182, 219, 230*b*, 233, 245, 254*t*, 264*t*, 267
Anti-infective agents, 74–75
Antiinflammatory drugs, 167–168, 192–193, 192*b*, 193*b*, 213. *See also* Nonsteroidal anti-inflammatory drugs
Antilipemics, 219
Antilipidemic drugs, 100–102, 101*b*
Antimetabolites, 199, 200–202
Antimigraine agents, 111–112, 112*b*, 223
Antimonilial preparations, 73–74, 74*f*
Antineoplastic drugs, 198–209, 198*b*, 207*t*, 209*b*
alkylating agents, 199–200
antimetabolites, 199–202
antitumor antibiotics, 199, 204–205
enzyme inhibitors, 199, 205
hormones, 199, 202–204
immunity and, 198*b*
immunomodulating agents, 199, 205–206
molecular medicine, 199, 206, 212, 214–215
platinum-containing agents, 199, 206
supportive agents used with, 208–209
targeted therapies, 199, 206, 212
vaccines, 199, 206
Antioxidants, 40
Antiparasitic agents, 62–63, 62*b*, 63*b*
Antiparkinsonian agents, 115–116, 116*b*, 116*t*, 230*b*, 264*t*
Antiplatelet therapy, 99–100, 100*b*
Antipsychotics, 131–132
Antisecretory agents, 155–156, 155*b*, 156*b*, 220
Antithyroid agents, 166, 166*b*, 232
Antitumor antibiotics, 199, 204–205
Antivert, 68, 158
Antiviral agents, 58–62, 58*t*, 63*b*, 186
for hepatitis, 58*t*, 59
for herpesvirus, 58*t*, 59
for HIV and AIDS, 59–62
for influenza, 58, 58*t*
Anxiety, 130–131, 130*b*, 136–137, 136*b*, 137*b*, 234, 238
Anxiolytic agents, 136, 136*b*
Anzemet, 209
Apidra, 170
Appetite stimulants, 157, 209
Aprepitant, 209
Aptivus, 61
AquaMEPHYTON, 97
Arabic numerals, 1–2
Ara-C, 200
Aramine, 147
Aranesp, 208
Arava, 214
ARBs. *See* Angiotensin receptor blockers
Ardeparin sodium injection, 98
Aredia, 125
Arformoterol tartrate, 84
Argatroban, 98
Aricept, 234*t*
Arimidex, 203
Aripiprazole, 131
Aristocort, 168
Armodafinil, 105
Armour Thyroid Tablets, 232
Arnica, 258
Aromasin, 203
Aromatase inhibitors, 203
Arranon, 207*t*
Arrhythmias, cardiac, 91–93
Arsenic trioxide, 207*t*
Artane, 116*t*
Arthritis, 214, 219–220, 231
Asafetida, 258
Ascorbic acid, 43
Asparaginase, 205
Aspirin, 69, 100, 111, 121–122, 139, 141, 141*b*, 142*b*, 143*b*, 219, 220–221, 228*b*, 231, 248*t*, 254*t*, 257, 266–267
Aspirin and extended-release dipyridamole, 100
Astelin, 68, 85
Astemizole, 76*b*
Asthma, 83, 83*b*
bronchodilators for, 83–85, 84*b*
environmental control for, 83
inhaled agents for, 84–85
preventive medications, 85–86
Astringents, 72
Atacand, 92
Atamet, 116
Atanazir sulfate, 61
Atarax, 132, 248*t*
Atenolol, 91, 147, 219
Athlete's foot, 73
Ativan, 130, 248*t*
Atomoxetine hydrochloride, 105
Atopic dermatitis, 77, 77*f*
Atorvastatin calcium, 101, 219
Atrial arrhythmias, 91–93
AtroPen, 150
Atropine, 109, 150, 230*b*
Atropine sulfate, 150, 161
Attention-deficit disorder (ADD), 105–106, 106*b*
Attention-deficit/hyperactivity disorder (ADHD), 105–106, 106*b*, 238
Augmentin, 51*t*
Autonomic nervous system, 145–151, 150*b*
neuromuscular blocking agents, 150–151
parasympatholytic (cholinergic blocking) agents, 150, 150*b*
parasympathomimetic (cholinergic) agents, 149, 149*f*
sympathetic and parasympathetic systems, 145–146, 146*f*, 146*t*
sympatholytic (adrenergic blocking) agents, 147–149
sympathomimetic (adrenergic) agents, 146–147, 147*f*
Avandamet, 172
Avandia, 171
Avapro, 92
Avastin, 215
Avelox, 54*t*
Aventyl, 135
Avitaminosis, 39
Avodart, 185
Avoirdupois measurement system, 14–15
Avonex, 193
Axert, 111–112
Axid, 156
Azacitidine, 200, 207*t*
Azactam, 52*t*
Azathioprine, 76*b*, 192, 192*b*, 213, 264*t*
Azelastine hydrochloride, 68, 85
Azithromycin, 53, 53*t*
Azmacort, 85
Aztreonam, 52*t*
Azulfidine, 56

B

Baclofen, 248*t*
Bactrim, 56, 184
Bactrim DS, 56, 184
Bactroban, 75
Baking soda, 156–157
Barbiturates, 76*b*, 107–108, 158, 230*b*, 255*t*
Basiliximab, 213
Beclomethasone dipropionate, 85
Beclovent, 85
Belladonna, 150, 161
Benadryl, 67–68
Benazepril, 90
Bendamustine HCl, 207*t*
Bendroflumethiazide, 57*b*
Benicar, 92, 219
Benign prostatic hypertrophy (BPH), 185–186, 185*b*
Bentyl, 150
Benzaclin, 76
Benzalkonium chloride, 74
Benzocaine, 72
Benzodiazepines, 108*b*, 124, 130–131, 130*b*, 221, 230*b*, 234, 264*t*
Benzoic acid, 72
Benzothiadiazine diuretics. *See* Thiazide diuretics
Benzoyl peroxide, 76
Benzoyl peroxide plus clindamycin, 76
Benzthiazide, 57*b*
Benztropine mesylate, 116*t*
Benzylpenicillin, 50
Beriberi, 42
Beta blockers, 91, 134*t*, 147, 150*b*, 219, 223–224, 228*b*, 233
Betadine, 75
17-Beta-estradiol, 202
Beta-lactam antibiotics, 51–52, 52*t*. *See also* Cephalosporins
Betamethasone, 167, 220
Betamethasone acetate, 220
Betamethasone dipropionate, augmented, 78*t*
Betamethasone sodium phosphate, 220
Betamethasone valerate, 78*t*
Betapace, 91
Betaseron, 193, 213
Betaxolol, 91
Bethanechol chloride, 149, 149*f*
Bevacizumab, 215
Bexarotene, 207*t*
Biaxin, 53*t*
Bicalutamide, 202
Bicillin, 50
Bicillin C-R, 50
Bicillin L-A, 50
BiCNU, 199
Biltricide, 62
Bioidentical hormone replacement therapy, 174
Bisacodyl, 160
Bismuth, 155
Bisoprolol fumarate, 91
Bisphosphonates, 125, 231–232
Bivalirudin, 98
Black cohosh, 174*b*, 258, 264*t*
Black root, 259
Blackthorn, 259
Blenoxane, 204
Bleomycin sulfate, 204
Blocadren, 91
Body surface area nomogram, 239*f*, 240
Boiled milk, 161
Boiled starch, 161
Bone marrow transplant patients, home therapy for, 243
Bone pain, 125
Bonine, 68, 158
Boniva, 220, 231
Bortezomib, 207*t*
Botulism immune globulin, 191
BPH. *See* Benign prostatic hypertrophy
Brethine, 84
Brevibloc, 91
Brevoxyl, 76
Bromides, 113, 158
Bromocriptine mesylate, 116*t*, 230*b*
Brompheniramine maleate, 67
Bronchodilators, 83–85, 84*b*, 267*t*
Brovana, 84
Budesonide, 85, 167
Bulk-increasing laxatives, 159, 228*b*
Bumetanide, 57*b*
Bupivacaine hydrochloride, 107*t*
Bupropion hydrochloride, 136, 254–255
BuSpar, 136, 136*b*, 234
Buspirone hydrochloride, 136, 136*b*, 234
Busulfan, 199
Butenafine hydrochloride, 73*t*
Butorphanol, 122
Butorphanol tartrate, 110

Byetta, 170
Bystolic, 91

C

Cabazitaxel, 207*t*
Caffeine, 83*b*, 221–225, 233, 261, 264*t*, 267*t*
Calan, 97
Calcimar, 231
Calcitonin, 220, 231
Calcium, 44–45, 45*b*, 220–222, 231
Calcium carbonate, 45, 90*b*
Calcium channel blockers, 96–97, 96*b*, 130*b*, 132*t*, 233, 267
Calcium chloride, 45, 97
Calcium citrate, 90*b*
Calcium gluconate, 45, 97
Calcium lactate, 45, 97
Calcium salts, 97, 220
Campath, 214–215
Camphor, 72
Camptosar, 205
Cancer
  drugs used to treat, 198–209, 198*b*, 207*t*, 209*b*
    alkylating agents, 199–200
    antimetabolites, 199–202
    antitumor antibiotics, 199, 204–205
    enzyme inhibitors, 199, 205
    hormones, 199, 202–204
    immunomodulating agents, 199, 205–206
    molecular medicine, 199, 206, 212, 214–215
    platinum-containing agents, 199, 206
    supportive agents, 208–209
    targeted therapies, 199, 206, 212
  immunizations against, 199, 206
  nutrition for, 230
Cancidas, 57*t*
Candesartan cilexetil, 92
Candidiasis, 73–74, 74*f*
Cannabis, 253
Capastat, 54*t*
Capecitabine, 200
Capoten, 90
Capreomycin sulfate, 54*t*
Capsaicin, 125, 259
Capsicum, 157*b*, 259, 264*t*
Captopril, 76*b*, 90
Carafate, 157
Carbamazepine, 76*b*, 113, 124, 134*t*, 136, 224, 248*t*
Carbamide, 177
Carbidopa, 116, 228*b*, 230*b*
Carbinoxamine maleate, 69
Carbocaine, 107*t*
Carbon dioxide, 82, 156–157
Carboplatin, 206
Cardene, 96
Cardiac arrhythmias, 91–93
Cardiac glycosides, 89–90, 90*b*
Cardiovascular disease, in women, 218–219
Cardizem, 96
Cardura, 96
Caregiver stress, 234–235
Carisoprodol, 125
Carmustine, 199
Carvedilol, 91
Casanthrol, 161
Casodex, 202
Caspofungin acetate, 57*t*
Castor oil, 160
Catapres, 95, 147
Catapres TTS, 95
Cathartics, 159–161, 162*b*
  irritant, 160
  saline, 160
Caverject Injections, 140
Cayenne, 157*b*, 259
CCNU, 199
2-Cda, 200
Cedax, 52*t*
Cefaclor, 52*t*
Cefadroxil, 52*t*
Cefazolin sodium, 52*t*
Cefdinir, 52*t*
Cefditoren pivoxil, 52*t*
Cefepime hydrochloride, 51, 52*t*
Cefixime, 52*t*
Cefotaxime sodium, 52*t*
Cefotetan disodium, 52*t*
Cefoxitin sodium, 52*t*
Cefpodoxime proxetil, 52*t*
Cefprozil, 52*t*
Ceftazidime sodium, 52*t*
Ceftibuten, 52*t*
Ceftin, 52*t*
Ceftriaxone sodium, 52*t*
Cefuroxime axetil, 52*t*
Cefuroxime sodium, 52*t*
Cefzil, 52*t*
Celebrex, 121, 142
Celecoxib, 121, 142
Celestone, 167, 220
Celexa, 134*t*
CellCept, 213
Celsius, 12–13, 12*f*
Central alpha-agonists, 95
Central nervous system depressants, 106–113, 106*t*, 107*t*, 108*b*, 112*b*, 117*b*
Central nervous system stimulants, 105–106, 105*b*, 106*b*, 117*b*
Centrum Silver, 230
Cephalexin, 52*t*
Cephalosporins, 51–52, 52*t*, 76*b*, 233
Cephamycins, 52*t*
Cerebyx, 114
Cerefolin NAC, 43
Cervidil Vaginal Insert, 140
Cetirizine hydrochloride, 68
Cetuximab, 215
Cevitamic acid, 43
Chamomile, 158*b*, 221–222, 259, 264*t*
Chantix, 255
Chaparral, 259
Charcoal, 161
Chemotherapy. *See* Antineoplastic drugs
Children, 237–240, 240*b*
  dosages for, 238–240, 239*f*
  home infusion for, 243
Chloral hydrate, 108
Chlorambucil, 199
Chloramphenicol, 54*t*, 99*b*, 183
Chlordiazepoxide, 76*b*, 150
Chlordiazepoxide hydrochloride, 130
Chloroform, 72
Chloromycetin, 54*t*
Chloroprocaine hydrochloride, 107*t*
Chloroquine, 76*b*
Chlorothiazide, 57*b*, 76*b*, 182
Chlorpheniramine maleate, 67
Chlorpromazine, 76*b*, 230*b*, 248*t*
Chlorpromazine hydrochloride, 131
Chlorpropamide, 57*b*, 171
Chlorthalidone, 57*b*, 76*b*, 89, 182, 219
Chlor-Trimeton, 67
Cholesterol, 100–102, 219
Cholestyramine, 101
Cholinergic agents, 149, 149*f*
Cholinergic blocking agents, 150, 150*b*
Chondroitin sulfate, 259
Chronic fatigue syndrome, 221
Cialis, 186
Ciclesonide, 85
Ciclopirox olamine, 72
Ciclopirox solution, 73
Cidofovir, 58*t*
Cilostazol, 100
Cimetidine, 100*b*, 134*t*, 155, 155*b*, 228*b*, 230*b*, 248*t*
Cipro, 54*t*
Ciprofloxacin hydrochloride, 54*t*, 233–234
Circulatory system, 88–102, 89*f*, 102*b*
  blood, drugs affecting, 97–102, 99*b*, 100*b*, 101*b*, 102*b*
  blood vessels, drugs affecting, 93–97, 93*b*, 95*b*, 96*b*
  heart, 88–89, 89*f*
    drugs affecting, 90*b*, 102*b*, 93–97
  prostaglandins and, 140
Cisplatin, 206
Citalopram, 124, 134*t*, 203
Citanest, 107*t*
Citracal, 90*b*
Citrate of magnesia, 160
Citrucel, 159
Cladribine, 200
Claforan, 52*t*
Clarinex, 68
Clarithromycin, 53, 53*t*, 155
Claritin, 68
Claritin-D, 68
Clark's rule, 240
Clearasil Medicated Astringent, 76
Clemastine fumarate, 69
Cleocin, 54*t*
Cleocin-T, 77
Clevidipine butyrate, 96
Cleviprex, 96
Clidinium bromide plus chlordiazepoxide, 150
Climara, 223
Clindagel, 77
Clindamycin hydrochloride, 54*t*
Clindamycin phosphate, 76–77
Clinoril, 122, 142
Clioquinol, 73
Clobetasol propionate, 78*t*
Clofarabine, 200
Clofibrate, 99*b*
Clolar, 200
Clomid, 176
Clomiphene citrate, 176
Clonazepam, 113, 124, 221
Clonidine, 95, 123–124, 230*b*
Clonidine hydrochloride, 95, 147
Clopamide, 57*b*
Clopidogrel bisulfate, 100, 266–267
Clorazepate dipotassium, 130
Clotrimazole, 73–74, 248*t*
Coagulants, 97
Coanalgesics, 124–125
Cocaine, 72, 251, 253–254, 255*t*
Cocaine hydrochloride, 107*t*
Codeine, 109, 123*t*, 230*b*, 248*t*
Codeine phosphate, 110
Codeine sulfate, 110, 122, 248*t*
Cogentin, 116*t*
Cognex, 234*t*
Cognitive impairment, 230*b*
Colace, 161, 248*t*
Colchicine, 142
Colcrys, 142
Colestid, 101
Colestipol granules, 101
Colistimethate sodium, 54*t*
Colistin sulfate, 54*t*
Coly-Mycin M, 54*t*
Coly-Mycin S, 54*t*
Comfrey, 154*b*, 259, 264*t*
Compazine, 131, 159, 208–209, 248*t*
Comvax, 189
Concerta, 106
Congestive heart failure, 90–92, 102*b*
Constipation, 159–161
Contac, 69
Contraceptives
  emergency, 176
  injectable, 175
  oral, 76*b*, 133*b*, 174–175, 175*t*, 176, 177*b*, 223–224, 264*t*
  transdermal, 175
Controlled Drugs and Substances Act, 22
Controlled substances, 20–21
Controlled Substances Act, 20
Copaxone, 193
Copper, 45–46
Cordarone, 92
Cordran, 167
Coreg, 91
Corgard, 91, 93, 148
Coricidin D, 69
Coronary artery disease, 230
Corpus luteum, 172–173, 173*f*
Correctol, 161
Cortef, 168
Corticosteroids, 167–168, 192, 201, 230*b*
  antineoplastic, 202
  inhaled agents, 84–85
  topical, 56, 78–79, 78*t*
Cortisone, 167
Cortogen, 167
Cortone, 167
Corvert, 93
Cosmegen, 204
Cotolone, 168
Co-trimoxazole, 56, 184
Cough, 82, 82*b*
Coumadin, 99, 99*b*, 134*t*, 263
Coumarin, 76*b*, 93*b*, 98–99, 99*b*, 133*b*, 155, 261, 264*t*, 266–267
COX-2 inhibitors. *See* Cyclooxygenase-2 inhibitors
Cozaar, 92
CPT-11, 205
Creamalin, 156
Creolin, 75
Creon, 157
Crestor, 102
Cretinism, 165
Crixivan, 61
CroFab, 191
Crohn's disease, 214

Cromolyn sodium, 86
Crotalidae polyvalent immune Fab, 191
Crotamiton, 62
Curare, 149
Cutivate, 78*t*
Cyanocobalamin (B_{12}), 43, 201
Cyclobenzaprine, 125
Cyclocort, 78*t*
Cyclooxygenase-2 (COX-2) inhibitors, 142, 142*b*, 143*b*
Cyclopenthiazide, 57*b*
Cyclophosphamide, 192, 199, 213
Cycloserine, 54*t*
Cyclosporine, 133*b*, 192*b*, 193, 193*b*, 213, 228*b*, 264*t*
Cymbalta, 134
Cyproheptadine hydrochloride, 67
Cytarabine, 200
CytoGam, 191
Cytomegalovirus immune globulin, 191
Cytomel, 166*t*
Cytosar-U, 200
Cytotec, 140, 155
Cytovene, 58*t*
Cytoxan, 192, 199, 213

D

Dacarbazine, 201
Daclizumab, 213
Dacogen, 201
Dactinomycin, 204
Dalmane, 108, 130, 248*t*
Dalteparin sodium injection, 98
Dapsone, 54*t*, 57*b*
Daptacel, 189
Darbopoetin alfa, 208
Darunavir, 61
Dasatinib, 207*t*
Daunomycin, 204
Daunorubicin hydrochloride, 204
Daunorubicin liposome, 204
Dauoxome, 204
Daypro, 142
Daytrana, 106
DDAVP, 238
DDAVP Nasal Spray, 184
DEA. *See* Drug Enforcement Administration
Decadron, 202, 209
Decimals, 7–10
  addition of, 8
  changing between fractions and, 10
  division of, 9–10
  multiplication of, 9
  reading and writing of, 7–8, 7*f*
  subtraction of, 8–9
Decitabine, 201
Declomycin, 53*t*
Decongestants, 264*t*, 267*t*
Delavirdine mesylate, 60
Delta-9-tetrahydrocannabinol (THC), 253
Deltasone, 168
Demadex, 183
Demeclocycline hydrochloride, 53*t*
Demerol, 110, 122, 248*t*
Demulcents, 71–72, 161
Demulen, 175*t*
Denavir, 59
Denileukin diftitox, 215
Denosumab, 231
Deoxycorticosterone, 167
Depakene, 115, 248*t*
Depakote, 136, 224, 248*t*
Depo-Provera, 175
Depression, 222
  drugs used to treat, 133–136, 133*b*
    MAOIs, 134–135
    SSRIs, 133–134, 134*b*, 134*t*
    tricyclic antidepressants, 135
  older adults and, 229, 232, 234
  pain and, 124
Dermatitis. *See* Atopic dermatitis
Desenex, 73
Desipramine, 76*b*, 125, 253–254
Desipramine hydrochloride, 135, 248*t*
Desloratadine, 68
Desmopressin acetate, 184, 238
Desonide, 78*t*
DesOwen, 78*t*
Desoximetasone, 78*t*
Desvenlafaxine succinate, 134, 203
Detrol, 185
Detrol LA, 185
Dexamethasone, 124, 192, 202, 209
Dexedrine, 105
Dextroamphetamine sulfate, 105
Diabeta, 171
Diabetes mellitus, 168–172, 168*t*, 169*t*, 219
  home care for, 243
  incretin mimetic for, 170
  insulin for, 168–170, 168*t*, 169*t*, 177*b*
  nutrition for, 230
  oral hypoglycemic agents for, 170–172
Diabinese, 171
Dial soap, 74–75
Diarrhea, 161–162
Diazepam, 107*t*, 114, 124, 130, 155, 234, 248*t*
Diazoxide, 57*b*, 99*b*
Dibucaine, 72
Dichlorphenamide, 57*b*
Diclofenac, 141
Dicloxacillin sodium, 51*t*
Dicyclomine hydrochloride, 150
Didanosine, 60
Didronel, 231
Dietary Reference Intakes (DRIs), 40
Differin, 76
Diflorasone diacetate, 78*t*
Diflucan, 57*t*
Diflunisal, 76*b*, 122, 141
Digestants, 157, 157*b*
Digestive system, 153–154, 154*f*
Digibind, 90
Digitalis preparations, 89–90, 90*b*, 156*b*, 257, 264*t*
Digitek, 90
Digoxin, 56, 89–90, 90*b*, 102*b*, 133*b*, 228*b*, 230*b*, 264*t*, 267
Digoxin immune Fab, 90
Dihydroxyphenylalanine, 116
Dilantin, 115, 134*t*, 248*t*
Dilaudid, 110, 122, 248*t*, 252
Diltiazem, 76*b*
Diltiazem hydrochloride, 96
Dimenhydrinate, 67, 158
Dinoprostone, 140, 176
Dinoprostone cervical gel, 176
Dioctal, 161
Diovan, 92
Diphenhydramine hydrochloride, 67–68, 76*b*, 230*b*
Diphenoxylate hydrochloride, 248*t*
Diphenoxylate hydrochloride plus atropine sulfate, 161
Diphtheria and tetanus toxoids, acellular pertussis, and inactivated poliovirus vaccine, 189
Diphtheria and tetanus toxoids, acellular pertussis, inactivated poliovirus, and *Haemophilus b* vaccine, 189
Diphtheria and tetanus toxoids, acellular pertussis, inactivated poliovirus, and hepatitis B vaccine, 189
Diphtheria and tetanus toxoids, adsorbed (DT, Td), 189
Diphtheria and tetanus toxoids and acellular pertussis vaccine (DTaP), 189, 194*f*
Diprolene, 78*t*
Direct inhibitors of thrombin, 98
Dirithromycin, 53
Disopyramide phosphate, 93
Disulfiram, 99*b*, 254*t*
Ditropan, 185
Ditropan XL, 185
Diuretics, 89, 132*t*, 142, 174*b*, 181–183, 182*b*, 183*b*, 186*b*, 219, 228*b*, 230*b*, 233, 264*t*
Diuril, 182
Divalproex, 136, 224, 248*t*
Docetaxel, 207, 207*t*
Docusate calcium, 161
Docusate sodium, 161
Docusate sodium plus casanthrol, 161
Dofetilide, 93
Dolasetron, 209
Dolobid, 122, 141
Dolophine, 110, 122, 248*t*, 252
Donepezil hydrochloride, 234*t*
Donnazyme, 157
Dopamine receptor agonists, 108
Dopaminergic agents, 116
Dopar, 116
Dopram, 105
Doribax, 52*t*
Doripenem, 52*t*
Dosage forms, 30
Dosage of drugs, 24–27
  for children, 238–240, 239*f*
  prescriptions, 26–27, 26*f*, 27*t*
  standardized units for, 25–26, 25*f*
Dove soap, 76
Doxapram hydrochloride, 105
Doxazosin mesylate, 96
Doxepin, 125, 221
Doxepin hydrochloride, 135
Doxidan, 161
Doxil, 204
Doxorubicin hydrochloride, 204
Doxorubicin liposome, 204
Doxycycline hyclate, 53, 53*t*, 76*b*
Dramamine, 67, 158
DRIs. *See* Dietary Reference Intakes
Dristan, 69
Dronabinol, 209, 253
Dronedarone hydrochloride, 93
Drug abuse, 251–255, 255*b*
  signs and symptoms of, 252, 255, 255*t*
Drug administration, 16–17, 16*f*, 29–37
  disposal of unwanted medications, 37
  inhaled, 32
  innovative drug delivery systems for, 36–37
  local effects and, 30
  methods of, 29–37, 31*f*, 32*f*, 33*f*, 34*f*, 35*f*
  mucous membrane, 30
  oral, 31–32, 31*f*
  parenteral, 32–36, 32*f*, 33*f*, 34*f*, 35*f*
  safety guidelines for, 29, 30*b*
  skin, 30
  sublingual, 32
  systemic effects and, 30–36, 31*f*, 32*f*, 33*f*, 34*f*, 35*f*
Drug allergies, 66
Drug Enforcement Administration (DEA), 20
Drug interactions, 266–268, 267*t*, 268*b*
Drug legislation, 20–22
Drug reactions, 66
Drug standards, 21–22
Drug-herb interactions, 257, 263–267, 264*t*
DT. *See* Diphtheria and tetanus toxoids, adsorbed
DTaP. *See* Diphtheria and tetanus toxoids and acellular pertussis vaccine
DTIC-Dome, 201
Duac, 76
Dulcolax, 160, 248*t*
Duloxetine hydrochloride, 134, 203, 222
Duragesic, 110, 122, 248*t*
Duranest, 107*t*
Duricef, 52*t*
Dutasteride, 185
Dyazide, 183
Dyrenium, 183
Dysmenorrhea, 224

E

EAR. *See* Estimated Average Requirement
Ear preparations, 30
Echinacea, 192*b*, 259, 264*t*
Econazole nitrate, 73, 73*f*
Eczema. *See* Atopic dermatitis
Edecrin, 183
Edema, 181–183
Edex Injections, 140
Edrophonium chloride, 149
EES, 53*t*
Efavirenz, 61
Effexor, 134
Effient, 100
Egg white, 71–72
Elavil, 135, 248*t*
Electrolytes for oral solution, 160
Eletriptan hydrobromide, 112
Elidel, 77
Eligard, 203
Elimite, 63
Ellence, 204
Elocon, 78*t*
Eloxatin, 206
Elspar, 205
Embeda, 123
Emcyt, 202
Emend, 209
Emergency contraception, 176

Emetics, 158
Emgel, 77
Emollients, 71
Emtricitabine, 60
Emtriva, 60
Enalapril, 91
Enbrel, 214
Endocrine glands, 164, 165*f*. *See also* Hormones
End-of-life care, 244–249, 246*t*, 248*t*, 249*b*
Energy stimulants, 209
Enflurane, 106*t*
Enfuvirtide, 61
Engerix-B, 190
Enovid, 175*t*
Enovid-E, 175*t*
Enoxaparin sodium injection, 98
Enrich, 229
Ensure, 229
Ensure Plus, 229
Entecavir, 59
Entocort, 167
Enuresis, 184–185, 238
Enzyme inhibitors, 199, 205
Ephedra, 83*b*, 259–260, 264*t*
Ephedrine sulfate, 83, 264*t*
Epilepsy, 113–115
Epinephrine, 146–147, 147*f*, 167
Epinephrine hydrochloride, 146–147, 147*f*
Epinephrine injection, 84, 84*b*, 94
Epinephrine solution, 94
Epi-Pen, 146–147, 147*f*
Epirubicin hydrochloride, 204
Epivir, 59, 60
Epivir-HBV, 59
Eplerenome, 92, 182
Epocrates.com, 22
Epoetin alfa, 208
Epogen, 208
Eprosartan mesylate, 92
Eptifibatide, 100
Equivalent fractions, 4
Eraxis, 57*t*
Erbitux, 215
Erectile dysfunction, 140, 186
Ergonovine, 148
Ergonovine maleate, 176
Ergot alkaloids, 148–149
Ergotamine, 148
Ergotamine tartrate, 149
Ergotrate, 176
Erlotinib hydrochloride, 215
Ertapenem sodium, 52*t*
Eryc, 53*t*
Erygel, 77
Ery-Ped, 53*t*
Ery-Tab, 53*t*
Erythrocin lactobionate, 53*t*
Erythromycins, 53, 53*t*
Erythromycin estolate, 53*t*
Erythromycin ethylsuccinate, 53*t*
Erythromycin lactobionate, 53*t*
Erythromycin stearate, 53*t*
Erythromycin topical gel, 77
Escitalopram, 134*t*, 203
Eskalith, 132, 132*b*, 132*t*
Esmolol, 91
Esomeprazole, 100*b*, 155
Essential fatty acids, 40, 46
Esterified estrogens tablets, 174
Estimated Average Requirement (EAR), 40
Estrace, 225
Estraderm, 223
Estradiol, 172–174, 223
Estramustine phosphate sodium, 202
Estratab, 174
Estrogens, 173–174, 219, 264*t*
  for cancer treatment, 202
Estrogens, conjugated, 174, 231
Estrogen agonist-antagonists, 174
Estrogen replacement therapy, 174, 219–220, 223, 225, 231
Estrone, 174
Eszopiclone, 132
Etanercept, 214
Ethacrynic acid, 183
Ethambutol hydrochloride, 54*t*
Ethchlorvynol, 21, 99*b*
Ether, 106*t*
Ethinyl estradiol, 174–175, 175*t*, 176
Ethinyl estradiol and etonogestrel ring, 175
Ethinyl estradiol plus levonorgestrel, 176
Ethionamide, 54*t*
Ethosuximide, 114
Ethotoin, 114
Ethrane, 106*t*
Ethyl alcohol, 74, 112–113
Ethynodiol diacetate, 175*t*
Etidocaine hydrochloride, 107*t*
Etidronate disodium, 231
Etodolac, 122, 141
Etonogestrel ring, 175
Etonogestrel subdermal implant, 175
Etoposide, 205
Etravirene, 61
Eulexin, 202
Eurax, 62
Everolimus, 207*t*
Evista, 174, 220, 232
Exelon, 234*t*
Exemestane, 203
Exenatide, 170
Ezetimibe, 101
Ezetimibe with simvastatin, 101

F

Factive, 54*t*
Fahrenheit, 12–13, 12*f*
Famciclovir, 58*t*, 59
Family care, of older adults, 234–235
Famotidine, 155, 248*t*
Famvir, 58*t*, 59
Fareston, 203
Faslodex, 202
Febuxostat, 143
Fecal softeners, 160–161, 248*t*
Felbamate, 114
Felbatol, 114
Feldene, 142
Felodipine, 96
Femara, 203
Fenofibrate, 101
Fenofibric acid, 101
Fenoprofen calcium, 141, 231
Fentanyl, 123*t*
Fentanyl citrate, 122, 248*t*
Fentanyl transdermal system, 110
Feosol, 44
Fergon, 44
Ferrous gluconate, 44
Ferrous sulfate, 44
Fetal development, medications and, 237–238
Feverfew, 112*b*, 260, 264*t*
Fexofenadine hydrochloride, 68
Fexofenadine plus pseudoephedrine, 68
Fiber, 40, 40*t*, 228*b*, 230
Fibromyalgia, 116–117, 220–221
Filgrastim, 208
Finasteride, 185
Fish oil capsules, 230
Flagyl, 54*t*, 155, 254*t*
Flomax, 186
Flonase, 85
Florinef, 167
Floxuridine, 201
Flu shot. *See* Influenza vaccine
Fluconazole, 57*t*
Flucytosine, 57*t*
Fludara, 201
Fludarabine phosphate, 201
Fludrocortisone acetate, 167
Flumadine, 58*t*
FluMist, 190, 196*f*
Flunisolide nasal solution, 85
Fluocinolone A, 167
Fluocinonide, 78*t*
Fluorescein, 76*b*
Fluoride, 46
Fluorouracil, 76*b*, 201
Fluothane, 106*t*
Fluoxetine, 124, 134*t*, 203, 221–222, 266
Fluphenazine hydrochloride, 131
Flurandrenolide ointment, 167
Flurazepam hydrochloride, 108, 130, 248*t*
Flurbiprofen, 141
Flutamide, 202
Fluticasone propionate, 78*t*, 85
Fluticasone propionate and salmeterol, 85
Fluvirin, 190
Fluvoxamine, 134*t*
Fluzone, 190
Folic acid, 42–43, 43*b*, 201
Follicle-stimulating hormone (FSH), 172, 177
Food, drug interactions with, 267
Food and Drugs Act, 22
Food Guide Pyramid, 46, 47*f*
Foradil, 85
Formoterol fumarate, 85
Fortaz, 52*t*
Forteo, 167
Fosamax, 220, 231
Fosamprenavir calcium, 61
Foscarnet sodium, 58*t*
Foscavir, 58*t*
Fosinopril sodium, 91
Fosphenytoin sodium, 114
Fractions, 2, 2*f*
  addition of, 5
  changing between decimals and, 10
  conversions of, 3–4
  division of, 7
  equivalent, 4
  finding lowest common denominator of, 4–5
  kinds of, 2, 3*f*
  multiplication of, 6
  ratios, 7
  subtraction of, 6
Fragmin, 98
Fried's rule, 240
Frova, 112
Frovatriptan succinate, 112
FSH. *See* Follicle-stimulating hormone
5-FU, 200–201, 205–206
FUDR, 201
Fulvestrant, 202
Fulvicin, 57*t*
Fungal infection, treatment of, 57, 57*t*, 63*b*, 72–73, 73*f*, 73*t*
Fungizone, 57*t*
Fungoid, 73*t*
Furadantin, 184
Furosemide, 57*b*, 76*b*, 89, 183
Fusion inhibitors, 61–62
Fuzeon, 61

G

Gabapentin, 114, 124, 136, 248*t*
Gabitril, 115
Gamophen soap, 74–75
Ganciclovir sodium, 58*t*
Garamycin, 54*t*, 55*b*
Gardasil, 190, 206, 214
Garlic, 95*b*, 260, 264*t*
Gastric secretion, 153–157, 155*b*, 156*b*
Gastroesophageal reflux disease (GERD), 155–156
G-CSF, 208
Gefitinib, 207*t*
Gemcitabine hydrochloride, 201
Gemfibrozil, 101
Gemifloxacin mesylate, 54*t*
Gemtuzumab, 213
Gemtuzumab ozogamicin, 215
Gemzar, 201
Gene therapy, 212
General anesthetics, 106–107, 106*t*, 107*t*, 117*b*
Genetics, of disease, 211–212
Genital herpes, 58*t*, 59
Gentamicin sulfate, 54*t*, 55*b*, 230*b*, 233
Gentian violet, 74
GERD. *See* Gastroesophageal reflux disease
Ginger, 156*b*, 221–222, 260, 264*t*
Ginkgo biloba, 99*b*, 260, 264*t*
Ginseng, 105*b*, 260, 264*t*
Glatiramer acetate, 193
Gleevec, 205, 215
Gliclazide, 57*b*
Glimepiride, 57*b*, 171
Glipizide, 57*b*, 171, 267
Glipizide plus metformin, 171
Glucagon, 99*b*
Glucocorticoids, 124–125, 220
Glucophage, 171
Glucosamine, 260
Glucotrol, 171
Glucovance, 171
Glutethimide, 99*b*
Glyburide, 57*b*, 76*b*, 171
Glyburide plus metformin, 171
Glycerin, 161
Glyceryl trinitrate, 94
Glycyrrhiza, 161
Glynase, 171
Glyset, 171
GM-CSF, 208
Goiter, 165–166
Goldenseal, 62*b*, 260–261, 264*t*
GoLYTELY, 160
Gonads, 172–178, 172*f*, 173*f*, 174*b*, 175*t*

Goserelin acetate, 203
Gotu kola, 261
Gout, 142–143
Graafian follicle, 172, 173*f*
Gramicidin, 74
Granisetron, 209
Granisetron hydrochloride, 158
Granisetron transdermal, 209
Grapefruit juice, 96*b*, 193, 193*b*, 228*b*, 267
Grapeseed extract, 261
Graves' disease, 165–166, 166*b*
Green tea, 261
Grifulvin, 57*t*
Grisactin, 57*t*
Griseofulvin, 57*t*, 72, 76*b*
Gums, 71–72
Gyne-Lotrimin, 74
Gynergen, 149

H

Haemophilus b and hepatitis B vaccine, 189
Haemophilus b conjugate vaccine (Hib), 189, 194*f*
Halcion, 131, 248*t*
Haldol, 131–132, 248*t*
Hallucinogens, 251, 255*t*
Halobetasol propionate, 78*t*
Haloperidol, 76*b*, 131, 230*b*, 248*t*
Haloperidol decanoate, 132
Halothane, 106*t*
HandiHaler, 85
Hashimoto's disease, 165
Havrix, 189
Hawthorn, 264*t*
Head lice, 62–63
Heart, 88–89, 89*f*
  drugs affecting, 87–91, 90*b*, 102*b*
Heart failure, drugs used to treat, 89, 91–92, 102*b*
  ACE inhibitors, 90–91
  beta blockers, 91
  inotropic drugs, 89–90, 90*b*
Helicobacter pylori, 154–155
Hematinic agents, 208
Heparin, 97–98, 260–261, 264*t*
  dosage of, 25
  low-molecular-weight, 98
Heparin-induced thrombocytopenia (HIT), 97–98
Hepatitis, 58*t*, 59
Hepatitis A vaccine, 189, 189*b*, 194*f*, 195*f*
Hepatitis B immune globulin, 191
Hepatitis B vaccine, 189, 189*b*, 190, 194*f*, 195*f*
Herbal remedies, 257–265, 258*b*, 263*b*
Herceptin, 215
Heroin, 252, 255*t*
Herpesvirus infections, 58*t*, 59
Hexachlorophene, 72*b*, 74–75
Hexalen, 207*t*
Hib. *See* Haemophilus b conjugate vaccine
HibTITER, 189
Histrelin acetate, 207*t*
HIT. *See* Heparin-induced thrombocytopenia
Hitrastuzumab, 213
HIV. *See* Human immunodeficiency virus
Home health care, 242–249, 249*b*
  for bone marrow transplant patients, 243
  for diabetic patients, 243
  infusion therapy, 242–243
  psychiatric, 244
Hops, 261
Hormone replacement therapy, 174, 219–220, 223, 231
Hormones, 164–178, 177*b*
  adrenal, 167–168
  adrenocorticotropic, 164, 165*f*, 167
  for cancer treatment, 199, 202–204
  female, 172–177, 172*f*, 173*f*, 174*b*, 175*t*
  gonadotropic, 172–178, 172*f*, 173*f*, 174*b*, 175*t*
  male, 177–178
  pancreatic, 168–172, 168*t*, 169*t*, 177*b*
  parathyroid, 166–167
  pituitary, 164
  thyroid, 164–166, 166*b*, 166*t*, 177*b*, 232–233
  thyrotropic, 164–165
  tropic, 164
Horse chestnut, 93*b*, 261, 264*t*
Hospice care, 244, 246–249, 246*t*, 248*t*, 249*b*
Household measurement system, 14–15
Humalog, 170
Human immunodeficiency virus (HIV)
  fungal infection with, 57
  treatment of, 59–62
    fusion inhibitors, 61–62
    NNRTIs, 60–61
    NRTIs, 60
    protease inhibitors, 61, 130*b*
Human insulin, 169, 169*t*
Human insulin, isophane, 169, 169*t*
Human papillomavirus vaccine, 190, 194*f*, 195*f*, 206, 214
Humira, 214
Humulin 50/50, 170
Humulin 70/30, 170
Humulin L, 169, 169*t*
Humulin N, 169, 169*t*
Humulin R, 169, 169*t*
Humulin U, 169, 169*t*
Hyaluronic acid, 220
Hycamtin, 205
Hycodan, 110
Hydralazine, 230*b*
Hydration, in end-of-life care, 246
Hydrea, 207
Hydrocet, 110
Hydrochloric acid, 153–157, 155*b*, 156*b*
Hydrochlorothiazide, 57*b*, 76*b*, 89, 148, 182, 219
Hydrochlorothiazide plus spironolactone, 182
Hydrocodone, 109, 123*t*, 248*t*
Hydrocodone bitartrate, 110
Hydrocodone bitartrate, combined, 122
Hydrocodone bitartrate and ibuprofen, 122
Hydrocortisone, 73, 78*t*, 167–168
Hydrocortisone butyrate, 78*t*
Hydrocortisone valerate, 78*t*
Hydrocortone, 168
HydroDIURIL, 89, 182
Hydroflumethiazide, 57*b*
Hydrogen peroxide solution, 75
Hydromorphone, 109, 123–124, 123*t*, 252
Hydromorphone hydrochloride, 110, 122, 248*t*
Hydrous wool fat, 71
Hydroxyurea, 207
Hydroxyzine hydrochloride, 132, 230*b*, 248*t*
Hylan G-F, 220
Hyoscyamine, 150, 248*t*
Hyperglycemia, 168*t*
Hyperlipidemia, 100–102, 101*b*, 219
Hypertension, 92, 94–97, 95*b*, 96*b*, 174*b*, 182, 219, 230, 230*b*, 233
  drugs used to treat, 94–97
    ACE inhibitors, 90–91
    aldosterone inhibitors, 92
    alpha blockers, 95–96
    ARBs, 91–92
    beta blockers, 91
    calcium channel blockers, 96–97, 96*b*
    central alpha agonists, 95
    diuretics, 89
Hyperthyroidism, 165–166, 166*b*, 232–233
Hypnotics, 107–108, 108*b*, 116*b*, 117*b*, 221–222, 264*t*
  abuse of, 252
Hypoglycemia, 168*t*, 170
Hypoglycemic agents, 170–172, 230*b*, 254*t*
Hypothyroidism, 165–166, 166*t*, 232–233
Hypovitaminosis, 39
Hytone, 78*t*
Hytrin, 96
Hyzaar, 92

I

Ibandronate sodium, 220, 231
Ibritumomab tiuxetan, 215
Ibuprofen, 76*b*, 122, 141, 141*b*, 221, 224, 231, 248*t*, 266–267
Ibutilide fumarate, 93
Idamycin, 204
Idarubicin hydrochloride, 204
Ifex, 199
Ifosfamide, 199
IM injection. *See* Intramuscular injection
Imatinib mesylate, 205, 215
Imipenem and cilastatin sodium, 52*t*
Imipramine, 76*b*, 125, 253–254
Imipramine hydrochloride, 135, 185, 238
Imiquimod cream, 77–78
Imitrex, 112
Immune disorders, immunosuppressives for, 192–193, 192*b*
Immune human serum globulin, 191
Immunity, cancer and, 198*b*
Immunizations, 188–192, 188*b*, 189*b*, 193*b*, 194*f*, 195*f*, 196*f*, 238
  for cancer treatment, 199, 206
Immunology, prostaglandins and, 140
Immunomodulating agents
  for cancer treatment, 199, 205–206
  for multiple sclerosis, 193–194
Immunosuppressive agents, 192–193, 192*b*, 193*b*, 213, 264*t*
Immunotherapy, for allergic reactions, 69
Imodium, 161–162
Implanon, 175
Impotence therapy, 186
Imuran, 192, 213
Incontinence, 185
Incretin mimetic, 170
Indapamide, 57*b*, 182
Inderal, 91, 93, 148, 224
Indinavir, 133*b*, 264*t*
Indinavir sulfate, 61
Indocin, 122, 141, 248*t*
Indomethacin, 76*b*, 122, 141, 248*t*
Infanrix, 189
Infections. *See also* Antibiotics; Immunizations
  antifungal agents for, 57, 57*t*, 63*b*
  antiparasitic agents for, 62–63, 62*b*, 63*b*
  antiviral agents for, 58–62, 58*t*, 63*b*, 186
  cancer and, 214
  goldenseal for, 62*b*
  in older adults, 233–234
  sulfonamides for, 55–57, 57*b*, 63*b*, 76*b*
  urinary antiseptics for, 183–184
INFeD, 44
Inflammation, 81
Inflammatory conditions
  corticosteroids for, 167–168
  immunosuppressive agents for, 192–193, 192*b*, 193*b*, 213
  NSAIDs for, 76*b*, 93*b*, 95*b*, 99*b*, 105*b*, 112*b*, 121–122, 132*t*, 140–142, 155, 156*b*, 158*b*, 174*b*, 220–221, 223–224, 228, 228*b*, 230*b*, 231, 233, 260, 262–263, 264*t*, 267
    COX-2 inhibitors, 142, 142*b*, 143*b*
    gastric irritation by, 154–155
    prostaglandin inhibiting, 140–142, 141*b*, 142*b*, 143*b*
Infliximab, 213–214
Influenza, 58, 58*t*
Influenza vaccine, 189, 189*b*, 190, 194*f*, 195*f*, 196*f*
Influenza virus vaccine, 190
Influenza virus vaccine live, intranasal, 190, 196*f*
INH, 54*t*
Inhalants, 255*t*
Inhaled drug administration, 32
Injectable contraceptives, 175
Innohep, 98
Inotropic drugs, 89–90, 90*b*
Insomnia, 221–222
Inspra, 92, 182
Insulin, 168–170, 168*t*, 169*t*, 177*b*, 267
  analogs, 170
  combination products, 170
  dosage of, 25, 25*f*
  individual products, 169
  pump therapy, 170
  types of, 169*t*
Insulin aspart, 170
Insulin detemir, 170
Insulin glargine, 169*t*, 170
Insulin glulisine, 170
Insulin lispro, 169*t*, 170
Intal, 86
Integrilin, 100
Intelence, 61

Interferon alfa, 206
Interferon alfa-2b, 59
Interferon beta-1a, 193
Interferon beta-1b, 193, 213
Intra-arterial injection, 36
Intradermal injection, 33, 34*f*
Intramuscular (IM) injection, 33–35, 34*f*, 35*f*
Intrathecal pump implant, 125
Intravenous (IV) injection, 36
Intron A, 59, 206
Invanz, 36
Invirase, 61
Iodine, 165, 232
Iodine tincture, 75
Ionamin, 106
Ipecac syrup, 158
Ipilimumab, 207*t*
IPOL, 191
IPV, 191, 194*f*
Irbesartan, 92
Iressa, 207*t*
Irinotecan hydrochloride, 205
Iron, 43–44, 44*b*, 224, 228*b*
Iron dextran injection, 44
Irritant cathartics, 160
Irritants, 72
Islets of Langerhans, 168
Isoniazid, 54*t*, 230*b*
Isophane insulin, 169, 169*t*
Isopropyl alcohol, 75
Isoptin, 97
Isotretinoin, 77
Itraconazole, 57*t*
IV injection. *See* Intravenous injection
Ivermectin, 62
Ixabepilone, 207*t*
Ixempra, 207*t*

J
Jevtana, 207*t*
Juniper, 183*b*, 261, 264*t*

K
Kadian, 122
Kaletra, 61
Kanamycin sulfate, 54*t*, 55*b*, 233
Kantrex, 54*t*, 55*b*
Kaolin, 161
Kaolin-pectin, 161
Kaopectate, 161
Kava kava, 116*b*, 261, 264*t*
K-DUR 10, 45
Keflex, 52*t*
Kemadrin, 116*t*
Kenalog, 168
Keppra, 114
Keratolytics, 72
Kerlone, 91
Ketalar, 107*t*
Ketamine hydrochloride, 107*t*
Ketek, 53*t*
Ketoconazole, 57*t*, 73, 73*t*, 76*b*, 248*t*
Ketoprofen, 141
Ketorolac tromethamine, 122, 141, 248*t*
Kidneys, 180–181, 181*f*
Kineret, 214
Kinrix, 189
Klonopin, 113
Kutrase, 157
Ku-Zyme, 157
Kwell, 62
Kytril, 158, 209

L
Labetalol, 91
Lactaid, 157
Lactase enzyme, 157
Lactation, drug safety during, 222–223
Lactic acid, 72
Lamictal, 114
Lamisil, 57*t*, 73*t*
Lamivudine, 59–60
Lamotrigine, 114, 124
Lanolin. *See* Hydrous wool fat
Lanoxin, 90
Lansoprazole, 100*b*, 155
Lantus, 169*t*, 170
Lapatinib ditosylate, 207*t*
Larodopa, 116
Lasix, 89, 183
L-asparaginase, 205
Laudanum, 109
Laxatives, 124, 159–161, 162*b*, 267*t*
  bulk-increasing, 159, 228*b*
  lubricant, 159
Leflunomide, 214
Legislation. *See* Drug legislation
Lemon balm, 221–222
Lenalidomide, 207*t*
Lente insulin zinc, 169, 169*t*
Lepirudin, 98
Letrozole, 203
Leukeran, 199
Leukine, 208
Leuprolide acetate, 203
Leustatin, 200
Levalbuterol inhalation solution, 85
Levaquin, 54*t*
Levarterenol bitartrate injection, 147
Levemir, 170
Levetiracetam, 114
Levitra, 186
Levodopa, 116, 116*b*, 228*b*, 230*b*, 264*t*
Levodopa plus carbidopa, 116
Levo-Dromoran, 122, 248*t*
Levofloxacin, 54*t*, 233–234
Levonorgestrel, 176
Levonorgestrel intrauterine device, 175, 224
Levonorgestrel plus ethinyl estradiol, 174–176
Levophed, 147
Levorphanol, 123–124, 123*t*
Levorphanol tartrate, 122, 248*t*
Levothroid, 166*t*
Levothyroxine, 166*t*
Levoxine, 166*t*
Levsin, 248*t*
Lexapro, 134*t*
Lexiva, 61
LH. *See* Luteinizing hormone
Librax, 150
Librium, 130
Lice, 62–63
Licide, 63
Lidex, 78*t*
Lidex-E, 78*t*
Lidocaine, 125, 230*b*
Lidocaine hydrochloride, 93, 107*t*
Lidocaine patches, 124
Lidoderm, 124
Lindane, 62
Lioresal, 248*t*
Liothyronine, 166*t*
Lipase, 153–154
Lipitor, 101, 219
Lisdexamfetamine dimesylate, 105
Lisinopril, 91, 219
Lithane, 132, 132*b*, 132*t*
Lithium, 115–116, 132, 132*b*, 132*t*, 230*b*, 253–254, 264*t*, 267
Lithium carbonate, 132, 132*b*, 132*t*
Lithonate, 132, 132*b*, 132*t*
Local anesthetics, 72, 107, 107*t*, 117*b*, 125
Locoid, 78*t*
Lodine, 122
Lodosyn, 116
Lodrane, 67
Lomotil, 109, 161, 248*t*
Lomustine, 199
Lo/Ovral, 175*t*
Loperamide hydrochloride, 161–162
Lopid, 101
Lopinavir and ritonavir, 61
Lopressor, 148
Loprox, 72
Loratadine, 68
Loratadine plus pseudoephedrine, 68
Lorazepam, 124, 130, 248*t*
Lorcet Plus, 122
Lortab, 110, 248*t*
Losartan, 92
Lotensin, 90
Lotrel, 96
Lotrimin, 73–74
Lotronex, 161
Lovastatin, 101, 219
Lovenox, 98
Low-molecular-weight heparin, 98
Loxapine, 132
Loxitane, 132
Lozol, 182
LSD, 255*t*
Lubiprostone, 161
Lubricant laxatives, 159
Lucentis, 215–216
Luminal, 108
Lunesta, 132
Lupron, 203
Luteinizing hormone (LH), 172, 177
Luvox, 134*t*
Luxiq, 78*t*
Lyrica, 115–117, 124, 221
Lysodren, 207
Lysol, 75

M
Ma Huang, 83*b*, 259–260
Macrobid, 184
Macrodantin, 184
Macrolide antibiotics, 53, 53*t*, 130*b*. *See also* Erythromycins
Mafenide acetate cream, 75
Magnesia magma, 160
Magnesium, 221–222
Magnesium citrate solution, 160
Magnesium oxide, 156
Magnesium sulfate, 114
Malathion, 63
Mandelamine, 184
Mannitol, 183
MAOIs. *See* Monoamine oxidase inhibitors
Maraviroc, 62
Marcaine, 107*t*
Marijuana, 251–253, 255*t*
Marinol, 209, 253
Matulane, 200
Mavik, 91
Maxalt, 112
Maxipime, 51, 52*t*
Measles, mumps, and rubella virus vaccine, live, 190, 194*f*, 195*f*
Measurement systems, 13–15
Mebaral, 108
Mebendazole, 62
Meclizine hydrochloride, 68, 158
Meclofenamate, 141
Medication administration. *See* Drug administration
Medication use agreement, 126*f*, 125–127
Medrol, 168
Medroxyprogesterone acetate, 175
Mefenamic acid, 141
Mefoxin, 52*t*
Megace, 157, 202, 209
Megestrol acetate, 157, 202, 209
Mellaril, 131
Meloxicam, 141
Melphalan, 199
Memantine hydrochloride, 234*t*
Menactra, 190
Meningococcal vaccine, 190, 194*f*, 195*f*
Menomune, 190
Menopause, 173–174, 174*b*, 224–225
Menorrhagia, 224
Menstrual cycle, 172–173, 173*f*
  abnormalities in, 224
Menstrual migraines, 223–224
Mentax, 73*t*
Menthol, 72
Meperidine, 123*t*, 230*b*
Meperidine hydrochloride, 110, 122, 248*t*
Mephobarbital, 108
Mepivacaine hydrochloride, 107*t*
Meprobamate, 133
Mercaptopurine, 201
Meridia, 106
Meropenem, 52*t*
Merrem, 36
Mestranol, 175*t*
Metaglip, 171
Metaraminol bitartrate, 147
Metastatic bone pain, 125
Metformin, 171, 267
Metformin hydrochloride, 171
Methadone, 110, 123–124, 123*t*, 252
Methadone hydrochloride, 122, 248*t*, 252
Methenamine mandelate, 184
Methergine, 176
Methimazole, 165–166, 166*b*, 232
Methotrexate, 141*b*, 201, 214, 264*t*
Methoxyflurane, 106*t*
Methyclothiazide, 57*b*
Methylcellulose, 159
Methyldopa, 76*b*, 148, 230*b*
Methyldopa hydrochloride, 95
Methyldopa plus hydrochlorothiazide, 148
Methylergonovine maleate, 176
Methylphenidate, 95, 209
Methylphenidate hydrochloride, 105, 106*b*
Methylphenidate hydrochloride, extended-release tablets, 106
Methylphenidate transdermal system, 106
Methylprednisolone, 168
Metolazone, 57*b*, 89, 182–183
Metoprolol, 91

Metoprolol tartrate, 148
Metric system, 13–14
Metronidazole, 54*t*, 155, 254*t*
Mevacor, 101, 219
Miacalcin, 220, 231
Micafungin sodium, 57*t*
Micardis, 92
Miconazole, 57*t*
Miconazole nitrate tincture, 73*t*
Miconazole nitrate vaginal cream, 74
Micronase, 171
Midamor, 183
Midazolam hydrochloride, 107*t*, 130, 248*t*
Midodrine hydrochloride, 94
Mifeprex, 140, 177
Mifepristone, 140, 177
Miglitol, 171
Migraine headaches, 111–112, 112*b*
  drugs used to treat
    analgesics, 109–111, 123–124, 123*t*
    analgesics, nonnarcotic, 111
    triptans, 111–112, 112*b*
  menstrual and perimenopausal, 223–224
Milk, 71–72, 161, 267
Milk of magnesia, 160
Milk thistle, 261–262
Milnacipran, 116, 221
Milrinone lactate, 90
Mineral oil, 159
Minerals, 39–40, 43–46
  calcium, 44–45, 45*b*, 220, 221–222, 231
  copper, 45–46
  fluoride, 46
  iron, 43–44, 44*b*, 224, 228*b*
  phosphorus, 44–45
  potassium, 45, 181–182, 186*b*, 254*t*
  zinc, 39–40, 43, 45
Minipress, 96, 148
Minitran, 94
Minocin, 53*t*
Minocycline hydrochloride, 53*t*
Mintezol, 62
Mirapex, 108, 116*t*
Mirena, 175, 224
Mirtazapine, 136
Misoprostol, 121, 140, 155
Mitomycin-C, 205
Mitotane, 207
Mitoxantrone, 193–194
Mitoxantrone hydrochloride, 205
Mixed numbers, 3, 5–7
MMR, 190, 194*f*, 195*f*
M-M-R II, 190
Moban, 132
Mobic, 141
Modafinil, 106
Modane, 161
Moexipril hydrochloride, 91
Molecular medicine, 199, 206, 211–216, 211*f*, 216*b*
  for cancer, 199, 206, 212, 214–215
  gene therapy, 212
  genetic basis of disease and, 211–212
  immunosuppressants, 213
  monoclonal antibodies, 212–213
  rheumatoid arthritis and Crohn's disease treatments, 214
  stem cells, 212
  targeted therapies, 199, 206, 212
Molindone hydrochloride, 132
Mometasone furoate, 78*t*
Moniliasis, 73–74, 74*f*
Monistat, 57*t*, 74
Monoamine oxidase inhibitors (MAOIs), 105*b*, 133*b*, 134–135, 137*b*, 228*b*, 264*t*
Monoclonal antibodies, 212–213
Monopril, 91
Montelukast sodium, 86
Morphine, 123–124, 230*b*, 245–246, 252, 257
  opioid doses equivalent to, 123, 123*t*
Morphine sulfate, 109–110, 122, 248*t*
Morphine sulfate and naltrexone, 123
Morphine sulfate controlled release, 122, 248*t*
Motrin, 122, 141, 141*b*, 231, 248*t*
Moxifloxacin hydrochloride, 54*t*, 233–234
6-MP, 201
MS Contin, 109–110, 122, 248*t*
MSIR, 109–110
Mucilages, 71–72
Mucin, 153–154
Mucomyst, 86
Multaq, 93
Multiple sclerosis, 193–194
Mupirocin calcium, 75
Muscle relaxants, skeletal, 125
MUSE Suppositories, 140
Mustard, 72
Mutamycin, 205
Myambutol, 54*t*
Mycamine, 57*t*
Mycelex, 248*t*
Mycobutin, 54*t*
Mycolog cream/ointment, 74
Mycophenolate mofetil hydrochloride, 213
Mycophenolate sodium, 213
Mycostatin, 57*t*, 74, 248*t*
Myfortic, 213
Myleran, 199
Mylotarg, 215
Myocardial infarction, 91–92, 99–100
MyPlate, 46, 47*f*
Mysoline, 115
Myxedema, 165

N

Nab-paclitaxel, 208
Nabumetone, 142
Nadolol, 91, 93, 148
Nafcillin sodium, 51*t*
Nalbuphine, 123
Nalbuphine hydrochloride, 111
Nalfon, 141, 231
Nalidixic acid, 76*b*
Naloxone, 109–111
Naltrexone, 123
Namenda, 234*t*
Naprosyn, 122, 142, 248*t*
Naproxen, 76*b*, 142, 224
Naproxen sodium, 112, 122, 142, 248*t*
Naratriptan hydrochloride, 112
Narcan, 110
Narcotics, 109–111, 117*b*, 123–124, 123*t*, 127*b*, 255*t*, 266–267
  dependence on, 252
  tolerance to, 245–246
Nardil, 135
Nasalide, 85
Natalizumab, 213
Nateglinide, 171
Nausea, 158–159, 158*b*, 208–209
Navane, 132
Navelbine, 208
Nebcin, 54*t*
Nebivolol, 91
Nefazodone, 136
Nelarabine, 207*t*
Nelfinavir mesylate, 61
Neo-Fradin, 54*t*
Neomycin, 74
Neomycin sulfate, 54*t*
Neostigmine bromide, 149
Neostigmine methylsulfate, 149
Neo-Synephrine, 147
Nervous system, 104, 145–146, 146*f*, 146*t*
Nesacaine, 107*t*
Neulasta, 208
Neupogen, 208
Neupro, 116
Neuromuscular blocking agents, 150–151
Neurons, 145–146, 146*f*
Neurontin, 114, 124, 136, 248*t*
Neuropathic pain, 124
Neutrogena, 76
Nevirapine, 61
Nexavar, 207*t*
Nexium, 155
Niacin, 42, 101, 219
Niacor, 101, 219
Niaspan, 101, 219
Nicardipine, 96
Nicotinamide, 42
Nicotine, 251, 254–255, 267*t*
  inhaled, 255
Nicotinic acid, 42
Nicotrol, 255
Nifedipine, 76*b*, 96, 186
Nilandron, 202
Nilotinib, 207*t*
Nilutamide, 202
Nimodipine, 96
Nimotop, 96
Nipent, 205
Nisoldipine, 97
Nitrates, 94, 186
Nitrites, 94
Nitrodisc, 94
Nitro-Dur, 94
Nitrofurantoin, 76*b*, 233
Nitroglycerin, 94, 186
Nitrostat, 94
Nitrous oxide, 106*t*
Nix Creme Rinse, 63
Nizatidine, 156
Nizoral, 57*t*, 73, 73*t*, 248*t*
NNRTIs. *See* Nonnucleoside reverse transcriptase inhibitors
Nolvadex, 203
Nonnucleoside reverse transcriptase inhibitors (NNRTIs), 60–61
Nonphenothiazines, 131–132
Nonsteroidal anti-inflammatory drugs (NSAIDs), 76*b*, 93*b*, 95*b*, 99*b*, 105*b*, 112*b*, 121–122, 132*t*, 140–142, 155, 156*b*, 158*b*, 174*b*, 220–221, 223, 224, 228, 228*b*, 230*b*, 231, 233, 260, 262–263, 264*t*, 267
  COX-2 inhibitors, 142, 142*b*, 143*b*
  gastric irritation by, 154–155
  prostaglandin inhibiting, 140–142, 141*b*, 142*b*, 143*b*
Norelgestromin plus ethinyl estradiol, 175
Norepinephrine, 146, 167
Norepinephrine bitartrate, 147
Norethindrone, 175*t*
Norethindrone acetate, 175*t*
Norethynodrel, 175*t*
Norfloxacin, 54*t*, 233–234
Norgestrel, 175*t*
Norlestrin, 175*t*
Normiflo, 98
Normodyne, 91
Noroxin, 54*t*
Norpace, 93
Norpramin, 135, 248*t*
Nortriptyline, 76*b*, 125, 221
Nortriptyline hydrochloride, 135
Norvasc, 96
Norvir, 61
Novantrone, 193–194, 205
Novocain, 72, 107*t*
Novolin 70/30, 170
Novolin L, 169
Novolin N, 169
Novolin R, 169
Novolog, 170
Noxafil, 57*t*
NPH insulin, 168*t*, 169, 169*t*
NRTIs. *See* Nucleoside reverse transcriptase inhibitors
NSAIDs. *See* Nonsteroidal anti-inflammatory drugs
Nubain, 111, 123
Nucleoside reverse transcriptase inhibitors (NRTIs), 60
Nucynta, 122
NuLYTELY, 160
Numorphan, 111, 123, 248*t*
Nupercainal, 72
Nutrition, 39–46, 40*t*. *See also* Minerals; Vitamins
  changes in nutritional information, 46, 47*f*
  in end-of-life care, 246
  essential fatty acids, 40, 46
  fiber, 40, 40*t*, 228*b*, 230
  in older adults, 229–230
NuvaRing, 175
Nuvigil, 105
Nydrazid, 54*t*
Nystatin, 57*t*, 74, 248*t*
Nystatin vaginal tablets, 74

O

Obesity, 157–158, 158*b*
Ofloxacin, 54*t*, 76*b*, 233–234
Olanzapine, 132
Olmesartan, 92, 219
Olux, 78*t*
Olux-E, 78*t*
Omalizumab, 86, 213
Omega-3 fatty acids, 46
Omeprazole, 100*b*, 156, 266
Omnicef, 52*t*
Oncaspar, 205
Oncovin, 208
Ondansetron, 209
Ondansetron hydrochloride, 159
Ontak, 215
Opiates, 109–111, 123–124, 123*t*
  antidotes for, 110
Opioid analgesics, 109–111, 117*b*, 123–124, 123*t*, 127*b*, 221, 223
  equivalent doses of, 123, 123*t*

long-term effects of, 123–124
side effects of, 124
tolerance to, 245–246
OptiPen, 170
Oral contraceptives, 76*b*, 133*b*, 174–175, 175*t*, 176, 177*b*, 223–224, 264*t*
Oral drug administration, 31–32, 31*f*
Oral hypoglycemic agents, 170–172, 254*t*
Oramorph, 109–110
Oramorph SR, 122, 248*t*
Orap, 132
Orencia, 214
Orinase, 171
Orlistat, 157–158, 158*b*
Orphenadrine, 125
Ortho Evra, 175
Ortho Novum, 175*t*
Os-Cal, 90*b*
Oseltamivir, 58, 58*t*
Osmitrol, 183
Osteoarthritis, 219–220, 231
Osteomalacia, 41
Osteoporosis, 44, 167, 220, 230–232
Ototoxicity, of antibiotics, 55*b*
Ovary, 172, 172*f*
Ovide, 63
Ovral, 175*t*, 176
Ovulation, 172, 173*f*
promotion of, 176
Ovulen, 175*t*
Oxacillin sodium, 51*t*
Oxaliplatin, 206
Oxaprozin, 142
Oxazepam, 130
Oxcarbazepine, 114, 124
Oxiconazole nitrate, 73*t*
Oxistat, 73*t*
Oxybutynin, 230*b*
Oxybutynin chloride, 185
Oxycodone, 111, 123, 123*t*, 252
Oxycodone hydrochloride, 248*t*
combined, 122
OxyContin, 111, 123, 252
OxyFAST, 111, 123
OxyIR, 111, 123
Oxymorphone hydrochloride, 111, 123, 248*t*
Oxytocic agents, 176–177
Oxytocin injection, 177

P

PABA. *See* Para-aminobenzoic acid
Pacerone, 92
Paclitaxel, 207
Paclitaxel nanoparticle albumin, 208
Pain, 119–127, 127*b*. *See also* Analgesics; Anesthetics
antidepressants in treatment of, 136
assessment of, 120–121, 126*f*
depression and, 124
in end-of-life care, 244–246, 248*t*
etiology of, 120
investigating causes of, 120
levels of relief of, 121–123
metastatic bone, 125
mild, 121–122
moderate, 122
neuropathic, 124
in older adults, 232
patient medication use agreement for treatment of, 126*f*, 125–127
severe, 122–123
Painful conditions
analgesics, narcotic, 109–111, 123–124, 123*t*
analgesics, nonnarcotic, 111
in end-of-life care, 244–246, 248*t*
transdermal dosage forms, 110
Palgic, 69
Palivizumab, 58*t*
Palliative care. *See* End-of-life care
Palliative Performance Scale (PPS), 246, 246*t*
Palonosetron, 209
Pamelor, 135
Pamidronate disodium, 125
Pancreas, 168–172, 168*t*, 169*t*, 177*b*
Pancrease, 157
Pancreatin, 157
Pancrelipase, 157
Pancuronium bromide, 150
Panitumumab, 207*t*
Pantoprazole, 100*b*, 155–156
Pantothenic acid (B_5), 42
Para-aminobenzoic acid (PABA), 55–56, 75–76, 76*b*
Paraplatin, 206
Parasites, treatment of, 62–63, 62*b*, 63*b*
Parasympathetic nervous system, 145–146, 146*f*, 146*t*
Parasympatholytic agents, 150, 150*b*
Parasympathomimetic agents, 149, 149*f*
Parathyroid glands, 166–167
Paregoric, 109, 252
Parenteral drug administration, 32–36, 32*f*, 33*f*, 34*f*, 35*f*
Parkinsonism, 115–116, 116*b*, 116*t*
Parkinson's disease, 115–116, 116*b*, 116*t*
Parlodel, 116*t*
Parnate, 135
Paroxetine, 124, 134*b*, 134*t*, 203, 221, 248*t*
Passive immunity agents, 191–192
Patient medication use agreement, 126*f*, 125–127
Pavulon, 150
Paxil, 134*b*, 134*t*, 248*t*
PCP, 255*t*
Pediarix, 189
PedvaxHIB, 189
Peganone, 114
Pegaspargase, 205
Pegfilgrastim, 208
Peginterferon, 59
PEG-Intron, 59
Pellagra, 42
Pemetrexed, 201
Pemetrexed disodium, 207*t*
Penciclovir, 59
Penicillins, 50, 51*t*, 233
long-acting forms of penicillin G, 50
semisynthetic, 50, 51*t*
toxicity and side effects of, 50
Penicillin G, 50
Penicillin G benzathine, 50
Penicillin G procaine, 50
Penicillin V potassium, 50
Penlac Nail Lacquer, 73
Pentacel, 189
Pentazocine, 122, 230*b*
Pentazocine hydrochloride, 111
Pentazocine with acetaminophen, 111
Pentazocine with aspirin, 111
Pentazocine with naloxone, 111
Penthrane, 106*t*
Pentobarbital, 108
Pentostatin, 205
Pentothal, 107*t*
Pepcid, 155, 248*t*
Pepsin, 153–154
Peptic ulcer disease, 154–155, 154*b*
antacids for, 156–157, 156*b*
antisecretory agents for, 155–156, 155*b*, 156*b*
Helicobacter pylori treatments for, 154–155
Pepto-Bismol, 155
Percentage, 10–11
Percocet, 122, 248*t*
Percodan, 122, 248*t*
Pergolide mesylate, 116*t*
Periactin, 67
Peri-Colace, 161, 248*t*
Perimenopausal migraines, 223–224
Perindopril erbumine, 91
Permax, 116*t*
Permethrin cream rinse, 63
Permethrin topical cream, 63
Petrolatum, 71
Pharmaceutical preparations, 17–18
Pharmacology introduction, 16–18
terminology, 17–18
Phenazopyridine hydrochloride, 184
Phenelzine, 105*b*, 264*t*
Phenelzine sulfate, 135
Phenergan, 68, 208–209, 248*t*
Phenobarbital, 108, 113–115
Phenols, 72
Phenothiazines, 76*b*, 115–116, 131, 264*t*
Phentermine, 106
Phenylbutazone, 76*b*
Phenylephrine hydrochloride, 147
Phenytoin, 56, 113, 115, 124, 134*t*, 141*b*, 155, 228*b*, 230*b*, 248*t*, 264*t*, 267
pHisoHex, 74–75
Phosphorus, 44–45
Photosensitizers, 76, 76*b*
Physostigmine, 149
Phytonadione injection, 97
Pilocarpine, 150
Pilocarpine hydrochloride, 149
Pilocarpine nitrate, 149
Pimecrolimus, 77
Pimozide, 132
Pindolol, 91
Pioglitazone, 171
Piperacillin and tazobactam sodium, 51*t*
Piretanide, 57*b*
Piroxicam, 142
Pitocin, 177
Pituitary gland, 164
Pituitary hormone inhibitors, 203–204
Plan B, 176
Platinol-AQ, 206
Platinum-containing agents, 199, 206
Plavix, 100
Plendil, 96
Pletal, 100
PMDD. *See* Premenstrual dysphoria disorder
Pneumococcal 7-valent conjugate vaccine, 191
Pneumococcal vaccine, 189*b*, 194*f*, 195*f*
polyvalent, 190
Pneumovax 23, 190
Poliovirus vaccine, inactivated, 191, 192, 194*f*
Polymyxin B sulfate, 54*t*
Polythiazide, 57*b*
Ponstel, 141
Pontocaine, 107*t*
Posaconazole, 57*t*
Postpartum depression, 222
Potassium, 45, 181–182, 186*b*, 254*t*
Potassium chloride, 45
Povidone-iodine solution, 75
PPS. *See* Palliative Performance Scale
Pramipexole dihydrochloride, 108, 116*t*
Prandin, 171
Prasugrel hydrochloride, 100
Pravachol, 102
Pravastatin sodium, 102
Praziquantel, 62
Prazosin, 233
Prazosin hydrochloride, 96, 148
Precose, 171
Prednisolone, 168, 192
Prednisone, 124, 168, 192, 202
Pregabalin, 115–117, 124, 221
Pregnancy
depression during, 222
drug safety during, 222–223
medications and, 237–238
Prelone, 168
Premarin, 174, 225, 231
Premenstrual dysphoria disorder (PMDD), 222
Prepidil, 176
Prepidil Cervical Gel, 140
Prescriptions, 26–27, 26*f*, 27*t*
Prevacid, 155
Preven, 176
Prevnar, 191
Prevpac, 155
Prezista, 61
Priftin, 54*t*
Prilocaine hydrochloride, 107*t*
Prilosec, 156
Primacor, 90
Primaxin, 36
Primidone, 115
Prinivil, 91, 219
Pristiq, 134
ProAir HFA, 84
ProAmatine, 94
Probenecid, 57*b*, 141*b*, 142, 264*t*
Procainamide hydrochloride, 93, 186
Procaine, 72
Procaine hydrochloride, 107*t*
Procarbazine, 200
Procardia, 96
Prochlorperazine maleate, 131, 159, 208–209, 248*t*
Procrit, 208
Procyclidine hydrochloride, 116*t*
Progesterone, 172, 174
Prograf, 193, 213

ProHIBiT, 189
Proleukin, 206, 214
Prolia, 231
Prolixin, 131
Promazine, 76*b*
Promethazine, 76*b*, 208–209
Promethazine hydrochloride, 68, 248*t*
Pronestyl, 93
Proportion, 12
Propranolol hydrochloride, 91, 93, 148, 155, 224, 230*b*
Proprietary names. *See* Trade names
Propylthiouracil, 165–166, 166*b*, 232
Proscar, 185
Prostaglandins, 139–144
  actions of, 139–140
  allergy and, 140
  circulatory system and, 140
  gastrointestinal tract and, 140
  immunology and, 140
  inhibitors of, 140–143, 141*b*, 142*b*, 143*b*
  reproductive system and, 139–140
  urinary tract and, 140
Prostaglandin E, 140
Prostatic hypertrophy, 185–186, 185*b*
Prostigmin, 149
Prostin E_2, 176
Prostin E_2 Suppositories, 140
Prostin VR Pediatric Injection, 140
Protamine sulfate, 98
Protamine zinc, 168*t*
Protease inhibitors, 61, 130*b*
Prothrombin time (PT), 97, 98, 102*b*
Proton pump inhibitors, 100*b*, 121, 155
Protonix, 156
Protopic, 77
Protriptyline hydrochloride, 135, 253–254
Provenge, 206
Proventil, 84
Provigil, 106
Prozac, 134*t*
Pseudoaddiction, 123
Pseudoephedrine, 68–69, 233
Psorcon E, 78*t*
Psychiatric disease, 129–137, 137*b*
  anticonvulsants for, 136–137
  antidepressants for, 99*b*, 133–136, 133*b*, 134*b*, 134*t*, 137*b*
  anxiolytic agents for, 136, 136*b*
  home care for, 244
  tranquilizers for, 130–133, 130*b*, 132*b*, 132*t*, 137*b*
Psyllium seed, 159, 228*b*
PT. *See* Prothrombin time
Purinethol, 201
Pyrazinamide, 54*t*
Pyrethrins with piperonyl butoxide, 63
Pyridium, 184
Pyridoxine (B_6), 42, 221–222

Q

Questran, 101
Quetiapine fumarate, 132
Quinapril, 91
Quinethazone, 57*b*
Quinidine, 76*b*, 186, 230*b*
Quinidine sulfate, 93
Quinine, 257
Quinolones, 54, 54*t*, 228*b*, 233–234

R

Rabeprazole, 100*b*
Radioactive iodine, 165, 232
Radiotherapy, 125
Raloxifene hydrochloride, 174, 220, 232
Ramelteon, 108, 133
Ramipril, 91
Ranexa, 94
Ranibizumab, 215–216
Ranitidine, 100*b*, 156, 248*t*
Ranolazine, 94
Rapaflo, 186
Rapamune, 213
RDA. *See* Recommended Daily Allowance
Rebetol, 58*t*, 59
Rebetron, 59, 206
Rebif, 193
Reclast, 220, 232
Recombivax HB, 190
Recommended Daily Allowance (RDA), 40
Red clover, 82*b*, 262, 264*t*
Red yeast rice extract, 262
Refludan, 98
Relenza, 58, 58*t*
Relpax, 112
Remeron, 136
Remicade, 214
Renin inhibitors, 92, 219
Rennin, 153–154
ReoPro, 100, 215
Repaglinide, 171
Reproductive organs
  female, 172–177, 172*f*, 173*f*, 174*b*, 175*t*
  male, 172, 177–178
  prostaglandins and, 139–140
Requip, 108, 116*t*
Rescriptor, 60
Resorcinol, 72
Respiration, 81, 81*f*, 82*f*
Respiratory depressants, 82
Respiratory stimulants, 82
Respiratory system drugs, 81–87, 86*b*
  for asthma, 83–86, 83*b*, 84*b*
  drugs acting on respiratory center in brain, 82
  drugs acting on respiratory tract, 86
  drugs affecting mucous membranes of respiratory tract, 82, 82*b*
Restless leg syndrome (RLS), 108
Restoril, 248*t*
Retin-A, 77
Retinoic acid, 76*b*, 77
Retrovir, 60
Revlimid, 207*t*
Reyataz, 61
Rheumatic disorders, drugs used to treat, 214
  immune suppressive agents, 213
  monoclonal antibodies, 212–213
  NSAIDs, 140–142, 141*b*, 142*b*
Rheumatoid arthritis, 214
Rhinocort, 85
RhoGAM, 192
Rho(D) immune human globulin, 192
Ribavirin, 58*t*, 59
Riboflavin (B_2), 42
Rickets, 41, 44
Rifabutin, 54*t*
Rifadin, 54*t*
Rifamate, 54*t*
Rifampin, 54*t*
Rifapentine, 54*t*
Rimantadine hydrochloride, 58*t*
Risedronate, 220
Risedronate sodium, 232
Risperdal, 132
Risperidone, 132, 230*b*
Ritalin, 95, 105, 106*b*, 209
Ritonavir, 61
Rituxan, 215
Rituximab, 213, 215
Rivastigmine, 234*t*
Rizatriptan benzoate, 112, 223
RLS. *See* Restless leg syndrome
Rocephin, 52*t*
Roferon-A, 206
Roman numerals, 1–2
Ropinirole hydrochloride, 108, 116*t*
Rosewater ointment, 71
Rosiglitazone maleate, 171
Rosiglitazone plus metformin, 172
Rosuvastatin, 102
RotaTeq, 191
Rotavirus vaccine, live oral, 191, 194*f*
Rotigotine transdermal patch, 116
Roxanol, 109–110
Roxicodone, 111
Rozerem, 108, 133
rt-PA, 99
RU-486, 177

S

Saffron, 262
Salicylates, 99*b*
Salicylic acid, 72
Saline cathartics, 160
Salk vaccine, 191–192
Salmeterol, 85
Sancuso, 209
Sandimmune, 193, 213
Saponated cresol solution, 75
Saquinavir, 61
Sarafem, 134*t*
Sargramostim, 208
Sativex spray, 253
Savella, 116, 221
Saw palmetto, 185*b*, 262, 264*t*
Scabies, 62–63
Schedules of controlled substances, 20–21
Scopolamine, 150, 208–209, 248*t*
Scurvy, 43
Seasonale, 174
Secobarbital, 108
Seconal, 108
Secondary parkinsonism, 115–116
Sedatives, 107–108, 108*b*, 116*b*, 117*b*, 129–130, 158*b*, 221–222, 228, 228*b*, 245, 264*t*, 266–267, 267*t*. *See also* Tranquilizers
  abuse of, 252
  in end-of-life care, 245
Seizures, 113–115
Selective estrogen receptor modulators (SERMs), 203
Selective serotonin and norepinephrine reuptake inhibitors (SNRIs), 134, 203, 222
Selective serotonin reuptake inhibitors (SSRIs), 124, 130*b*, 133–134, 133*b*, 134*b*, 134*t*, 203, 221–223, 230*b*, 234, 264*t*
Selzentry, 62
Semprex-D, 69
Senna, 124, 160
Senokot, 160, 248*t*
Septisol, 74–75
Septra, 56, 184
Septra DS, 56, 184
Serevent Diskus, 85
SERMs. *See* Selective estrogen receptor modulators
Seromycin, 54*t*
Seroquel, 132
Sertraline, 134*t*, 203, 221–222, 248*t*
Shingles. *See* Varicella zoster
Sibutramine hydrochloride, 106
Sildenafil citrate, 186
Silodosin, 186
Silvadene cream, 75
Silver sulfadiazine, 75
Simulect, 213
Simvastatin, 101–102, 219
Sinemet, 116
Sinequan, 135
Singulair, 86
Sinutab, 69
Sipuleucel-T, 206
Sirolimus, 213
Skeletal muscle relaxants, 125
Skin
  drug administration via, 30
  drugs affecting, 71–79, 79*b*
    acne preparations, 76–77
    aloe, 75*b*
    antifungal agents, 72–73, 73*f*, 73*t*
    anti-infective agents, 74–75
    antimonilial preparations, 73–74, 74*f*
    astringents, 72
    atopic dermatitis agents, 77, 77*f*
    hexachlorophene, 72*b*
    irritants, 72
    keratolytics, 72
    local anesthetics, 72
    soothing substances, 71–72
    topical corticosteroids, 78–79, 78*t*
    wart treatments, 77–78, 78*f*
    wound care products, 75
  sun damage to, 75–76, 76*b*
Slippery elm, 262
Slow-K, 45
SNRIs. *See* Selective serotonin and norepinephrine reuptake inhibitors
Sodium bicarbonate, 156–157
Sodium chloride 20% injection, 177
Sodium heparin injection, 97–98
Sodium phosphate monobasic monohydrate, 160
Sodium valproate, 124
Solu-Cortef, 168
Solu-Medrol, 168
Sorafenib tosylate, 207*t*
Sotalol, 91
Spectazole, 73, 73*f*
Spectinomycin hydrochloride, 54*t*
Spectracef, 52*t*
Spinal cord stimulator implant, 125
Spiriva, 85
Spironolactone, 92, 182, 219

Sporanox, 57*t*
Sprycel, 207*t*
SSRIs. *See* Selective serotonin reuptake inhibitors
St. John's Wort, 133*b*, 222, 262, 264*t*
Stadol, 110, 122
Standards. *See* Drug standards
Starch, 71–72, 161
Starlix, 171
Stavudine, 60
Stelazine, 131
Stem cells, 212
Sterapred, 168
Steroid antagonists, 182
Steroids. *See* Corticosteroids; Glucocorticoids
Stimulants, 264*t*
  for children, 238
Stool softeners. *See* Fecal softeners
Strattera, 105
Streptokinase, 99*b*
Streptomycin, 54*t*
Streptomycin sulfate, 54*t*
Streptozocin, 205
Stri-Dex Pads, 76
Stroke, 99, 100
Stromectol, 62
Subcutaneous injection, 33, 34*f*
Sublingual drug administration, 32
Substance abuse, 251–255, 255*b*
  signs and symptoms of, 252, 255, 255*t*
Succinylcholine chloride, 150
Sucralfate, 157
Sufenta, 111
Sufentanil citrate, 111
Sular, 97
Sulfa drugs. *See* Sulfonamides
Sulfamethoxazole. *See* Trimethoprim-sulfamethoxazole
Sulfamylon cream, 75
Sulfasalazine, 56, 57*b*
Sulfonamides, 55–57, 63*b*, 76*b*
  allergic reactions to, 56–57
  cross-reactions with, 56–57, 57*b*
  long-acting, 56
Sulfonylureas, 230*b*
Sulindac, 122, 142
Sumatriptan succinate, 112, 223
Sumatriptan/naproxen sodium, 112
Sumycin, 53*t*
Sun damage to skin, 75–76, 76*b*
Sunitinib malate, 207*t*
Sunscreen, 75–76
Supportive agents, 208–209
Suprax, 52*t*
Surfak, 161
Surmontil, 135
Sustiva, 61
Sutent, 207*t*
Symmetrel, 58*t*
Sympathetic nervous system, 145–146, 146*f*, 146*t*
Sympatholytic agents, 147–149
Sympathomimetic agents, 146–147, 147*f*
Synagis, 58*t*
Synalar, 167
Synthetic thyroid preparations, 166, 166*t*
Synthroid, 166*t*, 232
Syntocinon, 177
Synvisc, 220

T

T_3. *See* Triiodothyronine
T_4. *See* Thyroxine
Tabloid, 202
Tacrine hydrochloride, 234*t*
Tacrolimus, 77, 193, 213
Tadalafil, 186
Tagamet, 134*t*, 155, 155*b*, 248*t*
Talacen, 111
Talwin, 111, 122
Talwin Compound, 111
Talwin NX, 111
Tamiflu, 58, 58*t*
Tamoxifen citrate, 203, 266
Tamsulosin hydrochloride, 186
Tannic acid, 72, 150
Tannins, 72
Tapazole, 166, 166*b*
Tapentadol, 122
Tarceva, 215
Targeted therapies, 199, 206, 212
Targretin, 207*t*
Tasigna, 207*t*
Tasmar, 116*t*
Tavist, 69
Taxol, 207
Taxotere, 207, 207*t*
Td. *See* Diphtheria and tetanus toxoids, adsorbed
Tdap. *See* Tetanus toxoid, reduced diphtheria toxoid, and acellular pertussis vaccine
Tea tree oil, 262
Tegretol, 113, 134*t*, 136, 224, 248*t*
Tekturna, 92
Teldrin, 67
Telithromycin, 53*t*
Telmisartan, 92
Temazepam, 248*t*
Temodar, 200
Temovate, 78*t*
Temovate E, 78*t*
Temozolomide, 200
Temperature, 12–13, 12*f*
Tempra, 111
Temsirolimus, 207*t*
TEN-K, 45
Tenormin, 91, 147, 219
Terazol, 74
Terazosin hydrochloride, 96
Terbinafine, 73*t*
Terbinafine hydrochloride, 57*t*
Terbutaline sulfate, 84
Terconazole, 74
Teriparatide, 167
Testes, 172
Testosterone, 177
Testosterone gel, 177
Testosterone transdermal system, 177–178
Tetanus immune human globulin, 192
Tetanus toxoid, 189*b*, 191
Tetanus toxoid, reduced diphtheria toxoid, and acellular pertussis vaccine (Tdap), 191, 194*f*, 195*f*
Tetanus vaccine, 191
Tetracaine hydrochloride, 107*t*
Tetracycline, 155, 228*b*, 267
Tetracycline hydrochloride, 53*t*, 76*b*
Tetracyclines, 53, 53*t*
Teveten, 92
6-TG, 202
Thalidomide, 207*t*, 222, 237–238
Thalitone, 89, 182
Thalomid, 207*t*
THC. *See* Delta-9-tetrahydrocannabinol
Theo-24, 84
Theolair, 84
Theophylline, 84, 133*b*, 263, 264*t*, 267
Theophylline ethylenediamine, 84
Thiabendazole, 62
Thiamine (B_1), 42
Thiazide diuretics, 132*t*, 142, 181–182, 182*b*, 228*b*
Thiazidelike diuretics, 182
Thiopental sodium, 107*t*
Thioridazine hydrochloride, 131
Thiotepa, 200
Thiothixene, 132
Thorazine, 131, 248*t*
Thrombin inhibitors, 98
Thromboembolic disorders, 97–99
Thrombolytic agents, 99
Thyroid, 166, 166*t*, 232
Thyroid disorders, drugs used to treat
  hyperthyroidism, 165–166, 166*b*
  hypothyroidism, 165–166, 166*t*
Thyroid gland, 164–166, 166*b*, 166*t*, 177*b*, 232–233
Thyroid preparations, 166, 166*b*, 166*t*
Thyroid-stimulating hormone (TSH), 164–165, 232–233
Thyrotropic hormone, 164–165
Thyrotropin. *See* Thyroid-stimulating hormone
Thyroxine (T_4), 164–165, 166*t*, 232
Tiagabine, 124
Tiagabine hydrochloride, 115
Ticarcillin disodium and clavulanate potassium, 51*t*
Ticlid, 100
Ticlopidine hydrochloride, 100
Tigan, 68, 159
Tigecycline, 53*t*
Tikosyn, 93
Timentin, 51*t*
Timolol maleate, 91, 224
Tinactin, 73
Tinzaparin sodium injection, 98
Tiotropium bromide, 85
Tipranavir, 61
Tirofiban, 100
Tisit Liquid, 63
TMP/SMX. *See* Trimethoprim-sulfamethoxazole
Tobramycin sulfate, 54*t*, 233
Tofranil, 135, 185, 238
Tolazamide, 57*b*, 76*b*, 171
Tolbutamide, 57*b*, 76*b*, 171
Tolcapone, 116*t*
Tolectin, 142
Tolmetin sodium, 142
Tolnaftate, 73
Tolterodine tartrate, 185, 230*b*
Topamax, 115, 136–137
Topical nitroglycerin, 94
Topicort, 78*t*
Topicort LP, 78*t*
Topiramate, 115, 124, 136–137
Topotecan, 205
Toprol, 91
Toprol-XL, 91
Toradol, 122, 248*t*
Toremifene citrate, 203
Torisel, 207*t*
Torsemide, 57*b*, 183
t-PA, 99
Trade names, 22
Tragacanth, 71–72
Tramadol hydrochloride, 111, 122, 221, 248*t*
Trandate, 91
Trandolapril, 91
Tranquilizers, 130–133, 130*b*, 132*b*, 132*t*, 137*b*, 254, 254*t*, 255*t*, 267, 267*t*
Transderm Scop, 248*t*
Transdermal contraceptives, 175
Transderm-Nitro, 94
Tranxene, 130
Tranylcypromine sulfate, 135
Trastuzumab, 215
Trazodone, 76*b*, 253–254
Treanda, 207*t*
Trecator, 54*t*
Trelstar, 204
Tretinoin, 77, 207*t*
Treximet, 112
Triamcinolone acetate, 74
Triamcinolone acetonide, 85, 168
Triamterene, 76*b*, 183
Triamterene plus hydrochlorothiazide, 183
Triazolam, 131, 234, 248*t*
Tricor, 101
Tricyclic antidepressants, 99*b*, 124–125, 133*b*, 135, 221, 230*b*, 264*t*
Tridione, 115
Triethanolamine, 76
Trifluoperazine hydrochloride, 131
Trifluridine, 58*t*
Trihexyphenidyl hydrochloride, 116*t*
Triiodothyronine (T_3), 164–165, 166*t*
Trileptal, 114
Trilipix, 101
Trimethadione, 115
Trimethobenzamide hydrochloride, 68, 159
Trimethoprim, 76*b*
Trimethoprim-sulfamethoxazole (TMP/SMX), 56, 184
Trimipramine maleate, 135
Tripedia, 189
Triphasil, 174–175
Triptans, 111–112, 223
Triptorelin pamoate, 204
Trisenox, 207*t*
Trobicin, 54*t*
Tropic hormones, 164
Tryptophan, 253–254
TSH. *See* Thyroid-stimulating hormone
Turmeric, 262–263
Tussend, 110
Tygacil, 53*t*
Tykerb, 207*t*
Tylenol, 111, 121, 248*t*
Tyrosine, 253–254
Tysabri, 213

U

Uloric, 143
Ultralente insulin, 169, 169*t*
Ultram, 111, 122, 248*t*
Ultrase, 157
Ultravate, 78*t*
Unasyn, 51*t*
Uniphyl, 84
Univasc, 91
Urea 40% to 50% injection, 177
Urecholine, 149, 149*f*
Urinary antiseptics, 183–184, 186*b*

Urinary tract infections, 183–184
  sulfonamides for, 55–57, 57*b*
  urinary antiseptics for, 183–184
Urokinase, 99
Uroxatral, 185

V

Vaccinations. *See* Immunizations
Valacyclovir hydrochloride, 58*t*, 59
Valerian, 108*b*, 263, 264*t*
Valium, 107*t*, 114, 130, 248*t*
Valproate sodium, 248*t*
Valproic acid, 115, 267
Valrubicin, 205
Valsartan, 92
Valstar, 205
Valtrex, 58*t*, 59
Valturna, 92, 219
Vancocin, 54*t*
Vancomycin hydrochloride, 54*t*
Vantas, 207*t*
Vantin, 52*t*
VAQTA, 189
Vardenafil, 186
Varenicline, 255
Varicella virus vaccine, live, 191, 194*f*, 195*f*
Varicella zoster, 58*t*, 59
Varivax, 191
Vasoconstrictors, 94
Vasodilators, 94
Vasotec, 91
Vectibix, 207*t*
Vecuronium bromide, 150–151
Velban, 208
Velcade, 207*t*
Venlafaxine hydrochloride, 134, 203, 222
Ventolin, 84
Ventricular arrhythmias, 91–93
VePesid, 205
Verapamil hydrochloride, 97
Verelan, 97
Vermox, 62
Versed, 107*t*, 130, 248*t*
Vesanoid, 207*t*
VFEND, 57*t*
Viadur, 203
Viagra, 186
Vibramycin, 53*t*
Vicodin, 110, 122, 248*t*
Vicoprofen, 122
Vidarabine, 58*t*
Vidaza, 200, 207*t*
Videx, 60
Vinblastine, 76*b*
Vinblastine sulfate, 208
Vincristine sulfate, 208
Vinethene, 106*t*
Vinorelbine, 208
Vinyl ether, 106*t*
Vioform, 73
Viokase, 157
Vira-A, 58*t*
Viracept, 61
Viral infection
  cancer and, 214
  treatment of, 58–62, 58*t*, 63*b*
Viramune, 61
Virazole, 58*t*, 59
Viroptic, 58*t*
Visicol, 160
Visken, 91
Vistaril, 132, 248*t*
Vistide, 58*t*
Vitamin deficiencies, 41–43, 43*b*
Vitamins, 39–40
  characteristics of, 41
  fat-soluble, 41–42
    A, 41
    D, 41–42, 45*b*, 220, 231
    E, 42, 228*b*
    K, 42, 97–98
  nomenclature of, 40
  preparations of multiple, 43
  water-soluble, 42–43
    C, 43
    cyanocobalamin (B_{12}), 43, 201
    folic acid, 42–43, 43*b*, 201
    niacin, 42, 101, 219
    nicotinamide, 42
    nicotinic acid, 42
    pantothenic acid (B_5), 42
    pyridoxine (B_6), 42, 221–222
    riboflavin (B_2), 42
    thiamine (B_1), 42
Vitaxin, 213
Vivactil, 135
Voltaren, 141
Vomiting, 158–159, 158*b*, 208–209
Voriconazole, 57*t*
VP-16, 205
Vytorin, 101
Vyvanse, 105

W

Warfarin, 56, 76*b*, 93*b*, 95*b*, 99, 99*b*, 102*b*, 105*b*, 112*b*, 134*t*, 141*b*, 156*b*, 158*b*, 174*b*, 228, 228*b*, 233–234, 260, 262–263, 264*t*, 267
Warts, 77–78, 78*f*
Weight loss aids, 157–158, 158*b*
Wellbutrin, 136
Westcort, 78*t*
White willow, 141*b*, 263, 264*t*
Wintergreen oil, 72
Witch hazel, 72
Worms, 62
Wound care products, 75
Wycillin, 50

X

Xanax, 130, 134*t*, 248*t*
Xeloda, 200
Xenical, 157–158, 158*b*
Xolair, 86, 213
Xopenex, 85
Xylocaine, 93, 107*t*

Y

Young's rule, 240

Z

Zafirlukast, 86
Zanamivir, 58, 58*t*
Zanosar, 205
Zantac, 156, 248*t*
Zarontin, 114
Zaroxolyn, 89, 182–183
Zebeta, 91
Zenapax, 213
Zephiran chloride, 74
Zerit, 60
Zestril, 91
Zetia, 101
Zevalin, 215
Ziac, 91
Ziagen, 60
Zidovudine, 60
Zinacef, 52*t*
Zinc, 39–40, 43, 45
Zinc salts, 72
Zinc undecylenate ointment, 73
Zithromax, 53*t*
Zocor, 102, 219
Zofran, 159, 209
Zoladex, 203
Zoledronic acid, 220, 232
Zolmitriptan, 112, 223
Zoloft, 134*t*, 248*t*
Zolpidem tartrate, 108
Zometa, 232
Zomig, 112
Zostavax, 191
Zoster vaccine live, 191, 195*f*
Zosyn, 51*t*
Zovirax, 58*t*, 59, 248*t*
Z-Pak, 53*t*
Zyban, 136, 254–255
Zyloprim, 142
Zyprexa, 132
Zyrtec, 68